The Johns Hopkins Manual of Gynecology and Obstetrics

Department of Gynecology
and Obstetrics
Johns Hopkins University
School of Medicine
Baltimore, Maryland

Nicholas C. Lambrou, M.D.
Abraham N. Morse, M.D.
Edward E. Wallach, M.D.
Editors

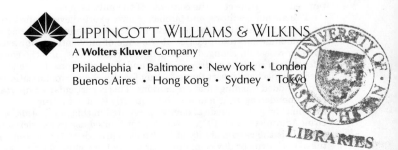

LIPPINCOTT WILLIAMS & WILKINS
A **Wolters Kluwer** Company
Philadelphia · Baltimore · New York · London
Buenos Aires · Hong Kong · Sydney · Tokyo

Acquisitions Editor: Lisa McAllister
Managing Editor: Susan R. Rhyner
Manufacturing Manager: Kevin Watt
Supervising Editor: Mary Ann McLaughlin
Editorial Coordinator: Brigitte P. Wilke
Production Service: Kim Langford, Silverchair Science + Communications
Cover Illustrator: Patricia Gast
Indexer: Linda Hallinger, Herr's Indexing Service
Compositor: Silverchair Science + Communications
Printer: RR Donnelley, Crawfordsville

Printed in the United States of America

9 8 7 6 5 4 3 2 1

Library of Congress Cataloging-in-Publication Data

The Johns Hopkins manual of gynecology and obstetrics / Department of Gynecology and Obstetrics, the Johns Hopkins University School of Medicine ; Nicholas C. Lambrou, Abraham N. Morse, Edward E. Wallach, editors.
    p.   cm.
Includes bibliographical references and index.
ISBN 0-316-46720-0
1. Obstetrics--Handbooks, manuals, etc. 2. Gynecology--Handbooks, manuals, etc. I. Lambrou, Nicholas C. II. Morse, Abraham N. III. Wallach, Edward E., 1933- . IV. Johns Hopkins University. Dept. of Gynecology and Obstetrics. V. Title: Manual of gynecology and obstetrics
    [DNLM: 1. Obstetrics. 2. Genital Diseases, Female. 3. Women's Health. WQ 100 J65 1999]
RG110.J64 1999
618--DC21
DNLM/DLC
for Library of Congress   98-47453
                                                                  CIP

This book is dedicated to the family members—spouses, parents, and children—of the house officers in the Department of Gynecology and Obstetrics at the Johns Hopkins University School of Medicine. The constant support and encouragement of these family members have enabled the development and productivity of these specialists in training.

Contents

Foreword

In these times of rapid change in gynecology and obstetrics and in women's health care, it is important to stay focused on our mission. For our department, that mission is to lead, promote, and advance the health and well-being of women through excellence and responsibility in patient care, honest and pioneering scholarship, and progressive and continuing education. This scholarly and practical work is a significant step toward that goal.

Harold E. Fox, M.D.
*Dr. Dorothy Edwards Professor of
    Gynecology and Obstetrics
Obstetrician and Gynecologist-in-
    Chief
Johns Hopkins University School
    of Medicine
Baltimore, Maryland*

Preface

The shelves of medical bookstores are replete with outstanding textbooks of obstetrics and gynecology and related subspecialties. Many of these books are authored or edited by leading educators in our field. This manual was not conceived to compete with such texts but to provide a practical synopsis of pathophysiology, diagnostic procedures, and management in obstetrics and gynecology. It targets the house officer who is on the front lines taking care of patients, the student with a desire to master the field of obstetrics and gynecology during the relatively short time provided for a clerkship or elective, and the busy practicing physician who must be both a jack-of-all-trades and a proficient practitioner.

The original concept for this manual arose during conversations with Dr. Timothy Johnson, then Director of Maternal-Fetal Medicine at the Johns Hopkins Hospital, now Chair of the Department of Obstetrics and Gynecology at the University of Michigan Medical School. Our master plan was to place responsibility for the preparation of each chapter in the hands of a resident physician partnered with a faculty member. Additional senior residents were appointed to serve as my associates in making assignments, reviewing chapter outlines, and transmitting manuscripts between authors and senior faculty members. Ms. Brigitte P. Wilke provided editorial assistance. In the final stages, Drs. Nicholas C. Lambrou and Abraham N. Morse worked diligently with me to review each of the 40 chapters in proof form. Lippincott Williams & Wilkins was most helpful in expediting the process of editing and printing the material. This team effort, with contributions from virtually every resident, fellow, and faculty member in the Department of Gynecology and Obstetrics at Johns Hopkins, has resulted in a book that should be, along with *The Harriet Lane Handbook* for pediatrics and *The Washington Manual of Medical Therapeutics* for medicine, a trusted companion for house officer, medical student, and practitioner. It is our hope that the practical material contained within the manual will also help the women who place their deepest trust in the skill and wisdom of their obstetricians and gynecologists.

Edward E. Wallach, M.D.
J. Donald Woodruff Professor
of Gynecology
Department of Gynecology
and Obstetrics
Johns Hopkins University
School of Medicine

Acknowledgments

The editors thank Laura Castleman, Robert Bristow, Greg Kaufman, Diljeet Singh, Jessica Bienstock, and Eva Pressman for their dedication and long hours of hard work. Without them this text could not have been completed.

The Johns Hopkins Manual of Gynecology and Obstetrics

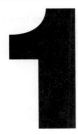

Pre-conception Counseling, Prenatal Care, and Breast-Feeding

Uma Reddy and
Judy Rossiter

I. Pre-conception care and counseling. Pre-conception care is important because it identifies women who can benefit from early intervention, such as those with diabetes mellitus, hypertension, and other metabolic and inherited disorders. Because organogenesis begins 17 days after fertilization, it is important to provide the optimal environment for the developing conceptus. Along with the possibility of prevention of some congenital anomalies and other complications of pregnancy, pre-conception counseling offers an ideal opportunity to educate women about the advantages of planning their pregnancies. Pre-conception care can be incorporated into any visit with a woman of childbearing age. The following issues should be discussed with both prospective parents:

A. Reproductive history
  1. Diagnosis and treatment of conditions such as uterine malformations, maternal autoimmune disease, and genital infection may lessen the risk of recurrent pregnancy loss.
  2. Review of an obstetric history when the woman is not pregnant may allow prospective parents to explore their fears, concerns, and questions.
  3. Recording the menstrual history provides an opportunity to evaluate a woman's knowledge of menstrual physiology and offer counseling about how she might use such knowledge to plan a pregnancy.

B. Pre-conception assessment of **family history** for genetic risks offers a number of advantages.
  1. **Carrier screening** based on family history or the ethnic or racial background of the couple allows for relevant counseling before the first potentially affected pregnancy. Pre-conception recognition of carrier status allows women and their partners to be informed of autosomal recessive risks outside the emotional context of pregnancy. Knowledge of carrier status also allows both informed decision making about conception and planning for desired testing should pregnancy occur.
     a. **Tay-Sachs disease** mainly affects families of European, Jewish, or French-Canadian ancestry.
     b. **Beta-thalassemia** mainly affects families of Mediterranean, Southeast Asian, Indian, Pakistani, or African ancestry.
     c. **Alpha-thalassemia** mainly affects families of Southeast Asian or African ancestry.
     d. **Sickle cell anemia** mainly affects families of African, Mediterranean, Middle Eastern, Caribbean, Latin American, or Indian descent.
     e. **Cystic fibrosis** screening may be offered to patients with a family history of the disease.
  2. Family history can reveal other risks for genetic diseases such as **fragile X** or **Down syndrome.** Risk may become apparent because of either parental age or familial occurrence. Genetic counseling should be offered to couples with identifiable risks so that they may understand the risks and, if desired, prepare for appropriate diagnostic tests such as chorionic villus sampling or amniocentesis in pregnancy. In some instances, genetic counseling may result in a decision to forgo pregnancy or to use assisted reproductive technologies that may obviate the risk.

Table 1-1. Pre-conception risk assessment: laboratory tests recommended for all women

1. Hemoglobin or hematocrit
2. Rh factor
3. Rubella titer
4. Urine dipstick (protein and sugar)
5. Pap smear
6. Gonococcal/chlamydia screen and pap screen
7. Syphilis test
8. Hepatitis B virus
9. Human immunodeficiency virus (offer)
10. Illicit drug screen (offer)

From U.S. Department of Health and Human Services. *Caring for our future: the content of prenatal care. A report of the PHS Export Panel.* Washington: U.S. Department of Health and Human Services, 1989. Adapted with permission.

C. **Medical assessment** (Tables 1-1 and 1-2). Pre-conception care for women with significant medical problems should include an assessment of potential risks not only to the fetus but also to the woman, should she become pregnant. Appropriate care may require close collaboration with other specialists. Risks include the following:
   1. **Primary pulmonary hypertension** has a maternal mortality rate that approaches 50% and a fetal mortality rate that exceeds 40%.
   2. The relatively high rate of congenital anomalies in infants of women with **insulin-dependent diabetes mellitus** is significantly reduced when these women maintain tight blood glucose control before and during pregnancy (during organogenesis).
   3. Women who experience recurrent spontaneous abortion as a result of **alloimmune or autoimmune disease** are more likely to carry a pregnancy to term when they receive pre-conception treatment.
D. **Infectious disease screening**
   1. **Patients at risk for congenital rubella syndrome** can be identified by pre-conception screening and prevented by vaccination. Providers sometimes hesitate to vaccinate women if they are not confident that the women will use effective contraceptives, as recommended, for three months after the vaccination. However, no case of congenital rubella syndrome has ever been reported after immunization within 3 months before or after conception.
   2. Universal screening of pregnant women for **hepatitis B virus** (HBV) has been recommended by the Centers for Disease Control and Prevention since 1988. Women with social or occupational risks for exposure to HBV should be counseled and offered vaccination. If they are not immunized appropriately, infants of HBV-infected women have a high probability of becoming chronic HBV carriers, and 25% of these children eventually die of liver-related disease.
   3. Patients at risk for **tuberculosis** should be tested if their histories of bacillus Calmette-Guérin vaccination do not meet the guidelines for screening or preventive therapy.
   4. **Cytomegalovirus** (CMV) screening should be offered to women who work in neonatal intensive care units, child care facilities, or dialysis units. Unlike rubella and other viral infections, past exposure to CMV, indicated by IgG antibodies in serum, does not confer complete immunity to pregnant women. Because no therapy or vaccine is effective against CMV and fetal risk is low, screening either before or during pregnancy is not cost-effective and is generally not recommended for the general population.

Table 1-2. Pre-conception risk assessment: laboratory tests recommended for some women

1. Tuberculosis screen
2. Toxoplasmosis
3. Cytomegalovirus
4. Herpes simplex
5. Varicella
6. Hemoglobinopathies
7. Tay-Sachs disease
8. Parental karyotype

From U.S. Department of Health and Human Services. *Caring for our future: the content of prenantal care. A report of the PHS Export Panel.* Washington: U.S. Department of Health and Human Services, 1989. Adapted with permission.

  5. **Toxoplasmosis** is of most concern to cat owners and people who eat or handle raw meat. Routine toxoplasmosis screening to determine antibody status before conception mainly provides reassurance to those who are already immune; a more prompt and definitive diagnosis can be made if seroconversion occurs during pregnancy. Counseling focuses on good hygiene. Someone other than the woman should dispose of cat litter daily. Women should wear gloves when gardening in a yard to which cats have access, avoid eating raw or undercooked meat, and wash their hands after handling such meat.
  6. Screening for **varicella** antibody should be performed if a positive history cannot be obtained. The varicella zoster virus vaccine is now available and recommended for all nonimmune adults.
  7. **Human immunodeficiency virus** (HIV) counseling and testing should be offered confidentially and voluntarily to all women.
  8. **Toxicologic examination** is a useful tool to encourage abstinence in women with a history of substance abuse. Standard informed consent and confidentiality restraints should be in effect.
  9. *Neisseria gonorrhea, Chlamydia trachomatis,* or *Treponema pallidum* testing should be performed.
E. **Determination of exposure to medications** includes over-the-counter and prescribed drugs. Ascertain drug use and provide information on the safest choices and how to avoid drugs associated with fetal risk.
  1. **Isotretinoin (Accutane),** an oral treatment approved by the U.S. Food and Drug Administration for severe, cystic acne, should be avoided before conception. Isotretinoin is highly teratogenic, causing craniofacial defects, malformations of the cardiovascular and central nervous systems, and defects of the thymus. For fetuses who survive until 20 weeks' gestation, the malformation rate is 23%.
  2. **Warfarin (Coumadin),** an anticoagulant, and its derivatives have been associated with warfarin embryopathy. Because heparin is not teratogenic, women requiring anticoagulation should be encouraged to switch to heparin therapy before conception.
  3. The offspring of women treated with **anticonvulsants** for epilepsy are at increased risk for congenital malformations. Debate continues as to whether the disease process, the medication, or a combination of both causes the malformations. Attempting a withdrawal from anticonvulsants for women who have not had a seizure in at least 2 years may eliminate one of the proposed contributing factors. For women who are not candidates for anticonvulsant withdrawal, the drug regimen that poses the least possible threat should be recommended.
  4. No evidence exists of teratogenicity from **oral contraceptive or contraceptive implant** use. It is best, however, for women to avoid systemic hor-

mones as they prepare for pregnancy. Women are advised to wait one full menstrual cycle after discontinuation of oral contraceptives or removal of contraceptive implants before attempting conception.

5. **Vaginal spermicides** are not teratogenic to the offspring of women who conceive while using them or immediately after discontinuing their use.

F. **Nutritional assessment**

1. The **body mass index,** defined as [weight in kilograms/(height in meters)^2], is the preferred indicator of nutritional status. Both overweight and underweight women are at risk for poor pregnancy outcomes. Women with a history of anorexia or bulimia may benefit from both nutritional and psychological counseling.

2. Discuss **eating habits** such as, fasting, pica, eating disorders, and the use of megavitamin supplementation. Excess use of multivitamin supplements containing vitamin A should be avoided. The teratogenicity of isotretinoin, a synthetic derivative of vitamin A, is well publicized. Retinoic acid also appears to be teratogenic. Because the estimated dietary intake of vitamin A for most women in the United States is sufficient, routine supplementation during pregnancy is not recommended.

3. Women with a history of phenylketonuria need close dietary supervision during their pregnancy. Infants born to women with classic **phenylketonuria** and a maternal blood phenylalanine level greater than 20 mg/dL are likely to have microcephaly and retardation. Dietary restrictions that result in lower levels of maternal phenylalanine during the earliest weeks of gestation appear to reduce the risk of fetal malformation.

4. Periconception intake of **folic acid** reduces the risk of neural tube defects (NTDs). The U.S. Public Health Service recommends daily supplementation with 0.4 mg of folic acid for all women capable of becoming pregnant. Unless contraindicated by pernicious anemia, women who have previously carried a fetus with an NTD should take 4.0 mg of folic acid daily, preferably starting 1 month before the time they plan to conceive and continuing through the first 3 months of pregnancy.

G. **Social assessment.** A social and **lifestyle history** should be obtained to identify behaviors and exposures that may compromise a good reproductive outcome and to identify social, financial, and psychological issues that could affect the optimal timing of conception.

1. **Environmental exposures** from hobbies, habits, and home or employment conditions that are associated with adverse reproductive outcomes should be identified and minimized in the periconception period. Examples include exposures to organic solvents, vinyl monomers used in the manufacturing of plastics, pesticides, and heavy metals such as lead and mercury. **Lead exposure** is still the most common pediatric problem in the United States. Some evidence has shown that exposure to elevated maternal blood levels of lead may be particularly deleterious to the fetus. If the answer to a screening question about lead is positive, a blood lead test should be ordered.

2. Assistance in answering questions about **reproductive toxicology** is available through the online database REPROTOX (http://reprotox.org). The Reproductive Toxicology Center at Columbia Hospital for Women Medical Center, one of the sponsors of REPROTOX, also offers a clinical inquiry program. Many states have teratogen hotlines or state-funded programs; the local March of Dimes is a good source for information about these and other resources.

3. Maternal use of **alcohol, tobacco, and other mood-altering substances** is more hazardous to a fetus than most other lifestyle choices. Alcohol is a known teratogen, and a clear dose-response relationship exists between alcohol use and fetal effects. The determination of how much alcohol causes harm varies. Increasing evidence suggests that cocaine is a teratogen as well as a cause of prematurity, abruptio placentae, and other complications. Tobacco use has been identified as the leading preventable cause of low birth weight. Although many women understand the risks of substance exposures after confirmation of pregnancy, they usually are

Table 1-3. Routine prenatal testing

Timing	Tests
Initial OB visit	Blood type, Rh type, antibody screen, CBC, rubella, VDRL/STS/RPR, HBSAg, HIV, Hgb electrophoresis, urine culture and sensitivity, Pap smear, gonorrhea and chlamydia testing; dating sonogram if questionable dating criteria
16–18 weeks' gestation (range: 15–22 weeks)	MSAFP/triple screen
16–20 weeks' gestation	Sonogram to rule out abnormalities
28 weeks' gestation	Blood type, Rh type, antibody screen, CBC, VDRL/STS/RPR, glucose screen. If high-risk OB patient repeat HBSAg, HIV, gonorrhea, and chlamydia cultures.
36 weeks' gestation	Group B streptococcus culture (optional)

CBC, complete blood cell count; HBSAg, hepatitis B surface antigen; Hgb, hemoglobin; HIV, human immunodeficiency virus; MSAFP, maternal serum alpha-fetoprotein; OB, obstetric; RPR, rapid plasma reagin; STS, serologic test for syphilis.

unaware of the risks of exposure during the earliest weeks of pregnancy. If substance addiction is present, structured recovery programs are needed to effect behavioral change. All patients should be asked about use of alcohol, tobacco, and illicit drugs. The pre-conception interview enables timely education about drug use and pregnancy, informed decision making about the risks while using these substances at the time of conception, and the introduction of interventions for women who abuse substances.

4. **Caffeine consumption.** Spontaneous abortion and intrauterine growth restriction (IUGR) are the most frequently reported consequences of caffeine intake during pregnancy. Some studies have implicated heavy caffeine use (more than 300 mg, or three cups of coffee, per day) in the 3 months before conception with an increased incidence of spontaneous abortion. The safest approach is the elimination of caffeine from the diet by 3 months before pregnancy. For women who cannot eliminate caffeine from their diets, restriction to less than 300 mg/day is clearly advisable.

5. Victims of **domestic violence** should be identified before they conceive, because they are more likely to be abused during pregnancy than at other times. Approximately 37% of obstetric patients are physically abused during their pregnancies. Such assaults can result in placental separation; antepartum hemorrhage; fetal fractures; rupture of the uterus, liver, or spleen; and preterm labor. Information about available community, social, and legal resources should be made available to women who are abused and a plan for dealing with the abusive partner devised.

6. **Financial difficulties.** The pre-conception interview is an appropriate time to discuss insurance coverage. Many women and couples do not know the eligibility requirements or amount of maternity coverage provided by their insurance carriers. Some women may have no medical insurance coverage. Also, many women are unaware of their employers' policies regarding benefits for complicated and uncomplicated pregnancies and the postpartum period. Facilitating enrollment in medical assistance programs should be part of pre-conception care for eligible women.

II. **Prenatal care.** Table 1-3 lists the tests to obtain during routine prenatal care, along with the recommended times for obtaining them.

Table 1-4. Range of accuracy of pregnancy dating by ultrasound according to gestational age

Gestational age	Ultrasound measurements	Range of accuracy
<8 wk	Sac size	±10 days
8–12 wk	CRL	±7 days
12–15 wk	CRL or BPD	±14 days
15–20 wk	BPD/HC/FL/AC	±10 days
20–28 wk	BPD/HC/FL/AC	±2 wk
>28 wk	BPD/HC/FL/AC	±3 wk

AC, abdominal circumference; BPD, biparietal diameter; CRL, crown-rump length; FL, femur length; HC, head circumference.

A. Pregnancy dating
   1. Clinical dating
      a. The average duration of human pregnancy is 280 days from the first day of the last menstrual period (LMP) until delivery. The 40-week gestational period is based on menstrual weeks (not conceptual weeks), with an assumption of ovulation and conception on the fourteenth day of a 28-day cycle.
      b. The most reliable clinical indicator of gestational age is an accurate LMP. Using Nägele's rule, the estimated date of delivery is calculated by subtracting 3 months from the first day of the LMP, then adding 1 week.
      c. A Doppler device allows detection of fetal heart tones by 11 to 12 weeks' gestation.
      d. A fetoscope can enable detection of heart tones at 19 to 20 weeks' gestation.
      e. Quickening is noted at about 19 weeks in the first pregnancy; in subsequent pregnancies, quickening usually is noted about 2 weeks earlier.
      f. The uterus reaches the umbilicus at 20 weeks.
   2. Ultrasound dating. Ultrasound dating is most accurate in the first 12 weeks of pregnancy. If LMP dating is consistent with ultrasound dating within the established range of accuracy for ultrasound (Table 1-4), the estimated date of delivery (EDD) is based on LMP. Before 20 weeks' gestation, if LMP dating is outside of the range of accuracy, then ultrasound dating is used.
B. Nutrition and weight gain
   1. Balanced nutrition
      a. Pregnant women should avoid uncooked meat because of the risk of toxoplasmosis.
      b. Pregnant women require 15% more kilocalories than nonpregnant women, usually 300 to 500 kcal more per day, depending on the patient's weight and activity.
      c. Dietary allowances for most minerals and vitamins increase with pregnancy. All of these nutrients, with the exception of iron, are supplied adequately by a well-balanced diet. Increased iron is needed both for the fetus and for the increase in maternal blood volume. Therefore, consumption of iron-containing foods should be encouraged. Iron is found in liver, red meats, eggs, dried beans, leafy green vegetables, whole grain–enriched bread and cereals, and dried fruits. Some physicians choose to give 30 mg of elemental ferrous iron supplements to pregnant women daily. The 30-mg iron supplement is

contained in approximately 150 mg of ferrous sulfate, 300 mg of ferrous gluconate, or 100 mg of ferrous fumarate. Taking iron between meals on an empty stomach or with orange juice facilitates its absorption.

2. The total **weight gain** recommended for pregnancy is based on the prepregnancy body mass index. The total weight gain recommended is 25 to 35 lb for women who fall within the normal range for prepregnancy weight.

   a. Underweight women may gain up to 40 lb, and overweight women should limit weight gain to less than 25 lb.

   b. Three to 6 lb are gained in the first trimester and 0.5 to 1.0 lb per week is gained in the last two trimesters of pregnancy.

   c. If a patient has not gained 10 lb by midpregnancy, her nutritional status should be carefully evaluated.

   d. Inadequate weight gain is associated with an increased risk of low birth weight in infants. Inadequate weight gain seems to have the greatest effect in women whose weight is low or normal before pregnancy.

   e. Patients should be warned against weight loss during pregnancy. Total weight gain in an obese patient can be as small as 15 lb, but weight gains of less than 15 lb are associated with a lack of expansion of plasma volume and a risk of intrauterine growth restriction.

3. **Nausea and vomiting**

   a. **Nonpharmacologic** recommendations for controlling nausea and vomiting in early pregnancy include the following:

      (1) Avoid eating greasy or spicy foods.

      (2) Keep some food in the stomach at all times by eating frequent, small meals or snacks.

      (3) Eat a protein snack at night; keep crackers at the bedside for consumption before rising in the morning.

   b. **Pharmacologic** therapy is discussed in Chap. 12, sec. **III.B.2–3.**

C. **Exercise.** In the absence of obstetric or medical complications, women who engage in a moderate level of physical activity can maintain cardiovascular and muscular fitness throughout pregnancy and the postpartum period. No data suggest that moderate aerobic exercise is harmful to mother or fetus. Women who engage in regular, non–weight-bearing exercise (cycling or swimming) are more likely to maintain their regimens throughout their pregnancies than women whose regular exercise before pregnancy is weight bearing. Women who wish to maintain body conditioning during their pregnancies may consider switching to non–weight-bearing exercise.

   1. Pregnancy induces alterations in **maternal hemodynamics,** including increases in blood volume, cardiac output, and resting pulse and a decrease in systemic vascular resistance.

   2. Because of **increased resting oxygen requirements** and the increased work of breathing brought about by the physical effects of an enlarged uterus on the diaphragm, a decreased amount of oxygen is available for the performance of aerobic exercise during pregnancy.

   3. For women who do not have any obstetric or medical contraindications, the following **exercise recommendations** may be made:

      a. Mild to moderate exercise routines are encouraged. Regular exercise (at least three times per week) is preferable to intermittent activity.

      b. Pregnant women should avoid exercise in the supine position after the first trimester. This position is associated with decreased cardiac output in most pregnant women, and the cardiac output is preferentially distributed away from splanchnic beds (including the uterus) during vigorous exercise; therefore, exercises performed supine are best avoided during pregnancy. Prolonged periods of stationary standing should also be avoided.

      c. Because of the decrease in oxygen available for aerobic exercise during pregnancy, pregnant women should modify the intensity of their exercise in response to symptoms of oxygen depletion such as shortness of breath. Pregnant women should stop exercising when fatigued and should not exercise to exhaustion.

   d. Physical maneuvers involving a shift in the physical center of gravity that may result in a loss of balance are contraindicated during pregnancy. Any type of exercise with the potential for even mild abdominal trauma should be avoided.

   e. Because pregnancy requires an additional 300 kcal/day to maintain metabolic homeostasis, women who exercise during pregnancy must be careful to ensure an adequate diet.

   f. Pregnant women who exercise in the first trimester should augment heat dissipation by maintaining adequate hydration, wearing appropriate clothing, and ensuring optimal environmental surroundings during exercise.

   g. Many of the physiologic and morphologic changes of pregnancy persist for 4 to 6 weeks postpartum. Therefore, prepregnancy exercise routines should be resumed gradually, based on a woman's individual physical capability.

4. The following conditions are **contraindications to exercise** during pregnancy:

   a. Pregnancy-induced hypertension
   b. Preterm rupture of membranes
   c. Preterm labor during a prior pregnancy, the current pregnancy, or both
   d. Incompetent cervix or cerclage
   e. Persistent second- or third-trimester bleeding
   f. Intrauterine growth restriction

5. Women with certain other conditions, including chronic hypertension or active thyroid, cardiac, vascular, or pulmonary disease, should be carefully evaluated to determine whether an exercise program is appropriate.

D. Smoking

1. Carbon monoxide and nicotine are believed to be the main ingredients in cigarette smoke responsible for adverse fetal effects. Compared with nonsmoking, smoking is associated with increased rates of occurrence of the following events:

   a. Spontaneous abortion (risk is 1.2 to 1.8 times greater in smokers than in nonsmokers)
   b. Abortion of a chromosomally normal fetus (39% more likely in smokers than in nonsmokers)
   c. Abruptio placentae, placenta previa, and premature rupture of membranes
   d. Preterm birth (risk is 1.2 to 1.5 times greater in smokers than in nonsmokers)
   e. Low infant birth weight
   f. Sudden infant death syndrome

2. **Smoking cessation** during pregnancy improves the birth weight of the infant, especially if cessation occurs before 16 weeks' gestation. If all pregnant women stopped smoking, it is estimated that a 10% reduction in fetal and infant deaths would be observed.

3. Prospective, randomized, controlled clinical trials have shown that intensive smoking reduction programs with frequent patient contact and close supervision aid in smoking cessation and result in increased infant birth weights. Successful interventions emphasize ways to stop smoking rather than merely providing antismoking advice.

4. **Nicotine replacement therapy** (chewing gum or transdermal patch). The package inserts of these therapies suggest that pregnant women should not use them because nicotine is considered an important cause of the adverse effects of smoking on mothers and fetuses. Nicotine, however, is only one of the toxins absorbed from tobacco smoke; cessation of smok-

ing with nicotine replacement reduces fetal exposure to carbon monoxide and other toxins. For women who smoke more than 20 cigarettes per day and who are unable to reduce their smoking otherwise, it may be reasonable to advise nicotine replacement as an adjunct to counseling during pregnancy.

E. Alcohol consumption

1. Ethanol freely crosses the placenta and the fetal blood–brain barrier.
2. Ethanol toxicity is dose related, and the exposure time of greatest risk is the first trimester.
3. Although an occasional drink during pregnancy has not been shown to be harmful, patients should be counseled that the threshold for adverse effects is unknown.
4. **Fetal alcohol syndrome** (FAS) is characterized by three findings: growth retardation (prenatally, postnatally, or both), facial abnormalities, and central nervous system dysfunction. In addition to a history of maternal alcohol use during pregnancy, at least one finding from each of these three categories must be present to confirm the diagnosis of FAS. Facial abnormalities include shortened palpebral fissures, low-set ears, midfacial hypoplasia, a smooth philtrum, and a thin upper lip. Central nervous system abnormalities of FAS include microcephaly, mental retardation, and behavioral disorders such as attention deficit disorder. Skeletal abnormalities and structural cardiac defects are also seen with greater frequency in the children of women who use alcohol during pregnancy than in those of women who do not, but these conditions are not required for the diagnosis of FAS. The most common cardiac structural anomalies are ventricular septal defects, but a number of others occur. Performance deficits in children with FAS include low IQ (average IQ for these children is 63) and fine motor dysfunction.

F. Illicit drug use

1. **Marijuana**
   a. The active ingredient is tetrahydrocannabinol.
   b. No evidence exists that marijuana is a significant teratogen in humans.
   c. Cannabinoid metabolites can be detected in urine of users for days to weeks, much longer than for alcohol and most other illicit drugs. The presence of cannabinoid metabolites in the urine may identify patients who are likely to be current users of other illicit substances as well.
2. **Cocaine**
   a. **Adverse maternal effects** include profound vasoconstriction leading to malignant hypertension, cardiac ischemia, and cerebral infarction. Cocaine may have a direct cardiotoxic effect, leading to sudden death.
   b. **Complications** of cocaine use in pregnancy include spontaneous abortion and fetal death *in utero*, premature rupture of membranes, preterm labor and delivery, intrauterine growth restriction, meconium-stained amniotic fluid, and abruptio placentae. Cocaine use also has been associated with cases of *in utero* fetal cerebral infarction. Increased incidence of microcephaly, limb reduction defects, and genitourinary malformations have been reported with first-trimester cocaine use.
   c. Infants born to women who use cocaine are at risk for neurobehavioral abnormalities and impairment in orientation, motor, and state regulation neurobehaviors.
3. **Opiates**
   a. Opiate use is associated with increased rates of stillbirth, fetal growth retardation, prematurity, and neonatal mortality.
   b. Treatment with methadone is associated with improved pregnancy outcomes.
   c. The newborn narcotic addict is at risk for a severe, potentially fatal, narcotic withdrawal syndrome. Although the incidence of clinically significant withdrawal is slightly lower among methadone-treated

addicts, it can be just as severe as in narcotic addicts. Neonatal withdrawal is characterized by a high-pitched cry, poor feeding, hypertonicity, tremors, irritability, sneezing, sweating, vomiting, diarrhea, and, occasionally, seizures.

   d. Frequent sharing of needles has resulted in extremely high rates of HIV infection (greater than 50%) and hepatitis among narcotic addicts.

4. **Amphetamines.** Crystal methamphetamine, a potent stimulant administered intravenously, has been associated with decreased head circumference and increased risk of abruptio placentae, intrauterine growth restriction, and fetal death *in utero.*

5. **Hallucinogens**
   a. No evidence has shown that lysergic acid diethylamide (LSD) or other hallucinogens cause chromosomal damage, as was once reported.
   b. Few studies exist on the possible deleterious effects of maternal hallucinogen use during pregnancy.

6. **Prenatal care for the substance abuser**
   a. Intensive prenatal care, involving a multidisciplinary team of health care and social service providers, to address the multiple problems of substance abusers has been shown to ameliorate the maternal and neonatal complications associated with substance abuse.
   b. At each prenatal visit, substance abuse treatment should be offered to substance abusers who have not quit.
   c. All substance abusers should be counseled about the potential risks of preterm delivery, fetal growth restriction, fetal death, and possible long-term neurobehavioral effects in the child.
   d. HIV testing should be encouraged.
   e. Periodic urine toxicology testing should be offered. The reliability of urine toxicology is limited by the rapid clearance of most substances. Overaggressive urine testing may be perceived by the patient as threatening and thus decrease patient compliance.
   f. Early ultrasound confirmation of gestational age is necessary, because growth restriction is a frequent finding among fetuses of substance abusers, and accurate assessment of gestational age is important in the management of IUGR.
   g. A fetal anatomic survey is necessary because of the increased frequency of structural anomalies among offspring of substance abusers.
   h. Antepartum testing is appropriate when a reason to suspect fetal compromise exists (e.g., size small for date, decreased fetal movement, suspected growth restriction). When normal growth and an active fetus are present, no evidence shows that regular antepartum testing is associated with improved perinatal outcome in substance-abusing patients.
   i. All patients should be screened for substance abuse (including alcohol and tobacco) at the time of their first prenatal visit. Several screening questionnaires to detect problem drinking (e.g., the T-ACE questions and the CAGE questionnaire) and substance abuse have been developed.
   j. Periodic urine testing is recommended to encourage and reinforce continued abstinence. Patients must give informed consent prior to testing. The requirements of consent vary from state to state. Universal toxicology screening is not recommended.

G. **Immunizations.** Pre-conception immunization of women to prevent disease in their offspring is preferred to vaccination of pregnant women; only live virus vaccines, however, carry any risk to the fetus.
   1. All women of childbearing age should be immune to measles, rubella, mumps, tetanus, diphtheria, and poliomyelitis through childhood immunization.
   2. Rubella infection during pregnancy is associated with congenital infection; measles with high risk of spontaneous abortion, preterm birth, and maternal morbidity; and tetanus with transplacental transfer of toxin, causing neonatal tetanus.

3. All pregnant women should be screened for hepatitis B surface antigen. Pregnancy is not a contraindication to the administration of an HBV vaccine or hepatitis B immune globulin (HBIG). Women at high risk for HBV infection who should be vaccinated during pregnancy include those with histories of the following:
   a. Intravenous drug use
   b. Acute episode of any sexually transmitted disease
   c. Multiple sexual partners
   d. Occupational exposure in a health care or public safety environment
   e. Household contact with a HBV carrier
   f. Occupational exposure or residence in an institution for the developmentally disabled
   g. Occupational exposure or treatment in a hemodialysis unit
   h. Receipt of clotting factor concentrates for bleeding disorders
4. Combined tetanus and diphtheria toxoids are the only immunobiological agents routinely indicated for susceptible pregnant women.
5. There is no evidence of fetal risk from inactivated virus vaccines, bacterial vaccines, or tetanus immunoglobulin, and these agents should be administered if appropriate.
6. Measles, mumps, and rubella single antigen vaccines, as well as the combined vaccine, are contraindicated during pregnancy but should be given at a pre-conception or postpartum visit. Despite theoretical risks, no evidence of congenital rubella syndrome in infants born to mothers inadvertently given rubella vaccine has been reported. Women who undergo immunization should be advised not to become pregnant for 3 months afterward. Measles, mumps, and rubella vaccines can be given to children of pregnant women as there is no evidence that the viruses can be transmitted by someone who has recently been vaccinated.
7. Immune globulin or vaccination against poliomyelitis, yellow fever, typhoid, or hepatitis may be indicated for travelers to areas where these diseases are endemic or epidemic.
8. Influenza and pneumococcal vaccines are recommended for women with special conditions that put them at high risk for infection. For example, women with certain chronic medical conditions should be given influenza vaccine, and patients who have undergone splenectomy should be given pneumococcal vaccine.
9. Immune globulin or a specific immune globulin may be indicated after exposure to measles, hepatitis A or B, tetanus, chickenpox, or rabies.
10. Varicella-zoster immune globulin (VZIG) should be administered to any newborn whose mother developed chickenpox within 5 days before or 2 days after delivery. No evidence shows that administration of VZIG to mothers reduces the rare occurrence of congenital varicella syndrome. VZIG can be considered for treating a pregnant woman to prevent the complications of chickenpox. (See Chap. 14, sec. **III.D.1.b.**)

H. Sexual intercourse
1. Generally, no restriction of sexual activity is necessary for pregnant women.
2. Instruct patients that pregnancy may cause changes in physical comfort and sexual desire.
3. Increased uterine activity after intercourse is common.
4. For women at risk for preterm labor or women with histories of previous pregnancy loss, avoidance of sexual activity may be recommended.

I. Employment
1. Most patients are able to work throughout their entire pregnancies.
2. Heavy lifting and excessive physical activity should be avoided.
3. Modification of occupational activities is rarely needed, unless the job involves physical danger.
4. Patients should be counseled to discontinue an activity whenever they experience discomfort.
5. Jobs that involve strenuous physical exercise, standing for prolonged periods, work on industrial machines, or other adverse environmental factors should be modified as necessary.

J. Travel. The following recommendations should be made to all pregnant women:
1. Avoid prolonged sitting because of the increased risk of venous thrombosis and thrombophlebitis during pregnancy.
2. Drive a maximum of 6 hours a day, stopping at least every 2 hours for 10 minutes to walk.
3. Wear support stockings for prolonged sitting in cars or airplanes.
4. Always wear a seat belt; place the belt under the abdomen as the pregnancy advances.

K. Carpal tunnel syndrome. In pregnancy, weight gain and edema can compress the median nerve, producing carpal tunnel syndrome. The syndrome consists of pain, numbness, or tingling in the thumb, index finger, middle finger, and radial side of the ring finger on the palmar aspect. Compressing the median nerve and percussing the wrist and forearm with a reflex hammer (Tinel's maneuver) often exacerbates the pain. The syndrome most often occurs in primigravidas over the age of 30 during the third trimester and usually recedes within 2 weeks of delivery. Treatment is conservative, with splinting of the wrist at night. Local injections of glucocorticoids may be necessary in severe cases.

L. Back pain
1. Back pain may be prevented by avoiding excessive weight gain.
2. Exercises to strengthen back muscles can help alleviate back pain.
3. Pregnant women should maintain good posture and wear low-heeled shoes.

M. Round ligament pain
1. Sharp groin pains are caused by spasm of round ligaments associated with movement.
2. The spasms more frequently are felt on the right side than the left because of the usual dextroversion of the uterus.
3. Round ligament pain is relieved by applying local heat: hot soaks, heating pad, or hot bath.
4. Patients sometimes awaken at night with round ligament pain after having suddenly rolled over in their sleep.
5. Modification of activity—rising and sitting down more gradually as well as avoiding sudden movement—can decrease the occurrence of round ligament pain.
6. Patients can use acetaminophen (Tylenol) for pain if necessary.

N. Hemorrhoids are varicose veins of the rectum.
1. Patients with hemorrhoids should avoid constipation, because straining during bowel movement aggravates hemorrhoids.
2. Patients should avoid prolonged sitting.
3. Hemorrhoids often regress after delivery but usually do not disappear completely.

O. Genetic screening. A summary of the indications for genetic counseling is provided in Table 1-5.
1. **Maternal serum alpha-fetoprotein**
   a. Alpha-fetoprotein (AFP) is a fetal glycoprotein that is synthesized sequentially in the embryonic yolk sac, gastrointestinal tract, and liver. Normally, a small amount of AFP enters the amniotic fluid via fetal urination, gastrointestinal secretions, and transudation from exposed blood vessels. AFP crosses the placenta and fetal membranes, appearing in low concentrations in maternal serum and detectable by the maternal serum AFP (MSAFP) test. The concentration of AFP in amniotic fluid is highest at 15 weeks of gestation and slowly declines during the remainder of pregnancy. MSAFP concentrations are low but peak at about 30 weeks' gestation. In the second trimester, the level of AFP in amniotic fluid is about 100 times that in maternal serum.
   b. The normal range of AFP values is established by each reference laboratory. Laboratories should provide interpretations of results and risk assessments that take into account race, maternal weight, mul-

Table 1-5. Indications for genetic counseling

1. Older parental age
    Mother 35 years of age or older
    Father 45 years of age or older
2. Fetal anomalies detected via ultrasound
3. Abnormal triple screen or abnormal alpha-fetoprotein results
4. Parental exposure to teratogens
    Drugs
    Radiation
    Infection
5. Family history of:
    Genetic disease (includes chromosome, single gene and multifactorial disorders)
    Birth defects
    Mental retardation
    Cancer, heart disease, hypertension, diabetes, and other common conditions
        (especially when onset occurs at an early age)
6. Members of ethnic groups in which certain genetic disorders are frequent, and for
    which disorders and appropriate screening or prenatal diagnosis is available (e.g.,
    sickle cell anemia, Tay-Sachs disease, thalassemia, cystic fibrosis)
7. Consanguinity
8. Reproductive failure
    Infertility
    Repeated spontaneous abortions
    Stillbirths and neonatal deaths
9. Infant, child, or adult with:
    Dysmorphic features
    Developmental and/or growth delay
    Mental or physical retardation
    Ambiguous genitalia or abnormal sexual development

tiple pregnancy, and insulin-dependent diabetes mellitus. Results are
reported in multiples of the median (MoM) to standardize interpretation of values among different laboratories. Rates of false-negative
and false-positive results vary from laboratory to laboratory because
of different cutoff levels defining an abnormal result.

2. **Amniocentesis**

   a. **Procedure.** Amniocentesis involves withdrawing a small sample of the
fluid that surrounds the fetus. Amniotic fluid contains cells that are
shed primarily from the fetal skin, bladder, gastrointestinal tract, and
amnion. Amniocentesis is performed at 15 to 18 weeks' gestation. In
the United States, the current standard of care is to offer chorionic
villus sampling (CVS) or amniocentesis to women who will be 35 years
or older when they give birth because older women are at increased
risk for giving birth to infants with Down syndrome and certain other
types of aneuploidy.

   b. **Karyotyping** of cells obtained by amniocentesis or CVS is the definitive way to diagnose aneuploidy in fetuses. The risk that a woman will
give birth to an infant with Down syndrome increases with age.
Among women 35 years old, the incidence of Down syndrome is one

in 385 births (0.3%), whereas for women 45 years old, the incidence is 1 in 30 births (3%). The baseline risk of major birth defects (with or without chromosomal abnormalities) in children born to women of all ages is approximately 3%.

    c. Ultrasound evaluation should include at least a search of the entire spinal column for any widening of the canal or abnormal vertebrae, as well as an evaluation of the head for skull and ventricle size, of the neck for cystic hygroma, and of the abdomen for ventral wall defects (e.g., gastroschisis). In some instances, no etiology for the elevated AFP level will be found. An elevated amniotic fluid acetylcholinesterase (AChE) level in the presence of an elevated AFP level indicates a strong possibility of an open NTD. A low or absent AChE level indicates that the cause of the AFP elevation is something other than an open NTD. In either case, the finding is followed up by a detailed ultrasound evaluation to define the nature and extent of the defect.

    d. Patients with a positive obstetric history for NTD should be appropriately counseled about the 2% to 3% risk of recurrence of NTD and offered amniocentesis at 15 to 16 weeks of gestation for amniotic fluid AFP testing; ultrasonographic evaluation of the fetus for NTD at 16 to 18 weeks' gestation should be performed. If the amniotic fluid AFP results and the ultrasonographic findings are normal, the likelihood of an open NTD is minimal. The amniocentesis site should be selected carefully; the placenta should be avoided to reduce the risk of contaminating the amniotic fluid specimen with fetal blood, which can result in falsely elevated amniotic fluid AFP levels. False-positive results due to contamination of amniotic fluid with fetal blood can be identified by the absence of AChE in amniotic fluid. After fetal blood contamination of the amniotic fluid has been excluded, elevated amniotic fluid AFP levels without elevated AChE levels should be investigated by detailed ultrasonographic examination.

    e. Risks and complications. The miscarriage rate from amniocentesis is 0.25% to 0.50% (1 in 400 to 1 in 200).

3. Chorionic villus sampling

    a. Procedure. CVS uses either a catheter or a needle to biopsy placental cells derived from the same fertilized egg as the fetus. CVS is performed at 10 to 12 weeks' gestation. CVS may be more acceptable than amniocentesis to some women because of the psychological and medical advantages provided by early diagnosis of abnormalities and first-trimester termination.

    b. Risks and complications. Rates of miscarriage after CVS vary widely by the center at which CVS is performed. Adjusting for confounding factors such as gestational age, the CVS-related miscarriage rate is approximately 0.5% to 1.0% (1 in 200 to 1 in 100). The overall rate of infection after CVS is less than 0.1%.

    c. Cytogenetically ambiguous results caused by maternal cell contamination or culture-related mosaicism are reported more often after CVS than after amniocentesis. In such instances, follow-up amniocentesis may be required to clarify results, increasing both the total cost of testing and the risk of miscarriage. Ambiguous CVS results, however, may indicate a condition (e.g., confined placental mosaicism) that has been associated with adverse outcomes for the fetus. In such situations, CVS may be more informative than amniocentesis alone.

    d. Reports of clusters of infants born with **limb deficiencies** after CVS were first published in 1991. Data from studies of CVS suggest that the severity of the outcome is associated with the specific time of CVS exposure. Therefore, CVS is not recommended before 10 weeks' gestation.

4. Significance of elevated AFP level findings

    a. Elevated AFP levels in maternal serum and amniotic fluid are usually (80% to 90% of cases) found with open NTDs (elevated value for MSAFP of 2.5 MoM). Closed defects, however, including those associated with hydrocephalus, are not associated with abnormal AFP findings.

b. Elevated AFP levels can also occur with multiple pregnancies, fetal abnormalities such as gastroschisis, congenital nephrosis, Turner syndrome with cystic hygroma, fetal bowel obstruction, and teratoma.

c. Fetal growth retardation, fetal death, and other adverse outcomes are also associated with elevated AFP levels.

d. Assignment of incorrect gestational age may lead to incorrect interpretation of AFP levels, particularly in maternal serum, because AFP levels change in relation to gestational age.

5. Neural tube defects. NTDs result from a failure of the neural tube to close in early embryogenesis. Among the most common major congenital malformations, NTDs include the fatal condition of anencephaly; various forms of spina bifida, such as the severely debilitating condition lumbar meningomyelocele; and lesions such as meningocele, which have the potential for surgical correction.

a. The incidence of NTDs in the United States is 1 to 2 per 1,000 live births.

b. A family history of NTD in either parent generally signifies an increased risk of an NTD in the offspring. If one partner has an NTD, this risk may be as high as 5%. In a couple with a prior affected child, the risk of recurrence is 2%; with two affected children, this risk increases to 6% to 10%. Ninety percent to 95% of NTDs occur in families without such histories. Therefore, all pregnant women should be offered MSAFP screening.

c. Prenatal diagnosis of an NTD allows for termination of pregnancy or preparation for the birth of an affected infant.

6. Down syndrome associated with trisomy 21 most often results from meiotic nondisjunction during chromosomal replication and division.

a. Down syndrome is characterized by mental retardation, cardiac defects, hypotonia, and characteristic facial features.

b. Incidence increases with maternal age (Table 1-6).

c. Prenatal diagnosis by chromosomal analysis currently is offered to women who will be 35 or older at the time of delivery. This approach detects only 20% of cases of Down syndrome; 80% of cases occur in women under 35 years of age.

d. The risk of recurrence in a couple who are both chromosomally normal and have had a prior child with Down syndrome is 1%.

e. Low MSAFP findings have been associated with fetuses with a chromosomal disorder, particularly Down syndrome. The extent to which a given low level of MSAFP increases the risk of a chromosomal disorder is estimated by considering maternal age in combination with MSAFP levels. For example, the risk of a 25-year-old woman carrying a fetus with Down syndrome, based on age alone, is 1 in 890. If her MSAFP level is 0.36 MoM at 16 weeks of gestation, however, then her risk of carrying a fetus with Down syndrome increases to 1 in 182, equivalent to the risk of a 35-year-old woman based on maternal age alone.

7. Because 90% of NTDs occur in the absence of a positive history of NTD, and 80% of cases of Down syndrome occur in women younger than 35 years, an **MSAFP screening program** for the entire obstetric population is necessary.

a. The first MSAFP screen is drawn at 16 to 18 weeks' gestation after informed consent and counseling are provided.

b. A second MSAFP screen is drawn within 1 to 2 weeks after the first screen from patients with a high initial test result. A second screen should not be drawn from patients with a positive low initial result because, due to the principle of regression to the mean, a second, more likely normal result may actually lower the detection rate for fetuses with Down syndrome.

Table 1-6. Chromosomal abnormalities in liveborns[a]

Maternal age	Risk for Down syndrome	Total risk for chromosomal abnormalities[b]
20	1/1,667	1/526
21	1/1,667	1/526
22	1/1,429	1/500
23	1/1,429	1/500
24	1/1,250	1/476
25	1/1,250	1/476
26	1/1,176	1/476
27	1/1,111	1/455
28	1/1,053	1/435
29	1/1,000	1/417
30	1/952	1/385
31	1/909	1/385
32	1/769	1/322
33	1/602	1/286
34	1/485	1/238
35	1/378	1/192
36	1/289	1/156
37	1/224	1/127
38	1/173	1/102
39	1/136	1/83
40	1/106	1/66
41	1/82	1/53
42	1/63	1/42
43	1/49	1/33
44	1/38	1/26
45	1/30	1/21
46	1/23	1/16
47	1/18	1/13
48	1/14	1/10
49	1/11	1/8

[a]Because sample size for some intervals is relatively small, 95% confidence limits are sometimes relatively large. Nonetheless, these figures are suitable for genetic counseling.
[b]Karyotype 47,XXX was excluded for ages 20–32 (data not available).
From Hook EB, Cross PK, Schreinemachers DM. Chromosomal abnormality rates at amniocentesis and in live-born infants. *JAMA* 1983;249:2034–2038. Modified with permission. Copyright 1983, American Medical Association. Modified with permission from Hook EB. Rates of chromosomal abnormalities at different maternal ages. *Obstet Gynecol* 1981;58:282–285. Copyright 1981, American College of Obstetricians and Gynecologists.

    c. Diagnostic ultrasound is performed on patients with elevated or low MSAFP results to determine gestational age, localize the placenta, and detect multiple pregnancies and fetal anomalies. Amniocentesis is indicated for patients found to have a single, living fetus of the expected gestational age without anomalies.

III. Breast-feeding. The American Academy of Pediatrics recommends exclusive breast-feeding for the first 4 to 6 months of life and gradual inclusion of solids in the diet no sooner than 4 months, and preferably at 6 months.

  A. Advantages of breast milk

    1. Antiinfective properties

      a. Bifidus factor in breast milk **protects against diarrhea** by promoting proliferation of *Lactobacillus bifidus* in infant intestines, which discourages colonization by pathogens.

      b. Breast milk protects against respiratory infections, including respiratory syncytial virus (RSV) and otitis media.

      c. Breast milk protects against necrotizing enterocolitis.

      d. Breast milk promotes phagocytosis by macrophages and leukocytes.

    2. Antiallergic properties

      a. A decreased incidence and severity of eczema has been demonstrated in breast-fed infants.

      b. Species-specific protein in breast milk delays introduction of foreign protein.

    3. Bonding

      a. Breast-feeding promotes special closeness between mother and baby.

      b. The prolactin response increases maternal relaxation.

      c. Breast-feeding increases maternal self-confidence.

      d. Breast-feeding meets an infant's need for safety, security, and cuddling.

    4. Lower solute load for newborn kidney

  B. Contraindications

    1. For women with breast cancer, the mother's need for treatment takes precedence over lactation.

    2. Women who have suffered acute HBV during pregnancy should not breast-feed; newborn infants of HBV-positive mothers who have received HBIG and vaccine, however, may be breast-fed.

    3. Hepatitis C infection is a contraindication to breast-feeding.

    4. Women with HIV infection should not breast-feed.

    5. A life-threatening illness in the mother precludes breast-feeding.

    6. Galactosemia in the infant is a contraindication to breast-feeding.

    7. For women with herpes simplex virus (HSV) infection, breast-feeding is contraindicated in the presence of active breast lesions.

    8. When a mother is an intravenous drug abuser, the infant can receive substantial amounts of the drug, as well as hepatitis or HIV, from the infected mother's breast milk.

  C. How to breast-feed

    1. Direct the mother to put the infant to breast as soon as feasible.

    2. Encourage rooming in. Glycogen stores in full-term infants generally are sufficient initially; avoid supplemental feeding unless medically indicated. Frequent breast-feeding helps establish a mother's milk supply, prevents excessive engorgement, and minimizes neonatal jaundice.

    3. Positioning

      a. Cradle position. The infant's head rests in the mother's antecubital fossa, with her body rotated so that the infant's abdomen is against the mother's chest; the infant's lower arm is behind the mother, and his or her head, chest, abdomen, and knees are in a horizontal line at the level of the breast (pillows may be needed for support).

      b. Clutch (football) position. The infant's body is positioned on pillows at the mother's side, with hips flexed and the back of his or her neck supported by the mother's hand.

    c. Side-lying position. The mother is positioned on her side in bed and the infant placed on his or her side facing the mother; the lower breast is offered first, then the mother rolls toward the baby or to her other side to offer the second breast.

  4. Latch-on

    a. The mother supports and lifts her breasts with her thumb on top and her fingers below, staying behind the areola; strokes the infant's lips gently with her nipple; waits for the baby to open the mouth wide; then, with the nipple directed toward the center of the mouth, the mother draws the baby in close. The tip of baby's nose should touch the breast; the airway can be maintained by lifting up the breast if necessary.

    b. Appropriate latch-on and nutritive sucking are achieved when the infant's jaw excursions are wide and swallows are audible. The infant's tongue should be visible coming forward to the lower gum (visualized by holding down its lower lip), and the baby should not be pulled easily off the breast. The infant's lips should be flanged outward and can be gently pulled out if necessary.

    c. If the baby latches on correctly and the mother does not report pain, there is no need for or benefit to limiting feeding time. Arbitrarily limiting feeding time can curtail intake by the infant as well as promote engorgement in the mother.

    d. Both breasts should be offered at each feeding; the breast offered should be alternated because the baby sucks more vigorously on the first breast at each feeding.

    e. The infant is removed from the breast by the mother's finger, inserted in the corner of the baby's mouth to release suction.

    f. The baby should be burped after each breast.

    g. To avoid drying and cracking of the nipple, a few drips of colostrum or milk should be expressed onto the nipple and areola after feeding, followed by air drying for several minutes.

D. Maternal diet. The mother should be encouraged to do the following:

  1. Consume an extra 500 kcal/day.

  2. Drink to thirst (there is no benefit to forcing fluids).

E. Plugged ducts

  1. A tender lump in a breast that is not softened by nursing suggests a plugged duct.

  2. No systemic symptoms accompany plugged ducts.

  3. Possible etiologic factors include a constricting bra, a missed feeding, fatigue, or the nursing of twins.

  4. Treatment consists of the following measures:

    a. Moist heat applied to the breast before nursing

    b. Frequent feeding

    c. Removal of bra, if too tight

    d. Massage of breast during feeding

    e. Positioning of the infant with his or her chin toward the lump to improve drainage of the affected area

    f. Vigilance for symptoms of mastitis

F. Mastitis

  1. Mastitis is an **infectious process** in the breast, producing localized tenderness, redness, and heat along with systemic reactions of fever, malaise, body aches, nausea, and vomiting. Mastitis usually is unilateral, and rarely bilateral.

  2. The most common infectious **organisms** implicated in mastitis include *Staphylococcus aureus*, *Escherichia coli*, and, rarely, *Streptococcus*.

  3. The highest **incidence** of mastitis occurs 2 to 6 weeks postpartum.

  4. Treatment consists of the following measures:

    a. Bed rest

    b. Warm compresses

    c. Frequent nursing to empty ducts

    d. Feedings begun on the unaffected breast

    e. Increased maternal fluid intake

    f. Analgesics such as aspirin or acetaminophen

    g. Support bra

    h. Antibiotic therapy for 10 days. The choice of antibiotic is based on local sensitivities and the length of time since delivery or exposure to resistant flora. Avoid sulfa drugs when the infant is younger than 1 month. For staphylococcal disease, amoxicillin, dicloxacillin, and nafcillin are the drugs of choice. For streptococcal disease, penicillin is preferable. For uncomplicated mastitis after 1 month postpartum, penicillin, ampicillin, or erythromycin is used initially. Regardless of the course of disease, the antibiotic should be given for at least 10 to 14 days. Shorter courses are associated with a high incidence of relapse.

G. Abscess formation can result from inadequate or delayed treatment of mastitis.

    1. Affected mothers may breast-feed unless the abscess drains into the ductal system.

    2. Treatment consists of the following measures:

        a. Incision and drainage if necessary

        b. Monitoring of the infant for infection

H. Drugs contraindicated for use by nursing mothers include (brief list according to the American Academy of Pediatrics):

    1. Bromocriptine

    2. Cyclosporine

    3. Lithium

    4. Phenindione

    5. Marijuana

    6. Cocaine

    7. Doxorubicin

    8. Methotrexate

    9. Amphetamine

    10. Nicotine (smoking)

    11. Cyclophosphamide

    12. Ergotamine

    13. Phencyclidine

    14. Heroin

    15. Certain radiopharmaceutical preparations

I. Hormonal contraception

    1. After a term delivery, oral contraceptives (OCs) may be taken when the milk flow has become established. Use of combination OCs can reduce the quantity and duration of lactation.

    2. Progestin-only OCs and injectable progestin do not impair lactation. When initiated within 1 week postpartum, progestin-only OCs have not been shown to adversely affect infant development.

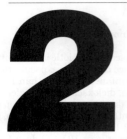

Fetal Assessment, Normal Labor, and Delivery

Emma Robinson and
Jessica Bienstock

Fetal Assessment

I. **Contraction stress test (CST), or oxytocin challenge test (OCT),** is the most specific test for fetal well-being used in obstetrics. The mother is placed in a supine position with a slight left tilt to avoid vena cava compression. External fetal Doppler is applied as well as an external tocodynamometer. During the initial observation period, baseline fetal heart rate and contraction patterns are noted. Uterine contractions lasting 40 to 60 seconds with a frequency of 3 in 10 minutes define an adequate test. If this result is not achieved spontaneously, then either nipple stimulation or oxytocin is used to stimulate contractions. A concentration of 0.5 mU/minute of oxytocin is given intravenously, and the infusion rate is doubled every 20 to 30 minutes until adequate contractions are achieved. Nipple stimulation is performed by the patient, who massages a nipple through her clothes for 10 minutes, then stops for 5 minutes. This cycle is repeated if necessary to achieve an adequate test. The patient is observed off oxytocin for resolution to baseline when the test is complete. A negative test finding is no late decelerations with adequate contractions. A positive test finding is late decelerations in greater than 50% of the contractions with adequate contractions. An unsatisfactory test is a tracing that is inadequate for interpretation. A suspicious test is a tracing that reveals late decelerations that are not consistent.

II. **Nonstress test (NST).** A reactive NST is defined as at least two accelerations of fetal heart rate 15 beats/minute above baseline for a 15-second duration during a 20-minute observation period. If this criterion is not achieved, then the test is nonreactive. The most common reasons for a negative test finding is a fetal sleep cycle or period of fetal inactivity. If the test is nonreactive, then the observation period can be extended to 40 minutes. If the test remains nonreactive, additional testing such as a CST or a biophysical profile (BPP) is indicated.

III. **Biophysical profile** incorporates real-time sonography with the NST. Five components constitute the scoring system: fetal breathing movements, fetal tone, gross body movement, amniotic fluid volume, and NST. Each component is given a score of 0 or 2, based on whether its criteria are achieved. Fetal breathing movement is one episode of breathing lasting longer than 30 seconds during a 30-minute observation period. Fetal tone is one episode of active extension or flexion of limbs or trunk, or opening or closing a hand. Gross movement is three discrete body or limb movements during the observation period. Amniotic fluid volume is at least one pocket of fluid measuring 2 cm in two perpendicular planes. NST is reactive as previously defined. Scoring ranges from 0 to 10. A score of 8 or higher is indicative of fetal well-being.

Normal Labor and Delivery

I. **Labor** is defined as repetitive uterine contractions of sufficient frequency, intensity, and duration to cause cervical effacement and dilation.

II. **Stages and phases**
   A. The **first stage** of labor is the interval between the onset of labor and full cervical dilation, defined by convention as 10 cm. The first stage is further divided into a latent and an active phase.
      1. The **latent phase** extends from the onset of labor to the point at which an upward inflection in the slope of cervical dilation occurs and is associated with a small incremental change in dilation. During this phase, uterine contractions typically begin as mild and irregular, becoming more intense, frequent, and regular as the latent phase progresses. Although the onset of the latent phase is often difficult to define precisely, and the duration of this phase varies, a latent phase is considered to be prolonged if it exceeds 20 hours in a nullipara and 14 hours in a multipara.
      2. The active phase is characterized by an increased rate of cervical dilation and, ultimately, by descent of the presenting fetal part. This phase is further subdivided into an acceleration phase, a phase of maximum slope, and a deceleration phase.
         a. **Acceleration phase.** A gradual increase in dilation initiates the active phase (usually beginning at about 2 to 3 cm of dilation) and leads, typically in about an hour, to a period of rapid dilation.
         b. **The phase of maximum slope** is defined as that period of labor when the rate of cervical dilation is maximal. Once established, this rate tends to be constant for each individual until the deceleration phase is reached. Primary dysfunctional labor is defined as active-phase dilation that occurs at a rate less than the fifth percentile of the general obstetric population. This value is 1.2 cm/hour for nulliparas and 1.5 cm/hour for multiparas (Table 2-1).
         c. **Deceleration phase.** During the terminal portion of the active phase, dilation appears to slow, terminating at full cervical dilation. Not all investigators accept the validity of a separate deceleration phase.
   B. The **second stage** of labor is the interval between full cervical dilation and the delivery of the infant. The duration of the second stage averages 50 minutes for nulliparas and 20 minutes for multiparas. Descent of the fetal presenting part begins in the late active phase and continues during the second stage. For nulliparous patients, the definition of a prolonged second stage of labor is 2 hours, or 3 hours if epidural anesthesia is used. For multiparous patients, the definition is 1 hour without and 2 hours with the use of an epidural. Studies show that the duration of the second stage of labor is unrelated to perinatal outcome in the absence of a nonreassuring fetal heart rate pattern or traumatic delivery. Therefore, a prolonged second stage alone usually is not considered an indication for operative intervention.
   C. The **third stage** of labor is the interval between delivery of the infant and delivery of the placenta, umbilical cord, and fetal membranes and lasts less than 10 minutes in most women. A prolonged third stage of labor is defined as greater than 30 minutes. Separation of the placenta is a result of continued uterine contractions after delivery of the infant. These contractions reduce the area of the uterine placental bed, with placental separation occurring along a plane in the spongiosa layer of the decidua vera (also known as *Nitabuch's layer*). Blood loss is controlled by compression of spiral arteries by the continued contractions, which transport the placenta from the fundus into the lower uterine segment and through the cervix.
   D. The **fourth stage,** or **puerperium,** is the time from delivery until complete resolution of the physiologic changes of pregnancy, considered by most to be the first 6 weeks postpartum. During this time, the reproductive tract returns to the nonpregnant state, and ovulation resumes.
III. **Mechanisms of labor.** The mechanisms of labor, or seven cardinal movements of labor, refer to the changes in position of the fetal head during passage through the birth canal. The vertex presentation is the most common, occurring in 95% of all term labors.

Table 2-1. Progression of spontaneous labor parameter

Parameter	Mean or median	Fifth centile
Nulliparas		
Total duration	10.1 hr	25.8 hr
Stages		
First	9.7 hr	24.7 hr
Second	33.0 min	117.5 min
Third	5.0 min	30 min
Latent phase (duration)	6.4 hr	20.6 hr
Maximal dilation (rate)	3.0 cm/hr	1.2 cm/hr
Descent (rate)	3.3 cm/hr	1.0 cm/hr
Multiparas		
Total duration	6.2 hr	19.5 hr
Stages		
First	8.0 hr	18.8 hr
Second	8.5 min	46.5 min
Third	5.0 min	30 min
Latent phase (duration)	4.8 hr	13.6 hr
Maximal dilation (rate)	5.7 cm/hr	1.5 cm/hr
Descent (rate)	6.6 cm/hr	2.1 cm/hr

From Friedman EA. *Labor: clinical evaluation and management.* East Norwalk, CT: Appleton-Century-Crofts, 1978:49. Reprinted with permission.

A. **Engagement** is the descent of the biparietal diameter of the fetal head below the plane of the pelvic inlet. Clinically, if the lowest portion of the occiput is at or below the level of the maternal ischial spines, station 0, engagement has usually taken place. Note that engagement often occurs before the onset of true labor, especially in nulliparas. Patients may experience a sense of decreased shortness of breath, referred to as lightening.

B. **Descent** of the fetal head to the pelvic floor is the most important event of labor. The highest rate of descent occurs in the deceleration phase of the first stage of labor and during the second stage of labor.

C. **Flexion** of the fetal head onto the chest is a passive movement that permits the smallest diameter of the fetal head (suboccipitobregmatic diameter averaging 9.5 cm) to be presented first to the maternal pelvis.

D. **Internal rotation.** The fetal occiput rotates from its original position (usually transverse with regard to the birth canal) toward the symphysis pubis or, less commonly, toward the hollow of the sacrum. As in flexion, this rotation allows the smallest possible diameters of the fetal head to lead into the birth canal.

E. **Extension** occurs after the fetus descends to the level of the perineum. The fetal head is delivered by extension from the flexed to the extended position, rotating around the symphysis pubis.

F. **External rotation.** After delivery of the head, the forces of the fetal musculature, now unopposed by the maternal bony pelvis and its musculature, cause the fetus to resume its face-forward position, with the occiput and spine lying in the same plane.

G. **Expulsion.** Further descent brings the anterior shoulder of the fetus to the level of the symphysis pubis. After delivery of the shoulder under the symphysis pubis, the rest of the body usually is expelled quickly.

Table 2-2. Pelvic types and characteristics

Type	Shape	Posterior sagittal diameter	Prognosis
Gynecoid	Round	Average	Good
Anthropoid	Long, oval	Long	Good
Android	Heart shaped	Short	Poor
Platypelloid	Flat, oval	Short	Poor

From Gabbe SG, Niebyl JK, Simpson JL. *Obstetrics: normal and problem pregnancies*, 3rd ed. New York: Churchill Livingstone, 1996:433. Reprinted with permission.

IV. Pelvimetry and labor

A. Pelvic shapes, planes, and diameters. The most commonly measured pelvic planes are the pelvic inlet and the midplane. The inlet (obstetric conjugate) is bounded anteriorly by the posterior border of the symphysis pubis, posteriorly by the sacral promontory, and laterally by the linea terminalis. Measurement of the inlet's transverse diameter is taken at its widest point. The midplane is bounded anteriorly by the lower margin of the symphysis, posteriorly by the sacrum (S-4 or S-5), and laterally by the inferior margins of the ischial spines.

Based on the general bony architecture, pelvises may be classified into four basic types. Gynecoid and anthropoid pelvises are amenable to childbirth, while android and platypelloid pelvises, which, because of a smaller amount of space in the posterior pelvis (measured by the posterior sagittal diameter taken from the sacral promontory to the greatest transverse diameter; Table 2-2), are less amenable to childbirth.

B. Clinical pelvimetry. The most important measurement is the diagonal conjugate, taken by placing the tip of the middle finger at the sacral promontory and measuring to the point on the hand that contacts the symphysis. The diagonal conjugate is the closest clinical estimate of the obstetric conjugate and is about 1.5 to 2.0 cm longer than the obstetric conjugate.

The second most important measurement, the bi-ischial diameter, is the distance between the ischial tuberosities (more than 8 cm is adequate). Other qualitative pelvic characteristics include angulation of the pubic arch, size of the ischial spines, size of the sacrospinous notch, and curvature of the sacrum and coccyx.

C. Radiographic pelvimetry

1. X-ray pelvimetry. Indications for performing x-ray pelvimetry to obtain more precise pelvic measurements include clinical evidence or obstetric history suggestive of pelvic abnormalities, history of pelvic trauma, and breech presentation for which a vaginal delivery is being contemplated. The most commonly used measurements are the anteroposterior and transverse diameters of the inlet and midplane (Table 2-3). A high likelihood of cephalopelvic disproportion exists if measurements are less than the established critical values. The main concern about x-ray pelvimetry is exposure of the fetus to ionizing radiation (0.5 to 1.0 rad). Current opinion is that, given the small risk of malignancy compared to the hazards associated with cephalopelvic disproportion, the risk to the fetus is justifiable if clinical circumstances dictate the procedure.

2. Other modalities. Computed tomography (CT) pelvimetry has been used but, like x-ray pelvimetry, exposes the fetus to ionizing radiation (up to 1.5 rad). CT is superior to x-ray pelvimetry for assessing the exact position of the fetal head relative to the maternal pelvis. Magnetic resonance imaging (MRI) also has been used successfully to assess maternal pelvic structure and has the advantage of better definition of soft-tissue structures, given that soft-tissue dystocia is a more frequent cause of fetopelvic disproportion than bony dystocia. MRI does not require the use of ionizing radiation.

Table 2-3. Average and critical limit values for pelvic measurements by x-ray pelvimetry

Diameter	Average value	Critical value
Inlet		
Anteroposterior (cm)	12.5	10.0
Transverse (cm)	13.0	12.0
Total (cm)	25.5	22.0
Area (cm^2)	145.0	123.0
Midplane		
Anteroposterior (cm)	11.5	10.0
Transverse (cm)	10.5	9.5
Total (cm)	22.0	20.0
Area (cm^2)	125.0	106.0

From Gabbe SG, Niebyl JK, Simpson JL. *Obstetrics: normal and problem pregnancies*, 3rd ed. New York: Churchill Livingstone, 1996:434. Reprinted with permission.

V. Management of normal labor and delivery

A. **Initial assessment** of labor includes an appropriate history, physical examination, review of the prenatal data, and necessary laboratory testing. Of special importance are time of onset of contractions, status of the fetal membranes, presence or absence of vaginal bleeding, fetal activity, maternal allergies, time of last food or fluid intake, and use of any medications. The admitting physical examination should include the patient's initial vital signs; fetal presentation; fetal heart rate; and frequency, duration, and character of uterine contractions. If no contraindications to pelvic examination exist, the amount of cervical dilation, effacement, status of the membranes, presence of meconium if membranes are ruptured, and nature and position of the presenting part should be determined.

B. **Leopold's maneuvers** consist of a series of four abdominal palpations of the gravid uterus to ascertain fetal lie and presentation. Although Leopold's maneuvers are limited by several factors (maternal obesity, polyhydramnios, multiple gestations), the procedure is a valuable adjunct to the vaginal examination.

1. First, the fundus is palpated to ascertain the presence or absence of a fetal pole (vertical vs. transverse lie) and the nature of the fetal pole (cranium vs. breech).

2. Second, the lateral walls of the uterus are examined using one hand to palpate and the other to fix the fetus. In vertical lies, the sides are usually occupied by the fetal spine (long, firm, and linear) and small parts or extremities.

3. Third, by palpating above the symphysis pubis, the nature of the presenting part is determined. In addition, determining the degree of descent of the presenting part below the pubic bone indicates the station of the presenting part.

4. Fourth, the cephalic prominence is palpated. In cephalic presentations, provided that the head is not too deep in the pelvis, the chin will be prominent if the head is neither flexed nor extended, as in a military presentation. If the head is not flexed, as in face presentation, the occiput will be felt below the spine. If the head is well flexed, neither chin nor occiput will be prominent.

C. Cervical examination. Three main components constitute a complete cervical examination.

1. **Dilation** (or dilatation) is the degree of patency of the cervix. The diameter of the internal os of the cervix is measured in centimeters, with 10 cm corresponding to complete cervical dilation.

2. **Effacement** is a shortening and thinning of the intravaginal portion of the cervix as it is drawn toward the abdomen by the uterine contractions. Effacement is expressed as a percentage, ranging from 0% (no reduction in length) to 100% (no cervix palpable below the fetal presenting part).

3. **Station** is the degree of descent of the presenting part of the fetus through the birth canal, measured as the estimated distance, in cm, between the leading bony portion of the fetal head and the level of the ischial spines. The level of the spines is station 0. The stations below the spines are +1 for 1 cm below the spines to +5 at the perineum. The stations above the spines are –1 for 1 cm above the spines to –5 at the level of the pelvic inlet.

D. Assignment of risk status. Based on prenatal history as well as initial assessment on admission, a patient should be assigned a high-risk or low-risk status. Approximately 20% of women who are identified antenatally as high risk account for 55% of poor pregnancy outcomes. In addition, the 5% to 10% of women who are identified as high risk only during labor account for 20% to 25% of poor outcomes. Twenty percent of perinatal morbidity and mortality, however, occurs in the group of patients considered to be low risk. Therefore, all women must be monitored carefully during labor and delivery.

E. Standard admission procedures. Upon admission, patients who have had no prenatal care should be considered at risk for syphilis, hepatitis B, and human immunodeficiency virus (HIV). Laboratory studies for these disorders as well as blood type, urine sample, rubella status, hematocrit, and Rh and antibody screen for atypical antibodies should be obtained for all unregistered patients. Patients who have had prenatal care require only a urine sample (to be tested for protein and glucose), hematocrit, blood count, and blood bank sample to be available for crossmatching if needed. Decisions regarding perineal hair shaving, enemas, showers, intravenous catheters, and positioning during labor and delivery should involve the patient, her family, and informed and prudent guidelines set forth by her health care team. Signed informed consent for management of labor and delivery should also be obtained from the patient upon admission.

F. Management of labor in low-risk patients. The quality of uterine contractions should be assessed. Cervical examinations should be kept to the minimum required to detect abnormalities in the progression of labor. Maternal blood pressure and pulse should be recorded every 10 minutes during the second stage of labor.

1. Well-controlled studies have shown that intermittent auscultation of the fetal heart is equivalent to continuous electronic monitoring in assessing fetal well-being when performed at specific intervals with a 1 to 1 nurse-to-patient ratio. The fetal heart rate should be recorded at least every 30 minutes during the active phase of the first stage of labor. The heart rate should be auscultated immediately after each uterine contraction. During the second stage of labor, the fetal heart rate should be recorded every 15 minutes.

2. Gastric emptying time increases in pregnant women, resulting in an increased risk of regurgitation and subsequent aspiration. Aspiration pneumonitis is a major cause of anesthesia-related maternal mortality and is related to the acidity of gastric contents. The use of an antacid such as sodium citrate (30 ml of 0.3 M solution orally) during the course of labor has been recommended by many authors.

3. For low-risk patients, delivery may take place in birthing rooms or traditional delivery areas. Consideration should be given to the patient's parity, the progression of labor, fetal presentation, and complications of labor. The lithotomy position is most frequently assumed for vaginal delivery in the United States, although alternative birthing positions, such as the lateral or Sims position or the partial sitting or squatting positions, are preferred by some patients, physicians, and midwives.

G. **Management of labor in high-risk patients.** Monitoring is intensified in high-risk labors.

   1. The fetal heart rate should be assessed according to the following guidelines:

      a. During the active phase of the first stage of labor, if intermittent auscultation is used, the fetal heart rate should be recorded at least every 15 minutes after a contraction. If continuous electronic fetal monitoring is used, the tracing should be evaluated every 15 minutes.

      b. During the second stage of labor, either the fetal heart rate should be auscultated and recorded every 5 minutes or, if continuous monitoring is used, the tracing evaluated every 5 minutes.

   2. Internal uterine pressure monitoring provides information about the quantity and quality of uterine contractions. Measurement of fetal scalp capillary pH can help to clarify confusing fetal heart rate patterns when fetal distress is suspected.

   3. Management of high-risk patients with no specific problems identified during labor may proceed in a manner similar to that previously outlined for low-risk patients.

H. **Induction of labor**

   1. **Indications.** Induction of labor is indicated when the benefits to the mother or fetus of delivery outweigh the benefits of continuing the pregnancy. Indications include:

      a. Pregnancy-induced hypertension, preeclampsia, or eclampsia

      b. Premature rupture of membranes at or near term

      c. Chorioamnionitis

      d. Fetal compromise (severe fetal growth restriction, isoimmunization)

      e. Maternal medical problems (e.g., diabetes, renal disease, chronic pulmonary disease, heart disease)

      f. Fetal demise

      g. Logistical issues (e.g., history of precipitous labor, distance from hospital, psychosocial conditions)

      h. Postterm pregnancies

   2. An assessment of **fetal lung maturity** is necessary before induction of labor can begin. If any one of the following criteria is met, amniocentesis is unnecessary:

      a. Documented fetal heart tones for 20 weeks by fetoscope or for 30 weeks by Doppler ultrasound

      b. Positive serum or urine pregnancy test at least 36 weeks previously

      c. Ultrasound obtained between 6 and 11 weeks that supports a gestational age of 39 weeks or more

      d. Ultrasound obtained between 12 and 20 weeks that confirms a gestational age of 39 weeks determined by clinical history and physical examination

   3. The **state of the cervix** is related to the success of labor induction. Using the Bishop scoring system (Table 2-4), when the total cervical score exceeds 8, the likelihood of vaginal delivery after labor induction is similar to that after spontaneous labor. Induction of labor in patients with a lower cervical score has been associated with a higher rate of failed induction, prolonged labor, and a higher cesarean section rate. The Bishop scoring system was originally designed for multiparas, although now it is applied to nulliparas as well.

I. **Cervical ripening** is a complex process that ultimately results in physical softening and distensibility of the cervix. Some degree of spontaneous cervical ripening usually precedes spontaneous labor at term. In many postterm preg-

Table 2-4. Bishop's scoring index

	Rating			
Factor	0	1	2	3
Dilation	Closed	1–2 cm	3–4 cm	5 cm +
Effacement	0–30%	40–50%	60–70%	80%+
Station	–3	–1, –2	–1, 0	+1, +2
Consistency	Firm	Medium	Soft	—
Position	Posterior	Middle	Anterior	—

From The American College of Obstetricians and Gynecologists, Bishop EH. Pelvic scoring for elective induction. *Obstet Gynecol* 1964;24:266. Reprinted with permission.

nancies, however, the cervix is unripe. Agents used for cervical ripening include prostaglandins (E_1, E_2, F_2) that appear to play a role in spontaneous maturation of the cervix by causing dissolution of collagen bundles and increasing submucosal water content.

    1. Prostaglandin E_2. Studies show that prostaglandin E_2 is superior to placebo in promoting cervical effacement and dilation. Prostaglandin E_2 also enhances sensitivity to oxytocin.

        a. Prepidil gel contains 0.5 mg of dinoprostone in a 2.5-ml syringe; the gel is injected intracervically up to every 6 hours for up to three doses in a 24-hour period.

        b. Cervidil is a vaginal insert containing 10 mg of dinoprostone. It provides a lower rate of release of medication (0.3 mg/hour) than the gel but has the advantage that it can be removed should hyperstimulation occur.

    2. Side effects. The major complication associated with the use of prostaglandin E_2 to induce cervical ripening is uterine hyperstimulation, which is usually reversible with a beta-adrenergic agent (e.g., terbutaline). Maternal systemic effects such as fever, vomiting, and diarrhea are possible but infrequent.

    3. Contraindications. Candidates for prostaglandin E_2 administration should not have a fever, an allergy to prostaglandins, or active vaginal bleeding. Caution should be exercised when using prostaglandin E_2 in patients with glaucoma or severe hepatic or renal impairment. Prostaglandin E_2 is a bronchodilator, so it is safe to use in asthmatic patients.

J. Oxytocin

    1. Indications. Oxytocin is used for both induction and augmentation of labor. Augmentation should be considered for slow progression through the latent phase, protraction or arrest disorders of labor, or the presence of a hypotonic uterine contraction pattern. Many studies have shown that the range of successful dosages and administration frequencies is wide, and that no method of administration is clearly superior to all others. In general, starting doses of 0.5 to 2.0 mIU/minute, with incremental increases of 1.0 to 2.0 mIU/minute every 30 to 60 minutes, are reasonable. Cervical dilation of 1 cm/hour in the active phase indicates that oxytocin dosing is adequate.

    2. Complications. Adverse effects of oxytocin are primarily dose related. The most common effect is fetal heart rate deceleration due to uterine hyperstimulation and resultant uteroplacental hypoperfusion. Hypotension can result from rapid intravenous infusion. Natural and synthetic oxytocins structurally resemble antidiuretic hormone; therefore, water intoxication and hyponatremia can develop with prolonged administration.

K. Fetal heart rate patterns correlate with fetal conditions such as hypoxia, umbilical cord compression, and acidosis, and examining heart rate patterns allows physicians to institute appropriate interventions. The two most important parameters of baseline fetal heart rate are rate and variability. Normal baseline heart rate at term is between 120 and 160 beats/minute. The presence or absence of variability—variation in the timing of successive beats in the fetal heart rate—is a useful indicator of central nervous system (CNS) integrity. The fetal CNS is very sensitive to hypoxia. In some instances of decreased oxygenation, the pattern of deceleration of the fetal heart rate can identify the mechanism causing the decrease.

1. **Variable decelerations** usually show an abrupt onset and return, giving them a characteristic V shape. These patterns coincide with the timing and duration of the uterine contraction and are caused by umbilical cord compression. Their severity (mild/moderate/severe) is graded by the drop in fetal heart rate and the duration of the deceleration.

2. **Early decelerations** are shallow and symmetric and reach their nadir at the peak of the contraction. They are benign patterns caused by fetal head compression.

3. **Late decelerations** are more ominous than early or variable decelerations. Late decelerations are U-shaped decelerations of gradual onset and gradual return that are usually shallow (10 to 30 beats/minute), reach their nadir after the peak of the contraction, and do not return to the baseline until after the contraction is over. They result from uteroplacental insufficiency and fetal hypoxia.

L. **Management of nonreassuring fetal heart rate patterns.** Studies have shown that although abnormal fetal heart rate patterns do correlate with neonatal depression at birth, they do not predict or prevent long-term adverse neurologic outcomes such as cerebral palsy. Several retrospective and prospective randomized trials have shown an increase in cesarean delivery rate as a result of electronic fetal heart rate monitoring. Such monitoring is nonetheless the best tool currently available for ensuring an optimal perinatal outcome, especially in high-risk patients.

1. **Noninvasive management**

   a. **Oxygen.** Administration of supplemental oxygen to the mother results in improved fetal oxygenation, assuming that placental exchange is adequate and umbilical cord circulation is unobstructed.

   b. **Maternal position.** Left lateral positioning releases vena caval compression by the gravid uterus, allowing increased venous return, increased cardiac output, increased blood pressure, and therefore improved uterine blood flow.

   c. **Oxytocin.** Oxytocin should be discontinued until fetal heart rate and uterine activity return to acceptable levels.

   d. **Vibroacoustic stimulation (VAS) or fetal scalp stimulation** may be used to induce accelerations in fetal heart rate that indicate the absence of acidosis. A 5-second VAS resulting in an acceleration of greater than 10 to 15 beats/minute lasting at least 10 or 15 seconds correlates with a mean pH value of 7.29 ± 0.07. Conversely, about a 50% chance of acidosis exists in the fetus who fails to respond to VAS in the setting of an otherwise nonreassuring heart rate pattern.

2. **Invasive management**

   a. **Amniotomy.** If the chorioamniotic membranes are intact, an amniotomy should be performed in the setting of fetal distress to allow access for internal monitoring. The vertex should be well applied to the cervix and engaged in the pelvis. The amount and character of fluid should be noted. A thorough examination should be performed after amniotomy to rule out cord prolapse.

   b. **Fetal scalp electrode.** Direct application of a fetal scalp electrode records the fetal electrocardiogram and thus allows the fetal heart rate to be determined on a beat-by-beat basis. This greater physiologic detail is useful when trying to evaluate effects of intrapartum stress on the fetus.

   c. **Intrauterine pressure catheter and amnioinfusion.** A catheter is inserted into the chorioamniotic sac and attached to a pressure gauge. Accurate pressure readings provide quantitative data on the strength, or amplitude, and duration of contractions. Amnioinfusion through the catheter of room-temperature normal saline can be used to replace amniotic fluid volume in the presence of variable decelerations in patients with oligohydramnios. This technique also should be used in patients with meconium in the amniotic fluid. Studies have shown a decrease in newborn respiratory complications in fetuses with moderate to heavy meconium-stained fluid with amnioinfusion, probably due to the dilutional effect of amnioinfusion. Either bolus infusion or continuous infusion can be used. Care should be taken to avoid overdistension of the uterine cavity.

   d. **Tocolytic agents.** Beta-adrenergic agonists (e.g., terbutaline, 0.25 mg s.q. or 0.125 to 0.25 mg i.v.) can be administered to decrease uterine activity in the presence of uterine hypertonus or nonreassuring fetal heart rate patterns that occur in response to uterine contractions. Potential side effects of beta-adrenergic agonists include both elevated serum glucose levels and increased maternal and fetal heart rates.

   e. **Epidural block.** Maternal hypotension, as a complication of epidural block, can lead to uteroplacental insufficiency and fetal heart rate decelerations. Management of hypotension includes intravenous fluid administration, left uterine displacement, and ephedrine administration (2.5 to 10.0 mg i.v. or i.m.).

   f. **Fetal scalp blood pH.** Determining fetal scalp blood pH can clarify the acid-base state of the fetus. A pH value of 7.25 or greater is normal for a fetus during labor. A pH range of 7.20 to 7.24 is a preacidotic range. A pH of less than 7.20 on two collections 5 to 10 minutes apart is thought by many investigators to indicate sufficient fetal acidosis to warrant immediate delivery, though some studies have shown that significant compromise is uncommon until a pH of less than 7.10 is noted.

   g. **Other procedures.** Newer techniques such as continuous fetal pulse oximetry to monitor fetal oxygenation on a minute-by-minute basis may become more popular in the clinical setting.

M. The goals of **assisted spontaneous delivery** are reduction of maternal trauma, prevention of fetal injury, and initial support of the newborn.

   1. **Episiotomy** is an incision into the perineal body to enlarge the area of the outlet and facilitate delivery. Episiotomy is indicated in cases of arrested or protracted descent or to accompany forceps or vacuum delivery. The role of prophylactic episiotomy, however, is debated.

      a. Proponents of prophylactic episiotomy cite the **advantages** of straight surgical incisions compared with ragged spontaneous lacerations; reduction in duration of the second stage of labor; and reduction in the incidence of trauma to pelvic floor musculature, with concomitant reduction in subsequent pelvic relaxation. Association of the latter advantage with episiotomy has never been proved.

      b. **Disadvantages** of prophylactic episiotomy include increased blood loss and, possibly, increased trauma.

      c. Although **mediolateral episiotomies** are associated with less damage to the anal sphincter and rectal mucosa than are medial episiotomies; they are more difficult to repair, result in greater blood loss and are more painful for the patient. They are performed by making an incision starting at the 4 or 8 o'clock position using Mayo scissors at a 45-degree angle from the interior portion of the hymeneal ring into the perineum, then extending the incision up the vaginal mucosa for about 2 to 3 cm.

      d. In the absence of complicating factors such as rectal or perineal lesions from inflammatory bowel disease or previous surgery, **medial episiotomies** are preferred. After the fetal head has distended the vulva to 2 to 3 cm, a midline incision half the length of the perineum is made and then extended up the vaginal mucosa for 2 to 3 cm. Medial episiotomies are classified by degree (first to fourth). First-degree episiotomies involve the vaginal mucosa, second-degree episiotomies involve the submucosa, third-degree episiotomies involve the anal sphincter, and fourth-degree episiotomies involve the rectal mucosa.

2. **Delivery of the head.** The goal of assisted delivery of the head is to prevent excessively rapid delivery. If extension of the head does not occur easily, a modified Ritgen maneuver can be performed by palpating the fetal chin through the perineum and pressing upward. After delivery of the head, external rotation is possible. If a nuchal cord is palpable, it is looped over the head; if it is irreducible, the cord is double clamped and cut. Mucus and amniotic fluid is aspirated from the infant's mouth and nose using bulb suction, or a De Lee suction catheter in the presence of meconium (to reduce the risk of meconium aspiration).

3. **Delivery of the shoulders and body.** After the fetal airway has been cleared, two hands are placed along the parietal bones of the fetal head, and the mother is asked to bear down. The fetus is directed posteriorly until the anterior shoulder has passed beneath the pubic bone. The fetus is then directed anteriorly until the posterior shoulder passes the perineum. After the shoulders are delivered, the fetus is grasped with one hand supporting the head and neck and the other hand along the spine. The infant is cradled as delivery is completed spontaneously or with a maternal push. Once delivered, the infant is dried off with a sterile towel and any remaining mucus is suctioned from the airway.

4. **Cord clamping.** After delivery, a net transfer of blood from the placenta to the infant occurs via the umbilical vein, which permits passage of blood for up to 3 minutes after birth. Spasm of the umbilical artery occurs within 1 minute of birth. Because the pressure gradient for blood flow in the umbilical vein depends on intrauterine and neonatal venous pressures, and these pressures are fairly low in the immediate postdelivery period, gravitational forces are important in maintaining flow. Altering the height at which the infant is held therefore can influence the degree of postnatal transfusion. The cord is generally double clamped and cut shortly after delivery of the infant.

5. **Delivery of the placenta.** As a result of continued uterine contractions after delivery of the fetus, placental separation occurs within 15 minutes in 95% of all deliveries. During the interval between delivery of the fetus and separation of the placenta, a thorough inspection of the cervix, vagina, and perineum is performed. Classic signs of **placental detachment** are a gush of blood from the vagina; descent of the umbilical cord; a change in shape of the uterine fundus from discoid to globular; and an increase in the height of the fundus as the lower uterine segment is distended by the placenta. After separation, the placenta, cord, and membranes are delivered by gentle traction on the cord and maternal expulsion efforts. Adherent membranes may be removed with a ring forceps. The placenta and membranes are examined for integrity. The cord is examined for length, presence of knots, and number of vessels. If retained tissue is suspected or excessive uterine bleeding is present, intrauterine exploration is necessary.

VI. **Obstetric anesthesia and analgesia.** Analgesia is defined as relief of pain without loss of consciousness. Anesthesia is defined as loss of feeling or sensation and includes loss of consciousness, motor power, and reflex activity.

  A. **Labor**

  1. **Systemic analgesics.** General recommendations for use of systemic analgesia during labor include use of the smallest dosage possible and keeping repeated doses to a minimum to reduce accumulation of drugs and metabolites in the fetus.

    a. **Meperidine (Demerol)** is a commonly used systemic analgesic agent. The usual dose is 25 to 50 mg i.v. or 50 to 75 mg i.m. every 3 to 4 hours. Demerol rapidly crosses the placenta, achieving equilibrium within 6 minutes. The duration of analgesia is 2 to 4 hours. Demerol's half-life is 2.5 hours in the mother but about seven times longer in the newborn because of underdeveloped neonatal hepatic metabolism.

    b. **Butorphanol (Stadol)** and **nalbuphine (Nubain),** synthetic narcotic agonist-antagonists, are used for analgesia during labor. Like Demerol, Stadol rapidly crosses the placenta; because its major metabolites are inactive, however, neonatal depression may occur less often than with Demerol.

   c. A wide variety of sedatives or tranquilizers such as promethazine, a phenothiazine, often are used to supplement narcotic analgesia. Maternal and neonatal respiratory depression secondary to use of narcotics can be antagonized by naloxone (Narcan). The usual dose of Narcan is 0.4 mg i.v. for adults, and 0.01 to 0.02 mg/kg body weight i.v. for neonates.

  2. **Epidural block** is the most widely used form of regional analgesia during labor. Segmental analgesia of spinal nerve roots T-10 to T-12 eliminates the pain of contractions while preserving sensations from pelvic structures. Epidural block can be achieved by either administration of a single dose or insertion of a catheter for repeated or continuous low-dose infusion. The most commonly used anesthetic agents are lidocaine (1%), bupivacaine (0.25% to 0.50%), and chloroprocaine (1% to 2%).

   a. The most common complication of epidural block is **maternal hypotension,** which causes uteroplacental insufficiency and can lead to fetal distress. Prophylactic intravascular volume expansion with 500 to 1,000 mL of Ringer's lactate solution is done before placing an epidural. If hypotension occurs despite intravascular volume expansion, it is corrected by additional intravenous fluids, ephedrine (2.5 to 10.0 mg), or both. Left uterus displacement is helpful in preventing and treating hypotension.

   b. **Other complications** include ineffective analgesia; dural puncture causing inadvertent spinal block; and CNS toxicity from intravascular injection of anesthetic causing dizziness, slurred speech, metallic taste, tinnitus, convulsions, and rarely cardiac arrest. Treatment of CNS toxicity involves establishing an airway, administering oxygen, correcting hypotension, treating convulsions with short-acting barbiturates or benzodiazepines, and respiratory support.

   c. Evidence suggests that labor may be slowed when epidural analgesia is begun before the active phase of the first stage. Active labor also may be transiently inhibited, usually for not longer than 30 minutes. An increased rate of forceps delivery occurs with epidural blocks because of the patient's diminished ability to push effectively in the second stage of labor.

   d. Relative **contraindications** to regional anesthesia are hemorrhage, coagulation disorders, neurologic disease, maternal spinal malformation, infection near the site of injection, and fetal distress.

B. Vaginal delivery

  1. **Local and pudendal blocks.** Local infiltration and pudendal blocks are commonly used to provide perineal analgesia for vaginal delivery. One percent lidocaine (Xylocaine) is the agent most commonly used, although 2% chloroprocaine (Nesacaine) is an effective alternative.

  2. **Spinal (saddle) block.** The main advantages of spinal blocks are that only small doses of local anesthetic are needed. The onset of anesthesia is rapid, and a spinal block is easier to administer and more reliable than an epidural block. The major complications are hypotension and high spinal blockade with resultant respiratory compromise. Left uterine displacement and intravascular preloading with Ringer's lactate solution help prevent hypotension, and careful positioning reduces the risk of high spinal blockade. The hyperbaric characteristics of the anesthetic agent and gravity are the main determinants of the degree of spinal analgesia.

  3. **Epidural block.** Epidural analgesia may be given *de novo* for vaginal delivery, though more commonly segmental epidural analgesia is augmented by administering a larger dose of anesthetic to achieve perineal analgesia. Chloroprocaine is often used for the perineal dose because it has a rapid onset of action and produces a more profound motor block.

  4. **General anesthesia** is rarely necessary for normal vaginal deliveries. When indicated, a rapid-sequence induction technique with prompt endotracheal intubation should be performed. Inhalational agents such as

halothane, enflurane, or isoflurane can be used to produce uterine relaxation, if needed.

C. Cesarean delivery

1. **Regional anesthesia.** Spinal and continuous lumbar epidural blocks commonly are used for cesarean delivery. With these techniques, the patient is awake and can receive oxygen in high concentrations, and the risk of gastric aspiration is reduced. To achieve an adequate surgical block, an anesthetized level of T-4 to T-8 is necessary. One percent tetracaine (8 to 10 mg) or 0.75% bupivacaine (10 to 15 mg) provide anesthesia for 1.5 to 2.0 hours. With 5% lidocaine (60 to 75 mg), the duration of anesthesia is 45 minutes to 1 hour. Continuous epidural block, in particular, has become one of the most popular forms of obstetric anesthesia. Two percent lidocaine with epinephrine is often used for this type of block. Both spinal and epidural blocks may be complicated by hypotension; the methods used to treat this problem are discussed in sec. **VI.A.2.a.**

2. **General anesthesia.** To reduce the degree of newborn depression, light general anesthesia with systemic analgesics and muscle relaxants are used.

    a. The most popular regimen is sodium pentothal (3 to 4 mg/kg) as the induction agent, followed by succinylcholine (60 to 100 mg) for muscle relaxation to facilitate intubation. Nitrous oxide and oxygen maintain anesthesia until delivery of the fetus. Preoxygenation with 100% oxygen increases oxygen stores in the maternal lungs. Additional inhalation agents (halothane, enflurane, isoflurane) are commonly used. Because these agents cause uterine relaxation, their use may result in increased blood loss, though several studies have shown no increased blood loss when these agents are used appropriately.

    b. The major **complications** of general anesthesia are hypertension associated with intubation, aspiration, and failed intubation. To reduce the risk of aspiration, cricoid pressure is applied until the endotracheal tube is inserted and the cuff inflated. An antacid is also administered 30 to 60 minutes before anesthesia to increase the pH of the stomach contents.

3. **Local anesthesia.** Occasionally, cesarean delivery must be performed under local anesthesia. Dilute concentrations of an agent such as lidocaine (0.5% to 1.0%) to a maximum dose of 7 mg/kg is used to infiltrate the skin and bathe the parietal and visceral peritoneum, which are the principal pain-sensitive structures. Manipulation of the pelvic organs will produce pain and a vasovagal response that can cause bradycardia, hypotension, or emesis. Local anesthesia is probably inadequate if difficult surgical manipulations are necessary.

VII. Postpartum analgesia

A. Nonsteroidal antiinflammatory drugs (NSAIDs). Analgesia can be accomplished in most patients who have undergone an uncomplicated vaginal delivery with NSAIDs such as ibuprofen. These drugs have been shown to be more effective than acetaminophen for episiotomy pain and uterine cramping. Ibuprofen is safe for nursing mothers.

B. Sitz baths provide additional relief of perineal pain resulting from a laceration or an episiotomy repair. Hot or cold sitz baths can be administered several times a day for 20 to 30 minutes. Sometimes a prolapsed hemorrhoid is mistaken for perineal pain. Local anesthetic sprays, witch hazel compresses, and suppositories containing corticosteroids provide relief from hemorrhoids.

C. Intravenous and epidural patient-controlled analgesia (PCA) is useful in managing postoperative pain in patients who have undergone cesarean delivery and require more relief than ibuprofen provides. The patient self-administers boluses of narcotic through either an intravenous or epidural catheter using a controlled infusion device. A continuous basal infusion rate can be instituted if pain is severe enough. One major advantage of PCA is that it eliminates the need for repeated parenteral injections as well as allowing the patient to exert control over her own pain management rather than depending completely on the nursing staff.

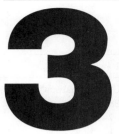

Malpresentations, Operative Deliveries, and Procedures

Amanda Lieb and
Frank Witter

I. Malpresentations

   A. A **normal presentation** is defined by a longitudinal lie, cephalic presentation, and flexion of the fetal neck. All other presentations are malpresentations. Malpresentations comprise approximately 5% of all deliveries and may lead to abnormalities of labor and endanger the mother or fetus.

   B. Factors that increase the risk of **malpresentation** include conditions that decrease the polarity of the uterus, increase or decrease fetal mobility, and block the presenting part from the pelvis.

   1. Maternal factors include grand multiparity, pelvic tumors, pelvic contracture, and uterine malformations.

   2. Fetal factors include prematurity, multiple gestation, hydramnios, macrosomatia, placenta previa, hydrocephaly, trisomy, anencephaly, and myotic dystrophy.

   C. Breech presentation occurs when the cephalic pole is in the uterine fundus.

   1. Incidence. Breech presentation is present in 25% of pregnancies at less than 28 weeks' gestation, 7% of pregnancies at 32 weeks' gestation, and 3% to 4% of patients in labor.

   2. There are three **types** of breech presentations:

   a. Complete breech, in which the fetus is flexed at the hips and flexed at the knees

   b. Incomplete, or footling, breech, in which the fetus has one or both hips extended

   c. Frank breech, in which both hips are flexed and both knees extended

   3. Risks

   a. Risks associated with specific presentations. The footling breech presentation increases the risk of cord prolapse and head entrapment. If the fetal neck is hyperextended, a risk of spinal cord injury exists.

   b. Risks of vaginal delivery. Patients with a complete or frank breech should be **counseled** as to the risks of each type of delivery. Cesarean section poses the risk of increased maternal morbidity and mortality. Vaginal breech delivery, however, poses increased risk to the fetus of the following:

   (1) Mortality (three to five times greater mortality rate than cesarean section if the fetus is heavier than 2,500 g and does not have a lethal anomaly)

   (2) Asphyxia (3.8 times greater risk than cesarean section)

   (3) Cord prolapse (5 to 20 times greater risk than cesarean section)

   (4) Birth trauma (13 times greater risk than cesarean section)

   (5) Spinal cord injuries (occur in 21% of vaginal deliveries if deflexion is present)

   c. Evaluation of risk based on fetal weight. The following recommendations for vaginal breech delivery are based on estimated fetal weight:

   (1) Less than 1,000 g. Most fetal mortality is due to prematurity or lethal anomalies. Because the potential for poor fetal outcome

Table 3-1. Zatuchni-Andros scoring system

Factor at presentation	Points		
	0	1	2
Parity		G1 multiparous*	
Gestational age	39	38	37
Estimated fetal weight (lb)	>8	7–8	<7
Previous breech	0	1	>2
Station	>–3	–3/–2	<–1

*A patient who has had at least one vaginal delivery.

resulting from prematurity exists regardless of the mode of delivery, vaginal delivery is recommended.

   (2) 1,000 to 1,500 g. Cesarean section is recommended.
   (3) 1,500 to 2,500 g. Management is controversial.
   (4) More than 2,500 to 3,800 g. The mother may attempt a vaginal delivery.

   d. **Zatuchni-Andros scoring system.** The Zatuchni-Andros system presented in Table 3-1 is used to determine appropriate candidates for breech vaginal delivery. A score lower than 4 represents a poor prognosis for successful vaginal delivery.

4. **Vaginal delivery.** A trial of labor may be attempted if the breech is complete or frank; the estimated fetal weight is between 2,500 and 3,800 g; the Zatuchni-Andros score is higher than 4; anesthesia is immediately available and a prompt cesarean section may be performed; the fetus is monitored continuously; and two obstetricians experienced with vaginal breech delivery and two pediatricians are present. A cesarean section should be performed in the event of any arrest of labor.

   a. The goal in vaginal delivery of breech presentations is to maximize cervical dilatation and maternal expulsion efforts in order to maintain flexion of the fetal vertex.

   b. The breech usually emerges in the sacrum transverse or oblique position. As crowning occurs (bitrochanteric diameter passes under the symphysis), perform a large episiotomy. Do not assist the delivery yet.

   c. When the umbilicus appears, place fingers medial to each thigh and press out laterally to deliver the legs. The fetus should then be rotated to the sacrum anterior position, and the trunk can be wrapped in a towel for traction.

   d. When the scapulae appear, place fingers over the shoulders from the back. Follow the humerus down, and rotate each arm across the chest and out. To deliver the *right arm,* turn the fetus in a *counterclockwise* direction; to deliver the *left arm,* turn in a *clockwise* direction. Clear and suction the airway.

   e. If the head does not deliver spontaneously, it is necessary to flex the vertex by placing downward traction and pressure on the maxillary ridge. Suprapubic pressure may also be applied. Piper **forceps** may be applied directly to the fetal vertex. The operator kneels down and places the blades from below the fetus. See sec. **IV.E** for description of forceps application.

   f. For delivery of a **breech second twin,** ultrasound should be available in the delivery room. The operator reaches into the uterus and grasps both feet, trying to leave the membranes intact. The feet are brought down to the introitus. Once the level of the scapula is reached, the remainder of the delivery is the same as that described above for a singleton breech.

g. Entrapment of the head during breech vaginal delivery may be managed by one of the following procedures:

   (1) Dührssen's incisions are made in the cervix at the 2, 6, and 10 o'clock positions. Either two or three incisions can be made. The 3 and 9 o'clock positions should be avoided because of the risk of entering the cervical vessels and causing hemorrhage.

   (2) Cephalocentesis can be performed if the fetus is no longer viable. The procedure is performed by perforating the base of the skull and suctioning the cranial contents.

5. External cephalic version

   a. Indications. Version is performed to avoid breech presentation in labor.

   b. Risks include cord compression and placental separation.

   c. Technique. Preferably, the procedure is performed as a forward roll. Alternatively, a back flip can be performed. Continuous fetal monitoring should be used, either with fetal heart rate monitoring or ultrasound. Tocolysis may be used. The use of spinal or epidural anesthesia for the procedure is controversial. Although anesthesia is beneficial if an emergency cesarean section is necessary, studies investigating the success rate of version when anesthesia is used have shown conflicting results. Anesthesia does allow the physician to apply more pressure on the abdomen than might otherwise be tolerated by the patient.

   d. Rh negative patients should receive $Rh_0(D)$ immune globulin (Rhogam) after the procedure.

   e. Factors associated with **failure** include obesity, oligohydramnios, deep engagement of the presenting part, and fetal back posterior. Nulliparity and an anterior placenta may also reduce the likelihood of success.

   f. Contraindications. Placenta previa and cephalopelvic disproportion are considered to be contraindications to external cephalic version. Version is not recommended if membranes have ruptured or labor has begun.

D. Abnormal lie. "Lie" refers to the alignment of the fetal spine in relation to the maternal spine. Longitudinal lie is considered normal. Oblique and transverse lies are considered abnormal. Abnormal lie is associated with multiparity, prematurity, pelvic contraction, and disorders of the placenta.

   1. Incidence of abnormal lie is 1 in 300, or 0.33%, of pregnancies at term. At 32 weeks' gestation, incidence is less than 2%.

   2. Risk. The greatest risk of abnormal lie is cord prolapse, because the fetal parts do not fill the pelvic inlet.

   3. Management. If abnormal lie persists beyond 35 to 38 weeks, hospitalization or external version is recommended.

E. Abnormal attitude and deflexion. Full flexion of the fetal neck is considered normal. Abnormalities range from partial deflexion to full extension.

   1. Face presentation results from extension of the fetal neck. The chin is the presenting part.

   a. Incidence of face presentation is between 0.14% and 0.54%. In 60% of cases, face presentation is associated with a fetal malformation. Anencephaly accounts for 33% of all cases.

   b. Diagnosis. Face presentation may be diagnosed by vaginal examination, ultrasound, or palpating the cephalic prominence and the fetal back on the same side of the abdomen.

   c. Risk. Perinatal mortality ranges from 0.6% to 5.0%.

   d. Management. The fetus must be mentum anterior for a vaginal delivery to be performed.

   2. Brow presentation results from partial deflexion of the fetal neck. The frontal bone is the point of designation; that is, the fetus is frontum anterior.

      a. Incidence is 1 in 670 to 1 in 3,433 pregnancies. Causes of brow presentation are similar to those of face presentation.

      b. Risks. Perinatal mortality ranges from 1.28% to 8.00%.

      c. Management. The majority of cases spontaneously convert to a flexed attitude. A vaginal delivery is indicated only if the maternal pelvis is large and, possibly, if the fetus is small. Forceps delivery is contraindicated.

F. Compound presentation occurs when an extremity prolapses beside the presenting part.

    1. Incidence is 1 in 377 to 1 in 1,213 pregnancies. Compound presentation usually is associated with prematurity.

    2. Diagnosis. Suspicion of compound presentation should be aroused if active labor is arrested or if the fetus fails to engage, as well as if the prolapsing extremity is palpated directly.

    3. Management. Do not manipulate the prolapsing extremity. Fetal monitoring is necessary because compound presentation can be associated with occult cord prolapse. Cesarean section is indicated for cord prolapse and failure of labor to progress.

II. Shoulder dystocia

A. Shoulder dystocia occurs in 0.15% to 1.70% of all vaginal deliveries. It is defined as impaction of the fetal shoulders after delivery of the head. The "turtle sign," in which the fetal chin is drawn up tightly against the perineum or maternal thighs, may be seen. Shoulder dystocia is associated with an increased incidence of fetal morbidity and mortality secondary to brachial plexus injuries and asphyxia.

B. Macrosomia is strongly associated with shoulder dystocia. In fact, the risk of shoulder dystocia is 11 times greater for infants weighing more than 4,000 g than for smaller infants, and 22 times greater in infants weighing more than 4,500 g. However, up to 50% of all cases of shoulder dystocia occur in infants weighing less than 4,000 g. Postterm and macrosomic infants are at risk because the trunk and shoulders grow more than the head in late pregnancy.

C. Other factors associated with shoulder dystocia include maternal obesity, previous birth of a macrosomic baby, diabetes mellitus, and gestational diabetes. Shoulder dystocia should be suspected in cases of prolonged second stage of labor or prolonged deceleration phase of first stage.

D. Management

    1. Anticipation and preparation. Perform the delivery in a delivery room. Call for help; extra hands will be needed during the delivery. If available, a pediatrician should be notified. Check the clock when the dystocia occurs, and follow the time elapsed. If necessary, it is possible to try and intubate the fetus while the head is still on the perineum.

    2. First-line measures

      a. Perform a generous episiotomy. Do not hesitate to extend it to a fourth-degree, a mediolateral, or even two mediolateral incisions.

      b. McRoberts maneuver. Hyperflex the maternal thighs and apply suprapubic pressure. This maneuver increases the posterior diameter. Do not apply fundal pressure, which may lead to uterine rupture.

      c. Apply pressure to the fetal sternum to decrease shoulder diameter.

    3. Second-line measures

      a. Place a hand into the vagina behind the fetal occiput, and push the anterior shoulder to oblique.

      b. Corkscrew. Turn the posterior shoulder 180 degrees and try to deliver it first.

      c. Flex the posterior arm and sweep it across the fetal chest, then deliver the arm.

      d. Fracture one or both clavicles. Use a thumb to fracture the clavicle outward to avoid lung or subclavian injury.

    4. Third-line measures

      a. Perform a symphysiotomy.

      b. Zavanelli maneuver. Replace the fetal head into the uterus, and proceed to cesarean section.

III. Episiotomy

A. Indications. Episiotomy is performed to increase the size of the outlet and to reduce maternal and fetal injury.

B. Benefits of episiotomy include shorter second stage of labor, a clean straight incision to repair (rather than more irregular lacerations), and reduced damage to the pelvic floor (although it has never been proven that episiotomy prevents pelvic relaxation). Mediolateral episiotomies may help avoid damage to the rectal sphincter. This type of episiotomy might benefit a patient with a history of inflammatory bowel disease or previous rectal surgery.

C. Risks of episiotomy include increased blood loss and, possibly, creation of more trauma than would have occurred with unassisted spontaneous vaginal delivery. Mediolateral episiotomies are more difficult to repair and more uncomfortable to the patient during recovery than median episiotomies.

D. Technique. An incision is made vertically in the perineal body, taking care to avoid the fetal presenting part. The incision should be approximately half the length of the perineal body. Mediolateral incisions should be made at a 45-degree angle to the midline of the perineum. The incision should extend into the vagina approximately 2 to 3 cm.

The episiotomy should be performed when approximately 3 cm of the fetal presenting part is visible between the labia. Excessive blood loss can result from performing the episiotomy too early. The episiotomy can be performed either before or after the application of forceps or a vacuum.

E. Repair. Most commonly, chromic suture is used for repair. First, the vaginal incision is closed with a running or running locking stitch until the hymenal ring is reached. The hymenal ring is then reapproximated. The suture may be cut and tied at this point, or carried down to the perineum. A few interrupted deep sutures may be placed in the fascia and muscles of the perineum. Next, a running suture is carried down to the apex of the incision, closing the superficial fascia. Finally, the perineal skin is closed with a running subcuticular stitch.

1. **Third-degree episiotomy.** The transected muscles of the external anal sphincter are isolated and the fascia on all four sides of the sphincter is reapproximated using interrupted sutures.

2. **Fourth-degree episiotomy.** The rectal mucosa is reapproximated by placing interrupted sutures through the submucosa approximately 0.5 cm apart. The suture line then may be reinforced with a layer of continuous stitches. The patient should be given stool softeners for at least 1 week after repair.

IV. Forceps delivery

A. Classification by station. Station is defined as the leading fetal bony part's position in relation to the ischial spines. Thus, station 0 is reached when the largest presenting diameter, or biparietal diameter (BPD), has reached the pelvic inlet (plane defined by the sacral promontory to the upper, inner aspect of the pubic symphysis), and the leading bony part of the skull is at the ischial spines. Each finger's breadth below the spines is a positive station: +1, +2, and so forth. The presenting part is said to be engaged when the BPD has passed through the pelvic inlet.

1. **High forceps.** The presenting part is at 0 station or above, or the cervix is not yet fully dilated.

2. **Mid forceps.** The presenting part is engaged, but above the level of +2 station.

3. **Low forceps.** The presenting part is at station +2 or below.

4. **Outlet forceps.** The presenting part is visible between the labia without the application of lateral traction, the station is at +4 or below, and the occiput is either directly anterior-posterior in alignment or does not require more than 45 degrees of rotation to place the sagittal suture in the anterior-posterior diameter.

B. Indications. There is no clinical indication for high forceps deliveries. Only mid to outlet forceps deliveries are justifiable. Indications include elective forceps, maternal exhaustion, fetal distress, or a maternal condition requiring a shortened second stage, such as cardiac or pulmonary disease.

C. Prerequisite criteria. Before performing forceps delivery, the following criteria should be met:

1. The fetal head must be engaged in the pelvis.
2. The cervix must be fully dilated.
3. The exact position of the fetal head should be known.
4. Maternal pelvis type should be known, and the pelvis must be adequate. Cephalopelvic disproportion is a contraindication for forceps delivery.
5. The patient should be given adequate anesthesia.
6. Someone who is able to perform neonatal resuscitation should be available.
7. The operator should have knowledge about, and experience with, the appropriate instrument and its proper application, and should be aware of possible complications.

D. Types of forceps

1. **Classic** forceps have been in use for years and follow a general style of construction. They have a blade with a toe at the end and a heel attached to the shank. The blade curves to accommodate the fetal head. This curve is known as the cephalic curve. The angle at which the blade connects to the shank defines the pelvic curve. The shank connects the blade to the handle. The shanks connect via a lock. Most forceps have an English lock.

    a. **Elliot type** forceps have overlapping shanks. Examples include Elliot and Tucker-McLane forceps.

    b. **Simpson type** forceps have parallel shanks and thus a more elongated cephalic curve. Examples include Simpson's, De Lee, and Hawks-Dennen forceps.

2. **Special forceps** are tailored to special clinical situations, such as Kielland's and Leff forceps for rotation of the vertex. Piper forceps are used for delivery of the head in a breech delivery. Zeplin forceps are used for outlet deliveries.

E. Techniques. A vaginal examination is performed to confirm the station and fetal position. If membranes are still intact, they must be ruptured. Adequate anesthesia is assured. The bladder is emptied.

1. The locked forceps are held close to the perineum in the position in which they will be applied. This enables the operator to visualize the final position of the forceps. Disarticulated forceps are designated left or right depending on their relation to the maternal left or right. The forceps are next disarticulated and the left half is held by its handle lightly in a pin grip by the left hand, while the right hand supports the blade. At the start of the application, the forceps should be perpendicular to the mother's abdomen with the internal surface of the blade against the fetal vertex and the external surface of the blade facing the operator. The right hand is then inserted into the vagina posterior to the fetal head and moved laterally to follow the path that the forceps will later take. The palm of the hand faces the fetal vertex and the back of the hand retracts and protects the posterior and left vaginal wall. The palm of the right hand forms a guide along which the left forceps blade traverses the vagina. The forceps blade rotates from vertical to horizontal relative to the maternal abdomen while rotating to the side of the fetal head. No force is required to achieve placement as the left hand gently brings the forceps handle down and around while the right hand provides retraction and a clear path for the blade to enter the left maternal pelvis. The blade should slide smoothly if properly placed and should not be forced. The right half of the forceps is next placed using the right hand to hold the handle and the left hand to provide the protective guide into the right maternal pelvis. The left blade should always be placed first to facilitate locking of the forceps.

2. Once the blades are in place and locked, the position of the forceps must be checked. The posterior fontanel should be midway between the blades and one finger's breadth above the shanks, the sagittal suture should be perpendicular to the plane of the shanks, and not more than a fingertip should be able to pass between the blade and the fetal head. If these criteria are not met, the blades should be readjusted or replaced.

3. When the placement of the blades is adequate, the head should be rotated to the direct occiput anterior (or posterior) position. Force is directed in a downward direction by a hand placed on the shanks and in an outward direction by the hand grasping the handles. The direction of traction should follow the path of the vertex through the pelvis; thus, as the occiput clears the pubic symphysis, the direction of traction should change to a more horizontal axis. A Bill's axis traction bar may be used to direct traction forces. Zeplin forceps have specially designed handles that are angled in the direction of proper traction for an outlet forceps delivery.

4. As the head extends over the perineum, the handles are elevated to no more than 45 degrees (to avoid sulcus tears), then first the right, and then the left, blade is removed. Sulcus tears occur less frequently when forceps with overlapping shanks are used than when forceps with parallel shanks are used.

F. **Complications**
   1. **Maternal.** Uterine, cervical, or vaginal lacerations, extension of the episiotomy, bladder or urethral injuries, and hematomas may occur.
   2. **Fetal.** Cephalohematoma, bruising, lacerations, facial nerve injury, and, rarely, skull fracture and intracranial hemorrhage may occur.

V. **Soft cup vacuum delivery.** Indications, contraindications, and complications are largely the same as for forceps. The suction cup is applied to the head over the posterior fontanel. Vacuum pressure to 0.7 to 0.8 kg/cc is reached, and traction is applied with one hand on the vacuum while the other hand maintains fetal flexion and ensures that the vacuum remains in place. Traction should be applied only during contractions. The vacuum pressure can be reduced between contractions.

VI. **Cesarean section**
A. **Indications.** Absolute indications for cesarean section are marked with an asterisk. The most common reasons that cesarean sections are performed are previous cesarean section, dystocia, breech presentation, and fetal distress.
   1. **Fetal** indications include
      a. Fetal distress or nonreassuring fetal heart rate tracing
      b. Nonvertex or breech presentation
      c. Maternal herpes simplex virus infection
      d. Major fetal anomalies, such as hydrocephalous
   2. **Maternal** indications include
      a. Obstruction of the lower genital tract (e.g., large condyloma)
      b. Abdominal cerclage*
      c. Conjoined twins*
      d. Previous cesarean section
   3. **Maternal and fetal** indications include
      a. Placenta previa*
      b. Abruptio placentae
      c. Labor dystocia or cephalopelvic disproportion
B. **Risks.** The patient should be counseled about the standard risks of surgery, such as discomfort, bleeding that may require transfusion, infection, and damage to nearby organs. In cases in which the cesarean section is being performed because of fetal indications, the patient should be informed of the increased fetal morbidity and mortality associated with surgical delivery.
C. **Procedure**
   1. The **abdominal incision** should be of sufficient length to allow for delivery.
      a. **Vertical** incisions are fastest to perform. In addition, if more room is needed to accommodate the delivery, the vertical incision can be extended above the umbilicus. Less dead space is present in the wound, which decreases the risk of infection. The resulting wound, however, is weaker than that from a transverse incision. The skin and subcutaneous tissue are dissected sharply down to the fascia. The fascia can be incised vertically with the knife, or a window can be created then the incision extended with Mayo scissors. The rectus and pyramidalis muscles are then separated in the midline, exposing the peritoneum. The peritoneum can be entered bluntly, or tented between two instruments and entered sharply, after transillumination demonstrates no

underlying bowel or omentum. The peritoneal incision is extended superiorly and inferiorly, taking care to avoid the bladder.

b. A sufficient **transverse** or **Pfannenstiel** incision is made approximately 2 fingers' breadths above the pubic symphysis. The tissue is divided sharply down to the fascia, which is transversely incised in a curvilinear fashion, either with the knife or with scissors. The superior and then inferior edges of the fascia are grasped and elevated, and the fascia is either bluntly or sharply separated from the underlying rectus muscles. Superiorly, dissection is continued to the level of the umbilicus, and inferiorly, to the pubic symphysis. The peritoneum is entered in the manner described in sec. **VI.C.1.a.**

2. **Bladder flap.** The vesicouterine serosa, which is a loose reflection of the peritoneum above the upper border of the bladder and covering the anterior lower uterine segment, is grasped, elevated, and sharply incised. Metzenbaum scissors are inserted and extended in a curvilinear fashion, then opened in each direction to undermine the serosa before sharply incising it. The bladder and lower portion of the peritoneum are then bluntly dissected off the lower uterine segment, and a bladder blade may be placed.

3. **Uterine incision**

   a. **Low transverse.** The transverse incision is used most commonly in cesarean sections. A curvilinear incision is made transversely in the lower uterine segment at least 1 to 2 cm above the upper margin of the bladder. The uterine cavity is entered carefully in the midline, taking care to avoid injury to the fetus. The incision is then extended bilaterally and cephalad, either with bandage scissors or bluntly. Curving the incision provides more length while helping to avoid the uterine vessels laterally. This type of incision is associated with less blood loss, fewer extensions into the bladder, decreased time of repair, and lower risk of rupture with subsequent pregnancies than other types of incision. Disadvantages are the limitation of the size of the incision, particularly if the lower uterine segment is not well developed, as in prematurity; and greater risk of extension into the uterine vessels.

   b. **Low vertical.** The advantage of the low vertical incision is that it can be extended if more room is needed; in so doing, however, the active segment of the uterus may be entered. Such an occurrence should be recorded in the operative notes, and the patient should be informed and counseled that vaginal birth trial is contraindicated thenceforth. Low vertical incisions are associated with extensions into the active segment more frequently than transverse incisions. In addition, the bladder must be dissected further for low vertical incisions than for transverse incisions to avoid injury.

   c. **Classic.** The classic type of incision extends from 1 to 2 cm above the bladder vertically up into the active segment of the uterus. Classic incisions are associated with more bleeding, longer repair time, greater risk of rupture with subsequent pregnancy, and greater incidence of adhesion of bowel or omentum than other types of uterine incisions. In cases of fetal prematurity, lower uterine segment fibroids, malpresentations, or fetal anomalies, however, it may be necessary to make this type of incision to provide adequate room for delivery.

   d. **T and J extensions.** If a low transverse incision is made, it may occasionally extend, or need to be extended, in a "T" or "J" fashion. If the active segment of the uterus is entered, the event should be recorded in the operative notes, and the patient should be informed and counseled that vaginal birth trial is contraindicated thenceforth. The J extension results in a stronger wound than the T extension, but neither type of extension is compatible with a subsequent trial of labor if the active segment is entered, which is usually the case.

4. **Delivery of the fetus**

   a. **Term, cephalic presentation.** Retractors are removed and a hand is inserted around the fetal head. The head is elevated through the incision. The remainder of the fetus is delivered using gentle traction on the head as well as fundal pressure. The infant is suctioned, the cord clamped and cut, and the infant delivered to the resuscitation team. If the head is deeply wedged in the pelvis, it may be necessary to insert a hand, in a sterile glove, into the vagina to elevate and disengage the head.

  b. Breech presentation. The fetal position should be confirmed before surgery. If the fetus lies transverse, back down or is preterm with a poorly developed maternal lower uterine segment, a classical cesarean section should be performed. Alternatively in cases of transverse, back down position, the fetus may be shifted to vertex or breech position by direct manipulation through the uterus after the abdomen is entered and the usual transverse incision is employed. The surgical assistant can manually maintain the fetus in the new position until delivery.

  c. Preterm delivery. If the lower uterine segment is inadequately developed, a low vertical or classical uterine incision should be made. Making a transverse incision under such circumstances risks injury to the uterine vessels, bladder, cervix, and vagina resulting from extension of the incision.

  d. Vacuum extraction or forceps in cesarean delivery. If the fetus is difficult to bring down to the low transverse incision and is in the vertex presentation, a vacuum extractor or forceps may be applied to assist in delivery without altering the uterine incision.

5. Uterine repair. After delivery of the placenta, either manually or by gentle traction on the umbilical cord, oxytocin is administered. The uterus may be removed through the abdominal incision or left in its anatomic position. The incision is inspected for extensions and the angles and points of bleeding are clamped with ring or Allis clamps. The uterine cavity is wiped with a laparotomy pad to remove retained membranes or placental fragments, and the uterus is wrapped in a moist laparotomy pad.

  a. Repair begins lateral to the angle of the incision, taking care to avoid the uterine vessels. A running or running locking stitch is placed. The entire myometrium should be included. Some surgeons advocate avoiding the endometrium in the repair to avoid future adenomyosis, but any benefit to this has not been proven. A second imbricated stitch, either horizontal or vertical, may then be placed. A second stitch, however, is not necessary because single layer closure is as strong as double layer closure and results in similar scar integrity. The incision is inspected, and further areas of bleeding may be controlled with figure-of-eight sutures.

  b. In classic cesarean sections, two or three layers may be required to close the myometrium. The serosa should then be closed with an inverting baseball stitch to decrease formation of adhesions of bowel and omentum to the uterine incision.

6. Abdominal closure. The tubes and ovaries are inspected. The posterior cul-de-sac and gutters are cleaned of blood and debris. The uterus is returned to the abdominal cavity and the incision reinspected with the tension off the vessels. The fascia then is closed with running or interrupted delayed-absorption sutures. The subcutaneous tissue is inspected for hemostasis, and the skin is closed with staples or subcuticular stitches. Subcutaneous dead space may also be closed with interrupted absorbable sutures.

D. Intraoperative complications

1. Uterine vessel injury usually occurs when a transverse incision is made. It may be necessary to open the broad ligament and identify the ureter before repairing the injury.

2. Bladder injury may occur when the dome of the bladder is injured upon entry into the peritoneum. The base is usually injured as the bladder is dissected from the lower uterine segment and vagina. The method of repair is controversial. The bladder usually is repaired in one or two layers, which may be interrupted, running, or both and may or may not include the mucosa. If the trigone or base is injured, it may be wise to visualize the ureteral orifices to ascertain that they were not damaged, by either extending the bladder defect or using cystoscopy. A large-caliber Foley catheter usually is left in place up to 7 days postoperatively.

3. **Bowel injury** usually occurs when previous surgery has caused adhesion formation. If only the bowel serosa is injured, the defect may be sewn over with interrupted sutures. If a full thickness injury has occurred, the bowel usually is repaired in two layers, running parallel to the lumen and avoiding the mucosa.

4. **Ureteral injury** usually occurs during repair of lateral extensions; therefore, opening the broad ligament to visualize the ureters before (or even after) a repair is recommended.

5. In cases of **atony,** the fundus should be massaged. Oxytocin (20 to 40 U/L), methylergonovine (Methergine) (0.2 mg i.m. or i.v.), 15-methyl $PGF_{2\alpha}$, (Hemabate) (250 μg in successive doses up to 1.0 to 1.5 mg i.m. or intramyometrially) may be given if contraindications, namely hypertension for Methergine, and asthma for 15-methyl $PGF_{2\alpha}$, do not exist. If pharmacologic treatment fails, uterine or hypogastric artery ligation or hysterectomy may be performed.

VII. Vaginal birth after cesarean. According to the American College of Obstetricians and Gynecologists, provided that no other contraindications exist, a woman who has undergone one previous low transverse cesarean section should be counseled to undergo a trial of labor in subsequent pregnancies. Even if she has had two previous cesarean sections, a trial of labor may be suggested. Recommendations for trial of labor after two or more cesarean sections are controversial.

A. Increased success of vaginal birth after cesarean section (VBAC) is seen when nonrecurrent conditions, such as malpresentation or fetal distress, prompted the previous cesarean section. Decreased success occurs when the conditions that prompted the previous cesarean section have a tendency to recur, such as failure to progress or cephalopelvic disproportion. Areas of controversy exist as to whether VBAC should be performed when multiple gestations are present, the estimated fetal weight is greater than 4,000 g, or the previous cesarean section was low vertical. VBAC is contraindicated after classic cesarean section.

B. When VBAC is attempted, epidural anesthesia and oxytocin may be used. Appropriate staffing, fetal monitoring, access to blood products, and a facility that can accommodate an emergency cesarean section should be available. Manual uterine exploration after delivery remains controversial, but probably is not indicated in VBAC.

VIII. Cesarean hysterectomy

A. The **indications** for cesarean hysterectomy include uterine atony that is unresponsive to massage, medication, or ligation of the uterine or hypogastric vessels; laceration of major vessels; severe cervical dysplasia or carcinoma *in situ*; and placenta accreta, increta, or percreta.

B. **Risks** of the procedure include increased operative time, increased blood loss, increased rate of infection, and increased incidence of damage to the bladder and ureters when compared with nongravid hysterectomy or cesarean section alone.

C. **Technique.** After delivery of the infant and the placenta, the uterine incision may or may not be approximated, depending on the degree of bleeding. The hysterectomy is performed in the standard fashion. If the hysterectomy is being performed because of bleeding, all pedicles may be clamped and cut and the uterus removed before suture ligation.

1. If a **supracervical** hysterectomy is performed, the uterus may be amputated from the cervix just below the level of the uterine vessels. The cervical stump is closed with interrupted sutures.

2. If a **total** hysterectomy is performed, it may be difficult to define the edges of the cervix if the cervix is dilated and effaced. An incision may be made in the lower uterine segment and a finger inserted into the incision to define the cervical edge. The glove on that hand should then be considered contaminated and discarded. After the cervix is removed, the vaginal vault is sutured using interrupted sutures or a continuous locking suture.

IX. Cerclage

    A. Indications. Cerclage is placed for surgical treatment of cervical incompetence.

    B. Risks include premature rupture of membranes (PROM), chorioamnionitis, and fibrous scarring of the cervix, which may result in abnormal dilatation or rupture at the time of labor. Before the cerclage is placed, cervical cultures should be obtained and any infections treated. Viability of the fetus should be confirmed via ultrasound. In cases of preterm labor and PROM, the cerclage should be cut promptly. A high index of suspicion for infection should be maintained.

    C. Procedures

        1. The **McDonald** cerclage is the most commonly performed and recommended technique. It involves placing a purse-string suture through the cervix as close as possible to the internal os. Care should be taken to avoid the vessels at the 3 and 9 o'clock positions on the cervix. Permanent suture material, such as mersilene tape or nylon, is used. A second stitch may be placed above the first. The knot usually is tied anteriorly to facilitate removal. The cerclage is removed at the time of labor, in the event of PROM, if infection is suspected, or at 37 weeks.

        2. In the **Shirodkar** cerclage, the suture is buried beneath the cervical mucosa. The suture may be left permanently in place, which necessitates cesarean section for delivery, or may be removed to allow for a vaginal delivery. This type of cerclage is associated with more blood loss during placement than the McDonald cerclage.

        3. In cases where a McDonald or Shirodkar cerclage have failed, an **abdominal** cerclage may be performed. Delivery via cesarean section is required after placement of this type of cerclage.

    D. Follow-up of the patient with a cerclage includes weekly cervical examinations and sonographic evaluation of cervical length. The patient should be placed on reduced activity or bed rest and should abstain from sexual intercourse.

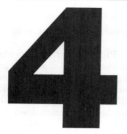

Complications of Labor and Delivery

Cynthia Holcroft and
Eva Pressman

I. Postpartum hemorrhage

A. Incidence. Defined as more than 500 mL of blood loss during the first 24 hours after a vaginal delivery or as more than 1 L of blood loss after a cesarean section, postpartum hemorrhage is the third most common cause of maternal mortality in the United States and accounts for 30% of maternal mortality in the developing world. The statistics are difficult to interpret, however, because the average blood loss during a vaginal delivery is 500 mL, and the average blood loss during a cesarean section is 1 L. In fact, the blood loss during most deliveries is underestimated.

B. Initial management. When a patient develops postpartum hemorrhage, action should be taken promptly; the uterus of a pregnant woman at term has a blood supply of 600 mL/minute, and a bleeding patient can rapidly become unstable. Furthermore, signs of hemorrhage in young, healthy women tend to be masked until serious intravascular depletion has occurred, so the clinical picture may be falsely reassuring in these patients. Large-bore intravenous access must be obtained and aggressive fluid resuscitation employed. In general, transfusion of blood products should be considered after 1 to 2 L of blood have been lost. Fresh frozen plasma (FFP) and platelets should be added after transfusion of six units of packed red blood cells to reduce the chances of dilutional and citrate-related coagulopathy. As soon as intravenous access is obtained, the physician must examine the patient to determine the cause of the hemorrhage and address the problem appropriately.

C. Causes of postpartum hemorrhage include uterine atony, lacerations, retained products of conception, uterine dehiscence or rupture, abruptio placentae, coagulopathy, and uterine inversion.

1. **Uterine atony** occurs in 90% of cases of postpartum hemorrhage. Predisposing factors include overdistension of the uterus from multiple gestation, polyhydramnios, or macrosomia; rapid or prolonged labor; grand multiparity; chorioamnionitis; general anesthesia or tocolytic agents; and use of oxytocin (Pitocin) during labor. Uterine contraction controls bleeding by compression of vessels, so atony leads to rapid blood loss.

   a. The first step in managing uterine atony is **bimanual massage** of the uterus, with evacuation of clot from the lower uterine segment to allow the uterus to clamp down.

   b. Next, **uterine contractile agents** such as Pitocin, methylergonovine (Methergine), 15-methyl $PGF_{2\alpha}$ (Hemabate), or dinoprostone can be administered. Ten units of Pitocin can be given i.m. or i.v., or 20 U/L can be added to maintenance intravenous fluid. Methergine can be administered as 0.2 mg p.o., i.v., or i.m. every 2 to 4 hours. Hemabate, 125 μg, can be administered i.m. every 15 to 90 minutes, and 20 mg of dinoprostone can be administered p.r. every 2 hours. Methylergonovine is contraindicated for patients with hypertension, and 15-methyl $PGF_{2\alpha}$ is contraindicated for patients with asthma.

   c. If uterine atony continues after administration of uterine contractile agents, **blunt curettage** may be performed to rule out retained products of conception as a cause. Preferably, ultrasound guidance is used to minimize the risk of uterine perforation.

d. Persistent hemorrhage resulting from uterine atony warrants more **invasive measures.** If interventional radiology is readily available, then embolization of pelvic vessels may be attempted; if not, the obstetrician must perform laparotomy. To save the uterus, bilateral uterine artery ligation, hypogastric artery ligation, or both may be attempted. Such measures decrease the pulse pressure to the uterus and help reduce blood loss, but because of the extent of collateral blood flow to the uterus, arterial ligation will not stop all bleeding. Because hypogastric artery ligation can be difficult technically, particularly if the surgical field is obscured by extensive bleeding, it may prove more prudent to proceed with hysterectomy instead of attempting arterial ligation. If hypogastric artery ligation is attempted, however, the hypogastric artery should be isolated and ligated approximately 2 cm distal to the origin of the posterior branch to avoid cutting off blood supply to the gluteal muscles. Care should be taken to avoid injury to the hypogastric vein that lies beneath the artery. Permanent suture, such as silk, is used for ligation. Aortic pressure may also be applied to control blood loss temporarily.

e. The definitive measure for controlling intractable uterine bleeding remains a **hysterectomy.** If the cervix is fully dilated at the time of hysterectomy, then a total abdominal hysterectomy must be performed, but if the cervix is not fully dilated, then supracervical hysterectomy may be considered to attempt to minimize blood loss. If total hysterectomy is performed, the surgeon's fingers can be placed in the vagina to help determine the location of the cervix. Often, patients must be monitored in an intensive care setting after peripartum hysterectomy because of massive blood loss and postoperative fluid shifts.

2. Lacerations cause approximately 6% of all postpartum hemorrhages and should be suspected particularly if an operative delivery or episiotomy was performed. Although lacerations often manifest as brisk vaginal bleeding, concealed pelvic hematomas, identified mainly by hypotension and pelvic pain, may also form.

a. Laceration of the vessels in the superficial fascia of the anterior or posterior triangle lead to **vulvar hematoma.** Constrained by Colles' fascia, the urogenital diaphragm, and the anal fascia, the hematoma may expand to the vulva, where it causes discomfort and swelling. Treatment of vulvar hematomas involves volume support and evacuation of the hematoma. A wide linear incision is made in the vulva, the blood clot is evacuated, and the dead space closed. Usually, the specific vessels that are bleeding are not identified, and packing leads only to further bleeding. After the incision is closed, a pressure dressing is applied and a Foley catheter is placed in the bladder.

b. Vaginal lacerations are associated with operative deliveries and can cause severe rectal pressure or a large mass in the vagina. A linear incision is made in the vagina over the clot, and the hematoma is evacuated. As in vulvar hematoma repair, it is unusual to identify the specific bleeding vessels, but in repair of vaginal lacerations the incision does not need to be closed because the vaginal wall folds together to reapproximate edges. A vaginal pack is inserted for 12 to 24 hours to stem bleeding, and a Foley catheter is placed in the bladder.

c. Retroperitoneal hematoma is a potentially life-threatening condition that may present as hypotension, cardiovascular shock, or flank pain. Although rare, retroperitoneal hematoma can result from laceration of the hypogastric artery that dissects up to the renal vasculature. Retroperitoneal hematoma also can result from uterine dehiscence or bleeding from the uterine arteries as a result of cesarean section. If a retroperitoneal bleed is stable, then it is safest to provide supportive care and allow the hematoma to stop itself in the retroperitoneum. If the hematoma continues to expand, however, then surgical exploration may be necessary. The retroperitoneum should be opened and bleeding vessels identified and ligated. If necessary, the hypogastric arteries may also be ligated. The retroperitoneum should then be closed, and the patient closely monitored.

3. **Retained products of conception** cause 3% to 4% of cases of postpartum hemorrhage. Risk factors include abnormal placentation such as placenta accreta, percreta, or increta, and the presence of accessory lobes of the placenta. After the placenta is delivered, it should be inspected carefully for missing cotyledons or vessels in the membranes that might indicate missing accessory lobes. Abnormal placentation should be suspected if the placenta fails to emerge spontaneously within 30 minutes after delivery of the infant. When the placenta is retained, manual exploration of the uterus is performed. If products of conception remain in the uterus after manual exploration, blunt curettage should be performed. Because of the high risk of perforation of the postpartum uterus during curettage, ultrasound guidance should be used if available. In cases of placenta accreta, increta, or percreta, it may be impossible to remove all of the placenta without injury to the uterus. In these cases, part of the placenta may be left in the uterus if the bleeding is adequately controlled with uterine contractile agents. Methotrexate can also be administered to help speed resorption of the remaining placenta. If bleeding persists despite curettage of the uterus and the use of contractile agents, then further invasive procedures, such as embolization of the uterine arteries or, possibly, laparotomy, must be performed.

4. **Coagulopathy** can also lead to postpartum hemorrhage. Risk factors include severe preeclampsia, abruptio placentae, idiopathic thrombocytopenia, amniotic fluid embolism, and hereditary coagulopathies such as von Willebrand's disease. If the cause of a patient's bleeding is coagulopathy, then supportive measures to correct the coagulopathy are required; surgical treatment does not address the problem and only leads to further hemorrhage. If coagulation factors are depleted, FFP or cryoprecipitate should be given; platelets should be given if the platelet count falls below 20,000, or if the patient's platelets are malfunctioning, regardless of the platelet count. Dexamethasone also has been shown to improve both platelet number and platelet function in patients with severe preeclampsia. Dexamethasone, 10 mg p.o. q.d., should be administered for 2 days, followed by 5 mg p.o. q.d. for 2 days.

II. **Uterine dehiscence or rupture.** Uterine dehiscence or rupture occurs in approximately 0.7% of patients during labor. Dehiscence is defined as a separation of a lower uterine scar that does not penetrate the serosa, and rarely causes significant hemorrhage. Rupture is defined as a complete separation of the uterine wall and may lead to significant hemorrhage and fetal distress.

A. **Risk factors** include a history of prior uterine surgery, including cesarean section, myomectomy, and ectopic surgery involving the cornua. Other risk factors are hyperstimulation of the uterus, internal version or extraction, operative delivery, cephalopelvic disproportion, and cocaine use. Approximately 1% of patients with a history of a prior low segment transverse cesarean section, and 5% of patients with a history of a cesarean section extending to the active segment of the uterus, experience rupture if allowed a trial of labor. One-third of women with a history of prior classic cesarean section who experience rupture do so before onset of labor.

B. If rupture occurs, severe hemorrhage can result, leading to a nonreassuring fetal heart tracing. On examination, the fetal heart position may move, and the station of the presenting part suddenly rises. The patient should undergo laparotomy, and the infant should be delivered. The rupture is then identified and repaired, and the patient should be counseled against trial of labor in future pregnancies. Occasionally, dehiscence or rupture of the uterus is found incidentally during cesarean section for failure to progress, and dehiscence or rupture may remain undiagnosed at vaginal delivery unless manual exploration of the uterus is performed.

III. **Uterine inversion**

   A. **Incidence.** Uterine inversion occurs in 1 in 2,000 deliveries and is diagnosed by partial delivery of the placenta that is followed by massive blood loss and hypotension. Inversion occurs most commonly with fundal placentas and is classified as incomplete if the corpus travels partially through the cervix, complete if the corpus travels entirely through the cervix, and prolapsed if the corpus travels through the vaginal introitus.

   B. **Treatment** of uterine inversion consists of manually replacing the uterus.

      1. If the uterus can be replaced easily without removing the placenta, less blood will be lost; if the bulk of the placenta prevents replacement of the uterus, however, the placenta should be removed to facilitate uterine replacement.

      2. If the cervix has contracted around the corpus of the uterus, uterine relaxant agents may be necessary to effect replacement. Several uterine relaxant agents are available including nitroglycerin, betamimetics such as terbutaline or ritodrine, magnesium, and halogenated general anesthetics such as halothane or isoflurane. If the patient is normotensive and has been given adequate analgesia, then nitroglycerin is the preferred agent because it has a rapid onset of 30 to 60 seconds and wears off within 5 minutes, which enables the uterus to contract again after it has been replaced, minimizing further blood loss. If nitroglycerin, betamimetics, or magnesium, alone or in combination, is unsuccessful in freeing the uterus, general anesthesia should be employed.

      3. After the uterus is replaced, uterine contractile agents should be used.

      4. If the obstetrician is unable to replace the uterus manually, it may be necessary to perform laparotomy. Traction can then be placed on the round ligaments, adding to vaginal pressure. If traction is unsuccessful, a vertical incision can be made on the posterior lower uterine segment to enable replacement of the uterus.

IV. **Amniotic fluid embolism.** Amniotic fluid embolism occurs during 1 in 30,000 deliveries and carries a 50% mortality rate.

   A. **Diagnosis and etiology.** Definitive diagnosis is made at postmortem autopsy, when fetal squames and lanugo are found in maternal pulmonary vasculature. The term *embolism* is a misnomer because the clinical findings are probably a result of anaphylactic shock, not massive pulmonary embolism. In fact, fetal squames and lanugo have been found in the pulmonary vasculature of postpartum women undergoing autopsy for reasons other than amniotic fluid embolism. Whatever its cause, amniotic fluid embolism is potentially catastrophic and should be suspected when sudden respiratory and cardiovascular collapse follows delivery of an infant. Cyanosis, hemorrhage, coma, and disseminated intravascular coagulation (DIC) rapidly ensues.

   B. **Management.** Aggressive supportive management is needed, and the patient should be intubated and monitored closely. Good intravenous access is essential, and invasive monitoring devices should be placed. Volume support, inotropic agents, and pressors should be given as needed to maintain adequate blood pressure. Packed red blood cells and FFP should also be available, because these patients are at high risk for developing DIC. Despite all efforts, approximately one-half of patients who develop amniotic fluid embolism die.

V. **Septic pelvic thrombophlebitis.** Septic pelvic thrombophlebitis (SPT) occurs in 1 in 2,000 deliveries, most commonly after cesarean section.

   A. **Diagnosis and etiology.** Thrombi form in the deep pelvic veins as a result of the hypercoagulability, increased predilection to injury, and relative venous stasis of pregnancy. The thrombi become superinfected and can cause septic emboli, particularly in the pulmonary system. SPT should be suspected when a patient's fever fails to respond to adequate antibiotic therapy for endomyometritis after 2 to 3 days. A pelvic examination should be performed to assess for masses or hematomas, and chest and abdominal radiographic studies should be obtained to rule out pneumonia or retained sponges. If such a workup is negative, pelvic ultrasound, pelvic and abdominal computed tomography (CT), or pelvic and abdominal magnetic resonance imaging (MRI) should be performed to locate abscesses or obvious thrombi in the inferior vena cava or iliac vessels. Unfortunately, imaging studies miss the majority of septic pelvic thrombi, and SPT remains largely a diagnosis of exclusion.

B. Management. If no other explanation of the persistent fever is found, the patient should be given heparin intravenously; patients with SPT who are treated with heparin typically experience fever reduction in 1 to 2 days, and should be maintained on heparin for 7 to 14 days. Long-term anticoagulation therapy is unnecessary unless deep venous thrombus or pulmonary embolus is present. If the patient remains febrile despite appropriate antibiotic and heparin therapy, surgical exploration may be necessary to identify and treat the cause of the hyperpyrexia.

VI. Chorioamnionitis. Chorioamnionitis occurs in 0.5% to 2.0% of all term pregnancies. Risk factors include low socioeconomic status; poor nutrition; invasive procedures, including vaginal examination and internal monitoring; prolonged rupture of membranes; preterm rupture of membranes; and infections such as gonorrhea and chlamydia.

A. Diagnosis. Chorioamnionitis is a polymicrobial infection and is usually diagnosed by clinical assessment. Signs and symptoms include maternal fever, tachycardia, leukocytosis, fundal tenderness, and fetal tachycardia. The definitive diagnosis, however, is made after amniocentesis with Gram's stain and culture of the amniotic fluid. If a preterm patient presents with fever and physical examination findings are inconclusive, amniocentesis may be performed to help distinguish chorioamnionitis from other causes of fever. Chorioamnionitis should be suspected in patients in preterm labor who are unresponsive to tocolytic therapy, and the pediatrics department should be informed of all patients with suspected chorioamnionitis.

B. Management. Definitive treatment of chorioamnionitis consists of delivery of the infant, with antibiotic coverage during labor. Usually ampicillin and gentamicin are administered during labor; if the patient is allergic to penicillins, clindamycin and gentamicin may be administered. If the patient is not in labor already, labor should be induced to help avoid sepsis in both the mother and the infant. A culture may be taken after delivery of the placenta and separation of the chorion and amnion, and the placenta should be sent to the pathology department to be examined for evidence of chorioamnionitis. No further antibiotic therapy is necessary after vaginal delivery. Patients who undergo cesarean section, however, should be given broad-spectrum antibiotics for prophylactic treatment of endomyometritis. Gentamicin and clindamycin can be administered, and ampicillin can be added. Although gentamicin should be administered every 8 hours before delivery, daily doses may be administered after delivery. If daily dosing is chosen, gentamicin levels do not require monitoring.

VII. Endomyometritis. In addition to the risk factors for chorioamnionitis, risk factors for endomyometritis also include cesarean section or pregnancy complicated by chorioamnionitis.

A. Diagnosis. Endomyometritis is a mainly clinical diagnosis that is based on findings of fever, fundal tenderness, and foul-smelling lochia accompanied by leukocytosis. Endometrial cultures tend to be unhelpful because they are usually contaminated by vaginal or cervical flora, and endomyometritis is a polymicrobial infection. If the patient's clinical picture is consistent with endomyometritis, blood cultures do not necessarily need to be performed because they have a low yield and do not affect the choice of antibiotics.

B. Management. Broad-spectrum antibiotics such as gentamicin and a course of clindamycin should be started. Ampicillin also can be added, particularly if the patient presents with a high fever within the first 24 to 48 hours after a delivery, because early temperature spikes are usually a result of streptococcal infection. If the patient continues to be febrile 24 to 48 hours after appropriate antibiotics are initiated, further workup to establish the source of the fever should be undertaken. Studies include urine and blood cultures, chest and abdominal radiography, pelvic examination, and, possibly, pelvic ultrasound, CT, or MRI. Patients with endomyometritis usually show improvement on physical examination and temperature curves 24 to 48 hours after beginning antibiotics. If the patient's examination findings show improvement, antibiotic therapy can be stopped after the patient has remained afebrile for 48 hours, and no further antibiotic treatment is necessary. It is worth noting that patients with endomyometritis carry an increased risk of secondary infertility as a result of scarring from inflammation.

VIII. Umbilical cord prolapse. Umbilical cord prolapse occurs when the umbilical cord slips past the presenting fetal part and passes through the open cervical os. The blood supply to the fetus is cut off when the fetus compresses the umbilical cord against the cervix. Risk factors include rupture of membranes when the fetus is not yet engaged in the pelvis, footling breech presentation, transverse lie, oblique lie, and unstable fetal presentations. These factors may be influenced by cephalopelvic disproportion, abnormal placentation, multiple gestation, polyhydramnios, and fetal and uterine anomalies.

    A. Diagnosis. Vaginal examination should be performed shortly after rupture of membranes is confirmed to evaluate the condition of the cervix and rule out the possibility of cord prolapse. Vaginal examination also should be performed promptly when fetal bradycardia occurs to investigate the possibility of cord prolapse.

    B. Management. If the umbilical cord is palpated on vaginal examination, the examiner should call for help and elevate the presenting fetal part to prevent compression of the umbilical cord. The examiner also can assess the fetal pulse by palpating the umbilical cord, taking care not to confuse his or her own pulse with that of the fetus. While the examiner continues to elevate the presenting fetal part, the patient should be transported to an operating room, where appropriate anesthesia should be initiated and urgent cesarean section performed. If a patient in labor presents with a prolapsed cord, viability of the fetus must be established before proceeding with cesarean section. If the fetus is dead, induction of labor for vaginal delivery should be performed.

IX. Meconium. Meconium complicates 8% to 16% of all deliveries and 25% to 30% of all postterm deliveries. Meconium passage by the fetus results from hypoxic stimulation of the parasympathetic system or from triggering of a mature vagal reflex.

    A. Uncommonly, meconium passage leads to **meconium aspiration syndrome,** which carries a mortality rate of 28%. Symptoms of meconium aspiration syndrome include tachypnea, chest retractions, cyanosis, barrel-shaped chest, and coarse breath sounds. Chest radiography shows coarse, irregular pulmonary densities with areas of decreased aeration. Persistent pulmonary hypertension also occurs. To prevent meconium aspiration, most physicians advocate amnioinfusion for moderate to thick meconium, in an effort to dilute the meconium in the uterus. Some believe, however, that amnioinfusion causes the meconium to become less viscous and therefore easier for the fetus to aspirate. Others note that meconium is often present before labor begins, so the damage from aspiration may be done before the efforts of the obstetrician or pediatrician to prevent it begin.

    B. Management. If meconium is present, De Lee suction should be used when the head is delivered before the body. Quickly and with minimal stimulation, the infant should be handed over to a pediatrician. Ideally, the pediatrician is able to perform laryngoscopy and suction below the vocal cords if meconium is present; laryngoscopy is deferred, however, if the infant is crying or breathing vigorously. At delivery, the placenta should be examined for meconium staining to determine whether the passage of meconium occurred recently or in the relatively distant past.

X. Fistulas

    A. Vesicovaginal fistulas occur when obstructed and prolonged labor causes pressure necrosis of the anterior vagina and vesicovaginal septum. The fistula usually becomes apparent by 1 week postpartum, when the patient presents with continuous, painless leakage of urine from the vagina that is unrelated to position. Diagnosis is confirmed when methylene blue is instilled into the bladder and either is observed draining from the vagina or stains a tampon placed in the vagina. To evaluate possible damage to the ureters, an intravenous pyelogram should be performed. An indwelling Foley catheter is placed to allow the fistula time to heal. If the fistula fails to heal despite placement of a urinary catheter, cystoscopy with biopsy of the tract margins should be performed. The fistula then can be closed in layers vaginally.

B. Rectovaginal fistulas usually involve the perineum, anal sphincter, anal canal, and distal rectum. On examination, the fistula is visible or palpable, and endoscopy can be performed to ensure that the colon or small bowel is not compromised. A fistulogram can help delineate anatomy; radiography is performed after barium is instilled into the vagina by Foley catheter. After the anatomy of the fistula is established, the patient receives a thorough bowel preparation and is taken to the operating room, where the fistula is debrided and closed in layers without tension. The anal sphincter and perineal body are reconstructed, and the patient is placed on stool softeners postoperatively to avoid excessive straining.

XI. Mastitis. Mastitis occurs in 1% to 2% of postpartum women and can appear in either an epidemic or nonepidemic form.

A. The **epidemic** form occurs 2 to 4 days after delivery and is associated with an outbreak in the nursery. The infant's nasopharynx is colonized with a virulent strain of *Staphylococcus aureus* and passes the bacteria to its mother while breast-feeding. This strain can cause deep breast abscess, and the mother presents with fever, breast tenderness, and purulent discharge from the breast. Gram's stain and culture of the nipple discharge may be performed to confirm the diagnosis. The mother and infant should be isolated from other patients, and penicillin should be administered to the mother. If an abscess is found, incision and drainage should be performed. The skin incision can be made either radially or parallel to the areola. If incision and drainage is performed, the contents of the abscess should undergo both culture and pathologic examination to rule out breast carcinoma.

B. The **nonepidemic** form of mastitis occurs weeks to months after delivery and usually occurs during the weaning period. Associated with milk stasis, this form of mastitis results in superficial cellulitis in periglandular connective tissue and rarely causes deep abscesses. The patient presents with fever, tachycardia, malaise, and breast tenderness; usually, however, she does not experience purulent drainage from the nipple. The diagnosis can be made clinically, or a white blood cell count can be performed on the milk from the affected breast. Culture can be performed and the patient treated with penicillin or dicloxacillin. The patient should continue to breast-feed or pump during the mastitis to help decrease milk stasis.

XII. Postpartum depression. Known colloquially as the *postpartum blues*, postpartum depression occurs after 10% to 15% of all deliveries. Manifestations range from transient tearfulness, anxiety, irritability, and restlessness to full-blown depression that can last up to 1 year. Risk factors include a prior history of depression, young age, and poor social support. Postpartum depression also tends to recur in future pregnancies. If a postpartum patient appears to be depressed, thyroid function tests should be performed and a course of tricyclic antidepressant can be started. Psychiatric follow-up should be arranged, and the patient should be questioned about suicidal or homicidal ideation. It may be necessary to involve social services to ensure that the baby is receiving adequate care. Postpartum psychosis also can occur, especially in patients with a prior psychiatric history. Such patients require close psychiatric follow-up as well as antipsychotic drug therapy.

Preterm Labor and Premature Rupture of Membranes

Karen Morrill and
Gina Hanna

I. **Preterm labor** (PTL) is defined as six to eight contractions per hour, or four in 20 minutes, that are associated with cervical change at less than 37 weeks' gestation. PTL also may be defined as cervical effacement greater than 80%, or dilation over 2 cm, at less than 37 weeks' gestation. The incidence of PTL has remained 9% of all live births despite such advances as the development and use of tocolytic agents.

A. **Risk factors** include infections, especially group B streptococcus, gonorrhea, *Chlamydia, Ureaplasma, Trichomonas,* bacterial vaginosis, *Treponema pallidum,* and *Mycoplasma;* low socioeconomic status; nonwhite race; maternal age of less than 18 or greater than 40; smoking; cocaine use; lack of prenatal care; low prepregnancy weight; history of PTL (recurrence rate of 17% to 37%); uterine malformations (i.e., bicornuate uterus or myoma); cervical incompetence; diethylstilbestrol (DES) exposure; placenta previa; premature rupture of membranes (PROM); abruptio placentae; hydramnios; multiple gestation; congenital anomalies of the fetus; and medical problems, including severe hypertension and severe diabetes mellitus. In most cases, the cause of PTL remains unknown.

B. **Possible fetal consequences** of preterm delivery include respiratory distress syndrome, bronchopulmonary dysplasia, patent ductus arteriosus, necrotizing enterocolitis, intraventricular hemorrhage, neurologic impairment, apnea, retrolental fibroplasia, neonatal sepsis, and death. Preterm birth is the cause of at least 75% of neonatal deaths that are not attributable to congenital malformations. Survival of infants born at 23 weeks' gestation is between zero and 8%. Of infants born at 24 weeks' gestation, 15% to 20% will survive long enough to be discharged from the hospital; of infants born at 25 weeks' gestation, 50% to 60% will survive; of infants born at 26 to 28 weeks' gestation, 85% will survive; and of infants born at 29 weeks' gestation, more than 90% will survive.

C. A number of approaches to **prevention** have been advocated; none, however, has proven effective. Education about PTL remains integral to prevention. Weekly cervical examinations have no demonstrated beneficial effect. The benefits of home uterine monitoring and daily nurse contact are the subject of controversy, except in cases of multiple gestation. Prophylactic oral tocolytic therapy also has no demonstrated beneficial effect overall; because of their side effects, tocolytic agents should be avoided before the onset of true PTL. Decreased activity or bed rest in the late second trimester and early third trimester commonly is recommended, although no studies of the efficacy of these measures have been done; similarly, no studies have demonstrated the efficacy of sexual abstinence, which is also a common recommendation. Prophylactic cervical cerclage is recommended only for women who have been diagnosed with cervical incompetence.

D. The **evaluation** of suspected PTL should include a thorough history, physical examination, laboratory studies, ultrasound, and evaluation of the continuous fetal heart rate tracing.

1. The **history** should elicit previous occurrences of preterm labor, preterm delivery, or both; infections during the present pregnancy or symptoms of current infection, including upper respiratory or urinary infection; recent intercourse; physical abuse or recent abdominal trauma; and recent drug use.

2. The **physical examination** should focus on vital signs (fever, maternal tachycardia, and fetal tachycardia), any potential source of infection, uterine tenderness, and contractions.

   a. **Sterile speculum examination** should include Nitrazine and fern test to rule out membrane rupture and procurement of specimens for cervical cultures, including *Chlamydia, Neisseria* gonorrhea (GC), and group B beta-hemolytic streptococcus (GBS), and wet preparations for bacterial vaginosis and *Trichomonas*. The advisability of obtaining cultures for *Ureaplasma* and *Mycoplasma* is a subject of controversy.

   b. If no evidence of membrane rupture is found, proceed with a **bimanual examination.** Repeat the examination at appropriate intervals to determine whether cervical change has occurred. If rupture has occurred, initiate treatment for PROM (see sec. II.B).

3. **Laboratory studies** include a complete blood cell count, cervical cultures, urine specimens for a toxicology screen, urinalysis, microscopic evaluation, culture, and sensitivity studies. Consider performing amniocentesis, especially if the patient does not respond well to tocolytic agents or is febrile without an obvious source of infection. If amniocentesis is performed, specimens should be designated for Gram's stain, cell count, glucose, culture, and fetal lung maturity studies if gestational age is between 30 and 35 weeks. Fetal fibronectin from cervicovaginal secretions is a marker for decidual disruption. The presence of this marker in serial specimens from high-risk patients or a single specimen from patients in whom the diagnosis of PTL is suspected holds promise as a diagnostic indicator.

4. **Ultrasound** studies are performed to assess fetal position, amniotic fluid index (AFI), estimated fetal weight, placental location, evidence of abruptio placentae (a rare finding on ultrasound even when abruptio placentae is the correct diagnosis), fetal or uterine anomalies, and biophysical profile if indicated.

5. **Continuous fetal heart rate monitoring** should be performed until the patient is stable and the rate of contractions remains less than six per hour for an extended period.

E. **Management**

1. **Intravenous hydration** with 500 mL of isotonic crystalloid solution is a common initial approach to treatment, although hydration is not a proven benefit for patients who are not dehydrated. Excessive hydration should be avoided because of its association with pulmonary edema during tocolytic therapy. Maintenance fluid should be Ringer's lactated solution or 0.9N saline, with or without dextrose to minimize the risk of pulmonary edema.

2. Patients should remain on strict **bed rest,** initially with continuous fetal monitoring.

3. **Antibiotic therapy** should be initiated for prophylaxis against GBS infection until all cervical and urine cultures return negative findings. Penicillin or ampicillin is recommended unless the patient is allergic to penicillin, in which case clindamycin is recommended. All specific infections implicated by positive culture findings should be treated appropriately.

4. **Corticosteroids** (12 mg i.m. of betamethasone, with a repeat dose in 24 hours) should be administered to induce fetal lung maturity between 24 and 34 weeks' gestation if no obvious signs of infection are present. Optimal benefit is achieved 24 hours after the second dose and lasts for 7 days. Corticosteroids accelerate the appearance of pulmonary surfactant and decrease the occurrence of neonatal deaths, cerebral hemorrhage, and necrotizing enterocolitis. The beneficial effects of corticosteroid therapy

in PTL and PROM are significant. Concerns about corticosteroid therapy include the increased risk of infection for both mother and infant and impaired maternal glucose tolerance, especially in diabetic patients. Diabetic mothers taking corticosteroids can slip easily into diabetic ketoacidosis and may require an insulin drip and careful monitoring. Weekly doses of steroids often are administered in the absence of infection; no beneficial effect, however, has been proven for this regimen.

F. Tocolytic therapy. In assessing whether a patient is a candidate for tocolysis, gestational age should be confirmed and fetal anomalies ruled out.

  1. General contraindications to tocolysis for PTL include acute fetal distress, chorioamnionitis, eclampsia or severe preeclampsia, fetal demise (singleton), fetal maturity, and maternal hemodynamic instability.

  2. Indications. Most physicians initiate tocolytic therapy when regular uterine contractions are present and cervical change is documented. Cervical dilation of at least 3 cm is associated with a decreased success rate for tocolytic therapy. Tocolytic therapy is, however, appropriate in some such cases to allow time for transfer to a tertiary medical center or treatment with a corticosteroid. Most physicians are willing to begin treatment with tocolytic agents until 34 weeks' gestation. Analysis of data from neonatal centers reveals that the survival rate of infants delivered at 34 weeks' gestation is within 1% of the survival rate of those delivered at 37 weeks' gestation. No studies have convincingly demonstrated an improvement in survival or in any index of long-term neonatal outcome with tocolytic therapy.

  3. Goals of tocolysis are similar regardless of which agent is chosen, and include decreasing uterine contractions and arresting cervical dilatation using the lowest effective dose, decreasing or stopping the drug if significant side effects develop, and stopping the drug or switching to an oral agent after intravenous or subcutaneous therapy has produced sustained clinical improvement for 12 to 48 hours.

  4. Once tocolysis has been achieved and maintained, the patient should be kept in the hospital for observation, initially on strict bed rest (which may be liberalized according to individual patient tolerance). Prophylactic penicillin should be administered until negative results of cervical and urine cultures are returned (if positive findings appear, the specific infection should be treated). Fetal heart tones should be obtained at least every 8 hours, and a physical therapy consult should be obtained if the possibility exists that bed rest will be prolonged. Fetal testing should be performed as indicated [i.e., by evidence of intrauterine growth retardation (IUGR) or oligohydramnios, or by maternal factors]. Penicillin should be administered during labor for patients with gestations of less than 37 weeks or with a history of a positive finding for GBS on cervical or urine culture.

  5. Terbutaline is a phenylethylamine derivative with beta$_2$ mimetic properties. Up to three doses of 0.25 mg are given s.q. every 20 minutes. Terbutaline is administered for contractions and is withheld if maternal heart rates are greater than 120 or fetal heart rates are greater than 160. It may be given every 1 to 4 hours for 24 hours. The total dose should not exceed 5 mg in 24 hours. No proven benefit is associated with the use of oral terbutaline.

    a. Relative **contraindications** include antepartum hemorrhage, cardiovascular disease, hyperthyroidism, and uncontrolled diabetes (even patients with well-controlled diabetes may require a concomitant insulin drip).

    b. Maternal side effects consist of tachycardia, tremor, palpitations, anxiety, shortness of breath, pulmonary edema, substernal pain, and mild hyperglycemia. In the patient whose initial test was negative, consider repeating the 50-g oral glucose screening test when a patient requires more than 1 week of therapy. The test may be repeated on a monthly or semimonthly basis.

      c. Fetal side effects include tachycardia (variability should be maintained) and hyperglycemia.

    6. Magnesium sulfate is thought to decrease uterine contractility by influencing the amplitude of motor plate potentials and interfering with calcium function at the myometrial neuronal junction. The initial dose is 4 to 6 g i.v. over 20 minutes, then 3 g/hour. The dose should be titrated to stop contractions, but usually 6 g/hour hour is not exceeded. Continue magnesium sulfate administration until the patient has had fewer than six contractions per hour for 12 hours.

      a. Absolute **contraindications** include myasthenia gravis and recent myocardial infarction. Magnesium is secreted by the kidney and its effects last significantly longer in patients with renal impairment than in patients with normal renal function.

      b. Maternal **side effects** include flushing, muscle weakness, hypotension, hyporeflexia, respiratory depression, pulmonary edema, cardiac arrest, tetany, nausea, and vomiting. Decreased variability is the only notable fetal side effect. The risk of side effects increases significantly if terbutaline and magnesium sulfate are administered together.

      c. Close **monitoring** is essential. Consider keeping a flow sheet with hourly documentation of symptoms, lung examination findings, deep tendon reflexes, and total intake and outputs. Limit i.v. fluids to 100 mL/hour.

      d. Watch for signs of **magnesium toxicity,** which include loss of patellar reflexes at magnesium levels of 8 to 12 mg/dL, respiratory depression at levels of 15 mg/dL, and cardiac collapse at levels of 30 mg/dL. It is not essential to check magnesium levels; the patient's examination record can be followed and the dose titrated accordingly to stop contractions. Magnesium levels often are checked, however, 6 hours after the initial bolus. If signs or symptoms of magnesium toxicity appear, administer calcium gluconate i.v. in a 1-g push.

    7. Indomethacin interferes with the synthesis of prostaglandins, primarily $PGF_{2\alpha}$, from fatty acid precursors. The usual course begins with a loading dose of 100 mg p.r., and therapeutic levels are maintained with doses of 25 mg p.o. or 50 mg p.r. every 4 to 6 hours for a maximum of 48 hours.

      a. Because indomethacin affects fetal kidneys, amniotic fluid volume may decrease. An **AFI** should be established before beginning therapy and should be checked after 48 hours. The effect of indomethacin on the fetal kidneys is reversible.

      b. Contraindications include peptic ulcer disease, estimated gestational age of greater than 32 weeks, renal disease, coagulopathy, and oligohydramnios.

      c. Headache, dizziness, gastrointestinal discomfort, fluid retention, nausea and vomiting, and pruritus are the primary **maternal side effects.**

      d. Oligohydramnios and potential ductal closure are the two most worrisome **fetal side effects.**

    8. Nifedipine blocks contraction of smooth muscle by inhibiting intracellular calcium entry. The recommended dose is 10 to 20 mg every 6 hours p.o. Nifedipine has been administered in a loading dose of 10 mg sublingually every 20 minutes up to three doses.

      a. Contraindications include congestive heart failure, aortic stenosis, and concomitant use of magnesium sulfate, which can precipitate severe hypotension.

      b. Side effects consist of hypotension, flushing, nasal congestion, tachycardia, dizziness, nausea, nervousness, bowel changes, and, in one case report, skeletal muscle blockade.

  G. Chorioamnionitis (see Chap. 3, sec. **VI**) is a frequent cause of PTL and should always be excluded before embarking on prolonged tocolytic therapy. It is characterized by maternal fever, leukocytosis, maternal and fetal tachycardia, uterine tenderness, and uterine contractions. PROM is commonly associated with this diagnosis. Amniocentesis can aid in the diagnosis. Polymorphonuclear neutrophil leukocytes in amniotic fluid are suggestive but not diagnostic of chorioamnionitis, as is a glucose level of less than 14 mg/dL; bacteria on Gram's stain specimen is specific but not sensitive, and culture results take more than 1 week to return. The usual treatment is ampicillin and gentamicin i.v. and delivery of the fetus. Tylenol is administered to reduce maternal fever after the diagnosis of chorioamnionitis has been made.

H. Proceed with **delivery** if signs or symptoms of chorioamnionitis or fetal distress are present. A fetal heart rate greater than 160 beats/min can indicate distress, especially in association with decreased variability. Anesthesia issues should be addressed early in the delivery process. During delivery, special care should be taken to avoid fetal asphyxia and birth trauma by controlling the second stage of labor. Episiotomy is indicated only when perineal resistance is present. Forceps should be employed as routinely indicated. Most obstetricians opt for delivery by cesarean section for nonvertex presentations at greater than 26 weeks' gestation. It is important to inform patients of the possibility that classical cesarean section will be performed under such circumstances. It is also important to inform patients of the possibility that classical cesarean section will be performed in cases of fetal distress, nonvertex presentations, or both at less than 26 weeks' gestation.

I. **Home management** of PTL is reserved for patients who have had stable cervical examination findings while taking no or oral tocolytics with at least bathroom privileges in the hospital. Candidates for home management must be able to comply with left-sided bed rest and pelvic rest instructions. Kick count charts should be utilized. Consider weekly betamethasone administration (see sec. **I.E.4**). Antenatal testing should be ordered as indicated. If IUGR is present, sonograms to track growth should be performed every 3 to 4 weeks.

II. **Premature rupture of membranes.** *Preterm* refers to an event that occurs before 37 weeks' gestation. When used to describe membrane rupture, *premature* signifies that the event occurred at least 1 hour before the onset of labor.

A. The **etiology** of PROM is unclear. Possible causative factors include local amniotic membrane defect; infection, including vaginal, cervical, or intraamniotic; colonization, especially with GBS; history of PROM; incompetent cervix; hydramnios; multiple gestation; trauma; fetal malformations; abruptio placentae; and placenta previa.

B. The **evaluation** for PROM is similar in many ways to that of PTL (see sec. **I.D**). In addition, it is important to note the time of the rupture and the color of the fluid. *Only* a sterile speculum examination is performed (no bimanual examination is performed unless delivery is anticipated within 24 hours) to procure specimens for nitrazine (false-positive results in the presence of *Trichomonas*, blood, semen, cervical mucus, and urine) and fern (false-positive results in the presence of cervical mucus, false-negative results in the presence of blood) test. Cervical specimens should also be obtained for culture. Consider testing vaginal pool fluid for fetal lung maturity (the Amniostat test is a rapid test used to detect the presence of phosphatidylglycerol). All of the commercially available methods of detecting fetal lung maturity using vaginal pool collections of fluid have been shown to be affected by the vaginal environment. These results should be used cautiously when there is evidence of maternal or intraamniotic infection.

C. **Management** of PROM usually is limited to conservative measures. Most obstetricians wait for signs or symptoms of infection or fetal distress to appear before intervening. Severe oligohydramnios and cessation of fetal breathing are associated with chorioamnionitis.

1. **Maternal testing and prophylaxis.** In all cases of PROM, it is important to assess the gestational age, weight, and position of the fetus. Betamethasone is given between 24 and 34 weeks' gestation only if no immediate signs of infection are present. Prophylaxis for GBS infection with penicillin G is recommended (clindamycin is used if the patient is allergic to penicillin) until negative results of cervical and urine cultures are received. Positive culture results should prompt appropriate treatment. Tocolytics generally are reserved for cases in which transport is neces-

sary, or to delay delivery in some cases for 48 hours so that steroids can produce a maximal effect on pulmonary maturation.

2. **Monitoring.** A neonatologist should be consulted. If the patient is not in labor, and the fetal heart rate tracing is stable, the patient may be kept under observation. Continue strict bed rest because of the risk of cord prolapse, and obtain fetal heart tones at least every 8 hours. Recommendations for fetal testing vary between daily nonstress tests and weekly biophysical profiles to semiweekly testing. If IUGR is identified, sonograms to track growth should be performed every 3 to 4 weeks.

3. **Indications for delivery** are identical to those for PTL.

4. Management of PROM in the setting of a **cerclage** is the subject of some controversy. Most obstetricians remove the cerclage and proceed with expectant management.

5. Consequences of **prolonged rupture** include increased risk of maternal and fetal infection, fetal limb contracture formation, and pulmonary hypoplasia of the fetus in addition to those listed for PTL. Prolonged bed rest leads to increased maternal risk of deep venous thrombosis and, possibly, pulmonary embolus. Therefore, patients on prolonged bed rest require physical therapy and thromboembolic disease stockings.

III. **Staff neonatologists** should be informed of all patients admitted to the hospital who are at risk for PTL. It is important for neonatologists to discuss the consequences of preterm delivery with the patient (see sec. **I.B**). Issues relating to cesarean delivery for fetal indications should be addressed with the patient. An effort should be made to specifically discuss the limits of viability; likely fetal outcome; and the high probability of a classic, instead of a low, transverse cesarean delivery during weeks 24 to 26.

Gestational Complications

Vanna Zanagnolo and
Eva Pressman

Amniotic Fluid Disorders

I. **Physiologic aspects of amniotic fluid.** Amniotic fluid volume (AFV) increases from a mean of 250 mL at 16 weeks' gestation to about 800 mL at about 22 weeks' gestation. Although considerable variability exists, the average volume of amniotic fluid remains stable from 22 weeks' to 39 weeks' gestation, then declines to about 500 mL at term. The steady-state volume of fluid in the amniotic cavity at any point in time represents a balance between the two sources that contribute bulk water (fetal urine and fetal alveolar fluid) and the two sources that remove bulk water (fetal swallowing and the amniotic chorionic interface with the maternal uterine wall).

II. **Technique for assessing amniotic fluid volume.** The amniotic fluid index (AFI) was developed in 1987 as a reproducible and quantitative technique for assessing amniotic volume. The maternal abdomen is divided into quadrants, with the umbilicus used as the reference point. The vertical depth of the largest amniotic fluid pocket in each quadrant is identified and measured. The sum of these measurements establishes the AFI in centimeters. AFI appears to be highly reproducible; it may be applied reliably at any gestational age using normative values. Finally, the AFI provides good sensitivity and predictive value in identifying oligohydramnios and polyhydramnios.

III. **Polyhydramnios** is the pathologic accumulation of amniotic fluid (volume excess of 2,000 mL at all gestational ages). It is associated with high maternal and perinatal morbidity and mortality. Currently, the diagnosis is most accurately based on an AFI greater than three standard deviations, or the ninety-fifth percentile, for gestational age. The incidence of polyhydramnios in the general population ranges from 0.2% to 1.6%. Mild increases in AFV usually are clinically insignificant.

   A. **Etiology.** Idiopathic polyhydramnios has been reported to represent between 16% and 66% of all cases. Commonly, polyhydramnios is associated with some impairment of the fetal swallowing mechanism.

   1. **Fetal structural malformations.** In cases of central nervous system abnormalities, the pathophysiologic mechanism may be related to transudation of fluid across the fetal meninges or to the lack of antidiuretic hormone and resultant polyuria in addition to impairment of the swallowing mechanism. In contrast, gastrointestinal tract abnormalities are not associated with an inability of the fetus to swallow but frequently are associated with an obstructive process. In cases of omphalocele or gastroschisis, the polyhydramnios is probably a result of transudation of fluid.

   2. In addition to fetal structural malformations, the incidence of **chromosomal and genetic abnormalities** is also increased in polyhydramnios patients. In fact, the incidence of chromosomal abnormalities may approach 35%. The most common chromosomal abnormalities involve trisomies 13, 18, and 21, in which impaired swallowing might contribute to amniotic fluid accumulation.

3. **Neuromuscular disorders** may also be manifested clinically as polyhydramnios.

4. **Other causes.** In the absence of a sonographically visible or chromosomal abnormality, the evaluation of polyhydramnios should also include screening tests for toxoplasmosis and cytomegalovirus, maternal diabetes mellitus, and Rh sensitization. Polyhydramnios that complicates maternal diabetes during the third trimester remains unexplained, but usually is associated with inadequate glycemic control or malformations. In the twin-to-twin transfusion syndrome, one twin develops polyhydramnios and, occasionally, hydrops fetalis, while the other twin develops growth retardation and oligohydramnios. Twin-to-twin transfusion syndrome is found in monozygotic twins with large arteriovenous anastomoses connecting their placentas.

B. **Diagnosis.** Clinical findings are uterine enlargement with difficulty palpating fetal small parts and hearing fetal heart tones. Ultrasound examination is necessary to better quantify amniotic fluid and to identify multiple fetuses and fetal abnormalities. Amniocentesis has become an indispensable diagnostic tool for viral cultures and, when indicated, karyotyping.

C. **Treatment.** Minor and moderate degrees of polyhydramnios with some discomfort usually can be managed without intervention until labor begins or until the membranes rupture spontaneously. If dyspnea or abdominal pain develops, or if ambulation is difficult, treatment becomes necessary.

1. **Amnioreduction** is the most common treatment. The principal purpose of amnioreduction is to relieve maternal discomfort, and to that end it is transiently successful. The volume of fluid removed at one time appears to be critical to success; the frequent removal of smaller volumes (rate of flow of amniotic fluid about 500 mL/hour, for a removal of approximately 1,500 to 2,000 mL) is associated less frequently with onset of preterm labor than the infrequent removal of larger volumes. The procedure is repeated every 1 to 3 weeks as needed until the fetus has achieved pulmonary maturity or delivery is required for another reason.

2. **Pharmacologic treatment** involves "manipulation" of fetal urine flow. Fetal renal blood flow is maintained under normal conditions chiefly by prostaglandins. The cyclooxygenase inhibitor indomethacin has been used to decrease fetal renal blood flow and to decrease AFV through reduction of urine production. Indomethacin acts by enhancing the action of vasopressin, which affects the autoregulation of renal blood flow. Data are available in the literature for treatment of polyhydramnios from 21 to 35 weeks' gestation with indomethacin (25 mg every 6 hours) for 2 to 11 weeks (1). The major concern about the use of indomethacin is the potential for closure of the fetal ductus arteriosus. Although closure of the fetal ductus arteriosus itself has not been described, ductal constriction detected by Doppler ultrasound has been reported, warranting close monitoring for ductal constriction. Treatment for twin-to-twin transfusion is discussed in Multiple Pregnancy, sec. **IV.H.**

IV. **Oligohydramnios** is quantitatively defined as an AFI less than the fifth percentile for gestational age. At term, oligohydramnios is considered whenever the AFI is less than 5 cm. Oligohydramnios is associated with an increase in perinatal morbidity and mortality at any gestational age but especially in the second trimester of pregnancy, when the risk of perinatal mortality reaches 80% to 90%. Prolonged oligohydramnios can lead to a deformation syndrome (10% to 15%), characterized by cranial, facial, or skeletal abnormalities, or to pulmonary hypoplasia (17%). The most probable cause of pulmonary hypoplasia is the lack of fluid available for inhalation into the terminal air sacs of the lungs; as a consequence of this deficit, lung growth is inhibited.

A. **Etiology.** The clinical conditions commonly associated with oligohydramnios are ruptured membranes, urinary tract malformations, intrauterine growth restriction (IUGR), postdate pregnancy, and placental insufficiency. Possible rupture of membranes always must be considered in the differential diagnosis for oligohydramnios at any gestational age. Renal agenesis or urinary tract obstruction often becomes apparent during the second trimester of pregnancy, when fetal urine flow begins to contribute significantly to the formation of amniotic fluid. IUGR often is associated with oligohydramnios; the fetal vascular volume deficit leads to a decrease in glomerular filtration and urinary flow rates. AFV also decreases in the postterm fetus; although the mechanism is unclear, the deterioration in placental function may cause a less efficient transfer of water from the mother to the fetus in the postdate gestation.

B. Diagnosis. Clinical findings, such as a lag in fundal height measurements or a reduction in fetal movements, can be unreliable. Ultrasound examination is necessary to better quantify amniotic fluid and to identify fetuses with IUGR or fetal abnormalities.

C. Treatment. Therapeutic options for the patient with oligohydramnios are limited. Maternal intravascular fluid status appears to be closely tied to that of the fetus. When the oligohydramnios is caused by a structural defect such as urinary tract obstruction, *in utero* surgical diversion of urine flow has produced promising results. To achieve optimal benefit, urinary diversion must be accomplished before the development of renal dysplasia and early enough in gestation to allow for lung development.

Intrauterine Growth Restriction

I. Description. Birth weight below the tenth percentile is the definition most widely used in describing IUGR. The incidence of IUGR varies according to the population under investigation; it is estimated to be approximately 4% to 8% in developed countries and 6% to 30% in developing countries. Growth restriction is classified as symmetric and asymmetric.

A. Symmetric growth restriction has an earlier onset than asymmetric growth restriction, and all body organs tend to be proportionally reduced in size. Factors typically associated with symmetric restriction include chromosomal abnormalities; anatomic (especially cardiac) malformations; congenital infection with rubella, cytomegalovirus, or toxoplasma; severe chronic maternal malnutrition; and smoking.

B. Asymmetric growth restriction has a late onset, and some body organs are more affected than others. Head size is the last fetal dimension to be affected, if it is affected at all, by impaired intrauterine growth. Asymmetric growth restriction is attributed to placental insufficiency caused by a variety of hypertensive complications of pregnancy and advanced diabetes mellitus, which is associated with impaired uteroplacental perfusion.

II. Etiology. Approximately 75% of small-for-gestational-age infants are constitutionally small; 15% to 20% have suffered from uteroplacental insufficiency resulting from various causes; and 5% to 10% have intrinsic impaired growth resulting from perinatal infection or malformation.

A. Maternal causes

1. **Constitutionally small mothers.** Maternal familial factors appear to significantly affect birth weight (2).

2. **Poor maternal weight gain.** If a woman weighs less than 100 lb at conception, her risk for delivering a small-for-gestational-age infant is increased by a factor of at least two. Inadequate weight gain throughout pregnancy or arrested weight gain after 28 weeks often is associated with fetal growth restriction. If the mother is above ideal body weight and otherwise healthy, below-average maternal weight gain is unlikely to be associated with fetal growth restriction.

3. **Chronic maternal disease.** Chronic maternal disease, including hypertension, cyanotic heart disease, long-standing diabetes, and collagen vas-

cular disease commonly cause growth restriction, especially when complicated by superimposed preeclampsia.

B. Fetal causes
1. **Fetal infection.** Viral, bacterial, protozoan, and spirochetal infections all have been associated with fetal growth restriction. Rubella and cytomegalovirus are among the best-known infectious antecedents of IUGR. Hepatitis A and B may cause restricted fetal growth. Varicella, influenza, listeriosis, tuberculosis, syphilis, toxoplasmosis, parvovirus B19, and congenital malaria may produce fetal growth restriction.
2. **Congenital malformations and chromosomal abnormalities.** Fetuses with chromosomal abnormalities, especially trisomy and triploidy, or those with serious cardiovascular malformations are most likely to have restricted growth. Trisomy 18 is associated with severe and early symmetric fetal growth restriction and polyhydramnios, whereas fetal growth restriction caused by trisomy 21 is often minimal. Trisomy 13 and Turner's syndrome also are associated with some degree of restricted fetal growth.
3. **Teratogens.** Any agent that causes a teratogenic injury is capable of producing fetal growth restriction. Anticonvulsants, tobacco, narcotics, and especially alcohol may impair fetal growth.

C. Placental causes
1. **Placental abnormalities.** Chronic abruptio placentae, extensive infarction, chorioangioma, and velamentous insertion of the cord are possible causes of restricted fetal growth. A circumvallate placenta or placenta previa also may impair growth.
2. **Multiple fetuses.** Pregnancy with two or more fetuses is likely to be complicated by appreciable impairment in growth of one or both fetuses (12% to 47%).

III. Diagnosis. Early establishment of gestational age and careful measurements of uterine height throughout pregnancy should help to identify most instances of abnormal fetal growth.
A. History of risk factors, a previously growth-restricted fetus, or fetal or neonatal death may alert the prenatal care provider to possible IUGR.
B. Clinical diagnosis may be unreliable. If the measurement of uterine fundal height differs more than 2 cm from the expected height, inappropriate fetal growth is suspected and ultrasound examination performed.
C. Ultrasound diagnosis. The most reliable method of estimating gestational age is the certain date of the patient's last menstrual period (LMP). Twenty percent to 40% of pregnant women, however, fail to recall the exact date of their LMP. Therefore, sonography may be of help in dating a pregnancy. Once a fetus is suspected of being growth restricted, an extensive ultrasonic survey should be done to look for structural abnormalities. See Chap. 1, sec. **II.A** for information on clinical dating.
1. **Third trimester** measurements are the least reliable for determining gestational age because growth restriction may already have occurred. Transverse cerebellar diameter (TCD) has been shown to correlate with gestational age in weeks up to 24 weeks, and it is not significantly affected by restricted fetal growth. The abdominal circumference (AC) has been reported to be the fetal biometric parameter that correlates best with fetal weight, and it is a sensitive tool for detecting IUGR (3). In contrast to BPD, AC is smaller in both symmetric and asymmetric types of IUGR; therefore, its measurement has high sensitivity. Unfortunately, AC is subject to more intraobserver and interobserver variation than either BPD or FL. Further AC variability may result from fetal breathing movements, compression, or position of the fetus. FL generally is decreased in symmetrically growth-restricted fetuses, but the femur may be of normal length in asymmetric IUGR. In fact, fetal head circumference and long bone length in asymmetric IUGR tend to be affected late in gestation. An elevated FL to AC ratio is suspicious for IUGR.

2. **Other associated findings.** An association between oligohydramnios and fetal growth restriction has long been recognized, in which IUGR is preceded by oligohydramnios. Grade III placenta before 34 weeks' gestation is suspicious for IUGR.

IV. **Management.** Perinatal morbidity and mortality are increased two to six times over the general population in patients with IUGR.

A. **Growth-restricted fetuses near term.** The best outcome for affected fetuses is achieved by prompt delivery.

B. **Growth-restricted fetuses remote from term** should be subject to a search for fetal anomalies, and if a chromosomal anomaly is suspected, amniocentesis, chorionic villus sampling (CVS), or fetal blood sampling for karyotyping and viral studies should be considered. Though it may be too late for abortion, the information gained from such studies may be important for parents, obstetricians, and pediatricians to have in planning delivery and newborn care. In some cases that involve fetuses who have multiple congenital anomalies associated with low life expectancy, such as fetuses with trisomy 13 or 18, cesarean section can be avoided.

1. **General management.** After ruling out structural and chromosomal abnormalities and possible congenital infection as completely as possible, hospitalization should be considered, physical activity restricted, adequate diet ensured, and fetal surveillance started. Fetal assessment should include fetal movement counting, sonographic assessment of fetal growth every 2 to 3 weeks, and nonstress test or biophysical profile (BPP) or both once or twice per week. In particular, AFV assessment is an important component of the profile because oligohydramnios is such a frequent finding in the IUGR-complicated pregnancy. Doppler flow studies of the umbilical artery are suggestive of a compromised fetus when they show elevated systolic to diastolic ratio or absent or reversed end-diastolic flow.

2. **Specific treatment.** In most cases of fetal growth restriction remote from term, no specific treatment exists. Possible exceptions are inadequate maternal nutrition, heavy smoking, use of street drugs, and, possibly, chronic alcoholism. It has been hypothesized that early antiplatelet therapy with low-dose aspirin (80 mg p.o. q.d.) may prevent uteroplacental thrombosis, placental infarction, and idiopathic fetal growth restriction in women with a history of recurrent, severe fetal growth restriction.

3. **Delivery.** For the fetus who is severely growth restricted but remote from term, the decision to proceed with delivery is a matter of comparing the degree of risk from further exposure to the intrauterine environment with the risks of preterm delivery. Confirmation of a lecithin-sphingomyelin (L-S) ratio of 2 or more or identification of phosphatidylglycerol in amniotic fluid is an indication for delivery. Close monitoring during labor to avoid further fetal compromise, with delivery accomplished by cesarean section whenever fetal distress is identified, and excellent neonatal care are mandatory for a successful outcome. The likelihood of severe fetal distress during labor is increased considerably because fetal growth restriction is commonly the result of insufficient placental function, which is likely to be aggravated by labor and is associated with lack of amniotic fluid, which predisposes to cord compression.

V. **Fetal outcome.** The growth-restricted fetus is at high risk for perinatal hypoxia and meconium aspiration. It is essential that care of the newborn infant be provided by someone who is skillful at clearing the airway below the vocal cords of meconium. The severely growth-restricted newborn is particularly susceptible to hypothermia and also may develop other metabolic abnormalities, especially severe hypoglycemia. In general, prolonged symmetrical growth restriction *in utero* is likely to be followed by slow growth after birth, whereas the asymmetric growth-restricted fetus is more likely to recuperate with fast growth after birth. The subsequent neurologic and intellectual capabilities of the infant who was growth restricted *in utero* cannot be predicted precisely. Data by Low and colleagues (4) show that fetal growth restriction has a deleterious effect on cognitive function, independent of other variables; almost 50% of children born small for gestational age had learning deficits at 9 to 11 years of age.

Congenital Anomalies

I. **Description.** Congenital malformation and genetic disorders play an important role in neonatal morbidity and mortality. Two percent of newborns have a serious malformation that has surgical or cosmetic significance. Birth defects or genetic disorders are caused by a multitude of conditions, including chromosomal abnormalities, single gene disorders, environmental agents, multifactorial disorders, and many still classified as unknown. Some of the factors that may raise the index of suspicion, prompting a careful anatomic survey of the fetus, include a positive family history, advanced maternal age, exposure to teratogens during pregnancy, or the detection of abnormalities in the volume of amniotic fluid, abnormal maternal serum marker screen, or fetal growth restriction.

II. **Methods of evaluation**
   A. **Ultrasound examination** should include evaluation and documentation of the following: fetal number, fetal presentation, fetal lie, placental location, amniotic fluid volume, gestational age, presence or absence and evaluation of maternal pelvic mass, survey of fetal anatomy for gross examination. A targeted ultrasound to exclude congenital anomalies should be deferred until midgestation, when organogenesis is complete and the structures of interest are large enough to permit accurate evaluation. Structures to be evaluated include:
      1. BPD of the **head.** Intracranial anatomy should be examined to ascertain that midline structures are present and ventricular anatomy normal.
      2. In a targeted examination for neural tube defects, the fetal **spine** should be examined in both longitudinal and transverse planes.
      3. A four-chamber image of the fetal **heart** and examination of the ventricular outflow tracts should be part of all examinations after 18 to 20 weeks' gestation.
      4. Ventral wall defects of the **abdomen** can be excluded by the demonstration of an intact abdomen in the area of the umbilical cord insertion. Other normal structures that should be sought are the single cystic area representing the stomach on the left side of the abdomen and the umbilical vein, which hooks toward the right in the liver. Kidneys can be visualized as early as at 14 weeks' gestation. The fetal bladder is usually visible as a fluid-filled structure in the midline, low in the pelvis; in fact, the bladder may visibly fill and empty during the course of an examination.
      5. While examining the **extremities,** the four fetal limbs should be identified and measured routinely during any second- or third-trimester examination. Both bones of the distal extremities should be present.
   B. **Maternal AFP determination and triple screen** have been used to screen for neural tube defects, abdominal wall defects, and chromosomal abnormalities.
   C. **Amniocentesis** for amniotic fluid AFP determination and karyotyping when indicated is a part of antenatal diagnosis of congenital anomalies (see Chap. 1, sec. I.O.2).

III. **Anomalies of the head and neck and central nervous system.** The most common head and neck abnormalities are neural tube defects and hydrocephalus.
   A. **Neural tube defects** result from failure of the anterior (anencephaly) or posterior (spina bifida) neural tube to close during the third to fourth week of gestation.
      1. The **etiology** is multifactorial. In anencephaly, the cranial vault is absent, as well as the telencephalic and encephalic structures. Associated malformations are common, and polyhydramnios frequently is found. Spina

bifida is subdivided into occult (characterized by vertebral schisis covered by normal soft tissue) and open (characterized by a defect in the skin, underlying soft tissues, and vertebral arches that exposes the neural canal). Open spina bifida almost always is associated with a typical intracranial malformation (Arnold-Chiari, type II). Hydrocephalus occurs in 60% to 85% of low lumbar and sacral defects and in 96% of high lumbar and thoracic lesions. Outcome is poor, with high lumbar or thoracic defects, severe hydrocephalus (less than 1 cm of frontal cerebral mantle), or other brain malformations or associated anomalies. The term cephalocele indicates a protrusion of intracranial contents through a bony defect of the skull; cephalocele may occur either as an isolated defect or as a part of genetic (Meckel syndrome) or nongenetic syndromes (amniotic band syndrome).

2. **Diagnosis.** The combined use of AFP determination and ultrasound as a screening tool for the prenatal diagnosis of neural tube defects is presently a routine part of antenatal care. Targeted ultrasound examinations of patients at risk because of either family history or elevated AFP are recommended. Typical cranial signs such as frontal cranial narrowing (the "lemon sign") and abnormal convex configuration of the cerebellum (the "banana sign") consistently are found in fetuses with spina bifida, in addition to splaying of the vertebral arches.

3. **Management.** Anencephaly is invariably fatal. Birth injury is frequent in fetuses with spina bifida, and, although disagreement exists, cesarean delivery commonly is recommended. The outcome for infants with spina bifida is dictated by the site and extension of the lesion. The mortality rate has been reported to be as high as 40%, and many of the survivors suffer disability, mainly from lower limb paralysis or dysfunction and incontinence. Pre-conception folic acid supplementation (4 mg daily), in accordance with the Centers for Disease Control and Prevention guidelines, may decrease recurrences of neural tube defects in offspring of women with prior affected infants.

B. **Hydrocephalus.** Possible etiologies include isolated aqueductal stenosis, intracranial hemorrhage, and other cerebral anomalies. Incidence ranges from 0.3 to 1.5 per 1,000 births in different series. Both congenital infection and genetic factors are involved in the pathogenesis of aqueductal stenosis. Infectious antecedents include toxoplasmosis, syphilis, cytomegalovirus, mumps, and influenza virus. Many familial cases indicate an X-linked pattern of transmission that is thought to account for 25% of lesions occurring in males. Multifactorial etiology also has been suggested. Communicating hydrocephalus usually results from nonreabsorption of cerebrospinal fluid. A multifactorial etiology with a recurrence risk of 1% to 2% has been suggested. The etiology of Dandy-Walker deformity (hydrocephalus, retrocerebellar cyst, and abnormal cerebellar vermis) is still unclear. Dandy-Walker deformity frequently is associated with other nervous system abnormalities and systemic anomalies such as congenital heart disease.

1. **Diagnosis** of hydrocephalus by sonography is based on direct demonstration of the enlargement of the ventricular system. After hydrocephalus has been recognized, the site of obstruction may be determined by identifying the enlarged and normal portions of the ventricular system. An incidence of almost 30% has been reported for severe associated anomalies, including chromosomal aberrations and other anatomic malformations. Detailed examination of the entire fetal anatomy by high-resolution ultrasound, echocardiography, and karyotyping is strongly recommended.

2. **Management.** Intrauterine treatment of congenital obstructive hydrocephalus by ventriculoamniotic shunting has been performed in animal models and in human fetuses, with discouraging results in terms of procedure-related mortality and residual neurologic morbidity. Fetuses with progressive hydrocephalus should be delivered as soon as fetal maturity is achieved in order to perform prompt neurologic treatment to maximize the

chances of survival and normal development. A cesarean section is recommended in cases of hydrocephalus with associated macrocrania. Neurologic studies of infants with aqueductal stenosis indicate that 50% of infants developed normal intelligence after surgical correction. Isolated communicating hydrocephalus carries a good prognosis. Infants with Dandy-Walker deformity have a mortality risk of 12% to 26% and IQ above 80 in 30% to 40% of cases.

IV. **Fetal thoracic malformations.** The most common thoracic malformations are congenital diaphragmatic hernia (CDH) and cystic adenomatoid malformation.

   A. **CDH** is an anatomical diaphragmatic defect characterized by herniation of abdominal contents into the thoracic cavity. Despite optimal postnatal medical management and surgical repair, many infants with CDH die of pulmonary hypoplasia, which appears to be secondary to compression of the developing fetal lungs by the herniated abdominal viscera. In general, the mortality rates for neonates with prenatally diagnosed CDH have been reported to range from 70% to 90%, especially if polyhydramnios is present (15,16). In contrast, the mortality rate for neonates without a prenatal diagnosis generally has been reported to be 50%.

      1. **Diagnosis.** Prenatal sonographic evaluation reveals the presence of an echolucent mass or masses, which represent the fetal stomach or loops of small bowel, in the fetal chest. A number of poor prognostic indicators have been identified, including diagnosis before 25 weeks' gestation, polyhydramnios, associated anomalies, and the presence of stomach or liver in the chest.

      2. **Management.** All fetuses with CDH diagnosed before 28 weeks' gestation should undergo a detailed ultrasonography, amniocentesis or percutaneous umbilical blood sampling for karyotype determination, and fetal cardiac echocardiography to exclude other anomalies. If an isolated CDH with poor prognostic indicators are present, the fetus is placed in an early or severe category with poor prognosis. In these cases, fetal surgical repair is recommended in the context of a controlled and randomized trial to establish efficacy. When the fetal prognosis is equivocal according to the prognostic criteria, appropriate parental counseling should be provided to help parents choose between fetal surgery and conventional management. Fetuses in the less severe category are managed conservatively and undergo postpartum surgical correction. Although early experience with intrauterine surgery was compromised by significant technical difficulties, Harrison and colleagues reported that four of ten fetuses who underwent intrauterine surgery survived and were doing well at home postpartum (5).

   B. **Congenital cystic adenomatoid malformation (CCAM)** represents a disease spectrum characterized by cystic lesions of the lung. In most cases, CCAM manifests after birth and is treated easily *ex utero*. In these cases, patients present with pulmonary masses causing either respiratory difficulty or recurrent pulmonary infections in infancy or childhood. At the severe end of the spectrum is a lesion that results in fetal hydrops, pulmonary hypoplasia, and fetal death.

      1. **Types of lesions.** CCAM can be divided into macrocystic or microcystic types, based on the presence or absence of single or multiple cysts greater than 5 mm in diameter. The macrocystic lesion usually is not associated with hydrops and has a more favorable prognosis than the microcystic lesion. The microcystic, or solid, lesion more frequently induces fetal hydrops, which is caused by vena cava obstruction or cardiac compression from extreme mediastinal shift. Once this occurs, rapid fetal demise may ensue.

      2. **Management.** The majority of affected fetuses have isolated small lesions, without hydrops, and are best treated by surgical resection after term delivery. Fetuses diagnosed in early gestation with a large CCAM should undergo serial sonographic examinations to evaluate fetal growth and

monitor for onset of hydrops. If pulmonary maturity is documented and hydrops develops, the fetus should be delivered, and the lesion may immediately be resected ex utero. Affected fetuses between 28 weeks' gestation and documented lung maturity with evolving hydrops should undergo an attempt at steroid-induced lung maturation, followed by immediate delivery with surfactant administration and emergent surgical resection. An immature fetus with a large CCAM and hydrops should be considered as a candidate for *in utero* resection of the tumor. *In utero* therapy has been attempted in selected cases of CCAM; best results were obtained by open fetal surgery.

V. **Cardiovascular anomalies.** Congenital heart defects (CHDs) are the malformations most frequently observed at birth. Incidence has been estimated at about 0.5% to 1.0%. CHD probably results from a wide variety of causes. Chromosomal anomalies are found in 4% to 5% of cases. Associated extracardiac structural abnormalities are present in 25% to 45% of affected fetuses with chromosomal anomalies. Women with any of the following risk factors should undergo a detailed ultrasound examination of the fetal heart: nonimmune hydrops, suspected abnormalities observed on screening sonogram, teratogen exposure, parental or sibling heart defects, aneuploidy, diabetes, and fetal arrhythmias.

   A. **Diagnosis.** A four-chamber view of the heart during ultrasound examination is central to fetal cardiac assessment. Up to 96% of fetuses with sonographically detectable heart defects had abnormal findings on four-chamber views. Examination of four-chamber views had a sensitivity of 92% and a 99.7% specificity. M-mode echocardiography may be required to measure chamber size, wall thickness, and wall and valve motion, and to facilitate assessment of cardiac arrhythmias. Real-time Doppler color flow mapping has been used to assess blood flow in the fetal cardiovascular system. In all cases of prenatally diagnosed congenital heart disease, further evaluation should include CVS, amniocentesis, or fetal blood sampling for chromosome analysis. The incidence of aneuploidy in fetuses diagnosed with CHD was found to be 28.5% in a recent study performed at Yale Fetal Cardiovascular Center (6). Evaluation of ventricular outflow tracts enables identification of cardiac malformations that may exhibit normal four-chamber views, such as transposition of the great vessels.

   B. **Management.** Some cardiovascular anomalies are incompatible with life (those associated with severe nonimmune fetal hydrops), and parents can be given the option of terminating the pregnancy. For many cardiac diagnoses, accurate prenatal diagnosis allows counseling for the parents and adequate medical planning for delivery and neonatal medical and surgical management. Survival statistics for fetuses with severe congenital heart disease are still unencouraging because prenatal diagnosis usually is made in relatively severe forms of disease.

   C. **Types of defects**
      1. **Tetralogy of Fallot** is defined as the association of a ventricular septal defect, infundibular pulmonic stenosis, aortic valve overriding the ventricular septum, and hypertrophy of the right ventricle. Enlargement of the ascending aorta is usually present. Study of the right ventricular outflow tract and pulmonary artery provides information about the degree of infundibular stenosis. Doppler ultrasound is valuable in establishing the presence of blood flow in the pulmonary artery.
      2. **Transposition of the great arteries (TGA)** has two anatomic forms: complete TGA (aorta arises from the right ventricles and pulmonary artery arises from the left ventricles) and corrected TGA (association of atrioventricular and ventriculoarterial discordance). Fetal echocardiography enables identification of abnormalities of the ventriculoarterial connection, but meticulous scanning is required to identify the aorta and pulmonary artery and their relationships with each ventricle. Fetuses with uncomplicated complete transposition should not be subjected to

hemodynamic compromise *in utero*; survival after birth depends on the persistence of fetal circulation. In cases of corrected transposition, ideally no hemodynamic imbalance should be present.

3. **Hypoplastic left heart syndrome (HLHS)** is characterized by a very small left ventricle, with mitral or aortic atresia or both. HLHS frequently is associated with intrauterine heart failure. Ultrasound recognition of HLHS in a fetus depends on the demonstration of small left ventricle; the ascending aorta is severely hypoplastic and the right ventricle, right atrium, and pulmonary artery are usually enlarged. The prognosis is extremely poor; palliative procedures and, recently, cardiac transplantation have been attempted, however, and long-term survivors have been reported.

4. **Fetal arrhythmia** encompasses irregular patterns of fetal heart rhythm. Brief periods of tachycardia, bradycardia, and ectopic beats are a frequent finding. A clear differentiation between physiologic variations and pathologic alteration can be difficult but must be attempted. A sustained bradycardia of less than 100 beats/minute, a sustained tachycardia of more than 200 beats/minute, and irregular rhythms occurring more than once in 10 beats must be considered abnormal. M-mode echocardiographic recordings of cardiac motion, pulsed Doppler ultrasound, and color-encoded M-mode echocardiography are the most suitable techniques for the assessment of irregular fetal heart rhythm.

   a. **Premature atrial and ventricular contractions** are the most frequent fetal arrhythmia. Premature contraction is a benign condition and usually disappears *in utero* or soon after birth. Serial monitoring of the fetal heartbeat during pregnancy is suggested because at least a theoretical possibility exists that an ectopic beat could trigger a reentrant tachyrhythmia.

   b. **Supraventricular tachyrhythmia** includes supraventricular paroxysmal tachycardia (SVT), atrial flutter, and atrial fibrillation. Diagnosis of fetal tachyrhythmia can be accomplished easily by direct auscultation or continuous Doppler examination. M-mode, pulsed Doppler ultrasound, or both enable identification of the precise heart rate and recognition of the atrioventricular sequence of contraction. The association of fetal tachyrhythmia with nonimmune hydrops is well established. The fast ventricular rate results in suboptimal filling of the ventricle, decreased cardiac output, right atrial overload, and congestive heart failure. Intrauterine pharmacologic cardioversion of fetal tachyrhythmia by administration (intravenously or orally) of drugs (digoxin, verapamil, propranolol, quinidine, procainamide, amiodarone, flecainide) to the mother has been attempted with success in many cases. Direct administration of medications to the fetus via umbilical venous puncture has been also advocated if no response to maternal treatment occurs. The optimal approach to treating this condition is still uncertain.

   c. **Atrioventricular (AV) block** can result from immaturity of the fetal conduction system, absence of connection to the AV node, or abnormal anatomical position of the AV node. This anomaly is commonly classified into three types: first-, second-, and third-degree AV block. Third-degree AV block may lead to significant bradycardia, decreased cardiac output, and congestive heart failure *in utero*. More than half of cases of third-degree AV block are accompanied by an anomaly. Although the etiology of the AV block in cases without structural cardiac disease is unknown, growing evidence suggests an association with the presence of maternal antibodies against SSA and SSB antigens (RO and LA). Transplacental passage of these antibodies can lead to inflammation and damage of the conduction system. Anti-SSA antibodies have been reported in more than 80% of mothers who delivered infants with AV block, although only 30% showed clinical evidence of connective tissue disease. Intrauterine ventricular pacing has been attempted. First- and second-degree AV block usually are not associated with any significant hemodynamic perturbation.

VI. **Gastrointestinal (GI) anomalies** are relatively common. Fetuses with GI anomalies, which often allow a good quality of life after postnatal surgical correction, benefit greatly from prenatal diagnosis. Anomalies can be divided into two groups: intestinal obstructions and ventral wall defects.

A. **Intestinal obstructions**

1. **Esophageal atresia** is a relatively frequent anomaly, occurring in 1 in 3,000 to 3,500 live births. In the most common type (90% to 95%), the upper portion of the esophagus ends blindly (esophageal atresia), and the lower portion develops from the trachea near the bifurcation. Severe structural anomalies are associated with esophageal atresia in nearly 50% of cases and include heart, GI, and genitourinary (GU) tract anomalies; skeletal deformity; cleft defects of the face; and central nervous system disorders (meningocele or hydrocephalus). Because the prognosis of affected newborns is worse if severe congenital anomalies are present, an accurate ultrasound examination of the entire fetal anatomy should be performed. Because chromosomal anomalies, particularly trisomy 21, are also commonly present in cases of esophageal atresia, fetal karyotype determination is indicated. Prenatal diagnosis is based on indirect findings: polyhydramnios, failure to visualize the stomach, and, rarely, an enlarged upper mediastinal and retrocardiac anechoic structure (dilated proximal esophageal pouch). In the majority of cases, a fistula between the respiratory and the GI tracts distal to the obstruction allows ingestion of amniotic fluid.

2. **Duodenal obstruction** occurs in approximately 1 in 7,500 to 10,000 live births. The anomaly can be either intrinsic or extrinsic. Nearly 30% of affected fetuses have trisomy 21; other common associated anomalies include structural cardiac anomaly (20%), malrotation of the colon (22%), and, less frequently, tracheoesophageal fistula or renal malformation. Detection of two echo-free areas inside the abdomen, which represent the dilated stomach and the first portion of the duodenum ("double-bubble" sign), is a crucial ultrasound examination finding in prenatal diagnosis. Polyhydramnios is almost always an associated finding. Complete survey of the entire fetal anatomy and fetal karyotyping are indicated in fetuses with duodenal obstruction. If the anomaly is isolated, a good quality of life may be anticipated after postnatal surgical correction. Spontaneous premature labor resulting from polyhydramnios is a frequent complication. Prenatal detection prevents neonatal vomiting and aspiration pneumonia caused by aspiration of gastric contents.

3. **Small or large bowel obstructions** are common congenital anomalies, occurring in 1 in 300 to 1,500 live births. Obstruction can be intrinsic or extrinsic. In cases of GI obstruction below the duodenum, multiple echo-free areas within the fetal abdomen are usually seen on ultrasound examination. Associated structural or chromosomal anomalies are rare. "High" bowel obstructions often are associated with a certain degree of polyhydramnios, whereas obstruction of the colon generally is characterized by normal AFV. Bowel perforation is a possible consequence of impaired blood supply to the distended bowel; suspicion of perforation can be aroused when ultrasound examination reveals ascites that was absent on previous examination. Because meconium begins to accumulate in the fetal bowel at 4 months' gestation, any perforation occurring after that time could cause meconium peritonitis. Fetuses with uncomplicated intestinal obstruction can be delivered vaginally at term. Induction of preterm delivery should be considered when perforation occurs and ascites is seen. In these cases, fetal paracentesis should be performed to decrease abdominal pressure on the diaphragm, thus allowing expansion of the lungs.

B. **Abdominal wall defects**
   1. **Gastroschisis** is caused by the herniation of some of the intraabdominal contents through a paraumbilical defect of the abdominal wall. The umbilical cord is inserted normally and no sac is visible; the wall defect is on the right side of the abdomen. In most cases, all segments of the small and large intestine protrude. Stomach, gallbladder, urinary bladder, and adnexa may also prolapse. Chemical peritonitis is a serious complication that results from exposure of amniotic fluid to eviscerated abdominal contents. The intestine can show marked dilatation of the lumen and increased thickness of the wall, with single or multiple atretic sites. The extruded structures are not covered by amnioperitoneal membrane, and the umbilical cord is inserted normally. Polyhydramnios and increased amniotic fluid AFP levels are common findings. Unlike omphalocele, gastroschisis often is associated with IUGR and oligohydramnios. As with omphalocele, a fetus affected by gastroschisis commonly is delivered in a medical center where the neonate can receive intensive care and undergo prompt neonatal surgical correction. Long-term follow-up of survivors demonstrates excellent outcomes. Unlike omphalocele, no association with chromosomal abnormality is found.
   2. **Omphalocele** is a sporadic anomaly with an occurrence rate of 1 in 6,000 live births. A protrusion of intraabdominal contents is covered by a translucent, avascular membrane, consisting of peritoneum inside and amniotic membrane outside. The defect varies greatly in size, from a small opening through which only one or two loops of small intestine protrude to a large defect containing all abdominal contents. A dense, echogenic mass outside the abdomen and covered by amnioperitoneal membrane can be seen on ultrasound examination. In small defects, umbilical cord insertion is on the top of the mass, whereas in large lesions, the cord is attached to the lower border of the mass. Polyhydramnios is often present and amniotic fluid levels of AFP are significantly elevated. Omphalocele, unlike gastroschisis, often is associated with additional structural or chromosomal anomalies (45% vs. 5%); the mortality rate for omphalocele is therefore higher than that for gastroschisis (34% vs. 12.7%). Thorough sonographic evaluation of the fetus and fetal karyotyping should be performed. The volume of the protruded viscera is also a critical factor in fetal prognosis; giant defects frequently are associated with liver evisceration and ectopia cordis and have a worse prognosis than small defects. When giant omphalocele or multiple malformations are diagnosed prenatally, termination of the pregnancy may be considered. In cases of ruptured omphalocele, preterm delivery to avoid the pathologic alterations of the bowel exposed to amniotic fluid may be considered. Delivery should be performed in a medical center with neonatal intensive care and pediatric surgery facilities.
VII. **Urinary tract anomalies.** Congenital malformations of the GU tract are relatively frequent anomalies that are classified as either primary renal dysgenesis of variable type and severity, or obstructive disorder.
   A. **Renal dysgenesis.** The most severe variant of renal dysgenesis is usually bilateral and characterized by absence of recognizable renal tissue, absent fetal bladder, extreme oligohydramnios (invariably present after 16 weeks), and lethal pulmonary hypoplasia. Prognosis is poor because bilateral renal agenesis is incompatible with life; affected fetuses die either in utero or soon after birth from pulmonary hypoplasia. Less severe variants of renal dysgenesis may manifest as unilateral (usual) or bilateral (uncommon) multicystic dysplasia, characterized by an increase in renal volume; distortion of renal architecture; multiple, echolucent renal cysts of various sizes; and areas of increased echogenicity. Bilateral disease may be associated with oligohydramnios and is always fatal. Unilateral disease is associated with normal or increased AFV and evidence of contralateral renal function (bladder filling), and has a favorable prognosis.

B. **Congenital urinary tract obstruction.** Fetal GU lesions are the most important cause of abdominal masses, and obstruction may occur at several sites. The most common site of obstruction is the ureteropelvic junction; obstructions at this site produce renal pelvis dilatation in mild cases and renal calyceal dilatation (hydronephrosis) in more severe cases. Most often the disease progresses slowly, and early delivery usually is not indicated. Outlet tract obstruction may be caused by posterior urethral valve syndrome, urethral atresia, or persistent cloacal syndrome. Outlet obstruction produces megalocystis, hydroureter, and hydronephrosis. Oligohydramnios is common. For the fetus in whom good renal function is predicted, management options depend on fetal lung maturity. Persistent outlet obstruction, particularly when caused by posterior urethral valve syndrome, can be treated with in utero diversion therapy. Antenatal ultrasonography permits accurate identification of the fetal urinary tract; therefore, most urinary tract lesions can be reliably detected. The antenatal diagnosis of such anomalies provides important information for choosing appropriate prenatal and postnatal management. If the fetus's gestational age is 28 weeks or older but inadequate lung maturity is indicated, temporary decompression can be achieved with percutaneous placement of a fetal vesicoamniotic shunt catheter.

VIII. **Fetal skeletal anomalies,** or skeletal dysplasias, are a complex group of anomalies with a variety of morphometric characteristics and prognoses. The diagnosis of skeletal dysplasia is based on objective morphometric data pertaining to limb length and growth and on subjective assessment of skeletal shape, density, and proportion. Nomograms for individual bone length and growth have been published (7).

A. **Thanatophoric dysplasia,** a fatal condition, manifests as extreme shortening of limbs, thoracic cage deformity, and relative cephalomegaly.

B. **Camptomelic dysplasia** is characterized by limb reduction and extreme bowing of the long bones; perinatal death is the usual outcome.

C. **Diastrophic dysplasia,** an autosomal recessive condition, is characterized by severe limb shortening and, frequently, radical displacement of the thumbs.

D. **Osteogenesis imperfecta** is a disease spectrum; characteristics range from mild bowing to extreme demineralization, fracture, and short limbs. Spontaneous intrauterine fracture, indicated by displacement of bone elements and seen most often in the ribs, is diagnostic of a severe form of disease.

E. **Achondroplasia** manifests as short limbs with marked flaring and enlargement of the metaphyses. Malrotation and malflexion of the feet (equinovalgus or equinovarus) may be diagnosed *in utero.*

Multiple Pregnancy

I. **Epidemiology.** The incidence of multiple pregnancy in the United States is about 1.5% of all births. Approximately one-third of multiple gestations are monozygotic, the result of cleavage of a single fertilized ovum. The incidence of monozygotic twins is constant at about 4 in 1,000 births and is unrelated to maternal age, race, or parity. The incidence of dizygotic twins, the result of two fertilized ova, is higher in certain families, is more common in blacks and less common in Asians than in other races, and increases with maternal age, parity, weight, and height. Women taking fertility medications that result in multiple ovulations also have a higher risk for dizygotic twins. Women who have undergone ovulation induction are at greatest risk; the incidence of multiple gestations after clomiphene therapy is 5% to 10%, and it is significantly higher (10% to 30%) when gonadotropins are used. In the absence of fertility agents, triplet pregnancies occur at a rate of about 1 in 10,000 births, and births of higher order are more rare. Multiple pregnancy remains a high-risk situation; maternal mortality and morbidity rates are increased, with published perinatal mortality rates in developed countries ranging between 47 and 120 per 1,000 births for twins and between 93 and 203 per 1,000 births for triplets.

II. **Clinical characteristics.** Clinical findings such as size-date disparity, palpation, and auscultation of two fetal heart tones are insufficient to diagnose multiple gestation. If multiple gestation is suspected, an ultrasound examination should be performed. Maternal serum AFP levels are elevated (more than four times the median) in multiple pregnancies. Patients should be referred to high-risk perinatal units early in their pregnancies.

III. **Placentation.** There are two principally different placenta types in multiple pregnancy: monochorionic and dichorionic. All monochorionic twins are monozygotic, but some monozygotic twins (20% to 30%) may have dichorionic placentas (twins who separated in the first two days after fertilization). The majority of monozygotic twins have a placenta with diamniotic (the dividing membranes consist of two translucent amnions only) and monochorionic membranes. The incidence of monoamniotic twins is about 1%, and conjoined twins are less common still. Dizygotic twins always have dichorionic placentation; their placentas may be separated or intimately fused, but blood vessels never cross from one side to the other, and the dividing membranes consist of one amnion on either side and two chorions in the middle. Monoamniotic twins carry a mortality rate of approximately 50% to 60%, and death usually occurs before 32 weeks' gestation. The perinatal mortality rate of diamniotic monochorionic twins is about 25% because of the high frequency of the twin-to-twin transfusion syndrome in this placenta type. Dichorionic twins have the lowest mortality rate (8.9%) of all placenta types. The relationship of placentae among triplets, quadruplets, and higher orders generally follows the same principles, except that monochorionic and dichorionic placentation may coexist and placental anomalies, particularly marginal and velamentous insertions of the cord and single umbilical artery, are more frequently associated with higher orders.

IV. **Complications**
   A. **Miscarriage** is at least twice as common in multiple pregnancy as in singleton pregnancy, and a continued pregnancy with resorption of one or more of the embryos may be even more common. Fewer than 50% of twin pregnancies diagnosed via ultrasound during the first trimester are delivered as twins (8). Some twins may be resorbed silently, whereas the demise of others is associated with bleeding and uterine activity.
   B. **Congenital anomalies** and malformations are approximately twice as common in twin infants as in singleton infants and four times as common in triplets. Monozygotic twins have a risk of 2% to 10% for developmental defects, twice the incidence of fetal abnormalities in dizygotic twins. Diagnostic amniocentesis should be considered at an earlier maternal age for multiple than for singleton pregnancy.
   C. **Nausea and vomiting** are often worse in twin pregnancies than in singleton pregnancies.
   D. **Preeclampsia** in multiple pregnancy is more common (threefold increase), occurs earlier, and is more severe than in singleton pregnancy. Approximately 40% of twin pregnancies and 60% of triplet pregnancies are affected.
   E. **Polyhydramnios** occurs in 5% to 8% of multiple pregnancies, particularly with monoamniotic twins. Acute polyhydramnios before 28 weeks' gestation has been reported to occur in 1.7% of all twin pregnancies; the perinatal mortality in such cases approaches 90%.
   F. **Preterm delivery.** Approximately 10% of preterm deliveries are twin gestations, which account for 25% of perinatal deaths in preterm deliveries. The incidence of preterm delivery in twin gestations approaches 50%. Most neonatal deaths in multiple premature births are associated with gestations of less than 32 weeks and birth weight under 1,500 g. The average length of gestation decreases inversely with the number of fetuses present.
   G. **Intrauterine growth restriction.** Two-thirds (12% to 14%) of twin infants show clinical and objective signs of IUGR. Disparity in growth rates between twins *in utero* often can be great, especially with twin-to-twin transfusion syndrome. Most studies of twin pregnancies show that more than 50% of twins are born weighing less than 2,500 g. The high rate of prematurity and IUGR in multiple gestation also is associated with a significant increase in neonatal morbidity.

Follow-up studies of growth-restricted twins show a tendency for persistence of short stature and lower weight percentiles.

H. Twin-to-twin transfusion syndrome. Approximately 15% of monochorionic twin pregnancies show clinical evidence of twin-to-twin transfusion, with high perinatal mortality rates for both twins. Single or multiple placental arteriovenous shunts may exist, some in opposing directions. When they are not accompanied by artery-to-artery or vein-to-vein anastomoses, one fetus continuously donates blood into the other, leading to hydrops and hypervolemia in the recipient and anemia in the donor. A common maternal symptom is rapid uterine growth between 20 and 30 weeks' gestation due to the hydramnios of the recipient twin, which frequently is the cause of premature delivery. The severity and time of observable growth discrepancy probably depends on the size and the number as well as the direction of arteriovenous shunts. Fetal hydrops is usually a terminal sign. Prenatal diagnosis of twin-to-twin transfusion syndrome usually can be made when ultrasonographic examination suggests single placentation and a single chorion, disparity in fetal size, polyhydramnios in the sac of the larger twin, and little or no fluid around the smaller fetus ("stuck twin" sign). If extreme prematurity prevents delivery, several radical interventions can be considered in view of the high mortality associated with expectant management. Repeated decompression amniocentesis has been shown to improve outcome in some cases. Intrauterine transfusion of the anemic twin risks congestive cardiac failure in the donor twin. Fetoscopically guided laser ablation anastomosis of placental vessels may be an option in the future because such an approach addresses the cause of the syndrome, but it is not yet an established and proven technique.

I. Hemorrhage. The risk of uterine atony and of postpartum hemorrhage is significantly increased in multiple pregnancy, presumably because of overdistension of the uterus.

J. Intrapartum complications, including malpresentation, cord prolapse, cord entanglement, incoordinated uterine action, fetal distress, and surgical intervention are more common during labor in multiple gestations than in singleton gestations. Locking of twins is extremely rare.

V. Antenatal management

A. Clinical management should include adequate nutrition (daily intake of about 300 kcal more than for a singleton pregnancy), diminished activity, frequent prenatal visits, ultrasonic assessment of fetal growth, assessment of fetal well-being, and prompt hospital admission for preterm labor (PTL) or other obstetric complications. The role of bed rest in prevention of PTL in women with multiple gestations remains controversial. Prophylactic tocolytic agents have not been shown to prevent preterm birth in twin gestations.

B. Ultrasound assessments should be conducted every 3 to 4 weeks from 23 weeks' gestation to delivery, to monitor the growth of each fetus and to detect evidence of twin-to-twin transfusion syndrome. Discordant growth is described as a fetal weight discrepancy of 20% to 25%. When weight discordance exceeds 25%, the fetal death rate increases 6.5-fold and the neonatal death rate 2.5-fold. Other criteria for discordant growth include a 5-mm difference in biparietal diameter, a 5% difference in head circumference, or a 20-mm difference in abdominal circumference.

C. Fetal surveillance. Performance of a nonstress test before 34 weeks' gestation is not indicated unless clinical or ultrasonographic measurements suggest IUGR or discordant growth. Although the practice of routine cardiotocography after 34 weeks' gestation is debatable from a cost-efficiency point of view, it certainly should be considered if any risk factors are present. A major difficulty arises when the results of the nonstress test are discordant. Additional testing, such as biophysical profile (BPP), may be necessary to better define fetal condition. The use of a contraction stress test is debatable because it might precipitate preterm delivery.

D. Amniocentesis should be performed in both sacs if indicated for prenatal diagnosis of a fetal condition, including genetic disorders or isoimmunization. To ensure aspiration from both sacs, 1 to 5 mL of indigo carmine is injected into the first sac. Blue-tinged fluid obtained at the time of the second aspiration indicates that the first sac has been reentered, and another attempt is necessary. In general, a L-S ratio in amniotic fluid of 2 or more obtained from one fetal sac is consistent with fetal lung maturity. When twins are concordant, the L-S ratio in one sac is usually similar to that obtained from the other. When twins are discordant, amniotic fluid should be obtained from the sac of the larger twin because pulmonary maturation of the larger twin usually occurs after pulmonary maturation of the smaller.

  E. **Death of one fetus,** once diagnosed, is managed based on the gestational age and the condition of the surviving fetus. Until evidence of fetal lung maturity in the surviving fetus is exhibited, weekly fetal surveillance and weekly maternal clotting profiles may be performed. Delivery should be considered if evidence of fetal lung maturity or fetal compromise appears.

VI. **Intrapartum management.** The optimal route of delivery of twin gestations remains the subject of controversy, and no prospective studies apply in all situations. The method of delivery must be assessed on a case-by-case basis and must take into account the presentation of the twins, the gestational age, the presence of maternal or fetal complications, the experience of the obstetrician, and the availability of anesthesia and neonatal intensive care. Various presentations of twins and their incidence are twin A–vertex, twin B–vertex (43%); twin A–vertex, twin B–nonvertex (38%); and twin A–nonvertex (19%).

  A. **Twin A–vertex, twin B–vertex.** Successful vaginal delivery has been reported in 70% to 80% of vertex-vertex twins. Surveillance of twin B with real-time ultrasound or continuous monitoring is advised during the time interval between vaginal delivery of the twins. After the vertex is in the pelvic outlet, amniotomy is performed. If twin B is in jeopardy or shows evidence of distress before atraumatic vaginal delivery is possible, cesarean delivery is performed.

  B. **Twin A–vertex, twin B–nonvertex.** Routine cesarean delivery is not always necessary for vertex-nonvertex twins. If vaginal delivery is planned, external cephalic version of twin B may be attempted (success rate of approximately 70%). Vaginal delivery of twin B in nonvertex presentation (podalic extraction) is reasonable to consider for infants with an estimated weight of more than 1,500 to 2,000 g. Insufficient data exist to advocate a specific route of delivery of a twin B whose birth weight is less than 1,500 g (9).

  C. **Twin A–nonvertex.** Cesarean delivery appears to be preferable to vaginal delivery; data documenting the safety of vaginal delivery for this group are insufficient to recommend it.

  D. **Locked twins** is a rare condition, occurring in approximately one in 817 twin gestations. Hypertonicity, monoamniotic twinning, or a reduced amount of amniotic fluid may contribute to the interlocking of the fetal heads.

VII. **Multifetal pregnancy reduction.** The presence of three, four, and more fetuses in one pregnancy is associated with increased maternal and perinatal mortality and morbidity. Although moral, ethical, and psychological concerns exist about reducing the number of fetuses in early pregnancy, reduction is now a reasonable option. The procedure usually is performed transabdominally between 10 and 12 weeks' gestation by means of potassium chloride injection into the pericardiums of the most accessible fetuses. Composite data from the centers with the most experience with reduction suggest an ultimate live birth rate after multifetal reduction of 75% to 80%.

Other Complications
of Pregnancy

  I. **Postterm pregnancy,** by definition, extends beyond 294 days or 42 weeks from the first day of the last menstrual cycle. An increase in perinatal morbidity and mortality has been documented when pregnancy extends beyond 42 weeks' gestation. The incidence of congenital anomalies is also increased in postdate pregnancies.

A. **Epidemiology.** The incidence of prolonged pregnancy has been reported to range between 7% and 12% of all pregnancies. Approximately 4% of all pregnancies extend beyond 43 weeks. Recurrence risk is 50%.

B. **Diagnosis** of prolonged pregnancy must be based on an accurate estimate of gestational age. Obstetric dates should be considered valid if two or more of the following criteria are met: last menstrual period known with certainty; positive urinary pregnancy test at 6 weeks from last menstrual period; fetal heart tone with Doppler at 10 to 12 weeks' gestation or with De Lee stethoscope at 18 to 20 weeks' gestation; fundal height at the umbilicus at 20 weeks' gestation; early registration, with estimated dates consistent with examination before 13 weeks' gestation; and ultrasound dating by crown–rump length between 6 and 14 weeks' gestation or by BPD before 26 weeks' gestation. The best obstetrical estimates of gestational age are based on a composite of as many criteria as possible.

C. **Complications**
   1. **Postmature or dysmature neonates** exhibit some of the following findings, most likely because of decreased placental reserve: wasting of subcutaneous tissue, failure of intrauterine growth, meconium staining, dehydration, absence of vernix caseosa and lanugo hair, oligohydramnios, and peeling of skin. Such findings are described in about 10% to 20% of true postterm fetuses.
   2. **Macrosomia** is a far more common complication of postterm pregnancy than term pregnancy because, under most circumstances, the fetus continues to grow *in utero*. Twice as many postterm fetuses as term fetuses weigh more than 4,000 g, and the occurrence of birth injuries caused by difficult forceps deliveries and shoulder dystocia is increased in postterm pregnancy.
   3. **Oligohydramnios.** Amniotic fluid tends to decrease in postterm gestation. Diminished AFV is associated with increased rates of intrapartum fetal distress and cesarean section.
   4. **Meconium.** Most studies of postterm gestations report a significantly increased incidence of meconium-stained amniotic fluid and an increased risk of meconium aspiration syndrome. The presence of oligohydramnios increases the risks of meconium-stained amniotic fluid, because of the lack of fluid to dilute the meconium.

D. **Management.** Postdate patients should keep daily fetal motion charts, beginning at 40 weeks' gestation. It is generally accepted that careful anti- and intrapartum fetal monitoring can reduce the risk of perinatal mortality for the postterm fetus virtually to that for the term fetus. Which fetal testing modality provides the greatest prognostic accuracy, and whether patients who reach 41 to 42 weeks' gestation with an unripe cervix are better managed by cervical ripening and induction or by continuous antenatal testing, are controversial questions.
   1. The use of the nonstress test as a single technique to evaluate the postterm gestation is not recommended, based on reports of poor outcome after a reactive nonstress test. In contrast, the contraction stress test, although more time consuming to perform, appears to be an earlier and more sensitive indicator of fetal hypoxia.
   2. Many experts recommend twice-weekly BPP testing, with delivery if oligohydramnios or BPP ≤6 develops, beginning at 41 weeks.
   3. Despite the fact that antenatal monitoring can almost entirely eliminate perinatal mortality in the postterm gestation, concern about morbidity persists. This concern has been addressed in an alternative approach: to achieve cervical ripening and induction of labor with prostaglandin gel at 41 weeks' gestation. A study (10) demonstrated that among 1,701 women induced with intracervical PGE_2 gel, the cesarean section rate was 21.2%, compared with 24.5% in patients followed by fetal monitoring. There was

no difference in the perinatal mortality and morbidity rate exists between the two groups, although the statistical power was low.

4. The data from studies of routine induction of labor rather than antenatal monitoring between 41 and 42 weeks' gestation remain the subject of some controversy. It seems appropriate, in evaluating and managing the postterm gestation, to perform weekly cervical examination starting at 41 weeks and to induce labor if the Bishop score is 5 or higher. If the cervix is unfavorable, it seems appropriate to accomplish delivery by the safest route for the fetus.

II. **Fetal demise *in utero*** (FDIU) describes stillborn infants, with no signs of life present at birth.

A. **Epidemiology.** About 50% of perinatal deaths are stillbirths. In the past few years the recorded incidence of fetal death (deaths at 28 or more weeks' gestation) has fallen from 9.2 to 7.7 per 1,000. Of all fetal deaths in the United States, the majority occur before 32 weeks' gestation, 22% occur between 36 and 40 weeks' gestation, and approximately 10% occur beyond 41 weeks gestation. With improvement in prenatal care and proper hospitalization, some of these deaths are preventable.

B. **Etiology.** For a large proportion of fetal deaths, no obvious explanation is found. Fetal deaths may be divided into those that occur during the antepartum period and those that occur during labor (intrapartum stillbirths). The antepartum fetal death rate in an unmonitored population is approximately 8 in 1,000, and represents 86% of fetal deaths. Antepartum death can be divided into four broad categories: chronic hypoxia of diverse origin; congenital malformation; superimposed complication of pregnancy, such as Rh isoimmunization, abruptio placentae, and fetal infection; and deaths of unexplained cause. Approximately 30% of antepartum fetal deaths may result from hypoxia; 25% from maternal complication, especially hypertension, preeclampsia, and abruptio placentae; 20% from congenital malformation; and 5% from infection. At least 25% of fetal deaths have no obvious etiology.

C. **Management.** The overriding question in this area is whether antepartum fetal deaths can be prevented. Studies (11) have been performed to identify any avoidable factors contributing to the fetal deaths. Failure of the patient management team to respond appropriately to abnormalities detected during pregnancy and labor, such as abnormal results from the monitoring of fetal growth or intrapartum fetal well being, significant weight loss, or reported reduction in fetal movements, constitutes the largest group of avoidable obstetric factors. Extensive clinical experience has demonstrated that antepartum fetal assessment can have a significant impact on the frequency and causes of antenatal fetal deaths. Schneider and colleagues (12) reviewed a decade of experience with antepartum fetal health monitoring and reported that the stillbirth rate in the nonmonitored population, 11.1 per 1,000, was twice that of patients who were followed with antepartum surveillance. When corrected for congenital anomalies, the stillbirth rate in the monitored high-risk population was only 2.2 per 1,000. In selecting the population of patients for antepartum fetal evaluation, inclusion criteria should be uteroplacental insufficiency such as in prolonged pregnancy, diabetes mellitus, hypertension, previous stillbirth, suspected IUGR, decreased fetal movement, and Rh disease.

References

1. Moise KJ Jr. Indomethacin therapy in the treatment of symptomatic polyhydramnios. *Clin Obstet Gynecol* 1991;34(2):310–318.
2. Emanuel I, Filakti H, Alberman E, Evans SJ. Intergenerational studies of human birthweight from the 1958 birth cohort. 1. Evidence for a multigenerational effect. *Br J Obstet Gynaecol* 1992;99(1):67–74.

3. Warsof SL, Cooper DJ, Little D, Campbell S. Routine ultrasound screening for antenatal detection of intrauterine growth retardation. *Obstet Gynecol* 1986;67(1):33–39.
4. Low JA, Handley-Derry MH, Burke SO, et al. Association of intrauterine fetal growth retardation and learning deficits at age 9 to 11 years. *Am J Obstet Gynecol* 1992;167(6):1499–1505.
5. Flake AW, Harrison MR. Fetal therapy: medical and surgical approaches. In: Creasy RK, Resnik R, eds. *Maternal fetal medicine,* 3rd ed. Philadelphia: WB Saunders, 1994:370–381.
6. Kleinman CS, Copel JA. Prenatal diagnosis of structural heart disease. In: Creasy RK, Resnik R, eds. *Maternal fetal medicine,* 3rd ed. Philadelphia: WB Saunders, 1994:233–242.
7. Jeanty P, Kirkpatrick C, Dramaix-Wilmet M, Struyven J. Ultrasonic evaluation of fetal limb growth. *Radiology* 1981;140(1):165–168.
8. Reddy KS, Petersen MB, Antonarakis SE, Blakemore KJ. The vanishing twin: an explanation for discordance between chorionic villus karyotype and fetal phenotype. *Prenat Diagn* 1991;11(9):679–684.
9. Chervenak FA, Johnson RE, Youcha S, Hobbins JC, Berkowitz RL. Intrapartum management of twin gestation. *Obstet Gynecol* 1985;65(1):119–124.
10. Hannah ME, Hannah WJ, Hellmann J, Hewson S, Milner R, Willan A. Induction of labor as compared with serial antenatal monitoring in post-term pregnancy. A randomized controlled trial. The Canadian Multicenter Post-term Pregnancy Trial Group. *N Engl J Med* 1992;326(24):1587–1592.
11. Druzin ML, Gabbe SG. Antepartum fetal evaluation. In: Gabbe SG, Niebyl JR, Simpson JL, eds. *Obstetrics: normal & problem pregnancies,* 3rd ed. New York: Churchill Livingstone, 1996:327–367.
12. Schneider EP, Hutson JM, Petrie RH. An assessment of the first decade's experience with antepartum fetal heart rate testing. *Am J Perinatol* 1988;5(2):134–141.

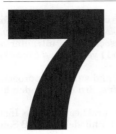

Endocrine Disorders in Pregnancy

Sylvia Abularach and
Nancy Callan

Diabetes Mellitus

Diabetes mellitus (DM) is the most common medical disorder encountered during pregnancy, affecting 2% to 3% of all pregnancies. Of those pregnancies complicated by diabetes, 90% are cases of gestational diabetes mellitus (GDM).

I. The **White classification** is specific to diabetes in pregnancy and was developed as a means of establishing a prognosis for pregnancy outcome and directing the planning of delivery. Cases are classified as follows:
   A. **Class A1.** Diet-controlled gestational diabetes
   B. **Class A2.** Gestational diabetes requiring insulin
   C. **Class B.** Diabetes onset at age older than 20 years or less than 10 years' duration
   D. **Class C.** Diabetes onset at age 10 to 19 years or 10 to 19 years' duration
   E. **Class D.** Diabetes onset at age younger than 10 years or longer than 20 years' duration
   F. **Class F.** Nephropathy
   G. **Class R.** Proliferative retinopathy
   H. **Class H.** Heart disease
   I. **Class T.** Renal transplantation

II. **Diagnosis.** Gestational diabetes is a state of carbohydrate intolerance of variable severity characterized by onset or first recognition during pregnancy.
   A. **Screening.** In some populations, almost 50% of women diagnosed with GDM lack specific risk factors. Selective screening based on criteria such as maternal age of at least 30 has been proposed, but currently the American College of Obstetricians and Gynecologists (ACOG) advocates universal screening. Patients with certain risk factors, including a history of GDM in a previous pregnancy, may benefit from screening at an earlier gestational age. If normal results are found on an early screening test, a follow-up test should still be performed at 24 to 28 weeks' gestation. Screening is performed by administering a 50-g oral glucose load (GCT) and measuring the serum glucose level 1 hour later. The test can be performed without regard for the time of day or the time of the patient's last meal; the sensitivity of the test improves, however, if it is administered to patients in the fasting state.
   B. **Follow-up.** Glucose levels that are equal or are greater than 140 mg/dL, 1 hour after GCT administration are considered abnormal and require further evaluation with a 3-hour glucose tolerance test (GTT). Some centers use 130 or 135 mg/dL as the cutoff value. Additionally, a level of 185 mg/dL or greater is diagnostic of GDM and a 3-hour GTT is not required. This test is performed by administering 100 g of glucose orally in at least 400 mL of water after an overnight fast of 8 to 14 hours. Normal values for the GTT not to be exceeded are: fasting glucose level of 105 mg/dL, 1-hour glucose level of 190 mg/dL, 2-hour glucose level of 165 mg/dL, and 3-hour glucose level of 145 mg/dL. The findings are considered diagnostic of GDM if at least two abnormally high values are obtained.

III. Physiology of glucose metabolism in normal pregnancy. Maternal metabolism changes during pregnancy to provide adequate nutrition for both the mother and the fetus. Glucose is transported to the fetus by means of facilitated diffusion; active transport is needed for the transport of amino acids to the fetus. In the fasting state, maternal glucose levels are lower in pregnancy than in the nonpregnant state (55 to 65 mg/dL), whereas the concentrations of free fatty acids, triglycerides, and plasma ketones increase. Therefore, a state of relative starvation exists, in which glucose is spared for fetal consumption while alternative fuels are used by the mother. During the second half of pregnancy, insulin levels increase, in part as a result of antiinsulin hormonal activity (human placental lactogen, estrogen, progesterone, cortisol, and prolactin). Degradation of insulin is also increased in pregnancy.

IV. Management

    A. Pregestational diabetes

        1. Pre-conception counseling and care. The incidence of congenital anomalies in infants of diabetic women is related to the presence of hyperglycemia early in gestation. Therefore, optimal glycemic control should be achieved before conception. Glycosylated hemoglobin (Hgb A_{1C}) levels can be monitored as a reflection of the patient's degree of glycemic control during the preceding 4 to 8 weeks. Normal levels are associated with an incidence of congenital malformations similar to that seen in nondiabetic women, and, although normal values vary among different laboratories, Hgb A_{1C} levels greater than 10% indicate the most significant risk of malformation development. Although the rate of congenital malformations has been found to be increased in infants of patients with elevated Hgb A_{1C} levels, it must be emphasized that fetal embryopathy may also occur in patients with normal Hgb A_{1C} levels. In addition to glycemic control, the patient's general medical status, including the presence or absence of retinopathy, nephropathy, hypertension, and ischemic heart disease must be assessed.

        2. Dietary therapy. The average caloric intake for diabetic patients of average height and normal weight should range between 2,200 and 2,400 kcal/day. Protein should constitute 12% to 20% of the total energy intake, with carbohydrates accounting for 50% to 60%, and fat constituting the remainder. Approximately 25% of daily calories should be consumed at breakfast, 30% at lunch, 30% at dinner, and 15% as a bedtime snack. Caloric intake should be based on prepregnancy weight (measured as body mass index) and weight gain.

        3. Insulin therapy

            a. Insulin preparations

                (1) The American Diabetes Association recommends the use of **human insulin** for pregnant women with diabetes and diabetics considering pregnancy.

                (2) Insulin is available in **three different forms,** which may be mixed in one syringe or injected separately. Short-acting insulins (regular and Semilente) have peak action at 2 to 4 hours postinjection. Intermediate-acting insulins (Lente and NPH) have peak action at 5 to 12 hours. Long-acting insulins (protamine zinc and Ultralente) have peak action of 12 to 24 hours.

            b. Insulin requirements increase throughout gestation, from approximately 0.7 U/kg body weight per day during weeks 6 to 18, to 0.8 U/kg during weeks 18 to 26, to 0.9 U/kg during weeks 26 to 36, to 1.0 U/kg during weeks 36 to 41.

            c. Regimens. Recommended regimens should be considered starting places and must be adjusted to each patient's specific needs. Generally, for a patient who is familiar with her diabetes, it is best to maintain the form of administration that she used before pregnancy, if possible.

                (1) Two-injection regimen. Two-thirds of the total daily dose is given in the morning (2:1 ratio of NPH to regular insulin) and one-third in the evening (1:1 ratio of NPH to regular).

(2) Three-injection regimen. Administration of NPH or Lente insulin at bedtime, rather than with dinner, has been found to prevent nocturnal hypoglycemia and result in improved control of fasting morning glucose levels.

(3) Four-injection regimen. Fifty percent to 60% of the total daily insulin requirement is given as Ultralente, together with regular insulin at premeal times.

(4) Continuous subcutaneous insulin infusion. A pump system, which is usually attached to the patient's abdominal wall, delivers regular insulin continuously to maintain basal blood glucose levels, with additional boluses administered at mealtimes. The same total insulin dose that would be administered in multiple injection therapy is administered in continuous infusion therapy. Fifty percent of this total dose is administered as the basal rate infusion, with the remainder administered as boluses before meals. Breakfast usually requires a larger bolus than other meals. Women who have maintained good metabolic control before pregnancy using this method can generally use it during gestation. The pump has not been shown to be superior to multiple injection regimens as a means of glycemic control.

4. Monitoring blood glucose levels. Portable glucose meters have made it possible for diabetic patients to monitor their blood glucose at home. When these glucose meters are standardized and used carefully, glucose values within 10% of values from a reference laboratory can be obtained. Most insulin regimens require glucose level monitoring at least four times a day: fasting (i.e., in the morning before breakfast) and either before or after each meal (either 1 or 2 hours postprandial). Postprandial monitoring is preferred to preprandial for tight glucose control in pregnant diabetics.

a. Recommended levels. The following glucose levels are recommended as therapeutic objectives for pregnant women: fasting levels between 60 and 90 mg/dL; before lunch, dinner, or bedtime snack levels between 60 and 105 mg/dL; after meals, 1-hour levels no higher than 130 to 140 mg/dL and 2-hour levels no higher than 120 mg/dL; and from 2 to 6 a.m., levels of 60 to 90 mg/dL. Monitoring during the night should be instituted if nocturnal hypoglycemia is suspected. Patients should be instructed to check their glucose levels whenever they experience symptoms of hypoglycemia, the most common of which include sweating, tremors, blurred or double vision, weakness, hunger, confusion, paresthesias of lips and tongue, anxiety, palpitations, nausea, headache, and stupor. Patients and family members must be instructed in the treatment of hypoglycemia, including the administration of glucagon.

b. Supervision. Hospitalization may be required early in gestation to provide intensive education and counseling and to improve glycemic control; in all cases, however, conscientious outpatient care, including frequent visits and phone calls, is essential to ensure optimal glucose control. Hospitalization is recommended for patients whose glycemic control is poor, such as those whose blood sugar levels consistently exceed 200 mg/dL or those who experience significant hypoglycemic episodes.

5. Antepartum assessment

a. Maternal assessment. Because approximately 25% of diabetic patients develop preeclampsia, it is imperative to monitor blood pressure, proteinuria, and the development of nondependent edema closely. Ophthalmologic, cardiac, and renal function should be assessed at the initial visit and reassessed during gestation as indicated. A urine specimen should be submitted for culture every trimester so that asymptomatic bacteriuria can be treated in a timely fashion.

b. **Fetal assessment.** Determination of maternal serum alpha-fetoprotein level should be carried out at 16 to 20 weeks' gestation. Normal levels are lower in diabetic patients when compared with nondiabetics. A sonogram should be obtained at 18 to 20 weeks' gestation to rule out fetal anomalies. A fetal echocardiogram also should be performed at 20 to 22 weeks' gestation for patients with class B or greater diabetes. Because infants of diabetic mothers are at risk for both macrosomia and intrauterine growth retardation (IUGR), serial sonograms should be performed as clinically indicated. Because diabetic patients carry an increased risk of stillbirth, particularly in the third trimester, fetal testing is recommended. The timing and frequency of testing depend on the degree of risk present; nonstress tests, biophysical profiles, and contraction stress tests are the modalities most commonly employed. Maternal monitoring of fetal activity also can be a useful means of fetal surveillance. Additionally, Doppler ultrasound is being used at some institutions as a means of detecting changes in vascular resistance that may precede fetal compromise.

6. **Timing of delivery.** Present recommendations are that appropriate timing of delivery should be based on both maternal and fetal risk factors. In general, delivery can be delayed until term or until the onset of spontaneous labor as long as good metabolic control and adequate antenatal surveillance are maintained.

   Other practitioners schedule labor induction for certain diabetic patients, including those in poor glycemic control, those with worsening hypertensive disorders, and those with suspected macrosomia, IUGR, or polyhydramnios between 37 and 40 weeks.

   Amniocentesis to document fetal pulmonary maturity should be performed before elective delivery for patients who are at less than 39 weeks' gestation by accurate and reliable dating or for patients with either poor or undocumented glycemic control. In some cases, delivery may be necessary despite immaturity of the fetal lungs; indications for such delivery include preeclampsia that is unresponsive to more conservative management strategies, worsening diabetic nephropathy leading to renal failure, and progressive retinopathy unresponsive to laser therapy. Assessment of lung maturity may be inaccurate in poorly controlled diabetes. In the well-controlled diabetic, phosphatidly glycerol should be positive to assure lung maturity.

7. **Method of delivery** is a controversial issue in pregnancies complicated by diabetes. Vaginal delivery of large infants of diabetic women is associated with increased risk of shoulder dystocia, and traumatic birth injury. The risk of these complications increases dramatically when the infant's birth weight is higher than 4,000 g. Birth injury is more likely to occur in large infants of diabetic women than in infants of similar weight born to nondiabetic women because of the excessive fat deposition on the trunk and shoulders of these infants. Induction of labor therefore is not recommended when the estimated fetal weight is 4,500 g or more; in these cases, elective cesarean delivery is preferred.

8. **Maternal euglycemia during labor and delivery** is necessary to avoid neonatal hypoglycemia. The target glucose levels should be between 80 and 100 mg/dL because an increased incidence of neonatal hypoglycemia has been associated with elevated maternal glucose levels. Maternal blood glucose levels should be checked on an hourly basis and adequate levels maintained with judicious continuous infusion of both glucose and insulin as necessary. A decrease in maternal insulin requirements during labor has been documented, particularly during the first stage. For patients who undergo elective labor induction or an elective cesarean section, it is recommended that the usual dose of insulin be administered at bedtime and that the morning dose of insulin be halved or withheld. When active

labor begins, a constant infusion of dextrose is started to meet maternal caloric requirements, with insulin added if the patient becomes hyperglycemic.

9. **Postpartum glycemic management.** Insulin requirements decrease after delivery, leading to a "honeymoon period" during which insulin doses significantly lower than those required during the third trimester of pregnancy are adequate for reasonable glycemic control. Because strict glucose control is no longer mandatory after delivery, blood glucose levels of 200 mg/dL or less are acceptable. Breast-feeding should not be discouraged for diabetic women; patients should be instructed to increase caloric intake just before nursing (e.g., by drinking a glass of milk), however, because hypoglycemia may occur after breast-feeding. The caloric intake requirement for a nursing mother is approximately 27 kcal/kg/day. It is important to bear in mind that normoglycemia should still be the ultimate goal for nursing patients.

B. **Gestational diabetes.** Women who develop GDM have a 50% chance of developing DM within 20 years. Timely detection and treatment can reduce the risks of potential complications, including macrosomia, birth trauma, intrauterine demise, and neonatal hypoglycemia and hyperbilirubinemia. Women with GDM usually can be managed on an outpatient basis without hospitalization for dietary instruction and glycemic management.

1. **Dietary therapy.** Dietary therapy is the mainstay of management of GDM. The daily caloric intake requirement for women whose weight is less than 80% of their ideal body weight (IBW) is 35 to 40 kcal/kg. This requirement decreases to 30 kcal/kg/day for women whose weight is 80% to 120% of their IBW and further decreases to 24 and 12 to 15 kcal/kg/day for women whose weights are 120% to 150% and greater than 150% of IBW, respectively.

2. **Insulin therapy.** Even with strict adherence to dietary therapy and close monitoring, 15% to 20% of GDM patients will require insulin for adequate glucose control. The institution of insulin therapy is recommended when dietary management is insufficient to maintain fasting glucose levels of less than 105 mg/dL or 2-hour postprandial glucose levels of 120 mg/dL. The level of glycemia that must be achieved to reduce the incidence of fetal and neonatal complications in patients with GDM has not been established. Infants of mothers whose glycemic levels do not conform to the above criteria are at greatest risk of perinatal morbidity and mortality. Evidence suggests that prophylactic insulin therapy of women with GDM according to postprandial, rather than preprandial, glucose levels improves glycemic control and decreases the risk of neonatal hypoglycemia, macrosomia, and cesarean delivery.

3. **Glucose monitoring.** Fasting and postprandial glucose levels in women with GDM are recommended once a week. Some clinicians advocate self-monitoring of levels at home in addition to regular weekly visits. Daily self-monitoring should be mandatory for patients who require insulin therapy for glycemic control.

4. **Antenatal testing.** Patients who achieve good control are at low risk for intrauterine fetal death. Patients who require insulin therapy should undergo fetal surveillance similar to that recommended for patients with pregestational diabetes. No consensus exists regarding the initiation and timing of fetal testing in well-controlled GDM. Some clinicians believe that fetal surveillance may be delayed until 40 weeks' gestation for patients who maintain fasting euglycemia throughout pregnancy, whereas others recommend weekly biophysical testing beginning as early as 34 weeks' gestation. Earlier testing (32 to 34 weeks' gestation) should be reserved for patients whose GDM is poorly controlled, patients who require insulin for glycemic control, and patients with additional risk factors, including preeclampsia, chronic hypertension, and history of a previous stillbirth.

5. **Timing of delivery.** In patients with well-controlled GDM, delivery may be delayed until the spontaneous onset of labor or a term gestation. In patients with poorly controlled GDM, however, induction of labor as soon as pulmonary maturity is documented is recommended.

6. **Method of delivery.** Because the risk of macrosomia is increased in patients with GDM, a careful estimate of the fetal weight should be performed before attempting a vaginal delivery. If the estimated fetal weight (EFW) is between 4,000 and 4,500 g, the patient's management should be based on the adequacy of the maternal pelvis and the previous obstetric history. A cesarean section should almost always be performed if the EFW is greater than 4,500 g.

7. **Labor and delivery.** Maintenance of maternal euglycemia is important during labor. Glucose levels should be monitored at 1- to 2-hour intervals in women with GDM who require insulin.

8. **Postpartum follow-up.** Because patients with GDM are at increased risk for developing overt DM, follow-up testing using fasting glucose values or a 2-hour, 75-g oral GTT is recommended 12 weeks or later postpartum and yearly thereafter. The diagnosis of diabetes is made if a fasting plasma glucose level of 140 mg/dL or greater or two postchallenge glucose measurements of 200 mg/dL or greater are obtained. This test can also identify impaired glucose tolerance (fasting glucose level of less than 140 mg/dL; postchallenge level at either 0.5, 1.0, or 1.5 hours of 200 mg/dL or more; and 2-hour postchallenge level of between 140 and 199 mg/dL). When it is impossible to perform a complete test easily and reliably, a fasting glucose level of 115 mg/dL can be used as a cutoff point for requiring the full test to be performed.

V. **Maternal complications**

A. **Diabetic ketoacidosis** (DKA) is a metabolic emergency that can be life threatening to both mother and fetus. In pregnant patients, DKA can occur at lower blood glucose levels and more rapidly than in nonpregnant diabetic patients. Although maternal death is rare with proper treatment, fetal mortality as high as 50% after a single episode of ketoacidosis has been reported. Medical illness, usually in the form of infection, is responsible for 50% of cases of DKA, with an additional 20% resulting from neglect of insulin therapy; in the remaining 30% of cases, no precipitating cause is identified. Antenatal steroid administration to promote fetal lung maturity can precipitate or exacerbate DKA in pregnant diabetic women. DKA results from either a relative or an absolute deficiency of insulin and an excess of antiinsulin hormones. The resulting hyperglycemia and glucosuria lead to an osmotic diuresis, which results in the loss of urinary potassium and sodium as well as water. The insulin deficiency increases lipolysis and therefore hepatic oxidation of fatty acids, which leads to the formation of ketones and the subsequent development of metabolic acidosis.

1. **Diagnosis.** Symptoms on presentation include abdominal pain, nausea and vomiting, polydipsia, and polyuria. Examination may reveal hypotension, rapid and deep respirations, a smell of acetone, and impaired mental status that can vary from mild drowsiness to profound lethargy. The diagnosis is made by documenting the presence of hyperglycemia, acidosis, ketonemia, and ketonuria. Ketoacidosis usually is defined as a plasma glucose of more than 300 mg/dL (although effects have appeared at lower levels during pregnancy), plasma bicarbonate of less than 15mEq/L, and arterial pH of less than 7.3.

2. **Management.** Initial treatment consists of vigorous intravenous hydration. One L of normal saline can be administered in the first hour, followed by 250 mL/hour thereafter; 3 to 5 L can be required in the first 24 hours. Initial insulin therapy consists of regular insulin at 0.1 U/kg i.v. push, then begin an i.v. infusion at 5 to 10 U/hour. The infusion rate should be decreased to 1 to 2 U/hour when the serum glucose level is found to be below 150 mg/dL. If glucose levels do not decrease by 25% in the first 2 hours of treatment, the amount of insulin infused should be doubled. Five percent dextrose in water should be started when glucose levels reach 250 mg/dL. Intravenous

insulin and glucose administration should be continued until urine ketones are cleared. Potassium replacement (20 to 40 mEq/L) should be started with the initial insulin therapy unless potassium levels are above 5.5 mEq/L or urine output is inadequate. Sodium bicarbonate may be added to the regimen for patients with a pH lower than 7.10. Plasma glucose, electrolytes, and arterial blood gases need to be monitored approximately every 4 hours. When the patient is able to tolerate oral food intake, subcutaneous NPH insulin twice a day with regular insulin at mealtimes can be administered.

B. Hypoglycemia. The strict glycemic control that is enforced during pregnancies complicated by diabetes places patients at increased risk for hypoglycemic episodes. Studies have reported that up to 45% of pregnant patients with insulin-dependent diabetes mellitus (IDDM) experienced episodes of hypoglycemia that were serious enough to require emergency room care or hospitalization. The most common symptoms on presentation include sweating, tremors, blurred or double vision, weakness, hunger, confusion, paresthesias of tongue and lips, anxiety, palpitations, nausea, headache, and stupor. Hypoglycemia may have a teratogenic effect in early gestation; the potential adverse effects that it may have on the developing fetus have not been fully elucidated and require further investigation.

C. Retinopathy. Retinopathy is the most common manifestation of vascular disease in diabetics and is one of the principal causes of blindness in adults in the United States. Diabetic retinopathy is believed to be a direct consequence of hyperglycemia, and it is related to the duration of the disease process; the prevalence of any retinopathy has been found to be approximately 2% within 2 years of the onset of IDDM and 98% among patients who have been diabetic for at least 15 years. It is classified as either background simple retinopathy or proliferative diabetic retinopathy. Progression to proliferative disease during pregnancy rarely occurs in patients who either have no retinal disease or only background changes. If benign retinopathy is diagnosed early in gestation, ophthalmologic follow-up should be performed in each trimester. Proliferative changes require more frequent examinations or therapy or both; photocoagulation of diabetic retinopathy can be accomplished safely during pregnancy.

D. Diabetic nephropathy is a progressive disease characterized by increased glomerular permeability to protein, glomerular scarring, and eventually, renal failure. It develops slowly, appearing an average of 17 years after the onset of IDDM, and has an estimated prevalence among pregnant women of 6%. The diagnosis is made in the presence of persistent proteinuria of greater than 300 mg/day during the first half of pregnancy in the absence of bacteriuria. Factors that may predict poor perinatal outcome include proteinuria greater than 3 g/day, serum creatinine greater than 1.5 mg/dL, hematocrit less than 25%, and hypertension with mean arterial pressure greater than 107 mm Hg. Creatinine clearance is also an important prognostic indicator because a clearance of less than 50 mL/minute has been associated with a high incidence of pregnancy-induced hypertension and fetal loss. Diabetic nephropathy is of particular concern in the pregnant patient because of its association with chronic hypertension, preeclampsia, fetal growth retardation, fetal distress, preterm delivery, and perinatal death. Patients with diabetic nephropathy require intensive maternal and fetal surveillance throughout gestation; with proper monitoring, a fetal survival rate of over 90% has been reported.

E. Atherosclerosis is present in many diabetic patients. A complete history and physical examination should be performed to elicit any signs or symptoms of ischemic heart disease, heart failure, peripheral vascular disease, or cerebral ischemia; evaluation should always include an ECG. Echocardiograms and cardiology consultations should be obtained if clinically indicated. Maternal mortality among diabetic patients with ischemic heart disease has been reported to be high; therefore, preconceptual counselling is essential and if conception occurs, termination of pregnancy may be considered.

F. Spontaneous abortion. The rate of miscarriage among patients with pregestational diabetes has been reported to range between 6% and 29%. Although some reports have suggested that no difference exists in the incidence of spontaneous abortion among diabetic and nondiabetic women, others have found up to a twofold incidence among diabetics. This increased incidence was associated with poor glucose control during the period following conception.

G. Polyhydramnios is a common complication during diabetic pregnancies, with a reported incidence of 3% to 32%. Up to a thirtyfold increase in incidence has been found among diabetic patients, compared with nondiabetic controls. Even though polyhydramnios can be associated with abnormalities of the fetal central nervous and gastrointestinal systems, no etiology is identified in almost 90% of diabetic patients. The pathogenesis of this polyhydramnios is not clear; among the possible mechanisms that have been proposed are increased glycemic loads, decreased fetal swallowing, fetal gastrointestinal obstructions, and fetal polyuria secondary to hyperglycemia. Higher perinatal morbidity and mortality rates have been associated with polyhydramnios; these higher rates can be attributed in part to the increased incidence of congenital anomalies and preterm delivery that also are associated with this condition.

H. Chronic hypertension can be found in diabetic pregnant patients, particularly in those with diabetic nephropathy. Bed rest, sodium restriction, and antihypertensive therapy are the principal management strategies employed. Affected patients must be monitored carefully for the potential development of pregnancy-induced hypertension, preeclampsia, and fetal growth restriction.

I. Preterm labor. One study revealed that the incidence of spontaneous preterm labor is three to four times higher among diabetic patients than in the general obstetric population. Moreover, those patients who had poor glycemic control during the second trimester were found to have increased rates of preterm delivery. Magnesium sulfate is the tocolytic of choice for women with diabetes mellitus because this drug has no effect on glycemic control. Beta-mimetic agents, on the other hand, are best avoided because they may worsen maternal glucose control, thus inducing hyperglycemia and possible ketoacidosis. Similar complications have been associated with the use of corticosteroids to promote fetal lung maturation. Careful monitoring of blood glucose levels is essential when administering betamethasone to diabetics. DKA precipitated by steroid administration has been reported.

VI. Neonatal morbidity. Complications during the neonatal period are common in infants of both gestational and pregestational diabetic mothers; the incidence of complications, however, is much higher among infants of pregestational diabetic patients, especially patients with poor glycemic control.

A. Congenital malformations. Because of reductions in intrauterine deaths, traumatic deliveries, and respiratory distress syndrome, congenital malformations are now the most important contributor to perinatal mortality in insulin-dependent diabetic pregnancies. Thirty percent to 50% of perinatal mortality can be attributed to malformations, which once accounted for no more than 10% of all deaths among these infants. A two- to fourfold increase in the incidence of major malformations has been documented among infants of IDDM patients as compared with the general population. Even though maternal hyperglycemia is considered the principal contributing factor, hypoglycemia and hyperketonemia have also been implicated. The single defect that is considered most characteristic of diabetic fetopathy is sacral agenesis or caudal regression. This rare malformation is diagnosed 200 to 400 times more frequently in diabetic gestations. A tenfold increase also exists in the incidence of central nervous system malformations, including anencephaly, holoprosencephaly, open spina bifida, microcephaly, encephalocele, and meningomyelocele. Cardiovascular anomalies are the most common and are increased fivefold in diabetic patients;

these defects include transposition of the great vessels, ventricular septal defects, atrial septal defects, hypoplastic left ventricle, situs inversus, and anomalies of the aorta. Malformations of the genitourinary and gastrointestinal systems are also found, including absent kidneys (Potter's syndrome), polycystic kidneys, double ureter, tracheoesophageal fistula, bowel atresia, and imperforate anus.

B. **Macrosomia,** which is defined as a birth weight greater than the ninetieth percentile or 4,000 g, occurs much more frequently among diabetic patients than among nondiabetic women (25% to 42% vs. 8% to 14%). Maternal diabetes is the most significant single risk factor for the development of macrosomia. Morbidity and mortality rates are higher in macrosomic infants than in smaller infants. Macrosomic infants are at risk for intrauterine death, hypertrophic cardiomyopathy, vascular thrombosis, neonatal hypoglycemia, and birth trauma. Their mothers are also more likely to undergo a cesarean delivery than mothers of smaller infants.

C. **Hypoglycemia.** Twenty-five percent to 40% of infants of diabetic mothers develop hypoglycemia during the first few hours of life. Poor maternal glycemic control during pregnancy and elevated maternal glucose levels at the time of delivery increase the risk of neonatal hypoglycemia. The pathogenesis of neonatal hypoglycemia involves the stimulation *in utero* of the fetal pancreas by the presence of significant hyperglycemia; this stimulation leads to islet cell hypertrophy and beta cell hyperplasia and consequently to hyperinsulinemia, which in turn results in hypoglycemia when the fetus's transplacental source of glucose is eliminated. The clinical signs of neonatal hypoglycemia include cyanosis, convulsions, tremor, apathy, sweating, and a weak or high-pitched cry. Severe and prolonged hypoglycemia is associated with neurological sequelae. Treatment should be instituted when the infant's glucose level drops below 40 mg/dL.

D. **Hypocalcemia and hypomagnesemia.** Alterations in mineral metabolism are common in infants of diabetic mothers. These alterations are related to the degree of maternal glycemic control.

E. **Polycythemia.** Thirty-three percent of infants born to diabetic mothers are polycythemic (hematocrit greater than 65%). It has been postulated that chronic intrauterine hypoxia leads to an increase in the production of erythropoietin, with a resultant increase in red blood cell production. Alternatively, elevated glucose may lead to the early and increased destruction of red blood cells, after which erythrocyte production must be increased by the erythropoietic system.

F. **Hyperbilirubinemia and neonatal jaundice** occur more commonly in the infants of diabetic mothers than among infants of nondiabetic patients of comparable gestational age.

G. **Respiratory distress syndrome (RDS).** The increased incidence of RDS in infants of diabetic mothers has been associated with delayed fetal lung maturation. Specifically, fetal hyperinsulinemia is thought to suppress the production and secretion of phosphatidylglycerol (PG), the major component of surfactant required for the lungs to remain inflated after the infant breathes. The reliability of the lecithin-sphingomyelin (L-S) ratio as an accurate predictor of lung maturity in diabetic pregnancies is the subject of controversy. For many infants, development of RDS is possible with an L-S ratio of at least 2. The presence of PG always should be established, because it is almost always associated with the absence of RDS in both normal and complicated pregnancies. Nevertheless, a low incidence of RDS can be expected in infants of patients whose disease is well controlled who have a mature L-S ratio, even in the absence of PG.

H. **Cardiomyopathy.** Infants of diabetic mothers are at increased risk for developing hypertrophic cardiomyopathies and congestive heart failure. One study reported that up to 10% of these infants may have evidence of hypertrophic changes. Several investigators have documented a strong correlation between the increased risk of cardiomyopathy and poor maternal glycemic control.

I. **Birth trauma and perinatal asphyxia.** Macrosomic infants are at increased risk for fractured clavicles, facial paralysis, Erb's palsy, phrenic nerve injury, and intracranial hemorrhage. Severe injuries may result in permanent morbidity and even death. Infants of diabetic mothers are also at increased risk for perinatal hypoxic sequlae.

Thyroid Disorders

After DM, thyroid disorders are the most common endocrinopathies found in pregnancy. Thyroid disorders are estimated to affect 0.2% of all pregnancies.

I. **Thyroid function in pregnancy.** The hypermetabolic symptoms that are often present in normal pregnancies may mimic the symptoms of some thyroid disorders. Moderate thyroid enlargement may result from glandular hyperplasia and increased vascularity. The thyroid gland responds to the increased renal excretion of iodine in pregnancy by increasing its uptake of iodine. The physiologic changes in thyroid function that occur during pregnancy result from hyperestrogenemia and increased hepatic biosynthesis. These changes are also evident in other hyperestrogenic states, including the use of oral contraceptives. The most dramatic alteration in thyroid function in pregnancy is the doubling of thyroxine-binding globulin (TBG) levels by approximately 12 weeks' gestation. The majority of thyroid hormone is bound to TBG; it is the unbound or free fraction, however, that is biologically active. The increase in TBG results in a decrease in triiodothyronine resin uptake (T_3RU) as well as increases in the total serum levels of thyroxine (T_4) and triiodothyronine (T_3). Free thyroid hormone concentrations, however, remain normal. Serum levels of T_4 increase in the first trimester and reach levels of 9 to 16 mg/dL (normal levels in nonpregnant euthyroid women are 5 to 12 mg/dL). Early in gestation, when levels of human chorionic gonadotropin (hCG) are at a maximum, free T_4 increases and thyroid-stimulating hormone (TSH) decreases. Nevertheless, during most of the pregnancy, normal levels of free T_4, free T_3, and TSH are found. Therefore, free T_4, TSH, and T_3 are the only useful measures of thyroid function in pregnancy.

II. **Hyperthyroidism.** Hyperthyroidism affects approximately 0.2% of pregnancies. No evidence exists that pregnancy worsens the disease process or makes it more difficult to treat. Most patients are found to have had symptoms before the beginning of pregnancy. Most women who have either mild or moderate disease tolerate pregnancy well. Despite the menstrual irregularities that sometimes are found among hyperthyroid women, fertility is usually not impaired. Patients whose thyroid disease is poorly controlled have an increased risk of maternal disease and adverse perinatal outcomes, which include preterm labor and intrauterine fetal demise.

A. **Etiology.** The most common cause of hyperthyroidism in pregnancy, accounting for more than 85% of all cases, is Graves' disease, an autoimmune condition associated with the presence of thyroid-stimulating antibodies. Less common etiologies include toxic nodular goiter, ingestion of thyroid hormone, subacute thyroiditis, and gestational trophoblastic disease. Hashimoto's thyroiditis may exhibit a hyperthyroid phase before the overt manifestation of hypothyroidism.

B. **Diagnosis**
   1. **Signs and symptoms.** The clinical findings of hyperthyroidism may mimic some of the signs and symptoms of normal pregnancy because both are hyperdynamic states; among these findings are heat intolerance, increased appetite, skin warmth, resting tachycardia with systolic flow murmurs, and a widened pulse pressure. Clinical features that are more indicative of hyperthyroidism than of normal pregnancy include thyromegaly, exophthalmos, onycholysis, failure of a nonobese woman to gain

weight despite normal or increased caloric intake, hyperemesis gravidarum, and resting tachycardia above 100 beats/minute that does not slow with the Valsalva maneuver.

2. **Laboratory evaluation.** Elevated free T_4 levels may be used to confirm the diagnosis. The TSH concentration is also useful for diagnosing and monitoring hyperthyroidism in pregnancy. The free T_4 index is also elevated because the characteristic decrease that is observed in T_3RU during normal pregnancy does not occur in patients with hyperthyroidism. In rare instances, hyperthyroidism can occur in the presence of a normal free T_4 index but elevated free T_3 levels. This condition, which is known as T_3 thyrotoxicosis, can be diagnosed by calculating the free T_3 index; T_3 thyrotoxicosis is more likely to occur in the presence than in the absence of a toxic nodular goiter and must be ruled out if symptoms of hyperthyroidism present with normal T_4 values. Thyroid-stimulating immunoglobulin levels may be established when Graves' disease is a concern. High levels of these antibodies may be associated with an increased risk of hyperthyroidism in the fetus. Markedly elevated hCG levels may indicate an ectopic source of thyroid hormone, such as a rare gestational tumor.

C. **Treatment**
   1. **Pharmacologic treatment**
      a. **Propylthiouracil** (PTU) and **methimazole** (Tapazole) are the principal medications used; they block the synthesis of thyroid hormone. Although they are equally effective, PTU generally is considered the agent of choice because some studies have found an association between *in utero* exposure to methimazole and aplasia cutis of the scalp in the newborn. The evidence that is currently available, however, has not demonstrated any definitive teratogenicity with either PTU or methimazole. Both of these agents cross the placenta; therefore, to avoid potential fetal complications such as the development of hypothyroidism and goiter, the lowest dose of medication required to achieve a state of clinical euthyroidism should be administered. Depending on the patient's symptoms, the recommended starting dose of PTU is 300 to 450 mg daily, usually in three divided doses. The dose is increased as needed to reduce T_4 to the upper normal range; the response to a given dose is revealed by laboratory values after approximately 3 to 4 weeks. Approximately 3% to 5% of patients who receive antithyroid medications experience minor side effects, including pruritus, a purpuric rash, arthralgias, or drug fever. Agranulocytosis is the most serious complication associated with these medications, affecting 1 in 300 patients.
      b. **Beta-blocking agents** may be used to treat the peripheral manifestations of hyperthyroidism, including tachycardia. The dose administered is titrated to maintain a maternal pulse of less than 100 beats/minute. The beta blocker most commonly used is propranolol, 20 to 40 mg every 6 to 8 hours. These agents may also be used in preparation for surgical intervention in certain pregnant patients.
   2. **Surgery.** Thyroidectomy may be performed after hyperthyroidism has been controlled medically. Subtotal thyroidectomy may be the treatment of choice for patients who either are unresponsive to or noncompliant with medical treatment or who develop severe side effects when treated with antithyroid agents. Administration of antithyroid medications should continue until surgery unless the patient is experiencing side effects.
   3. **Radioactive ablation.** The use of ^{131}I is contraindicated in pregnancy because after 10 weeks' gestation the fetus is able to concentrate this radioisotope, which may result in fetal hypothyroidism.
D. **Complications.** Patients with hyperthyroidism whose disease is poorly controlled are at greatest risk for both maternal and neonatal complications.

Maternal complications include pregnancy-induced hypertension, premature labor, spontaneous abortion, congestive heart failure, and thyroid storm. Fetuses may experience IUGR, prematurity, neonatal death, and neonatal thyroid dysfunction.

E. **Thyroid storm** is not well defined, but is a state of acute worsening of the effects of hyperthyroidism, especially tachycardia and hyperpyrexia. This complication rarely is diagnosed during pregnancy or the puerperium, even in untreated patients. Heart failure caused by the effects of T_4 on the myocardium is encountered more frequently than thyroid storm. In cases of either thyroid storm or cardiac failure, pharmacologic management consists of PTU and iodide given orally or by nasogastric tube. Beta blockers may be used to blunt peripheral manifestations but must be administered with great caution in patients with heart failure. Proper rehydration and thermoregulation are important adjuncts to the pharmacologic treatment. It is very important to conduct a comprehensive search for an infectious process in patients with these complications. Acetaminophen, not aspirin, should be used for fever reduction. In addition, these patients should be managed in an intensive care setting.

F. **Breast-feeding.** Antithyroid medications are not an absolute contraindication to breast-feeding. PTU is found in minute quantities in breast milk. Although methimazole is secreted in larger quantities than PTU, its concentration in breast milk is still low. The American Academy of Pediatrics has stated that neither of these drugs is a contraindication to nursing, however, the infant's thyroid function should be monitored closely.

G. **Effects on the neonate.** Fetal morbidity and mortality rates are highest among infants whose mothers remained hyperthyroid while pregnant. Neonates should undergo careful evaluation for hyperthyroidism. Approximately 1% of infants born to women with Graves' disease have hyperthyroidism related to the presence of thyroid-stimulating antibodies. The manifestation of neonatal disease may be delayed if the mother received antithyroid treatment during pregnancy. Affected infants may require treatment for several weeks until thyroid-stimulating antibodies passed through the placenta are cleared. Most cases of neonatal hyperthyroidism are transient; if the disease is unrecognized and allowed to progress, however, development of the infant's central nervous system may be impaired. Mortality in neonates with hyperthyroidism may be as high as 30%.

H. **Gestational trophoblastic disease and hyperthyroidism.** Clinically evident hyperthyroidism is diagnosed in approximately 2% of molar pregnancies. It has been postulated that, in addition to the estrogen-induced elevation in serum T_4 levels, free T_4 concentrations may be elevated as a result of the TSH-like action of chorionic gonadotropin.

III. **Hypothyroidism**

A. **Pathophysiology.** Overt hypothyroidism in pregnancy is rare because hypothyroidism often results in anovulation. The most common causes of hypothyroidism in women of childbearing age are thyroid ablation therapy, antithyroid medications, and autoimmune thyroid disease. Of the autoimmune processes, Hashimoto's thyroiditis is the most frequently encountered.

B. **Diagnosis**

1. **Signs and symptoms.** Hypothyroid patients frequently experience nonspecific symptoms such as weakness, lethargy, constipation, paresthesias, and cold sensitivity. Physical findings include hair loss, myxedematous changes, delayed deep tendon reflexes, and cool, dry skin; weight gain is also common.

2. **Laboratory evaluation.** The diagnosis is established by the findings of an elevated serum TSH level and a low T_4 or a free T_4 index value. An elevation of thyroid antimicrosomal and antithyroglobulin antibodies may be present in cases with an autoimmune etiology.

C. **Subclinical hypothyroidism** is more common than overt hypothyroidism and is characterized by the absence of symptoms in the presence of an elevated

TSH level and normal T_4 and T_3 levels. A high incidence of subclinical disease has been reported in patients with type I diabetes mellitus.

   D. Treatment consists of replacement therapy in sufficiently high doses to achieve a state of euthyroidism. L-Thyroxine (Synthroid) generally is administered in daily doses of 0.05 to 0.10 mg; it may be increased over several weeks to a maximum of 0.2 mg/day. It may take up to 2 months for serum TSH levels to return to baseline. Ferrous sulfate has been found to reduce the efficacy of thyroid hormone. This effect probably is mediated by the binding of iron to thyroxine. It is therefore recommended that these medications be taken at least 2 hours apart.

   E. Complications. Patients with untreated or inadequately treated hypothyroidism are at increased risk for intrauterine fetal death and infants with low birth weights. An increased incidence of preeclampsia, heart failure, and abruptio placentae also exists. Recent studies have not confirmed the findings of earlier research proposing a high incidence of congenital malformations and perinatal death among these patients.

   F. Effects on the neonate. Most infants of women with hypothyroidism show no evidence of thyroid dysfunction, however, when neonatal disease is diagnosed, replacement therapy should be initiated in a timely fashion.

IV. Postpartum thyroid dysfunction

   A. Pathophysiology. Postpartum thyroid dysfunction develops approximately 1 to 8 months postpartum and affects up to 5% of women. It is an autoimmune disorder characterized histologically by a destructive, lymphocytic thyroiditis in which microsomal autoantibodies play a key role. Ten percent to 30% of those who develop postpartum thyroid dysfunction eventually develop hypothyroidism. Spontaneous recovery occurs in 90% of cases. Postpartum thyroid dysfunction tends to recur in subsequent pregnancies.

   B. Treatment. In general, therapy depends on the stage and severity of the manifestations. PTU not only is ineffective in treating the hyperthyroid phase, but may actually precipitate the development of the hypothyroid phase.

V. Thyroid nodule. Solitary thyroid nodules require evaluation because of the possibility of malignancy. Because radioiodine scanning is contraindicated in pregnancy, ultrasonography is the diagnostic modality of choice. The likelihood of a solitary nodule being malignant ranges between 5% and 30% and is affected by risk factors such as a history of radiation exposure to the upper body, rapid growth of a painless mass, the presence of suspicious palpable nodes, and advanced patient age. Despite the fact that most thyroid carcinomas are well differentiated and associated with an indolent course and good prognosis, surgical treatment should not be deferred or delayed on the basis of pregnancy. Suppression therapy with thyroxine may be useful when a malignancy has been ruled out.

Parathyroid Disorders

I. Physiology

   A. During pregnancy, daily **calcium requirements** increase because increased concentrations are required for the proper development of the fetal skeleton. Recommended intake is 1,200 mg/day, which is higher than the nonpregnant requirement by approximately one-third. It is estimated that at term, 25 to 30 g of calcium has accumulated in a fetus. Fetal uptake is greatest in late gestation.

   B. Maternal physiology. No significant change occurs in the levels of ionized calcium found in the mother during pregnancy. Total calcium concentration, however, decreases progressively, beginning in the second or third month of pregnancy and reaching a nadir in the middle of the third trimester. This decrease reflects the declining levels of albumin that are observed throughout gestation. In addition to lower albumin levels, increased calcium excretion secondary to increased glomerular filtration rates as well as active placental transfer may contribute to the decrease in calcium levels. Maternal parathyroid hormone (PTH) levels are elevated, resulting in a state of "physiologic hyperparathyroidism" during pregnancy. Studies have reported increased concentrations of calcitonin in pregnancy as well as increases in 1,25-dihydroxyvitamin D, which promote increased absorption of maternal calcium from gastrointestinal sources.

C. **Fetal physiology.** Maternal PTH, calcitonin, and vitamin D do not cross the placenta; but the placenta is able to convert maternal 25-hydroxyvitamin D to 1,25-dihydroxyvitamin D.

II. Hyperparathyroidism

A. **Pathophysiology.** Hyperparathyroidism is diagnosed very rarely during gestation. It generally is caused by a single parathyroid adenoma. This condition is not known to affect fertility, although pregnancy can exacerbate preexisting disease.

B. **Diagnosis**
1. **Signs and symptoms.** Initial presenting symptoms are nonspecific and include fatigue, muscle weakness, constipation, and abdominal and back pain. Polyuria and polydipsia may develop as a consequence of impaired renal concentrating ability. Progressive disease is characterized by bone pain, fractures, and nephrolithiasis.
2. **Laboratory evaluation.** The diagnosis of hyperparathyroidism can be confirmed by elevated free serum calcium levels and decreased phosphorus levels. PTH concentrations are elevated out of proportion to the serum calcium level. If localization studies are required in the patient's evaluation, efforts should be made to minimize the amount of radiation exposure.

C. The preferred **treatment** for hyperparathyroidism is surgical excision of the abnormal parathyroid tissue. In cases of severe disease, medical control should be achieved before performing surgery. Medical therapy should be administered for only short periods of time, for example when it would enable delivery of the fetus before surgery.

D. The most commonly reported **complications** of hyperparathyroidism are increased rates of spontaneous abortion and intrauterine fetal death.

E. **Effects on the neonate.** A high percentage of infants born to hyperparathyroid mothers are found to have low calcium levels at 1 to 2 weeks of age. This hypocalcemia is transient and is thought to result from fetal parathyroid suppression secondary to elevated maternal calcium levels present in utero. Neonatal hypocalcemia may manifest as tetany or seizures.

III. Hypoparathyroidism

A. **Pathophysiology.** Hypoparathyroidism is a rare condition that most often results from the inadvertent removal of the parathyroid gland during thyroid surgery. Hypoparathyroidism also has been diagnosed in association with autoimmune disorders including Addison's disease, chronic lymphocytic thyroiditis, and premature ovarian failure. Pseudohypoparathyroidism is a related condition characterized by refractoriness to PTH in the presence of normal parathyroid glands.

B. **Diagnosis**
1. **Signs and symptoms** include weakness, lethargy, bone pain, paresthesias, muscle cramps, irritability, numbness and tingling, and tetany. The relatively alkalotic blood pH of pregnancy increases calcium binding, thus increasing the likelihood of tetany. Physical examination may reveal Trousseau's or Chvostek's signs.
2. **Laboratory evaluation.** The diagnosis is confirmed by the presence of low calcium and PTH levels and elevated serum phosphate levels.

C. **Treatment** consists of calcium and vitamin D supplementation.

D. **Complications.** If poorly controlled, hypoparathyroidism may lead to fetal hypocalcemia and skeletal demineralization. If calcium levels are very low during labor and delivery, it may be necessary to infuse calcium gluconate. Hyperventilation in labor may result in alkalosis, thus precipitating tetany.

E. Effects on the neonate. Infants of mothers with hypoparathyroidism have been found to have bone demineralization, subperiosteal resorption, and osteitis fibrosa cystica.

Pituitary Disorders

I. Anterior pituitary disorders

A. Pituitary adenomas. Spontaneous ovulation is rare in the presence of a pituitary tumor. Most patients with prolactin-producing adenomas present with symptoms of amenorrhea, galactorrhea, or anovulatory cycles and infertility. (See Chap. 29.)

The pituitary gland increases in size during normal gestation, in part because of the lactotrophic cells in the anterior pituitary. Although it is possible for this increase in pituitary size to result in the enlargement of adenomas, most patients with microadenomas (tumor less than 1 cm in size) have unremarkable pregnancies. Regression following delivery is typical for patients who become symptomatic during gestation. Prolactinomas larger than 10 cm in diameter are considered macroadenomas. Symptomatic tumors are treated with bromocriptine. Surgery should be reserved for women who do not respond to medical therapy. Transsphenoidal adenoma resection is the surgical treatment of choice.

B. Acromegaly. Although menstrual irregularities are common in acromegalic patients, pregnancy is possible. Pregnancy has not been reported to influence the course of the disease, and elevated levels of growth hormone have not been found to exert a deleterious effect on gestation. Symptomatic tumor enlargement may require treatment with bromocriptine or surgery.

II. Posterior pituitary disorders, including postpartum diabetes insipidus. Following delivery, central diabetes insipidus may develop in association with pituitary insufficiency, which may in turn result from either Sheehan's syndrome or lymphocytic hypophysitis.

Adrenal Disorders

I. Pheochromocytoma. This tumor rarely is diagnosed in pregnancy. It is situated in the adrenal gland in 90% of cases and is found to be malignant in 10% of cases. The tumor secretes norepinephrine and epinephrine.

A. Diagnosis. The signs and symptoms associated with pheochromocytomas can mimic those found in pregnancy-induced hypertension and include headaches, visual changes, and abdominal pain. Additional symptoms include paroxysmal hypertension, palpitations, flushing, and sweating attacks; hypoglycemia and postural hypotension are also associated clinical findings. Diagnosis is made by the presence of elevated catecholamines and their metabolites in a 24-hour urine collection.

B. Treatment. Some practitioners recommend surgical intervention regardless of gestational age, whereas others advocate the use of medical management, in the form of alpha-blockade, for women diagnosed after 24 weeks' gestation. Cesarean delivery is preferred for patients who are managed medically to minimize the risks associated with catecholamine surges during labor and vaginal delivery. The maternal and fetal mortality rates that have been reported for this condition are both high. When the tumor is diagnosed during pregnancy, maternal mortality is approximately 11% and fetal mortality is 46%. Maternal mortality increases to about 55% when the diagnosis is not made until the postpartum period. Catecholamines do not cross the placenta; therefore, adverse fetal effects occur indirectly and can be attributed to disturbances in the maternal environment. The neonate does not carry additional risks after delivery.

II. Adrenal insufficiency. This disorder may be either primary (Addison's disease) or secondary to pituitary failure or adrenal suppression resulting from steroid replacement. Primary failure affects the production of all steroid hormones, whereas secondary failure results in significant losses of glucocorticoids only. Treatment consists of replacement of glucocorticoids and mineralocorticoids. Properly treated patients can sustain an unremarkable pregnancy. Patients with Addison's disease need additional steroid replacement during labor and delivery as well as at times of stress or infection. Infants born to these patients have not been reported to exhibit adverse effects; no evidence of fetal or neonatal adrenal destruction has been found.

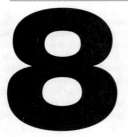

Hypertensive Disorders of Pregnancy

Uma Reddy and
Frank Witter

I. Classification and definitions

A. Chronic hypertension

1. Chronic hypertension is defined as hypertension diagnosed before pregnancy or before 20 weeks' gestation, or elevated blood pressure (BP) that is first diagnosed during pregnancy and persists after 42 days postpartum.
2. Hypertension is defined as BP greater than or equal to 140/90 mm Hg.

B. Preeclampsia and eclampsia

1. **Preeclampsia** is defined as elevated BP along with proteinuria, edema, or both after 20 weeks' gestation (except in the presence of trophoblastic disease or multiple gestation, in which cases preeclampsia may appear before 20 weeks' gestation).
2. **Mild preeclampsia.** The following criteria must be met to confirm the diagnosis of mild preeclampsia:
   a. **Blood pressure** of 140/90 mm Hg or greater after 20 weeks' gestation, measured on two occasions at least 6 hours apart
   b. **Proteinuria** greater than 300 mg in a 24-hour urine collection or a score of 1+ on a random urine dipstick test
   c. **Edema**
      (1) Edema must be generalized for diagnosis of preeclampsia; dependent edema (e.g., low back, legs) is not sufficient.
      (2) Fluid retention is evidenced by rapid weight gain (more than 5 lb in 1 week).
3. **Severe preeclampsia.** The following criteria must be met to confirm the diagnosis of severe preeclampsia:
   a. **Blood pressure** during bed rest of 160 mm Hg systolic or 110 mm Hg diastolic, measured on two occasions at least 6 hours apart
   b. **Proteinuria** greater than 5 g in a 24-hour collection or a score of 3+ to 4+ on random urine dipstick test
   c. **Oliguria,** indicated by a 24-hour urine output less than 400 mL, or serum creatinine level higher than 1.2 mg/dL (unless known to be higher previously)
   d. **Cerebral or visual disturbances,** including
      (1) Altered consciousness
      (2) Headache
      (3) Scotomata
      (4) Blurred vision
   e. **Pulmonary edema or cyanosis**
   f. **Epigastric or right upper quadrant pain**
   g. **Impaired liver function without a known etiology,** indicated by elevated aspartate aminotransferase (AST) of 70 U/L
   h. **Thrombocytopenia,** indicated by a platelet count lower than 100,000 mm^3 or evidence of microangiopathic hemolytic anemia such as abnormal findings on peripheral smear, increased bilirubin (1.2 mg/dL or higher), or elevated lactate dehydrogenase (LDH) (600 U/L or higher)
4. **Eclampsia** is preeclampsia accompanied by seizures.

C. Chronic hypertension with superimposed preeclampsia is defined as preeclampsia that occurs in a patient with preexisting chronic hypertension. It is often difficult to differentiate chronic hypertension with superimposed preeclampsia from an exacerbation of chronic hypertension. Superimposed preeclampsia is defined as a rise in BP of 30 mm Hg systolic or 15 mm Hg diastolic with generalized edema, proteinuria, or both.

D. Transient hypertension

1. Transient hypertension, also known as pregnancy-induced hypertension (PIH), is defined as elevated BP during pregnancy or the first 24 hours postpartum without other signs of preeclampsia or chronic hypertension.
2. Transient hypertension must be differentiated from preeclampsia because transient hypertension is associated with an increased risk of chronic hypertension, whereas preeclampsia, or eclampsia, is not associated with such a risk.

II. Preeclampsia

A. Epidemiology. Risk factors for preeclampsia and eclampsia include age of younger than 20 years or older than 40 years, nulliparous status, chronic hypertension, lupus, diabetes, renal disease, previous eclampsia as primigravida, previous preeclampsia as multipara, previous superimposed preeclampsia, positive family history for preeclampsia or eclampsia, multiple gestation, hydatidiform moles, and fetal hydrops.

B. Pathophysiology. The etiology of preeclampsia is unknown. The major pathophysiologic derangements are vasospasm and endothelial damage.

C. Diagnosis

1. **BP values** should be recorded with the woman sitting or in a semi-reclining position. Her right arm should be held consistently, roughly horizontally at heart level. Early timing of the baseline BP is important because BP normally declines in the second trimester.
2. **Symptoms** of preeclampsia or eclampsia include the following:
   a. Headache
   b. Visual symptoms: blurred vision, scotomata, and blindness (retinal detachment)
   c. Epigastric or right upper quadrant pain
   d. Nausea and vomiting
   e. Dyspnea (from pulmonary edema)
   f. Decreased urine output, hematuria, or rapid weight gain (greater than 5 lb in 1 week)
   g. Constant abdominal pain (resulting from abruptio placentae)
   h. Absence of fetal movement (resulting from fetal compromise)
   i. Premature labor
3. **Physical findings** include the following:
   a. Retinal vascular spasm on funduscopic examination
   b. Bibasilar rales on cardiovascular examination
   c. Right upper quadrant tenderness (secondary to hepatic edema causing stretching of the liver capsule), uterine tenderness, or uterine tetany secondary to abruptio placentae on abdominal examination
   d. Nondependent edema (face and hands)
4. **Laboratory findings** include the following:
   a. Increase in hematocrit (resulting from decreased intravascular volume)
   b. Proteinuria (1+ or greater on dipstick) greater than 300 mg/dL in a 24-hour collection
   c. Uric acid level higher than 5 mg/dL, which is abnormal in pregnancy but is not used to diagnose preeclampsia
   d. Creatinine level 0.9 mg/dL or higher, which is abnormal in pregnancy (see sec. **I.B.3.c**)
   e. Elevated liver enzymes, indicated by AST higher than 70 U/L
   f. Platelet count lower than 100,000
   g. Prolonged prothrombin and partial thromboplastin times, which may be a result of primary coagulopathy or abruptio placentae

      h. Decreased fibrinogen, fibrin degradation products, or both as a result of coagulopathy or abruptio placentae

D. Prevention

    1. Calcium supplementation. Ingestion of 2 g of elemental calcium per day may lower the risk of preeclampsia and also cause a mild decrease in BP in patients with chronic hypertension.

    2. Aspirin, once thought to decrease the risk of preeclampsia, now is not considered useful.

    3. Diuretics and salt restriction have no role in the prevention of preeclampsia.

E. Management. Definitive treatment for preeclampsia or eclampsia and transient hypertension is delivery. Patients presenting at more than 34 weeks' gestation with these conditions should undergo delivery. The urgency of delivery depends on severity.

    1. Mild preeclampsia. If the gestation is remote from term when mild preeclampsia is discovered, the patient may be managed expectantly. Salt restriction, sedatives, or antihypertensive therapy do not improve fetal outcome.

        a. Outpatient management. Some compliant patients with mild preeclampsia may be managed at home with home blood pressure monitoring and twice weekly fetal testing.

        b. Inpatient management consists of the following measures:

          (1) Bed rest

          (2) Regular diet (no salt restriction)

          (3) BP measurement every 4 hours while awake

          (4) Daily review of weight, urine output, and symptoms, with examination for edema, deep tendon reflex (DTR) check, and fetal movement count

          (5) Every other day 24-hour urine protein measurement

          (6) Twice weekly hematocrit, platelet count, AST, and nonstress test (NST)

          (7) Fetal growth sonogram no more frequently than every 2 weeks

          (8) Fetal surveillance with weekly or semiweekly NST or biophysical profiles

    2. Severe preeclampsia

        a. The mother's safety must be considered above all. The first priority is to assess and stabilize maternal condition, particularly coagulation abnormalities.

        b. At 34 weeks' or later gestation, delivery is the optimal treatment. Immediate delivery by cesarean section is not indicated in every case. Patients in labor, or with a cervical condition favorable to the initiation of labor with oxytocin, can deliver vaginally. Both maternal and fetal conditions, however, must be monitored continuously, with hourly assessments and careful attention to intake and output.

        c. Earlier than 34 weeks' gestation, patients may be managed expectantly if their blood pressure can be controlled adequately without antihypertensives, and if bed rest reduces their symptoms and produces diuresis.

          (1) Between 28 and 32 weeks' gestation, patients who are candidates for expectant management should receive an antenatal steroid course to induce fetal lung maturity.

          (2) At 24 weeks' gestation and earlier, the prognosis for perinatal survival is extremely poor, and termination of the pregnancy should be considered for maternal welfare.

          (3) Between 25 and 27 weeks' gestation, aggressive *in utero* therapy may give the fetus a better chance for perinatal survival than immediate delivery in selected cases. If the patient has none of the factors that necessitate delivery, aggressive antihypertensive therapy (see sec. **II.E.5** and **IV**) may be employed to keep the diastolic BP below 105 until hypertension can no longer be controlled

Table 8-1. Loading dose for phenytoin (Dilantin)

Maternal weight	Dose
<50 kg	1,000 mg
50–70 kg	1,250 mg
>70 kg	1,500 mg

or fetal testing (which may need to be done twice a day) shows increased fetal compromise.

d. **Inpatient management of severe preeclampsia.** Patients who are eligible to be followed expectantly should receive the following:
   (1) Bed rest
   (2) Seizure prophylaxis for first 24 hours of hospitalization
   (3) BP measurement every 4 hours
   (4) Daily examination to assess weight, review systems, check for edema, and check DTR; evaluation of 24-hour urine specimen for volume and protein level measurement; complete blood cell count (CBC) with platelet count; and measurement of AST, LDH, and bilirubin
   (5) Daily fetal surveillance including fetal movement counts; NST or biophysical profile

3. **Seizure prophylaxis** during labor and for 24 hours postpartum is necessary for all patients with preeclampsia. Some patients with severe preeclampsia will need seizure prophylaxis for longer periods before and after delivery than patients with less severe preeclampsia.
   a. **Intravenous magnesium sulfate (MgSO$_4$)**
      (1) Loading dose is 6 g administered over 15 to 20 minutes.
      (2) Maintenance is 2 g/hour and may be titrated to higher doses.
   b. **Intramuscular MgSO$_4$**
      (1) Loading dose is 10 g of a 50% solution in divided doses in the upper quadrant of each buttock.
      (2) Maintenance is 5 g as a 50% solution injected in alternate buttocks every 4 hours.
      (3) The therapeutic magnesium level is 4 to 6 mEq/L.
      (4) Check the magnesium level 4 hours after administering the loading dose, then every 6 hours as needed.
   c. **Phenytoin (Dilantin)**
      (1) Loading dose is based on maternal weight (Table 8-1).
      (2) The first 750 mg of the loading dose should be given at 25 mg/min and the remainder at 12.5 mg/minute. If the patient shows a normal cardiac rhythm and has no history of heart disease before initiation of therapy, electrocardiographic (ECG) monitoring is not necessary at this rate of infusion.
      (3) Thirty to 60 minutes after infusion, obtain serum phenytoin level. The therapeutic level is higher than 12 μg/mL. If the findings show levels lower than 10 μg/mL, reload with 500 mg and recheck the level in 30 to 60 minutes. If levels of 10 to 12 μg/mL are found, reload with 250 mg and recheck the level in 30 to 60 minutes.
      (4) If the serum phenytoin level is therapeutic at 30 to 60 minutes, recheck the level in 12 hours.
      (5) Phenytoin has no tocolytic effect.
   d. **Efficacy** of MgSO$_4$ in preventing seizures was shown to be superior to phenytoin in a landmark randomized, controlled trial (1).

4. **Conditions that necessitate delivery irrespective of gestational age** include the following:
   a. Eclampsia
   b. Thrombocytopenia of less than 100,000/mm^3

    c. Hemolysis (seen on peripheral blood smear)

    d. Elevated liver enzymes

    e. Pulmonary edema

    f. Oliguria

    g. Persistent need for antihypertensive medication, except in selected cases between 25 and 27 weeks' gestation

5. Antihypertensive therapy is indicated for antepartum, intrapartum, and postpartum patients with a **diastolic blood pressure of 105 mm Hg or higher.** Acute treatment for severe hypertension in pregnancy involves reducing BP in a controlled manner without reducing uteroplacental perfusion. The goal is not to make the patient normotensive, but rather to reduce the patient's diastolic BP to 90 to 100 mm Hg. A rapid or significant drop in BP interferes with uteroplacental perfusion and results in fetal heart rate decelerations.

    a. Hydralazine, administered intravenously, is the drug of choice for acute BP control.

        (1) The onset of action is 10 to 20 minutes, with a peak effect in 60 minutes and a duration of effect of 4 to 6 hours.

        (2) Intermittent bolus infusion should be used rather than continuous infusion.

        (3) Hydralazine decreases BP without sacrificing uteroplacental blood flow.

        (4) Dosing should begin with a 5-mg bolus, and if BP is not in the range of 150 to 140/100 to 90 mm Hg at 20 minutes, repeat the bolus at a dose of 5 to 10 mg. Boluses may be repeated every 20 minutes, and doses may be increased to a maximum of 20 mg if no response occurs.

        (5) A decrease in urine output may occur 2 to 3 hours after a bolus when diastolic BP is below 90 mm Hg.

    b. Labetalol, administered intravenously, is an alternative therapy to i.v. hydralazine for women who cannot be given or have not responded to hydralazine.

        (1) Labetalol has a more rapid onset than hydralazine and, like hydralazine, maintains uteroplacental perfusion.

        (2) Labetalol is contraindicated if maternal heart block of greater than first degree is present.

        (3) Given as escalating boluses or a continuous infusion. The escalating bolus protocol begins with boluses every 10 minutes of 20, 40, 80, 80, and 80 mg, to a maximum dose of 300 mg. The continuous infusion protocol starts at 0.5 mg/kg/hour and increases every 30 minutes by 0.5 mg/kg/hour to a maximum dose of 3 mg/kg/hour.

        (4) Conversion from intermittent boluses to infusion may be accomplished by beginning the continuous infusion after the BP has started to rise but not immediately after the last bolus. Start infusion at the lowest rate and titrate to the final infusion rate to avoid overdosing the patient.

    c. Intravenous trimethaphan (Arfonad)

        (1) Trimethaphan can be used for sudden onset extreme hypertension requiring minute to minute titration.

        (2) It is a ganglionic blocker and an extremely potent agent, and is best used for hypertensive emergencies that occur intraoperatively at the time of delivery. The dose is 5 to 30 μg/kg/minute.

6. Fluid management. Patients with preeclampsia frequently are hypovolemic because of loss of fluid into the interstitial spaces due to low serum oncotic pressure, increased capillary permeability. These same abnormalities, however, also put these patients at increased risk for pulmonary edema. Intravenous fluids should be restricted to 84 to 125 mL/hour.

    a. Oliguria is defined as urine output less than 100 mL in 4 hours; it is treated with a 500-mL bolus of crystalloid fluid if the lungs are clear. If no response to this treatment occurs, then another 500-mL bolus can be given. If there is still no response after a total of 1 L has been administered, central hemodynamic monitoring should guide further management.

   b. Pulmonary edema. A pulmonary artery catheter is required to guide therapy for pulmonary edema.

   c. Central venous pressure monitoring does not correlate with pulmonary capillary wedge pressure in all situations; therefore, a Swan-Ganz catheter may be required.

   d. Patients usually enter a diuresis phase 12 to 24 hours after delivery. In cases of severe renal compromise, diuresis may take 72 hours or more to appear.

F. Complications of severe preeclampsia include renal failure (acute tubular necrosis), acute cortical necrosis, cardiac failure, pulmonary edema, thrombocytopenia, disseminated intravascular coagulopathy (DIC), and cerebrovascular accidents.

G. Perinatal outcome. Pregnancies complicated by severe preeclampsia are associated with high perinatal mortality and morbidity rates. These high rates are attributable to extreme prematurity, intrauterine growth retardation (IUGR), abruptio placentae, and perinatal asphyxia. Patients whose onset of severe preeclampsia occurs in the second trimester and those with HELLP syndrome (see sec. **H**) and pulmonary edema are at significant risk of maternal morbidity.

H. HELLP syndrome, which consists of hemolysis, elevated liver enzymes, and low platelets, is a form of severe preeclampsia.

   1. Definition

   a. Thrombocytopenia. A platelet count of less than $100,000/mm^3$ is the most consistent finding in HELLP syndrome.

   b. Hemolysis is defined as the presence of an abnormal peripheral smear with burr cells and schistocytes, bilirubin level of 1.2 mg/dL or higher, and LDH greater than 600 U/L.

   c. Elevated liver enzymes are indicated by AST greater than 70 U/L.

   2. Presentation. Typically, HELLP syndrome occurs in a white multiparous patient older than 25 years. It may develop antepartum or postpartum. The majority of cases appear to develop antepartum. The patient usually is remote from term and complains of epigastric or right upper quadrant pain (90%), nausea and vomiting (50%), and sometimes a nonspecific virus-like syndrome. Ninety percent of patients give a history of malaise of several days' duration before presenting. Patients may present with hematuria or gastrointestinal bleeding. Hypertension may be absent (20%), mild (30%), or severe (50%).

   3. Physical examination may reveal right upper quadrant tenderness (80%) and significant weight gain with edema (60%).

   4. Differential diagnosis includes idiopathic thrombocytopenic purpura, thrombotic thrombocytopenic purpura, hemolytic uremic syndrome, gallbladder disease, viral hepatitis, pyelonephritis, acute fatty liver of pregnancy, kidney stones, glomerulonephritis, and gastroenteritis.

   5. Management is the same as for severe preeclampsia: delivery. The average time for resolution of symptoms is 4 days.

   6. Outcome. HELLP syndrome is associated with poor maternal and perinatal outcomes. The reported perinatal fetal mortality rate ranges from 7.7% to 60.0%, and the reported maternal mortality ranges from zero to 24%. Maternal morbidity is common. Many patients with HELLP syndrome require transfusions of blood and blood products and are at increased risk for acute renal failure, pulmonary edema, ascites, cerebral edema, and hepatic rupture. HELLP syndrome also is associated with high incidences of abruptio placentae and DIC.

III. Eclampsia is defined as the development of convulsions, coma, or both in a patient with preeclampsia. Eclampsia occurs in 1% of patients with preeclampsia. Although many other conditions can result in seizures during pregnancy, obstetric patients with seizures should be considered eclamptic until proven otherwise. Perinatal mortality in one U.S. series was 12%, attributable to extreme prematurity, abruptio placentae, and IUGR.

A. **Clinical presentation.** Maternal complications may include pulmonary edema, aspiration pneumonitis, abruptio placentae with hemorrhage, cardiac failure, intracranial hemorrhage, and transient blindness.

B. **Pathophysiology.** The etiology of eclamptic seizures is unknown. It is thought that eclampsia occurs when the patient's mean arterial pressure (MAP) exceeds the upper limit of cerebral autoregulation. The arterioles then fail to protect the cerebral capillaries from the systemic hypertension. Increased cerebral edema, increased intracranial pressure, or both may play a role. The eclamptic convulsion is part of a process that involves the central nervous, cardiovascular, hematologic, renal, and hepatic systems.

C. **Management.** Eclampsia is an obstetric emergency requiring immediate treatment.

　　1. **Goals of therapy** include the following:
　　　　a. Control of seizures
　　　　b. Correction of hypoxia and acidosis
　　　　c. Control of severe hypertension
　　　　d. Delivery

　　2. **Methods of therapy**
　　　　a. **Control seizures. Magnesium sulfate,** administered parenterally, is the treatment of choice for treatment of eclamptic seizures in the United States. The alternative treatment is **phenytoin.** Treatment protocols for both agents are the same as the protocols for seizure prophylaxis (see sec. **II.E.3**).

　　　　　　(1) **Magnesium levels** are checked 4 hours after administration of the loading dose, then every 6 hours to ensure therapeutic levels (4 to 6 mEq/L). Decrease the maintenance dose as indicated by clinical factors (absent deep tendon reflexes, decreased respiratory rate, oliguria, or renal insufficiency) or plasma magnesium levels.

　　　　　　(2) **Duration of therapy** is 24 hours postdelivery or 24 hours after a postpartum seizure.

　　　　　　(3) **Magnesium toxicity** may occur when therapeutic levels are exceeded. Loss of patellar reflexes occurs at 8 to 10 mEq/L, respiratory depression or arrest occurs at 12 mEq/L, and mental status changes may occur at levels higher than 12 mEq/L. To treat magnesium toxicity, discontinue magnesium administration and send off a plasma magnesium level. Therapy should begin, however, based on a clinical diagnosis. Maintain airway and oxygenation; mechanical ventilation may be necessary. Monitor ventilation and oxygenation by pulse oximetry. Intravenous calcium gluconate should be administered in a dose of 1 g i.v. over at least 3 minutes. ECG changes and arrhythmias may occur if toxicity is severe. Diuretic agents (furosemide, mannitol) may be administered.

　　　　　　(4) **Loading dose** of magnesium sulfate is 6 g over 15 to 20 minutes i.v. If the patient has a seizure after the loading dose, another bolus of 2 g of $MgSO_4$ can be administered over 3 to 5 minutes.

　　　　　　(5) If seizures occur while the patient is receiving magnesium prophylaxis, the magnesium level should be checked. If the level is subtherapeutic (therapeutic range 4 to 6 mEq/L), an additional 2-g bolus of $MgSO_4$ should be administered slowly, at a rate not to exceed 1 g/minute. An immediate plasma magnesium level should be obtained. If the level is therapeutic, i.v. phenytoin is used to treat seizures refractory to $MgSO_4$. The treatment protocol for phenytoin is same as the prophylaxis protocol (see sec. **II.E.3**).

　　　　　　(6) **Status epilepticus is treated with diazepam,** administered intravenously at a rate of 1 mg/minute, or up to 250 mg of **sodium amobarbital,** slowly administered i.v.

　　　　b. **Protect the patient from harm during seizures.** Never leave the patient unattended. Bedside rails should be elevated, and a padded tongue depressor should be available to prevent oral lacerations.

Table 8-2. Grades of chronic hypertension

Grade	Diastolic blood pressure (mm Hg)
Mild	90–104
Moderate	105–114
Severe	≥115

    c. Control airway and ventilation. Pulse oximetry should be performed or arterial blood gas levels obtained. The patient may require oxygen administration by mask or endotracheal tube. Difficulty in oxygenating patients with repetitive seizures warrants a chest x-ray examination to rule out aspiration pneumonia.

    d. Treat hypertension. Treatment of hypertension in eclampsia is the same as treatment in preeclampsia (see sec. **II.E.5**).

    e. Deliver the fetus. Induction of labor may begin, or a cesarean section may be performed, after the patient is stabilized. Although prompt delivery is desirable, vaginal delivery may be attempted in the absence of other maternal or fetal complications. During the acute eclamptic episode, fetal bradycardia is common and usually resolves spontaneously in 3 to 5 minutes. Immediate delivery for fetal bradycardia is unnecessary. Allowing the fetus to recover *in utero* from the maternal seizure, hypoxia, and hypercarbia before delivery is advantageous. If the fetal bradycardia persists beyond 10 minutes, however, abruptio placentae should be suspected. Preparation for emergency cesarean section should always be made in case maternal or fetal condition deteriorates.

    f. Limit fluids unless fluid loss is excessive. Frequent chest auscultation to rule out pulmonary edema and accurate monitoring of urine output using an indwelling Foley catheter are necessary. Pulmonary edema and refractory oliguria are indications for invasive hemodynamic monitoring.

  D. Outcome. Long-term neurologic sequelae of eclampsia are rare. Central nervous system imaging with computed tomography or magnetic resonance imaging should be performed if seizures are of late onset (longer than 48 hours postdelivery) or if neurologic deficits are clinically evident. The signs and symptoms of preeclampsia usually resolve within 1 to 2 weeks postpartum. About 25% of eclamptic patients develop preeclampsia in subsequent pregnancies, with a recurrence of eclampsia in 2% of cases.

IV. Chronic hypertension

  A. Chronic hypertension is defined and graded by diastolic pressure and carries increased risks of preterm delivery, superimposed preeclampsia, abruptio placentae, and IUGR.

  B. Grades of chronic hypertension are listed in Table 8-2.

  C. Management

    1. Gather baseline information, including the following data:

      a. History of the duration of hypertension

      b. History of current and previous treatments

      c. Other cardiovascular risk factors (smoking, increased plasma lipids, obesity, diabetes mellitus)

      d. Other complicating medical factors (e.g., headaches, myocardial infarction or chest pain, prior stroke, renal disease)

      e. Medication with vasoactive drugs (e.g., sympathomimetic amines, nasal decongestants, diet pills)

      f. Baseline blood values, including CBC, serum creatinine, serum urea nitrogen, uric acid, and serum calcium

g. Urinalysis findings

h. 24-hour urine test results for creatinine clearance and protein

i. ECG, if the patient has not had one in the past 6 months

j. 24-hour urine calcium measurement

2. **Differential diagnosis**

   a. Essential hypertension is the etiology in 90% of chronic hypertension cases. Other conditions should be ruled out, however, including renal disease; endocrine disorders such as adrenal disease (primary aldosteronism, congenital adrenal hyperplasia, Cushing's disease, pheochromocytoma), diabetes mellitus, and hyperthyroidism; new onset of a collagen vascular disease such as systemic lupus erythematosus; and cocaine abuse.

   b. Worsening chronic hypertension is difficult to distinguish from superimposed preeclampsia. If seizures, thrombocytopenia, pulmonary edema, unexplained hemolysis, or unexplained elevations in liver enzymes develop, superimposed preeclampsia should be presumed and the fetus delivered. If these findings are not present, a 24-hour urine calcium measurement may be useful. Patients with preeclampsia have significantly lower 24-hour urinary calcium findings (42 ± 29 mg/24 hours) than pregnant patients with chronic hypertension (223 ± 41 mg/24 hours).

3. **Treatment**

   a. Patients with mild hypertension, and some with moderate hypertension, may be managed initially without drug therapy, using the following measures:

   (1) Dietary sodium restriction to 4 g

   (2) Cessation of smoking and alcohol use

   (3) Decrease in activity

   (4) Sonograms at 18 weeks' gestation then every 4 to 6 weeks to follow fetal growth; sonograms may be more frequent if indicated, but no more frequent than every 2 weeks

   (5) Antepartum testing, to begin at 32 weeks' gestation (or earlier if hypertension is severe or IUGR is suspected)

   (6) NST or biophysical profile weekly or biweekly depending on the severity of the hypertension

   b. Angiotensin-converting enzyme (ACE) inhibitors and diuretics should be avoided in pregnancy. If, however, a diuretic is an essential component in maintaining control for a patient with severe hypertension, it may be continued.

   c. Drug therapy initiated during pregnancy. Choices for single-agent drug therapy for diastolic BP greater than 105 mm Hg include the following:

   (1) Methyldopa (Aldomet), 250 mg t.i.d. up to 2 g/day in four doses. Methyldopa is a centrally acting adrenergic inhibitor that decreases systemic vascular resistance and has been shown to be safe in pregnancy. It can produce hepatic damage, so liver enzymes should be checked at least once a trimester.

   (2) Hydralazine often is used as a second agent when maximum doses of Aldomet are reached. Hydralazine should not be used as first-line oral therapy. It is a peripheral direct vasodilator and can be used effectively in combination with Aldomet and a beta blocker. Hydralazine can produce a lupus-like syndrome, but usually only when used at doses higher than 200 mg/day for longer than 6 months. It can lead to fluid retention, so the dosage should be 10 mg four times a day initially and may be increased to a maximum of 200 mg/day.

   (3) Labetalol is safe for use in pregnancy and can be used in patients who cannot take methyldopa or in whom methyldopa is ineffective. Labetalol is a nonspecific beta and alpha blocker and is contraindicated in patients who have greater than first-degree heart block. Labetalol may be used as monotherapy but also works well in combination with hydralazine or a diuretic. The beginning dosage is usually 200 mg b.i.d. to t.i.d.; the usual therapeutic dose is 1,600 mg/day, and the maximum dose is 2,400 mg/day.

d. Drug therapy that was initiated before pregnancy. If necessary for adequate blood pressure control, most patients can continue to use the antihypertensive agents they used before pregnancy, with the exception of nifedipine and ACE inhibitors.

   (1) Thiazide diuretics must not be started late in pregnancy.

   (2) Clonidine withdrawal may produce acute hypertension. Clonidine may be used safely in pregnancy.

   (3) Beta blockers may be used safely in pregnancy.

   (4) Nifedipine is a calcium channel blocker that is teratogenic in animals but has been used in the third trimester of pregnancy in humans. Nifedipine is potentially hazardous because it may lead to acute hypotension. It is used as a tocolytic agent, and should not be used within 6 hours of $MgSO_4$ administration.

   (5) ACE inhibitors are contraindicated in pregnancy. They are associated with fetal death *in utero* and neonatal renal failure.

e. Emergency treatment for hypertensive crisis

   (1) Intravenous therapy for patients with hypertensive emergencies in pregnancy is the same as that for patients with preeclampsia (see sec. **II.E.5**).

   (2) Nitroprusside may cause fetal thiocyanate and cyanide poisoning and should be used only as a last resort and for no longer than 30 minutes before delivery.

Reference

1. Lucas MJ, Leveno KJ, Cunningham FG. A comparison of magnesium sulfate with phenytoin for the prevention of eclampsia. *N Engl J Med* 1995;333(4):201–205.

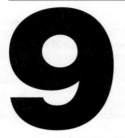

Third Trimester Bleeding

Karen Morrill and
Frank Witter

Third trimester bleeding complicates 2% to 6% of all pregnancies. The differential diagnosis is extensive and includes abruptio placentae, placenta previa, labor (bloody show), cervical erosion, cervicitis, cervical polyp, carcinoma, trauma, and uterine rupture.

I. **Abruptio placentae** is defined as premature separation of the normally implanted placenta from the uterine wall. Abruptio placentae occurs in approximately 1 in 120 pregnancies. Perinatal mortality is 4 in 1,000 affected pregnancies. As many as 80% of fetal deaths occur before the onset of labor.

A. The primary **etiology** of abruptio placentae is unknown. Increased incidence is associated with advanced maternal age and multiparity, maternal shock, poor nutrition, maternal hypertension, cocaine and tobacco use, and chorioamnionitis. An increased incidence of abruptio placentae also is associated with rapid contraction of an overdistended uterus, as in delivery of a multiple gestation or a singleton with polyhydramnios. One to two percent of all cases of abruptio placentae are caused by external trauma. Abruptio placentae has a recurrence rate of 5% to 17% after an episode in one previous pregnancy and 25% after episodes in two previous pregnancies.

B. **Diagnosis**

1. The diagnosis of abruptio placentae begins with the **history and physical examination.** It is important to elicit any history of abruptio placentae, abdominal trauma, or tobacco or cocaine use. The amount and appearance of the blood and whether the bleeding is painless or painful should be noted. Abruptio placentae tends to be sudden in onset, and pain is constant. Eighty percent of affected patients experience external vaginal bleeding. Maternal vital signs, fetal heart rate pattern, and uterine tone are the most important aspects of the physical examination. Fundal height also should be recorded serially to rule out a concealed hemorrhage.

2. **Ultrasound** should be used to rule out placenta previa before proceeding to the pelvic examination. Visualization of the placenta via ultrasound may reveal evidence of abruption (hypoechoic area between uterine wall and placenta). The sensitivity of ultrasound, however, is quite low. Ultrasound also should be used to assess fetal position and estimated fetal weight to rule out intrauterine growth restriction and prepare for a possible urgent operative delivery.

3. If placenta previa is ruled out, a **speculum examination** is performed to seek vaginal lacerations. The cervix also should be inspected. Consider obtaining wet prep and potassium hydroxide (KOH), and cervical cultures (gonococci, chlamydia, group B streptococci) if the discharge is suspicious or the cervix is friable.

4. **Laboratory tests** performed should include blood type and crossmatching, complete blood cell count, prothrombin time, partial thromboplastin time, and fibrinogen as well as the Kleihauer-Betke test to assess for fetomaternal hemorrhage. A "poor man's clot" consists of placing a specimen of whole blood in a red-top tube. The blood should clot in less than 10 minutes. Longer clotting times suggest disseminated intravascular coagula-

tion (DIC). The Apt test is used to determine whether fetal blood is a component of the vaginal blood. Mix vaginal blood with an equal amount of 0.25% sodium hydroxide (NaOH), and place the mixture on filter paper. Blood of fetal origin does not change color, whereas maternal blood turns light brown.

C. **Management** of abruptio placentae is based on its severity and the gestational age of the fetus. Fluids should be run through one or two large-bore intravenous lines. All patients should be typed and crossmatched.

1. **Delivery.** If the fetus is at term and the mother is stable, it is permissible to induce labor. Patients with abruptio placentae must be monitored closely during labor for signs of distress. A Foley catheter should be placed to monitor urine output (maintain 0.5 mL/kg/hour). Continuous fetal monitoring is necessary to assess for fetal distress and hyperstimulation. Serial hematocrit levels should be obtained, and hematocrit levels should be maintained at above 30%. Cesarean section is reserved for cases of fetal distress or maternal hemorrhage and for traditional obstetric indications.

2. **Expectant management.** If the fetus is preterm, the patient may be managed expectantly. Tocolysis may be performed when indicated if evidence of fetal or maternal distress is absent. If tocolysis is successful, continue with expectant management, with semiweekly fetal testing and ultrasound every 3 to 4 weeks to assess fetal growth. The patient should be on strict bed rest with an active type and screen at all times.

3. **Disseminated intravascular coagulation.** Abruptio placentae may stimulate the clotting cascade and lead to DIC. The normal plasma fibrinogen level in pregnancy is approximately 450 mg/dL; if the level of fibrinogen drops below 300 mg/dL, significant coagulation abnormalities usually are present, and blood product transfusion probably is required. Replenish 2 to 3 mL of crystalloid blood product for each mL of blood lost. Packed cells and fresh frozen plasma or whole blood should be used for transfusion. It is important to administer Rh_o(D) immune globulin to all Rh-negative mothers within 72 hours of abruption. Management of patients with severe coagulation disorders or fetal demise is the subject of controversy. Most obstetricians advocate induction of labor, with maintenance of maternal blood volume status, in such cases.

4. **Abdominal trauma.** Abruptio placentae must be ruled out after abdominal trauma. Abruptio placentae complicates 1% to 5% of minor injuries and 40% to 50% of major, life-threatening injuries to pregnant women. Management of these patients is the same as that previously described for abruptio placentae in the absence of trauma. Monitoring for periods of 2 to 6 hours is adequate if no uterine contractions, uterine tenderness, or bleeding is present. If any of these signs are present, 24 hours of observation is warranted. Fetomaternal hemorrhage increases four- to fivefold in pregnant women following trauma. Ninety percent will hemorrhage less than 30 mL of fetal whole blood; therefore, 1 ampule (300 g) of Rh_o(D) immune globulin should protect from Rh isoimmunization. If a Kleihauer-Betke test indicates a fetomaternal hemorrhage of greater than 30 mL, additional Rh_o(D) immune globulin should be given.

D. **Maternal complications** associated with abruptio placentae include hemorrhagic shock; DIC; ischemic necrosis of distant organs (primarily kidneys and the anterior pituitary); and Couvelaire uterus (extravasation of blood into uterine muscle), which results in a poorly contractile uterus. The maternal mortality rate is less than 1%.

E. **Fetal complications** include growth restriction, prematurity, neonatal anemia, asphyxia, and major malformations. The fetal mortality rate may be as high as 30% to 60%.

II. **Placenta previa** is defined as implantation of the placenta in the lower uterine segment, below the fetal presenting part. Classification is based on the location of the placenta relative to the cervical os. The placenta in a total previa (complete) covers the entire internal os. In a partial previa, the placenta covers part of the internal os. In a marginal previa, the placenta just reaches the internal cervical os, and a low-lying placenta previa is implanted in the lower uterine segment.

A. The **incidence** of placenta previa averages 1 in 200 to 250 pregnancies. The incidence is lower, at 1 in 1,500, in nulliparous patients and higher, at 1 in 20, in grand multiparous patients. Ten percent of placenta previa cases occur after four or more deliveries by cesarean section. Forty-five percent of all pregnant women exhibit a low-lying placenta in the second trimester; of these, 90% resolve without symptoms. The recurrence rate varies between 4% and 8%. The etiology of placenta previa is unknown, but its incidence increases with advancing maternal age and multiparity. The incidence of placenta previa is also increased in patients with a prior uterine scar.

B. **Diagnosis** of placenta previa is based on a history of sudden onset of painless vaginal bleeding in the second or third trimester of pregnancy. The blood is usually bright red. Ultrasound accurately confirms the diagnosis in is 95% to 98% of cases. Coexisting abruptio placentae is found in 10% of patients with placenta previa. Peak incidence occurs at 34 weeks' gestation.

C. **Management** decisions initially depend on maternal condition. The first priority is to stabilize the mother; when her condition is stable, management is based on gestational age, severity of the bleeding, and fetal condition and presentation.

   1. **After 37 weeks' gestation,** for patients with a complete previa or fetal malpresentation or who are unstable, a cesarean section is indicated. In cases of marginal or partial previa in which the fetus is at term and the mother is stable, a vaginal delivery can be attempted in a facility capable of supporting emergency cesarean section if required. The patient should be prepared and draped for surgery, and anesthesia should be available. A speculum should be used for initial examination, and if the examiner is unable to visualize the placenta, an attempt can be made to palpate the placental edge through the fornices or carefully to introduce a finger into the cervical os.

   2. **At 24 to 36 weeks' gestation,** patients should be managed expectantly as long as the mother and fetus remain stable. Management is similar to expectant management for abruptio placentae (see previous section). Maternal hematocrit should be maintained at levels above 30%, and a type and screen should be active at all times (crossmatch if bleeding is significant). $Rh_o(D)$ immune globulin should be administered to all Rh-negative patients within 72 hours of a bleeding episode.

     a. **Tocolytics** may be used to prevent labor if the condition of the mother and fetus is stable. Magnesium sulfate is the tocolytic of choice because beta-mimetic agents cause tachycardia and can mimic hypovolemia. The dose most often administered is a 4-g load, then 2 g/hour with titration to stop contractions. After adequate blood volume is achieved, beta-mimetic agents are safe and appropriate. Steroids should be given to patients between 24 and 34 weeks' gestation; consider weekly doses in those who do not deliver during that time. If the patient remains stable after tocolytic therapy, continue conservative therapy including bed rest, maintenance of a large-bore intravenous line, active type and screen, and hematocrit levels above 30%.

     b. **Fetal testing** is controversial, but often semiweekly testing is instituted. Amniocentesis should be considered at 36 weeks' gestation. If the fetal lecithin-sphingomyelin ratio is at least 2:1, or phosphatidyl-glycerol is present, proceed with delivery.

D. Three major **complications** occur with placenta previa.

   1. **Placenta accreta** is placental adherence to the uterine wall without the usual intervening decidua basalis. **Placenta increta** is placenta accreta that invades the myometrium, and **placenta percreta** is placenta accreta that penetrates the entire uterine wall. The risk of placenta accreta is increased (16% to 25%) in patients who have had a prior cesarean section or uterine surgery. The incidence in patients who have not had prior uterine surgery is approximately 4%.

2. **Vasa previa** is vaginal bleeding secondary to the rupture of a fetal blood vessel, usually due to a velamentous cord insertion. The incidence of vasa previa varies between 8% and 10%, with a fetal mortality rate of 50%. The Apt test is important in the diagnosis of vasa previa; usually, however, significant fetal distress is present and an emergency cesarean section is indicated.

3. **Hemorrhagic shock** can develop from significant vaginal bleeding. Close monitoring of maternal vital signs and urine output is required. A central venous pressure catheter or Swan-Ganz catheter may be necessary. If the patient is in shock, replace blood loss with transfusion of whole blood, if possible. Otherwise, packed cells, cryoprecipitate, or fresh frozen plasma is used.

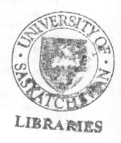

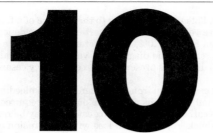

Isoimmunization

Uma Reddy and
Frank Witter

I. The Rh blood group system
   A. A high degree of **polymorphism** characterizes the Rh blood group. Five major antigens are identified with typing sera, and many variant antigens are known to exist.
   B. The **Fischer-Race nomenclature** is most commonly used to classify Rh antigens. The nomenclature assumes the presence of three genetic loci, each with two major alleles, C, c, D, E, e. No antiserum specific for the d antigen has been found. The Rh antigen complex is the final expression of a group of at least these five possible antigens. Because the vast majority of instances of Rh isoimmunizations causing severe hemolytic disease of the newborn are the result of incompatibility with respect to D antigen, an Rh-positive designation indicates the presence of D antigen and Rh-negative indicates the absence of D antigen.
   C. The **Du antigen** is one of the most common of approximately 36 antigenic variants. Du antigen is an incomplete form of D antigen, and some red blood cells (RBCs) that express the Du antigen bind anti-D typing sera; therefore, the Du antigen is capable of causing sensitization in Rh-negative mothers.
II. The Rh antigen. Rh antigens consist of polypeptides embedded in RBC membranes and appear by 52 days' gestation. At least three different D-antigen epitopes exist.
III. Rh isoimmunization requirements. All of the following criteria must be met for isoimmunization to occur:
   A. The fetus must have Rh-positive RBCs, and the mother must have Rh-negative RBCs.
   B. A sufficient number of fetal RBCs must gain access to maternal circulation.
   C. The mother must have the immunogenic capacity to produce antibody directed against D antigen.
IV. Incidence. The highest proportion of Rh-negative individuals is found among the Basque communities of France and Spain, with a prevalence of 25% to 40%. Overall, white Americans have an Rh-negative prevalence of 15%; black Americans, greater than 7%; and Hispanic Americans, 7%. In the white U.S. population, an Rh-negative woman has an 85% chance of mating with an Rh-positive man, and an Rh-positive man has a 70% chance of producing an Rh-positive fetus; thus, a 60% chance of an Rh-incompatible pregnancy exists for any Rh-negative woman. The incidence of Rh sensitization is 0.2%.
V. Fetomaternal hemorrhage (FMH) sufficient to cause isoimmunization most commonly occurs at delivery. Most hemorrhages are less than 0.1 mL; 0.2% to 1.0% are greater than 30 mL. The amount of FMH necessary to cause isoimmunization varies with the immunogenic capacity of the RBCs and the immune responsiveness of the mother. FMH is detected in 6.7% of first trimester pregnancies, 13.9% of second trimester pregnancies, and 29.0% of third trimester pregnancies. FMH also can be detected in 15% to 25% of amniocentesis procedures in the second and third trimesters, even with ultrasound guidance. The incidence of FMH is higher in terminated pregnancies than in spontaneous abortions. As many as 30% of Rh-negative individuals are immunogenic "nonresponders" and

do not appear to be at risk for Rh isoimmunization. ABO incompatibility between the mother and fetus has a protective effect against Rh sensitization.

VI. **$Rh_o(D)$ immune globulin**
   A. $Rh_o(D)$ immune globulin (RhoGAM) is administered intramuscularly to prevent active immunization. Three hunderd micrograms is administered within 72 hours of delivery or FMH. The 72-hour time limit is an artifact of study methodology. Administration RhoGAM as late as 14 to 28 days postpartum may be effective in preventing isoimmunization.
   B. Overall, 16% of Rh-negative women become isoimmunized by their first Rh-incompatible (ABO compatible) pregnancy if untreated with RhoGAM. This rate decreases to 1.5% if RhoGAM is administered within 72 hours after delivery, and further decreases to 0.1% if prophylaxis occurs at 28 weeks' gestation.
   C. Other indications for $Rh_o(D)$ immune globulin, and the recommended dose for each, include the following:
      1. First trimester abortion or chorionic villus sampling (CVS); administer 50 μg
      2. Ectopic pregnancy; administer 300 μg
      3. Amniocentesis or second trimester CVS; administer 300 μg
      4. Fetomaternal hemorrhage; administer 10 μg per estimated mL of whole fetal blood. Quantitation of FMH requires a Kleihauer-Betke smear of maternal blood. This test returns the percentage of fetal red blood cells in the maternal blood. To determine the amount of FMH, the percentage of fetal RBCs is multiplied by maternal blood volume; that product is then multiplied by the maternal hematocrit; the end product represents the volume of fetal RBCs in maternal circulation.

VII. **Management of unsensitized, Rh-negative pregnancies**
   A. **Patients who are Rh negative, Du negative**
      1. **At less than 20 weeks' gestation,** obtain the following tests: ABO blood group, Rh type, antibody screen.
      2. **At 28 weeks' gestation,** repeat the antibody screen. If the results are negative, administer 300 μg of RhoGAM. If the results are positive, management should be the same as in an Rh-immunized pregnancy.
      3. **After delivery,** repeat the antibody screen and test for excessive fetomaternal hemorrhage. If the antibody screen findings are negative and estimated FMH is less than 30 mL of whole blood, administer 300 μg of RhoGAM if the neonate is Rh positive or Du positive. If the antibody screen result is negative and the estimated FMH is greater than 30 mL, administer RhoGAM, 300 μg per 30 mL of estimated fetal blood if the neonate is Rh positive or Du positive. If the antibody screen result is positive (titer greater than 1:4), manage the next pregnancy as Rh immunized. Lower titers probably result from passively administered RhoGAM, and patients with low titers are candidates for RhoGAM in subsequent pregnancies.
   B. Infrequently, an Rh-negative woman is found to have **"weak" Rh antibody,** detectable only by very sensitive techniques. The majority of these women are not Rh immunized and should be given prophylactic RhoGAM according to protocol.

VIII. **Patients who are Du positive.** Treat Du-positive mothers as if they were Rh positive. Beware of previously typed Rh-negative mothers found to be Du positive during pregnancy or postpartum. Such a finding usually is the result of a large number of fetal cells in the maternal circulation; check for fetomaternal hemorrhage, and treat with RhoGAM.

IX. **Management of Rh-isoimmunized pregnancies.** Assess the fetus. Any patient with an anti-D antibody titer greater than 1:4 should be considered Rh sensitized (Fig. 10-1).
   A. **Obtain an accurate estimate of gestational age** (EGA). EGA is crucial to management, particularly to timing of amniocentesis, cordocentesis, and delivery.

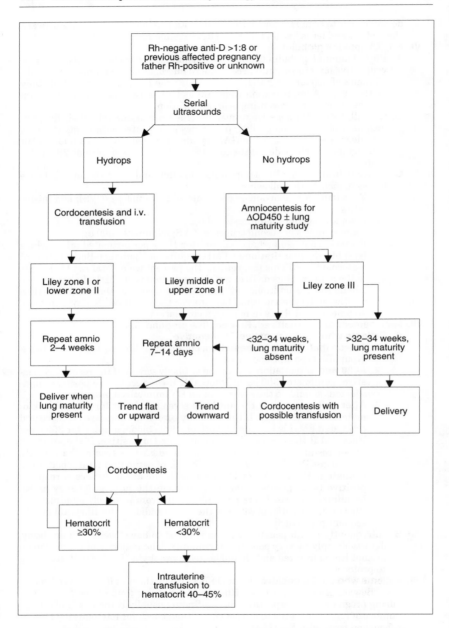

Figure 10-1. Flow diagram outlining the management of an Rh-sensitized pregnancy. The timing of the first amniocentesis is based on the history, maternal titer, and gestational age. In addition to assessment of amniotic fluid bilirubin or umbilical cord hematocrit, daily monitoring of fetal movements by patients after 26 to 28 weeks' gestation, nonstress tests one to two times weekly, and ultrasound examinations every 1 to 2 weeks are recommended. (From Gabbe SG, Niebly JK, Simpson JL. *Obstetrics: normal and problem pregnancies,* 3rd ed. New York: Churchill Livingstone, 1996. Reproduced with permission.)

B. **Determine the Rh antigen status of the baby's father.** If the father is Rh negative, no further intervention is needed. Confirm with the mother *in private* that the apparent father is the only possible father.

C. **Determine the antibody titer.** In first sensitized pregnancies, the antibody titer that determines the need for amniocentesis is called the *critical titer*; it varies from laboratory to laboratory but is usually 1:8 or 1:32. After the critical titer is reached and the need for amniocentesis established, titers are not useful in management. Eighty percent of severely affected patients have stable titers. A DNA probe now exists for Rh antigen, which enables determination of the Rh status of the fetus from amniocytes.

   1. If the antibody titer is less than critical titer in a first sensitized pregnancy, repeat the titer every 2 to 4 weeks, beginning at 16 to 18 weeks' gestation.
   2. If the titer is less than 1:8 and the patient has previously carried an infant with fetal hemolytic disease (FHD), repeat the titers every 2 to 4 weeks and follow fetal progress with serial ultrasound.
   3. If the titer is greater than critical titer, further evaluation with amniocentesis is necessary beginning at 26 weeks' gestation.

D. **Obtain an obstetric history.** A history of previous sensitized pregnancies is useful. FHD tends to be as severe or more severe in subsequent pregnancies than in the first. If a previous fetus is hydropic, an 80% chance exists that the next Rh-positive fetus will be hydropic. FHD also tends to develop at the same time or somewhat earlier in subsequent pregnancies. Obstetric history is not significant, however, if the previous pregnancy was the first sensitized pregnancy, because few fetuses in the first pregnancy develop hydrops.

E. **Analyze the amniotic fluid.** In 1956, Bevis determined that the bilirubin concentration of amniotic fluid in Rh-sensitized pregnancies correlated with severity of fetal hemolysis. In 1961, Liley showed that the spectrophotometric peak at 450 nm (OD450) was directly proportional to the concentration of bilirubin in amniotic fluid after the mid-second trimester.

   1. **Three prognostic zones** have been described: zone 3 (upper, severely affected) to zone 1 (lower, unaffected or mildly affected). Zone 2 encompasses a wide range of severity. It is important to establish the OD450 trend. Amniotic fluid bilirubin decreases as normal pregnancy advances, so a horizontal or rising trend is ominous (Fig. 10-2).
   2. **Interpretation of amniotic fluid findings**
      a. A single OD450 value is often insufficient for accurate analysis; a trend is more reliable.
      b. Relying solely on OD450 values may lead to a false impression of severity. Fetal blood sampling is indicated for rising OD450 values or upper zone II or zone III OD450 findings.
      c. Extrapolating Liley graph values before 26 weeks' gestation may lead to erroneous conclusions.

F. **Analyze fetal blood.** Fetoscopic or ultrasound-guided vascular puncture techniques were developed in the 1970s to determine fetal blood type, hematocrit, and blood gas concentrations; these techniques also enabled intravascular fetal blood transfusion. Fetal blood analysis is the first step in the care of the fetus at risk for severe hemolytic disease in many centers.

G. **Perform ultrasound and Doppler studies.** Ultrasound evidence of cardiac failure is a late sign of hydrops (hematocrit less than 15%). Findings suggesting a lesser degree of anemia include increased placental thickness, increased umbilical vein diameter, pericardial effusion, and bowel wall edema.

H. **Evaluate the need for intrauterine transfusion.** The need for intrauterine transfusion is based on OD450 values and trend. Severe anemia is suspected when OD450 values rise into the upper quarter of zone II before 30 weeks' gestation or into zone III before 32 weeks' gestation. A single OD450 value in zone III before 32 to 34 weeks' gestation also may indicate severe anemia. Sonographic evidence of hydrops implies a hematocrit of less than 15%.

X. **Intrauterine transfusion in Rh-isoimmunized pregnancy** offers an alternative to preterm delivery in severe FHD. The goals of intrauterine transfusion are to

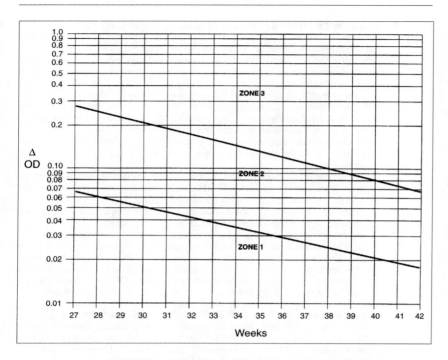

Figure 10-2. Liley graph depicting degrees of Rh sensitization. (From Liley AW. Liquor amnii analysis in management of pregnancy complicated by rhesus sensitization. *Am J Obstet Gynecol* 1961;82:1359–1370. Reproduced with permission.)

correct anemia, thus improving oxygenation, and to reduce extramedullary hematopoietic demand, thus decreasing portal venous pressure and improving hepatic function. Liley, in 1963, reported the first successful intraperitoneal intrauterine transfusion. Rodecke and colleagues in 1981 performed successful intravascular transfusions using a fetoscopic technique. Ultrasound-guided transfusion is now more common. The needle is placed into the umbilical vein at its insertion into the placenta. Type O-negative, leukocyte-poor packed erythrocytes that are crossmatched with the maternal serum are used.

A. Intraperitoneal versus intravascular transfusion
   1. Intravascular (i.v.) transfusion allows the degree of fetal anemia to be measured, thus allowing precise calculation of the amount of blood required.
   2. I.v. transfusion provides immediate correction of the anemia, reversing fetal hydrops more quickly.
   3. I.v. transfusion used alone increases the total number of procedures required, because the volume transfused is smaller than in intraperitoneal (i.p.) transfusion.
   4. The risk of fetal death for i.p. transfusion is 2% per procedure; that for i.v. transfusion is 4% per procedure.

B. General risks of intrauterine transfusion include rupture of membranes, fetomaternal hemorrhage, and infection.

XI. Timing of delivery. In cases of mild fetal hemolysis, fetal lung maturity is awaited, with delivery between 34 and 37 weeks' gestation. In severely sensitized pregnancies, the decision to deliver is individualized, with every attempt made to bring the fetus to 32 weeks' gestation using transfusions. Correcting hydrops *in utero* results in better neonatal outcome, regardless of gestational age.

XII. Perinatal outcome. The earlier a transfusion is required, the poorer the outcome. If transfusion is performed at earlier than 25 weeks' gestation, the perinatal mortality rate is 91%. Fetal hydrops at the time of first transfusion is associated with a poor outcome.

XIII. Sensitization caused by minor antigens. Today, maternal antibodies to minor antigens are detected as frequently as or more frequently than anti-D antibody. The incidence of sensitization caused by these minor antigens is increased in multiparas and in patients who received a blood transfusion in the past.

    A. Lewis antigens. Le^a and Le^b are not true RBC antigens but are secreted by other tissues and acquired by RBCs. Fetal RBCs acquire little antigen and react weakly with antibodies (a mnemonic is Lewis Lives).

    B. The most commonly encountered potentially serious antibodies are anti-E, **anti-Kell,** anti-c, anti-c+E and **anti-Fy^a** (mnemonics: Kell Kills, Duffy Dies).

        1. Anti-Kell sensitization

            a. Diagnosis. The fetal anemia produced by anti-Kell sensitization is qualitatively different from that of Rh disease. The primary cause of the anemia is suppression of fetal erythropoiesis rather than hemolysis; therefore, the OD450 value in cases of anti-Kell anemia may not be as elevated for a given degree of fetal anemia as it is in Rh disease because the test measures fetal bilirubin.

            b. Management should include the use of cordocentesis, rather than OD450, to determine fetal anemia. It is worth determining paternal antigen status because 90% of fathers of affected fetuses are Kell antigen-negative, and only 0.2% are homozygous.

XIV. ABO incompatibility occurs in 20% to 25% of pregnancies. This condition does not cause fetal hemolysis. It is a pediatric, not an obstetric, problem and manifests as mild to moderate hyperbilirubinemia during the first 24 hours of life.

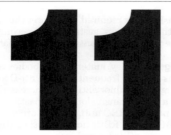

Cardiopulmonary Disorders and Pregnancy

Amanda Lieb and
Eva Pressman

Cardiac Disorders

Cardiovascular disorders, which complicate 1% of all pregnancies, may include preexisting disease, conditions that develop during pregnancy or in the postpartum period, congenital or acquired structural abnormalities, and arrhythmias.

I. **Hemodynamic changes during pregnancy.** The enormous changes in the cardiovascular system during pregnancy have many implications for the management of cardiac disease in the pregnant patient. These implications must be considered for labor management as well as for appropriate care during the antepartum and postpartum periods.

A. **Blood volume.** By 32 weeks' gestation, an increase in total blood volume of 40% has occurred, with an increase in the total plasma volume of up to 50%. Because the red cell mass only increases by 20%, a dilutional anemia exists at term.

B. **Cardiac output.** Because of increased stroke volume, cardiac output increases during pregnancy 30% to 50% by 20 to 24 weeks' gestation. A marked decrease in cardiac output, however, can occur when a pregnant woman is in the supine position because of caval compression.

C. **Systemic vascular resistance** decreases during pregnancy. It reaches its nadir during the second trimester, then slowly returns to prepregnancy levels by term.

D. **Redistribution of blood flow.** During pregnancy, blood flow to the kidneys, the skin, and the uterus increases. Uterine blood flow may be as high as 500 mL/minute at term.

E. **Hemodynamic changes during labor.** Venous pressure is increased during labor because of the increase in venous return from the uterine veins that occurs with contractions. This increase in venous pressure produces increases in cardiac output and right ventricular pressure, which in turn increase mean arterial pressure.

F. **Postpartum hemodynamic changes.** In the postpartum period, caval compression decreases, which results in an increase in the circulating blood volume. An increase in cardiac output ensues, and a reflex bradycardia may be observed. Because of increased blood loss, these hemodynamic changes are subtler in patients who undergo cesarean section.

II. **Epidural anesthesia** affects the cardiovascular system. The epidural anesthetic creates a functional sympathectomy. Peripheral vasodilatation occurs, resulting in decreased venous return to the heart. This decrease reduces preload; therefore, caution must be exercised in administering epidural anesthesia to patients with conditions in which effective management depends on adequate preload (e.g., pulmonary hypertension).

III. **Cardiac diseases in pregnancy**

A. **Diagnosis and evaluation**

1. **Signs and symptoms.** The signs and symptoms of cardiac disease may be difficult to distinguish from common complaints and findings in preg-

nancy and include fatigue, shortness of breath, orthopnea, palpitations, edema, systolic flow murmur, and a third heart sound.

2. **Warning signs.** Because it may be hard to distinguish the signs of cardiac disease from the changes associated with a normal, uncomplicated pregnancy, particular attention must be paid to warning signs, which include the following:

   a. Worsening dyspnea on exertion, or dyspnea at rest
   b. Chest pain with exercise or activity
   c. Syncope preceded by palpitations or exertion
   d. Loud systolic murmurs or a diastolic murmur
   e. Cyanosis or clubbing
   f. Jugular venous distension
   g. Cardiomegaly or a ventricular heave

3. **Evaluation** (workup) of cardiac disease must include a thorough history and physical examination. Tests may include a chest radiograph to assess cardiomegaly and pulmonary vascular prominence; an electrocardiogram (ECG) to assess ischemic, acute, or chronic changes in cardiac function; and an echocardiogram.

B. **Management of patients with known cardiac disease**

   1. An evaluation of a patient's cardiac status should be performed as early as possible in the pregnancy, or even pre-conception, if the opportunity exists.

   2. Patients should be monitored closely throughout their pregnancies, and ideally should be followed by both an obstetrician and a cardiologist. Clinicians should pay close attention to signs or symptoms of worsening congestive heart failure. Each visit should include the following:

      a. Cardiac examination and cardiac review of systems
      b. Documentation of weight, blood pressure, and pulse
      c. Evaluation of peripheral edema

   3. If a patient's symptoms worsen, hospitalization, bed rest, diuresis, or correction of an underlying arrhythmia may be required. If surgical correction of a cardiac defect is necessitated by a deteriorating condition, it is best performed early in pregnancy but after the period of fetal organogenesis.

   4. **Medical management**

      a. **Prophylaxis for endocarditis.** In 1997, the American Heart Association published a consensus of recommendations for the prevention of bacterial endocarditis. The consensus states that the majority of obstetrical and gynecological procedures do not require prophylactic antibiotic treatment because of the low likelihood of bacteremia (1% to 5% for a vaginal delivery). In cases in which an unanticipated bacteremia is suspected, i.v. antibiotics can be administered at the time the suspicion arises. For patients at high risk of developing endocarditis (Table 11-1), prophylaxis is optional, both for vaginal hysterectomies and for vaginal deliveries (Table 11-2). If antibiotic prophylaxis is required, the following doses should be administered: 2 g of ampicillin i.v. or i.m. and 1.5 mg/kg of gentamicin i.m. or i.v. during active labor, then one dose of ampicillin, 8 hours postpartum. If the patient is allergic to penicillin, 1 g of vancomycin i.v. can be substituted for ampicillin.

      b. Patients with **rheumatic heart disease** should receive 1.2 million units of penicillin G every month, or daily oral penicillin or erythromycin.

      c. If **anticoagulation** is necessary, heparin should be used rather than warfarin (Coumadin) because of the association of Coumadin exposure with fetal malformations. Heparin does not cross the placenta. Coumadin may be used in the third trimester, although a risk exists of fetal or placental hemorrhage or birth defects.

C. **Counseling.** When the patient's cardiac status is known, she should be appropriately informed about the maternal and fetal risks her cardiac disease causes during pregnancy. Ideally, this conversation would take place preconception, but if the patient is already pregnant, it should take place as early as possible in the pregnancy. If the pregnancy poses a serious threat to mater-

Table 11-1. Cardiac conditions associated with endocarditis for which prophylaxis is recommended

High-risk category
   Prosthetic cardiac valves, including bioprosthetic and homograft valves
   Previous bacterial endocarditis
   Complex cyanotic congenital heart disease (e.g., single ventricle states, transposition of the great arteries, tetralogy of Fallot)
   Surgically constructed systemic pulmonary shunts or conduits
Moderate-risk category
   Most other congenitial cardiac malformations (other than above and below)
   Acquired valvar dysfunction (e.g., rheumatic heart disease)
   Hypertrophic cardiomyopathy
   Mitral valve prolapse with valvar regurgitation and/or thickened leaflets

From Dajani AS, et al. Prevention of bacterial endocarditis. *JAMA* 1997;277(22):1795. Adapted with permission.

nal health, the patient should receive counseling to help her evaluate the option of terminating the pregnancy.

IV. **Valvular heart disease**
   A. **Mitral valve prolapse** is the most common congenital heart defect in young women and usually does not affect pregnancy in any way. A midsystolic click may be detected, or the patient may complain of palpitations. Antibiotic prophylaxis is still a subject of debate, but because it is relatively safe, it is suggested.
   B. **Mitral stenosis** is the most common rheumatic heart disease in pregnancy. This disorder follows a natural course in which mitral insufficiency progresses to mitral stenosis. Up to 10 years may elapse before the patient experiences symptoms arising from decreased cardiac output. Eventually, a left atrial outflow obstruction develops, which leads to increased atrial pressure, then to increased pulmonary capillary wedge pressure. Pulmonary congestion later leads to right heart failure and pulmonary hypertension. The increased plasma volume of pregnancy imposes great stress on the cardiovascular sys-

Table 11-2. Genitourinary tract procedures for which endocarditis prophylaxis is not recommended

Vaginal hysterectomy[a]
Vaginal delivery[a]
Cesarean section
Urethral catheterization[b]
Uterine dilatation and curettage[b]
Therapeutic abortion[b]
Sterilization procedures
Insertion or removal of intrauterine devices[b]

[a]Prophylaxis is optional for high-risk patients.
[b]In uninfected tissues.
From Dajani AS, et al. Prevention of bacterial endocarditis. *JAMA* 1997;277(22):1797. Adapted with permission.

tem of women with mitral stenosis because of their fixed cardiac output. Up to 20% of pregnant patients with mitral stenosis become symptomatic by 20 weeks' gestation, when cardiac output is at its maximum.

1. **Management.** During pregnancy, affected patients should limit their physical activity. If volume overload is present, they should be diuresed carefully. If arrhythmias exist, especially atrial fibrillation, the arrhythmias should be controlled to avoid decreased diastolic filling time, which leads to a further decrease in cardiac output. If mural thrombi are present and anticoagulation is required, the patient should be treated with heparin. If medical management fails, the patient may require a valve replacement or commissurotomy.

2. **Considerations during labor.** Cesarean section should be performed for obstetric indications only. If significant heart disease exists, especially with pulmonary hypertension, invasive cardiac monitoring with a Swan-Ganz catheter should be considered during labor. The patient should undergo labor in the left lateral position and receive supplemental oxygen.

   a. **Tachycardia should be prevented** because it may lead to decreased cardiac output caused by a decreased diastolic filling time. Verapamil or digoxin may be used to slow the ventricular contraction rate if an atrial arrhythmia is present. Anesthetics may be useful in slowing sinus tachycardia. If an epidural anesthetic is used, care must be taken to prevent hypotension, which may lead to decreased venous return to the ventricles or to tachycardia with decreased diastolic filling time. If necessary, alpha agonists may be used to maintain systemic vascular resistance.

   b. The second stage of labor may be shortened by performing a **forceps delivery or vacuum extraction** delivery. Hypotension should be prevented if possible because adequate blood return is critical to maintaining cardiac output.

C. **Mitral regurgitation** may occur in patients with a history of rheumatic fever; endocarditis; idiopathic hypertrophic subaortic stenosis; or, most commonly, mitral valve prolapse. Typically a decrescendo murmur is detected. This murmur, however, is often diminished during pregnancy. In most cases, mitral regurgitation is tolerated well during pregnancy.

   1. In severe cases, the onset of symptoms usually occurs later than in cases of mitral stenosis. Patients may present with symptoms of left heart failure such as fatigue and dyspnea. Atrial enlargement and fibrillation, as well as ventricular enlargement and dysfunction, may develop. Inotropic agents may be necessary if left ventricular dilatation and dysfunction are present.

   2. During labor, patients with advanced disease may require central monitoring. The pain of labor may lead to an increase in blood pressure, and consequently in afterload, causing pulmonary vascular congestion. Therefore, epidural anesthesia is recommended. Affected patients should receive antibiotic prophylaxis during labor.

D. **Aortic stenosis** is rarely seen in pregnancy. It is a late complication of rheumatic fever that develops over several decades. Patients are usually not symptomatic until the fifth or sixth decade of life. Symptoms arise from obstruction of the left ventricular outflow tract, which compromises cardiac output. Angina and syncope upon exertion are common symptoms of advanced disease. Sudden death caused by hypotension may occur. After symptoms appear, decompensation is usually rapid, with a 50% mortality in 5 years.

   1. During pregnancy, mortality for patients with aortic stenosis may be as high as 17%.

   2. Because this disorder is characterized by a fixed afterload, adequate end-diastolic volume, and therefore adequate filling pressure, is necessary to maintain cardiac output. Consequently, great care must be taken to prevent hypotension and tachycardia caused by blood loss, regional anes-

thesia, or other medications. Patients should be hydrated adequately and placed in the left lateral position to maximize venous return. Central monitoring with a Swan-Ganz catheter is recommended in severe cases. Affected patients should receive antibiotic prophylaxis.

E. Aortic regurgitation is often a late complication of rheumatic fever that appears 10 years after the acute disease episode. Aortic regurgitation also may be seen with congenital bifid aortic valves and secondary to dilatation of the aortic root, such as occurs in Marfan syndrome. Symptoms usually develop in the fourth or fifth decade of life. Typically, the patient has a high-pitched, blowing murmur. During pregnancy, because of decreased systemic vascular resistance, the murmur and the regurgitation may decrease. Therefore, the condition is usually well tolerated in pregnancy.

1. If a patient shows evidence of left heart failure and requires valve replacement, pregnancy should be delayed until after the repair has been completed. If a patient is not yet symptomatic, she should be encouraged to complete her childbearing early, before the onset of symptoms.

2. During labor, afterload reduction should be undertaken. Epidural anesthesia is recommended. Bradycardia is poorly tolerated because the increased time of diastole allows more time for regurgitation. Therefore, a target heart rate of 80 to 100 beats/minute should be maintained. Antibiotic prophylaxis during labor is required.

V. Congenital lesions

A. Left-to-right shunts usually are corrected during childhood. If the defect has been corrected, the outcome of pregnancy is usually good. If the defect has not been corrected, or if reversal of the shunt has developed as a result of pulmonary hypertension, the outcome of pregnancy is poor, with a high rate of maternal mortality. Usually pregnancy does not significantly alter the degree of shunting, but the shunt may increase somewhat because of increased intravascular volume.

1. **Atrial septal defects** are the most common congenital heart lesions in adults. Affected patients usually exhibit a pulmonary ejection murmur and a second heart sound that is split in both the inspiratory and expiratory phases. The defects are usually very well tolerated unless they are associated with pulmonary hypertension. If complications develop, such as atrial arrhythmias, pulmonary hypertension or heart failure, they usually do not arise until the fifth decade of life and therefore are seen uncommonly in pregnancy.

   a. For affected patients without complications, no special therapy or management is necessary during labor. Antibiotic prophylaxis may be given, but the risk of endocarditis is low.

   b. If the patient has advanced disease, careful monitoring throughout pregnancy by both an obstetrician and a cardiologist is recommended. Prolonged bed rest may be necessary during the pregnancy. In particular, the patient should be observed for the development of atrial dilatation, supraventricular arrhythmias, pulmonary hypertension, or heart failure. During labor, invasive cardiac monitoring should be considered, and arrhythmias and tachycardia should be promptly treated.

2. **Ventricular septal defects** (VSDs) often close spontaneously. Large lesions usually are corrected surgically in childhood. Therefore, significant VSDs rarely are seen in pregnancy. Occasionally, uncorrected lesions may lead to significant left-to-right shunts with pulmonary hypertension, right ventricular failure, or reversal of the shunt, but such complications are rare.

   a. Because of the increased systemic vascular resistance that occurs during labor, epidural anesthesia is recommended. If the patient has pulmonary hypertension or right-to-left shunt, however, the decrease in systemic vascular resistance caused by epidural anesthesia is poorly tolerated because of decreased perfusion of the lungs. The patient should undergo invasive cardiac monitoring via Swan-Ganz catheter and must be observed carefully for cyanosis in the presence of adequate

cardiac output, which signals a worsening of the right-to-left shunt.
   b. Affected patients require antibiotic prophylaxis during labor. In addition, the incidence of VSD in the offspring of affected parents is 4%, so fetal echocardiography should be considered. Small VSDs, however, are often difficult to detect on fetal echocardiograms.
   3. Patent ductus arteriosus (PDA) usually is tolerated well during pregnancy. If a large PDA is present, the patient usually develops pulmonary hypertension, which is associated with a very high maternal mortality rate and poor pregnancy outcomes. Because of increased volume, left heart failure and therefore pulmonary hypertension usually worsen during pregnancy. Therefore, pregnancy is not recommended for patients with large PDAs and associated complications. Patients with PDAs who continue their pregnancies should receive antibiotic prophylaxis.
B. Right-to-left shunts
   1. Tetralogy of Fallot is characterized by right ventricular outflow tract obstruction, a ventricular septal defect, right ventricular hypertrophy, and an overriding aorta. These conditions cause a right-to-left shunt and cyanosis. If the defect goes uncorrected, the afflicted patient rarely lives beyond childhood; pregnancy is therefore very rare. If pregnancy does occur, however, the incidence of heart failure during gestation is 40%. Affected patients should be observed carefully for evidence of left heart failure. The increased cardiac output associated with labor can lead to a worsening of the right-to-left shunt. The shunt also can worsen during the immediate postpartum period because of the decreases in systemic vascular resistance and in blood volume that occur at that time.
      a. During pregnancy, the fetus should be watched for evidence of intrauterine growth retardation (IUGR). In addition, maternal cyanosis is associated with spontaneous abortion and preterm birth, and the patient should be counseled accordingly.
      b. During labor, invasive cardiac monitoring should be employed. Adequate venous return must be maintained to enable adequate perfusion of the lungs. Therefore, the best choices for anesthesia are systemic inhalation agents or a pudendal block. Extreme caution must be exercised if an epidural or spinal anesthetic is used because of the risk of hypotension.
   2. Coarctation of the aorta. Severe cases of coarctation of the aorta usually are corrected in infancy, and consequently this condition rarely is seen in pregnancy. Surgical correction during pregnancy is recommended only if dissection occurs. Coarctation of the aorta is associated with other cardiac lesions as well as with Berry aneurysms.
      a. Coarctation of the aorta is characterized by a fixed cardiac output. Therefore, the patient's heart cannot meet the increased cardiac demands of pregnancy by increasing its heart rate, and extreme care must be taken to prevent hypotension, which leads to decompensation.
      b. The newborn should be evaluated carefully because 2% of infants of mothers with coarctation of the aorta may themselves exhibit cardiac lesions.
   3. Eisenmenger syndrome refers to a right-to-left shunt that forms secondary to an initial left-to-right lesion that results in pulmonary arterial obliteration and pulmonary hypertension. Eisenmenger syndrome is a very serious condition in pregnancy, with a maternal mortality rate of 50% and a fetal mortality rate of greater than 50% if cyanosis is present. In addition, 30% of fetuses in pregnancies complicated by this syndrome exhibit IUGR. Because of increased maternal mortality, termination of the pregnancy is advised. If the pregnancy is continued, special precautions must be taken during labor. The patient should be monitored with a Swan-Ganz catheter, and hypovolemia should be prevented.
C. Marfan syndrome. Marfan syndrome is an autosomal dominant disorder of the fibrillin gene characterized by weakness of the connective tissues. Car-

diovascular manifestations may include aortic root dilatation, mitral valve prolapse, and aneurysms. Genetic counseling is recommended.

1. Because great variability exists in the clinical expression of Marfan syndrome, affected patients' cardiovascular systems should be studied before recommendations about the safety and management of the pregnancy are made. If a patient's cardiovascular involvement is minor and her aortic root diameter is less than 40 mm, her risk of complications during pregnancy does not significantly exceed that of the general population. If cardiovascular involvement is more extensive or the aortic root is greater than 40 mm, the risks of complications during pregnancy and aortic dissection are significantly increased.

2. During the pregnancy and in labor, hypertension should be prevented or, if present, managed with beta blockers. Beta blockers should be considered for patients with Marfan syndrome from the second trimester until delivery. Regional anesthesia during labor is considered safe. Antibiotic prophylaxis is suggested.

D. **Idiopathic hypertrophic subaortic stenosis** (IHSS) is an autosomal dominant disorder; therefore, genetic counseling is advised for affected patients. IHSS manifests as left ventricular outflow tract obstruction secondary to a hypertrophic interventricular septum.

1. Patients' conditions improve when left ventricular end-diastolic volume is maximized; therefore, pregnant patients often fare quite well initially because of an increase in circulating blood volume. Later in pregnancy, however, decreased systemic vascular resistance and decreased venous return caused by caval compression by the gravid uterus may worsen the obstruction. This may cause left ventricular failure, or supraventricular arrhythmias from left atrial distension.

2. The following management points should be kept in mind during labor:
   a. Inotropic agents should not be administered because they may exacerbate the obstruction.
   b. The patient should labor in the left lateral decubitus position.
   c. Administration of drugs that decrease systemic vascular resistance should be avoided or limited.
   d. Monitoring for arrhythmias should be employed, and tachycardia should be treated promptly.
   e. The second stage of labor should be curtailed (i.e., forceps delivery) to avoid Valsalva's maneuver.

E. **Ebstein's anomaly** is a congenital malformation of the tricuspid valve, in which the tricuspid valve is either stenotic enough to cause obstruction or so incompetent that the right ventricle must act as both an atrium and a ventricle. If surgical correction is necessary, it should be performed prior to pregnancy.

F. **Congenital atrioventricular block.** Compared with acquired adult atrioventricular block, the ventricular rate in the congenital form is usually higher and the electrocardiographic wave complex normal, or only slightly widened. The use of a pacemaker may be indicated. With or without pacing, patients usually fare well and do not require special treatment during pregnancy.

VI. **Cardiomyopathy**

A. **Idiopathic** dilated cardiomyopathy may be caused by an autoimmune response to myocardial damage. The heart becomes uniformly dilated, so its walls are not thick even if some hypertrophy is present. Filling pressures increase, and cardiac output decreases. Eventually, heart failure develops and is often refractory to treatment. The five-year survival rate is poor, approximately 50%; therefore, consideration of pregnancy requires careful counseling, even if heart failure is absent.

B. **Peripartum** cardiomyopathy is a dilated cardiomyopathy of unknown etiology that develops in the third trimester of pregnancy or postpartum. Approximately 50% of patients recover, and the other 50% develop a permanently dilated cardiomyopathy. A risk of recurrence with future pregnancies exists for both groups of patients, but the risk is higher among patients with persistent dilated cardiomyopathy. Patients should be counseled accordingly.

1. Several factors have been identified that predispose patients to develop peripartum cardiomyopathy, including multiparity, increased maternal age, multiple gestations, and preeclampsia or eclampsia. Management of peripartum cardiomyopathy includes bed rest; sodium restriction; medical therapy with agents such as diuretics, inotropics, or anticoagulants; and, in cases of advanced disease, transplant.
   2. During labor, very careful cardiac monitoring with a Swan-Ganz catheter should be considered in cases of advanced disease. Monitoring should continue for at least 24 hours postpartum. Furosemide, digoxin, or hydralazine may be administered, as well as dopamine or dobutamine if necessary. The patient should be given supplemental oxygen and an epidural anesthetic for pain control, and the second stage of labor should be curtailed. Cesarean section should be performed for obstetric indications.
VII. Arrhythmias. Nonsustained arrhythmias in the absence of organic cardiac disease are best left untreated. Serious, life-threatening arrhythmias that are associated with an aberrant reentrant pathway should be treated prior to pregnancy by ablation. If medical therapy is necessary during pregnancy, established—rather than new or experimental—drugs should be used. Artificial pacing should not have any effect on the fetus, nor should electrical defibrillation or cardioversion of the maternal heart.
VIII. Ischemic heart disease is uncommon in women of childbearing age. However, the incidence of ischemic heart disease in pregnancy has increased because of larger numbers of older gravidas and smokers. Although myocardial infarction (MI) during pregnancy is rare, the most consistent risk factor for such an occurrence is age over 35. Usually ischemic heart disease is caused by atherosclerosis, but emboli and coronary vasospasm are other possible etiologies.
   A. About 67% of myocardial ischemia during pregnancy occurs during the third trimester. If an MI occurs before 24 weeks' gestation, termination of the pregnancy is recommended. If delivery takes place within 2 weeks of the acute event, the mortality rate reaches 50%. If delivery takes place more than 2 weeks after the event, however, the mortality rate is greatly decreased.
   B. Management of MI in a pregnant patient is the same as that in a nonpregnant patient. The patient should be monitored in an intensive care unit and should receive supplemental oxygen and appropriate analgesia. She should be observed carefully for the development of arrhythmias.
   C. During labor, a cesarean section should be performed for obstetric indications. Epidural pain control is considered safe. If another pregnancy is desired, the patient should receive thorough pre-conception counseling and evaluation.

Pulmonary Disorders

I. Physiologic changes during pregnancy. Because pregnancy imposes much less stress on the pulmonary system than on the cardiovascular system, patients with pulmonary disease are much less likely to experience a deterioration in their conditions during pregnancy than patients with cardiovascular disease.
   A. Structural alterations. The mucosa of the upper respiratory tract becomes edematous and mucus production increases, leading to a sensation of stuffiness and chronic cold symptoms. An increase in the subcostal angle occurs in pregnancy even before the uterus increases significantly in size. The transverse diameter and chest circumference also increase early in pregnancy. Later in pregnancy the diaphragm is elevated, but diaphragmatic excursion with each breath increases.
   B. Oxygen consumption
      1. **Partial pressure of oxygen.** Although minute ventilation increases by 30% to 40% during pregnancy, oxygen consumption increases by only 15% to 20%. Consequently, Po_2 and Pco_2 levels increase to an average of 104 to 108 mm Hg. The increase in oxygen consumption is attributable to

fetal oxygen consumption; increased oxygen consumption by the placenta and the maternal cardiovascular system (because of increased cardiac output) and kidneys; and increased tissue mass of the breasts and uterus.

2. **Partial pressure of carbon dioxide.** Although carbon dioxide production increases during pregnancy, Pco_2 and Po_2 levels decrease to an average of 27 to 32 mm Hg because of the increased minute ventilation. This decrease facilitates carbon dioxide exchange between the mother and the fetus. Arterial pH does not change significantly because the decrease in Pco_2 levels is offset by a decrease in serum bicarbonate levels to an average of 18 to 31 mEq/L as a result of an increased rate of renal excretion.

C. **Tidal volume** increases by 30% to 40% in pregnancy because of a progesterone effect. Progesterone lowers the carbon dioxide threshold in the respiratory center. The expiratory reserve volume and functional residual capacity decrease in pregnancy, but the respiratory rate and vital capacity remain the same. Therefore, the increase in tidal volume is solely responsible for the 30% to 40% increase in minute ventilation that occurs during pregnancy. Many women complain of dyspnea during pregnancy, sometimes as early as the first trimester. This subjective experience is most likely a result of the increase in tidal volume and the decreased levels of Pco_2.

D. **Resistance.** Forced expiratory volume and peak expiratory flow rate, which are indirect measures of airway resistance and lung compliance, are unchanged in pregnancy.

II. **Asthma**

A. Approximately 1% of pregnancies are complicated by asthma.

B. **Effect of pregnancy on asthma and of asthma on pregnancy**

1. **Maternal effects.** The course of asthma in pregnancy varies, and a patient may be affected differently in one pregnancy than in another. No change in severity of preexisting asthma occurs in 22% to 49% of pregnancies. The asthma worsens in 9% to 23% of pregnancies and improves in 29% to 69% of pregnancies. (These percentages may be easier to remember as a rule of thirds: one-third of patients get better, one-third get worse, and one-third remain the same.)

2. **Fetal effects.** No fetal malformations are associated with asthma. Some studies have shown an increased incidence of growth retardation, especially if the mother is on chronic steroid therapy.

C. **Surveillance.** At each visit, a pulmonary examination and review of symptoms should be performed. Peak flow can be evaluated at each visit. In addition, patients may monitor their peak flows at home and begin treatment before they become dangerously symptomatic. Influenza vaccines are recommended for patients with asthma.

D. **Management.** Asthma should be treated aggressively in symptomatic pregnant patients. Because of the increased demands on the respiratory system in pregnancy, an asthma exacerbation can become severe more quickly in pregnancy. Beta-mimetics, steroids, anticholinergics, and theophylline should not be withheld if indicated.

1. **Medications**

a. **Theophylline** inhibits phosphodiesterase, thereby increasing circulating levels of cyclic adenosine monophosphate (cAMP). When B_2 receptors are stimulated, cAMP is released, causing relaxation of the bronchi. Clearance of theophylline increases in the third trimester; therefore, theophylline levels should be rechecked during this period.

b. **Beta sympathomimetic** drugs are also useful for controlling asthma during pregnancy because of increased cAMP release. Preparations may be oral (such as terbutaline) or aerosolized. Aerosolized preparations cause fewer systemic side effects, such as tachycardia, than oral preparations. Albuterol (Proventil) and metaproterenol (Alupent) are frequently used.

c. **Anticholinergics** such as aerosolized glycopyrrolate are also useful in asthma control during pregnancy. Side effects include tachycardia.

d. **Steroids.** Aerosolized steroids such as beclomethasone (Beclovent, Vanceril) are very active locally with little systemic activity. Systemic steroids are indicated when patients do not respond adequately to theophylline, beta-mimetics, or aerosolized steroids. Oral prednisone may be used, or, in acute settings, intravenous hydrocortisone or methylprednisolone, typically hydrocortisone, 100 mg i.v. or methylpredisolone, 60 mg every 6 to 8 hours. Although studies have shown an increased incidence of cleft palate in rabbits with steroid use during pregnancy, this finding has not been demonstrated in humans. Fetal adrenal suppression with chronic steroid use is possible but very rare because most of the prednisone ingested by the mother is inactivated by the placenta. Consequently, the fetus only receives 10% to 30% of the ingested steroid.

2. **Upper respiratory infections** may cause acute asthma exacerbations and should therefore be treated aggressively. Patients should be instructed to present at the first sign of infection and should be treated with broad-spectrum antibiotics. Tetracyclines should be avoided because of teratogenic effects.

3. **Asthma attacks during labor** are rare, possibly because of an increase in endogenous cortisol production. Patients who were given long-term, systemic steroids during their pregnancies should receive stress-dose steroids during labor and delivery. Methylprednisolone, 60 mg i.v. every 6 to 8 hours, or hydrocortisone, 100 mg every 4 hours, may be administered. Epidural anesthesia is preferable to general endotracheal anesthesia because of the increased incidence of bronchospasm and atelectasis with general anesthetic use. If cervical ripening is necessary, prostaglandin E_2 (which has a bronchodilatory effect) should be used rather than prostaglandin $F_{2\alpha}$, which can cause bronchoconstriction. Dinoprostone (Prepidil or Cervidil) may be used with caution according to manufacturers' recommendations.

4. During **acute exacerbations** requiring hospital observation or admission, patients should be given 30% to 40% humidified oxygen. Systemic steroids, either methylprednisolone or hydrocortisone, should be considered. Arterial blood gas should be monitored, and in critical cases in which the Po_2 begins to fall and the Pco_2 begins to rise, intubation should be considered. Note that normal Pco_2 in pregnancy is 31 mm Hg. Asthmatic patients whose Pco_2 rises above 40 mm Hg are candidates for intubation.

III. **Sarcoidosis**
   A. **Description.** Sarcoidosis is a disease of noncaseating granulomas with multiorgan involvement. The etiology of the disease is unknown. It is usually diagnosed in patients between the ages of 20 and 40. The patient may present with bilateral hilar or palpable cervical adenopathy, cough, and interstitial lung disease seen on chest radiograph. Differential diagnosis includes non-Hodgkin's lymphoma and tuberculosis. Diagnosis may be confirmed by lymph node or liver biopsy. Two-thirds of patients show spontaneous improvement over a period of 2 to 3 years from the time of diagnosis. The remaining one-third of patients usually exhibit slow progression of their disease.
   B. **Effect of pregnancy on the disease and of the disease on pregnancy.** Pregnancy does not appear to have any adverse effects on the course of the disease, nor does the disease appear to have any adverse effects on pregnancy.
   C. **Prognosis.** Parenchymal pulmonary lesions on chest radiograph, advanced maternal age, low inflammatory activity on biopsies, extrapulmonary disease, and a need for medications other than steroids are factors associated with a relatively poor prognosis for sarcoidosis.
   D. **Evaluation and workup** include pulmonary function tests and an arterial blood gas at the first prenatal visit and again in the third trimester, and an ECG, 24-hour urine study, and liver function studies for assessment of possible extrapulmonary disease.
   E. **Management.** The mainstay of treatment of sarcoidosis is steroids.
IV. **Cystic fibrosis**
   A. **Incidence, natural course.** Cystic fibrosis is present in approximately 1 in 2,500 live births. Because of improved treatment of this disease, more and more affected women are reaching childbearing age.
   B. **Effect of pregnancy on the disease and of the disease on pregnancy.** Although the rate of spontaneous abortion is not increased in pregnant patients

with cystic fibrosis, the rate of maternal mortality in affected patients is significantly higher than that in the general population. This increased mortality rate, however, is no higher than that for nonpregnant cystic fibrosis patients.

C. Prenatal diagnosis and genetic counseling. For two-thirds of couples with one or more previous affected children, a prenatal diagnosis is possible. Many mutations can cause this disorder, however, which renders prenatal diagnosis difficult.

D. Poor prognostic factors include a vital capacity of less than 50% of predicted value, cor pulmonale, and pulmonary hypertension.

E. Other systemic manifestations. Affected patients may exhibit pancreatic insufficiency and cirrhosis of the liver.

F. Management
  1. **During labor,** careful attention to the following indicators is essential:
     a. **Fluid and electrolyte balance** should be monitored closely. Because of the increased sodium content of sweat in cystic fibrosis, affected patients are prone to hypovolemia during labor.
     b. **Oxygen levels.** Supplemental oxygen may be used if necessary.
     c. **Anesthesia.** Epidural or regional anesthesia is preferable to general endotracheal anesthesia for patients with cystic fibrosis.
  2. **Breast-feeding.** Breast milk should be evaluated for sodium content before the infant is allowed to breast-feed because the sodium content of the milk of mothers with cystic fibrosis may be elevated significantly. In such cases, breast-feeding may be contraindicated.

V. Infections
  A. Tuberculosis (TB). The incidence of TB is rising in urban areas.
    1. **Diagnosis.** Screening is performed by placing a purified protein derivative (PPD) subcutaneously. Drawbacks of this method are that only 80% of results are positive in the setting of reactivation of disease, and that if a patient has received a bacille Calmette-Guérin vaccine, the PPD results are positive for life. If the PPD is positive or TB is suspected, a chest x-ray study with abdominal shielding should be performed, preferably after 20 weeks' gestation. A definitive diagnosis of TB can be based on a positive culture for *Mycobacterium tuberculosis* or on the results of an acid-fast sputum stain. The first morning sputum should be collected for 3 days. A sputum sample may be induced using aerosolized saline.
    2. **Medical treatment.** If a sputum stain finding is positive for acid-fast bacilli, antibiotic therapy should be initiated while final culture and sensitivity results (which may take up to 6 weeks to return) are awaited. Standard treatment consists of the following: isoniazid (INH), 300 mg q.d.; plus ethambutol, 15 mg/kg/day; plus pyridoxine, 20 to 50 mg q.d. Streptomycin should be avoided because of the risk of fetal cranial nerve VIII damage. Rifampin should also be avoided during pregnancy unless INH and ethambutol cannot be used. Rifampin crosses the placenta and could theoretically cause fetal injury. INH prophylaxis for recent positive conversions of test results with no evidence of active disease is not recommended during pregnancy.
    3. **Effect of pregnancy on tuberculosis and of tuberculosis on pregnancy.** If the infection is treated, it should not have an effect on the pregnancy, and the pregnancy should not affect the course of the disease.
  B. Pneumonia
    1. **Signs and symptoms.** Bacterial pneumonia is usually caused by gram-positive diplococci, namely *Streptococcus pneumoniae*. Symptoms include sudden onset of productive cough, sputum production, fever, chills, and tachypnea. *Mycoplasma pneumoniae* usually is characterized by gradual onset; nonproductive cough; and diffuse, patchy infiltrate on chest radiograph, which may be unilateral or bilateral. The obstetrician must consider this pathogen if the patient does not respond to treatment with penicillin or a cephalosporin.
    2. **Diagnosis** is confirmed by examining a chest radiograph, sputum culture, and Gram's stain.

3. **Management.** Streptococcal pneumonia may be treated with i.v. penicillin G until several days after defervescence, then with oral penicillin for a 10- to 14-day total course. *Mycoplasma* pneumonia may be treated with erythromycin or azithromycin.

4. **Medical complications** include bacteremia, empyema, arrhythmias, and respiratory failure.

5. **Pregnancy complications** include preterm labor, which occurs in 44% of cases, and preterm delivery, which occurs in 36% of cases.

C. **Bronchitis** resulting from infection and subsequent airway obstruction should be managed the same way as asthma.

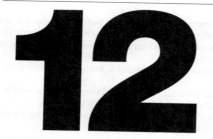

Renal, Hepatic, and Gastrointestinal Disease and Systemic Lupus Erythematosus in Pregnancy

Samuel Del Rio and
Eva Pressman

I. Renal disease

A. Renal physiology in pregnancy. A gradual accumulation of 500 to 900 mEq of sodium and 6 to 8 L of water occurs during pregnancy. During gestation, renal plasma flow increases by 60% to 80%, and glomerular filtration rate (GFR) by 30% to 50%. Because of these changes, creatinine clearance increases over 100 mL/minute, a change that must be taken into account when assessing a patient's renal function. The expansion of the plasma volume and the increase in the GFR result in lower normal values for blood urea nitrogen (BUN) and serum creatinine during pregnancy (8.5 mg/dL and 0.46 mg/dL, respectively). Therefore, during pregnancy, concentrations of BUN and serum creatinine exceeding 13 mg/dL and 0.8 mg/dL, respectively, suggest renal impairment. Tubular reabsorption of glucose, amino acids, and some proteins decreases during pregnancy, resulting in higher rates of urinary excretion. As a result, urinary protein excretion of about 150 to 180 mg/24 hours is commonly found in the second and third trimesters.

B. Morphologic changes to the urinary tract in pregnancy. The morphology of the urinary tract is altered considerably during gestation. Changes include an increase in the size of the kidneys, dilatations of the renal pelves and ureters, and increased incidence of vesicoureteral reflux.

C. Routine assessment of renal function. Each prenatal visit should include a urine dipstick test for proteinuria. A value of +1 should be followed up by collection of a clean-catch urine sample for culture and sensitivity testing as well as microscopic evaluation for pyuria. If the proteinuria persists with a negative urine culture finding, then a 24-hour urine collection should be obtained. Abnormal results should then be referred to a nephrologist for further evaluation unless preeclampsia is identified as the cause of the abnormalities.

D. Urinary tract infections, including asymptomatic bacteriuria, cystitis, and acute pyelonephritis, are common in both pregnant and nonpregnant women. Although pregnancy by itself does not increase the overall likelihood of these infections, a shift toward an increased incidence of acute symptomatic infection, particularly acute pyelonephritis, takes place in pregnant women.

    1. Asymptomatic bacteriuria (ASB) may be defined as the presence of actively multiplying bacteria within the urinary tract (excluding the distal urethra) at a time when the patient is experiencing no symptoms of infection. The prevalence of ASB during pregnancy ranges from 2% to 7%. In women with sickle cell trait, ASB is twice as common as in women without sickle cell trait. If left untreated, ASB progresses to acute pyelonephritis in approximately 20% to 30% of pregnant women; the use of antibiotics to treat ASB in pregnant women reduces this rate to approximately 3%. Therefore, all women should undergo screening for bacteriuria at their first prenatal visit.

        a. Management. Bacteriuria is managed with appropriate antimicrobial therapy and urine culture surveillance. If available, urine dipstick tests for protein, leukocyte esterase, and nitrites should be performed for patients with sickle cell trait at each prenatal visit, and urine cultures each trimester should be considered for these patients as well. The diagnosis of ASB is based on a clean-catch urine specimen yielding a colony count greater than 10^5 organisms/mL. *Escherichia coli* accounts for approximately 80% of all infections, while *Klebsiella* sp., *Proteus* sp., and *Enterobacter* sp. account for most of the remaining isolates. Initial therapy (7 to 10 days) is usually empiric, and a variety of agents, including sulfonamides, nitrofurantoin, ampicillin, and cephalosporins, have been shown to be both safe and effective. Test-of-cure urine cultures should be obtained 1 to 2 weeks after treatment and again each trimester for the remainder of the pregnancy.

  b. **Treatment failures.** Treatment should be repeated according to antibiotic sensitivity, and the appropriate antimicrobial should be administered for 2 to 3 weeks. After the second course of short-term, high-dose treatment, patients receive low-dose, long-term prophylactic therapy for the remainder of their pregnancies. Nitrofurantoin (100 mg q.d.), ampicillin (250 mg q.d.) or trimethoprim and sulfamethoxazole (160 mg/800 mg tablet q.d.) are usually effective chronic suppressive agents for urinary bacteria. Sulfonamides should be avoided during the last few weeks of pregnancy because they competitively inhibit the binding of bilirubin to albumin and theoretically may increase the risk of hyperbilirubinemia in the newborn. In patients with glucose-6-phosphate dehydrogenase enzyme deficiency, nitrofurantoin should be avoided because of the potential for exacerbation of hemolytic anemia.

2. **Acute cystitis** occurs in about 1% of pregnant women. The diagnosis of cystitis is based on the symptom complex of urinary frequency, urgency, dysuria, hematuria, and suprapubic discomfort, as well as a positive urine culture result. The bacteriology of acute cystitis is the same as that of ASB. Similar treatment is recommended, with the aims of abolishing symptoms and preventing progression to acute pyelonephritis.

3. **Acute pyelonephritis** is the most common major urinary tract complication of pregnancy, occurring in approximately 2% of all pregnancies. Its presentation in pregnant women is similar to that in nonpregnant women, with fever (often reaching 40°C or higher), flank pain, nausea, and vomiting with or without frequency, urgency, and dysuria. Acute pyelonephritis may mimic or precipitate premature labor. Bacteremia occurs in approximately 10% to 20% of all cases.

  a. **Treatment** consists of aggressive intravenous hydration and administration of intravenous antibiotics, cefazolin, and analgesics. Cefazolin or ampicillin and gentamicin are the first-line antibiotics and should be continued until the patient has been afebrile for at least 48 hours. The choice of first-line therapy depends on the incidence of cefazolin-resistant organisms (usually *E. coli*) in the patient population. If this incidence is greater than 10%, then ampicillin and gentamicin should be used. Urine should be strained to capture any stones, which could have been responsible for the initial infection. Urine culture findings must be monitored to determine speciation and sensitivities.

  b. **Treatment failures.** Patients who do not respond to appropriate antibiotic treatment and continue to experience either fever or costovertebral angle tenderness should have a renal ultrasound image for further evaluation. After resolution of the acute pyelonephritis, the patient should be kept on suppressive therapy for the remainder of the pregnancy. For patients with a history of multiple urinary tract infections or pyelonephritis, it may be helpful to initiate suppressive therapy as soon as a viable pregnancy is documented.

4. **Urolithiasis** should be considered for pregnant patients with negative urine culture findings in whom pyelonephritis, microscopic hematuria, or recurrent infection is suspected. Patients with a history of urolithiasis should be advised to keep themselves well hydrated.

a. **Treatment** depends on the patient's symptoms and the gestational age of the fetus. Initially, intravenous hydration and analgesics should be administered. Associated infections are treated aggressively. In over one-half of cases, the stone passes spontaneously. Ultrasonography can be used to assess for obstruction, but the usefulness of this modality is hampered by the gravid uterus and presence of baseline ureteral dilatation during pregnancy. An intravenous pyelogram (IVP) should be obtained for patients with urinary infection that does not respond to 48 hours of antibiotic therapy, declining renal function, massive hydronephrosis on renal ultrasonography, or pain and dehydration from vomiting.

b. **Indications for intervention** include calculous pyelonephritis, persistent massive hydronephrosis with impairment of renal function, and protracted pain or sepsis. Approximately one-third of pregnant women with symptomatic stones will require cytoscopy, ureteral catheterization, percutaneous nephrostomy, basket extraction, or surgical exploration. In certain cases, a ureteral double-J stent, placed cystoscopically, may be warranted until surgery can be performed safely postpartum.

E. **Chronic renal disease**

1. **Renal disease** can be categorized as **mild,** with a serum creatinine less than 1.4 mg/100 mL; **moderate,** with serum creatinine greater than 1.4 to less than 2.5 mg/100 mL; or **severe,** with serum creatinine greater than 2.5 mg/100 mL. In general, as renal disease progresses and function declines, the ability to conceive and to sustain a viable pregnancy decreases. Normal pregnancy is rare when renal function decreases to the point at which pre-conception serum creatinine and BUN exceed 3 mg/dL and 30 mg/dL, respectively (1). Pregnant patients with preexisting renal disease are at risk for deterioration of renal function, or even renal failure, and superimposed preeclampsia. In general, patients with mild renal dysfunction experience little or no disease progression during pregnancy, whereas patients with moderate to severe renal insufficiency are at greatest risk for worsening of their renal function.

2. **Pregnancy outcome** is affected by chronic renal disease, which is associated with increases in perinatal mortality, preterm delivery, and intrauterine growth retardation (IUGR). Outcomes for patients with chronic renal disease depend on the degree of associated hypertension and renal insufficiency in each case. Patients with glomerulonephritis or nephrosclerosis appear to be at greatest risk for poor pregnancy outcomes.

3. **Antepartum management** should include the following, with hospitalization when clinically indicated:

   a. Early pregnancy diagnosis and accurate dating

   b. Baseline laboratory studies, preferably performed pre-conception, including blood pressure; serum creatinine; serum electrolytes; blood urea nitrogen; 24-hour urine collection for protein excretion; and creatinine clearance, urinalysis, and urine culture

   c. Biweekly antenatal visits until 28 to 32 weeks' gestation, then weekly visits until delivery

   d. Laboratory studies repeated each trimester and when clinically indicated

   e. Serial ultrasound examinations for assessment of fetal growth

   f. Nonstress test or contraction stress test, fetal movement charting, biophysical profiles, and lung maturity studies as necessary to monitor fetal well-being and maturity. Antepartum fetal assessment usually should begin at 28 weeks' gestation for patients with severe disease and as late as 34 weeks' gestation for patients with mild disease.

4. Pregnancy occurs in only 1 in 200 women on **dialysis therapy.** As in managing nonpregnant patients with renal impairment, control of blood pressure is important, especially during dialysis, when blood pressure can fluctuate widely. Volume shifts during dialysis should be avoided, and particular attention must be paid to electrolyte balance. Later in pregnancy, the fetal heart rate should be continuously moni-

tored during dialysis. Patients should receive longer and more frequent dialysis sessions to maintain a blood urea nitrogen level of less than 50 mg/dL. Chronic anemia is a common problem in hemodialysis patients. Hematocrit should be maintained above 25% with transfusions or erythropoietin therapy. Successful pregnancies also have been achieved with the use of chronic ambulatory peritoneal dialysis or chronic cycling peritoneal dialysis. Unfortunately, high rates of preterm deliveries and IUGR are associated with these procedures. Preterm delivery usually occurs because of preterm labor (PTL), fetal distress, abruptio placentae, or maternal bleeding. Antepartum testing should begin at 28 weeks' gestation.

5. After successful **renal transplantation,** approximately 1 in 50 women becomes pregnant. Complications more likely to occur in these pregnancies include infections, preeclampsia, premature delivery, premature rupture of membranes, premature onset of labor, and small-for-gestational-age babies. Women contemplating pregnancy who have undergone renal transplantation should meet the following criteria:
   a. Serum creatinine less than 2 mg/dL
   b. Minimal or well-controlled hypertension
   c. Minimal or no proteinuria
   d. Good general health
   e. Elapsed time from transplant surgery of 18 to 24 months
   f. No evidence of pelvicaliceal distention on recent IVP
   g. Response to immunosuppressive therapy that is stable at 15 mg/day or less of prednisone and 2 mg/kg/day or less of azathioprine. If the patient is on prednisone, screening for gestational diabetes should be undertaken at 20 to 24 weeks' gestation, and repeated at 28 to 32 weeks' gestation if the results of the initial screen are negative. Antepartum testing should begin by 28 weeks' gestation.

II. **Hepatic disease**
   A. **Intrahepatic cholestasis of pregnancy** is the most common liver disorder unique to pregnancy. The disease is uncommon in the United States and almost nonexistent among black Americans; it has been reported to affect up to 10% of pregnancies in Chile, however, and is also common in the Swedish population. Studies have shown an increased risk of preterm birth and fetal death for patients who develop intrahepatic cholestasis of pregnancy; therefore, antepartum fetal testing should be undertaken in all cases. Labor should be induced at term or when amniotic fluid studies indicate fetal lung maturity. A recurrence rate of approximately 70% has been reported.
      1. **Diagnosis.** All patients with cholestasis complain of pruritus. A mild jaundice may develop in approximately 50% of patients. The differential diagnosis includes viral hepatitis and gallbladder disease. Usually no fever, abdominal pain, or nausea or emesis is present; these symptoms frequently are seen in hepatitis and gallbladder disease.
      2. **Laboratory studies** are remarkable for the following findings:
         a. Elevation in serum alkaline phosphatase, usually by five- to tenfold over normal levels
         b. Elevated total bilirubin, but rarely greater than 5 mg/dL and mostly direct
         c. Marked increase in serum bile acids, deoxycholic and chenodeoxycholic acids up to tenfold above normal; elevated serum bile acids with pruritus is considered diagnostic
         d. Moderate elevation in serum aminotransferase activity.
      3. **Management** is aimed at reducing the intense pruritus. Cholestyramine at 8 to 16 g/day in three to four divided doses has been shown to be effective in reducing pruritus. Diphenhydramine may provide some relief. Dexamethasone at a dose of 12 mg/day for 7 days has also been shown to be effective. In addition, phenobarbital at a dose of 90 mg at bedtime has been used when patients cannot tolerate cholestyramine. Because cholestyramine results in decreased absorption of vitamin K, patients

may develop a prolonged prothrombin time. The prothrombin time should be checked weekly, and parenteral vitamin K administered at a daily dose of 10 mg until the prothrombin time normalizes. After delivery, symptoms usually abate within 2 days. Oral contraceptives should be prescribed cautiously for these patients because cholestasis may develop postpartum when oral contraceptives are taken.

B. Chronic liver disease
  1. **Chronic active hepatitis** responds to immunosuppression with corticosteroids, often augmented with azathioprine. Pregnancy is associated with an increased incidence of stillbirths, prematurity, and preeclampsia. Immunosuppression must be continued during pregnancy to avoid relapse.
  2. Women with **cirrhosis** are likely to be infertile. Pregnancy in these patients is associated with high perinatal loss as well as a poor maternal prognosis. Fatal hemorrhage may occur from esophageal varices complicating portal venous hypertension.
  3. **Budd-Chiari syndrome** (venoocclusive disease of the hepatic veins of the liver) occasionally may occur in pregnancy, presumably as a result of the coagulopathy associated with pregnancy. The disease is marked by abdominal pain and the abrupt onset of ascites and hepatomegaly.

III. Gastrointestinal disease
  A. Gastroenteritis. Viral enteritis of the Norwalk variety is the most common infectious disease of the gastrointestinal tract during pregnancy. Patients usually present with nausea, cramping, vomiting, and diarrhea, which may be associated with headache and myalgia. Low-grade fever is common. The symptoms last 48 to 72 hours, and treatment is supportive. The mainstay of treatment is to keep patients well hydrated and to place the bowel at rest. In cases of severe dehydration, i.v. hydration is indicated.
  B. Nausea and emesis are common in pregnancy; true **hyperemesis gravidarum,** however, affects only a small number of pregnant women; the incidence is 0.5 to 10.0 per 1,000 pregnancies. The peak occurrence is between the eighth and twelfth weeks of pregnancy.
  1. The **etiology** of hyperemesis gravidarum is unknown but is believed to be multifactorial and to involve hormonal, neurological, metabolic, toxic, and psychosocial factors. Laboratory findings reveal ketonuria, increased urine specific gravity, elevated hematocrit and BUN, hyponatremia, hypokalemia, hypochloremia, and metabolic alkalosis. Serum beta human chorionic gonadotropin tests and thyroid function tests usually are performed because molar pregnancy and hyperthyroidism can cause hyperemesis. Some patients with hyperemesis gravidarum have transient hyperthyroidism. The treatment of the transient hyperthyroidism is controversial because in most cases both resolve spontaneously as pregnancy continues.
  2. **Treatment** should be tailored to the specific presentation and severity of symptoms. Initial therapy usually includes oral hydration with oral or rectal antiemetics. If ketonuria does not respond and emesis continues, intravenous hydration (Ringer's solution with 5% dextrose) with i.m. or i.v. antiemetics can be used. Patients may need to be hospitalized for intractable emesis, correction of any laboratory abnormalities, and hypovolemia. Nutrition consultation always should be obtained. In severe cases in which prolonged i.v. hydration is anticipated, parenteral nutrition and vitamins may be instituted for alimentation, including thiamine supplementation (100 mg q.d. i.m. or i.v.) to avoid Wernicke's encephalopathy. Oral feedings should be introduced slowly when tolerated, starting with clear liquids and progressing to a bland solid diet consisting of small, carbohydrate-rich meals. Greasy and spicy foods should be avoided. When pregnant women do not respond to the medical and supportive care of obstetric and nursing professionals, a psychiatric consultation is advisable.
  3. If possible, **medications** should be avoided during the first ten weeks of pregnancy, during the organogenesis phase. The risk-benefit ratio of medical therapy, however, should be determined on a case-by-case basis. Medicines commonly administered include the following (the FDA has approved no drugs for treatment of nausea and vomiting in pregnancy):

     a. Pyridoxine (vitamin B_6), 25 mg t.i.d. p.o.

     b. Phosphorylated carbohydrate solution (Emetrol), 15 to 30 mL every 15 minutes for a maximum of five doses

     c. Doxylamine (Unisom), one-half to one tablet q.h.s., p.o.

     d. Metoclopramide (Reglan), 5 to 10 mg t.i.d., p.o. or i.v.

     e. Promethazine (Phenergan), 12.5 to 25.0 mg b.i.d. to q.i.d., p.o., p.r., i.v., or i.m.

     f. Prochlorperazine (Compazine), 5 to 10 mg t.i.d., p.o., i.v., or p.r.

     g. Chlorpromazine (Thorazine), 10 to 25 mg q.i.d., p.o.; 25 to 50 mg t.i.d. to q.i.d., i.m. or i.v.; 50 to 100 mg b.i.d. to t.i.d., p.r.

     h. Ondansetron (Zofran), 4 to 8 mg every 8 hours (case reports only)

     i. Methylprednisolone (Medrol), 48 mg q.d., p.o. for 3 days, followed by a taper (uncontrolled studies) (2)

C. Gastroesophageal reflux disease, with resultant heartburn, is very common during pregnancy. Pathophysiology primarily involves a decrease in lower esophageal sphincter tone and increased pressure on the stomach from the gravid uterus. Heartburn usually is more severe after meals and is aggravated by recumbent positions. Treatment of reflux during pregnancy consists primarily of neutralizing or decreasing the acid material that is being regurgitated. Measures that may provide symptomatic relief include elevation of the head of the bed, small meals, reduced-fat diet, refraining from ingesting meals or liquids other than water within 3 hours of bedtime, smoking cessation, and avoidance of chocolate and caffeine. For relatively severe symptoms, treatment with over-the-counter antacids after meals and at bedtime, or the use of sucralfate (1 g t.i.d.) should be considered. In refractory cases, the H_2 blocker cimetidine should be administered, 400 mg after the evening meal (3).

D. Peptic ulcer disease (PUD) during pregnancy is uncommon. Patients who develop PUD before pregnancy frequently experience fewer symptoms during pregnancy and may even become totally asymptomatic.

     1. The **treatment** of PUD during pregnancy consists primarily of taking antacids after meals and at bedtime; avoiding fatty foods, caffeine, alcohol, chocolate, and nicotine, which may trigger gastric retention; avoiding aspirin and nonsteroidal antiinflammatory drugs (NSAIDs); and taking an H_2-receptor antagonist such as cimetidine or ranitidine. In addition, indomethacin should not be used as a tocolytic agent for patients with a history or current episode of PUD.

     2. Serious complications of PUD in pregnancy, although rare, may include hemorrhage, obstruction, and perforation. When serious complications occur, they should be managed as in the nonpregnant patient.

E. Inflammatory bowel disease (IBD). Because ulcerative colitis and Crohn's disease are predominantly diseases of young people, with peak incidence among people between 15 and 30 years for Crohn's disease and between 20 and 35 years for ulcerative colitis, these diseases frequently coincide with childbearing. General consensus has been reached that the fertility rate is unaffected in patients with ulcerative colitis; reduced fertility, however, has been associated with Crohn's disease, possibly because of the chronic pelvic adhesions that result from the inflammatory process.

     1. The **medical management** of IBD in pregnant patients is similar to its management in the nonpregnant patient, with a few exceptions. The mainstay of medical therapy for IBD is sulfasalazine and corticosteroids. Both of these agents have been shown to be safe in pregnancy. Because sulfasalazine may interfere with the absorption of folate, supplemental folate should be prescribed to pregnant women. Metronidazole, ciprofloxacin, azathioprine, and 6-mercaptopurine also are used occasionally in the medical therapy of IBD; their use in pregnancy, however, is limited. Decisions about the use of these agents during pregnancy should be made on a case-by-case basis.

     2. Surgical intervention is indicated for complications of severe IBD. Intestinal obstruction, perforation, unremitting gastrointestinal bleeding, and the development of toxic megacolon may necessitate surgical intervention. Indications for surgery in pregnant patients should be the same as in nonpregnant patients.

3. The method of **delivery** chosen may be affected by IBD. Vaginal delivery can be undertaken by most women with IBD unless severe perineal disease exists. Crohn's disease may be associated with perineal scarring, which may make vaginal delivery difficult. Active perineal disease or perineal fistula may prevent adequate healing of an episiotomy. If a patient has been on prolonged corticosteroid therapy, stress-dose i.v. corticosteroids should be administered during labor. When cesarean section is necessary, difficult intraperitoneal adhesions should be expected and preparations made accordingly.

F. **Acute pancreatitis** is an uncommon cause of abdominal pain in pregnancy, with an incidence of approximately 1 in 1,000 to 1 in 3,800 pregnancies.

1. The **clinical presentation** is similar to that of the nonpregnant patient: midepigastric or left upper quadrant pain with radiation to the back, nausea, vomiting, ileus, and low-grade fever. Whereas gallstones and alcohol abuse are equal contributors to the development of the disease in nonpregnant women, during pregnancy cholelithiasis is the most common cause. Elevation of serum amylase, lipase, or both remains the key finding in the diagnosis of acute pancreatitis. Ultrasonographic evaluation may be of limited use in the evaluation of acute pancreatitis in pregnant patients because of the enlarged uterus and overlying bowel gas.

2. **Management** is principally conservative and aimed at resting the gastrointestinal tract and preventing complications. Most cases of gallstone pancreatitis can be managed successfully with conservative treatment during pregnancy, with elective cholecystectomy postpartum if indicated; cholecystectomy, however, can be performed safely during pregnancy after the first trimester, if necessary. Exploratory laparotomy is indicated in women with unrelenting disease and in those in whom the diagnosis is uncertain. It is important to withhold definitive biliary surgery until the acute inflammation has subsided. Endoscopic retrograde cholangiopancreatography with shielding of the maternal abdomen can be performed under intravenous sedation during the second trimester, followed by definitive cholecystectomy postpartum.

G. **Acute appendicitis** is discussed in Chap.15, Acute Abdomen in Pregnancy, sec. I.

IV. **Systemic lupus erythematosus (SLE).** Women with SLE have a normal fertility rate; a higher rate of fetal loss and preterm birth, however, are associated with SLE. In general, women with SLE should not be advised against pregnancy. Patients should be counseled, however, that the optimal time to conceive is during remission. Exceptions are patients with major end-organ damage such as lupus nephropathy, which may be associated with disease exacerbation leading to permanent organ damage, or patients who are taking cyclophosphamide or warfarin.

A. **Diagnosis** of SLE is based on the history, physical examination, and laboratory tests. SLE should be ruled out in any pregnant women with a photosensitivity rash, polyarthritis, undiagnosed proteinuria, false-positive syphilis test finding, or multiple spontaneous abortions. Abnormal laboratory test findings include: positive antinuclear antibody (ANA) test results (greater than 1 in 160; patterns common in SLE include homogeneous, nucleolar, and rim-only); elevated anti–SS-A (anti-Ro) and anti–SS-B (anti-La) antibody titers; decreased C3 and C4 complement levels; positive lupus anticoagulant (LAC) (dilute activated partial thromboplastin time test, kaolin clotting time test, or a Russell viper venom time test); and elevated anticardiolipin (ACL) antibody or anti-dsDNA antibody titers.

B. **Effect of pregnancy on SLE.** Although the subject is controversial, pregnancy does not appear to alter the long-term prognosis of most SLE patients. Transient lupus flares are more likely during pregnancy than at other times. The risk of a flare increases threefold during the first trimester, one- to twofold during the second trimester, and sixfold postpartum.

C. **Effect of SLE on pregnancy.** Patients with SLE have a 15% risk of spontaneous abortion, a 25% risk of IUGR, and an increased risk of prematurity and cesarean section necessitated by fetal distress.

D. Management of SLE in pregnancy
   1. **First trimester.** Initial laboratory studies include complete blood cell count (CBC), creatinine, 24-hour urine collection for protein and creatinine, microscopic urinalysis, and a "lupus package" (ANA, anti-Ro and anti-La antibody titers, C3 and C4 complement levels, LAC, and ACL antibody and anti-dsDNA antibody titers). An obstetric ultrasound image should be obtained to determine gestational age and viability of the fetus. The patient should be seen at least every month.
   2. **Second trimester.** Repeated laboratory studies include CBC, creatinine, 24-hour urine collection for protein and creatinine, microscopic urinalysis, and serologic tests (C3 and C4 and anti-dsDNA). Obstetric ultrasound should be obtained every 4 weeks after 20 weeks' gestation to monitor fetal growth. In anti-Ro–positive women, careful fetal heart auscultation or serial fetal echocardiograms should begin at 16 to 18 weeks' gestation to assess for possible heart block.
   3. **Third trimester.** The patients should be seen at least every other week. After 26 weeks' gestation, fetal testing may be initiated, with weekly nonstress test and weekly biophysical profiles. In addition to serial growth ultrasounds and fetal echocardiograms, fetal Doppler studies should be obtained to identify abnormal uteroplacental flow in pregnant women with lupus who are at highest risk, such as those with antiphospholipid antibodies, who are anti-Ro and anti-La, or whose obstetric histories are poor. Treatment with dexamethasone or betamethasone should be initiated in patients with poor fetal test results or worsening maternal disease in anticipation of a preterm delivery.
   4. **Lupus flare.** Most lupus flares are diagnosed clinically when patients present with fever, malaise, and lymphadenopathy. Laboratory findings include low C3 or C4 complement levels, active sediment on urine microscopic analysis [defined by more than 20 red blood cells (RBCs) or white blood cells (WBCs) per high-power field or cellular casts], elevation in anti-dsDNA antibody titer, and hemolytic anemia, thrombocytopenia, and leukopenia. Distinguishing a lupus flare from preeclampsia in pregnant patients can be challenging. Factors that are unhelpful include the quantity of proteinuria and the presence of thrombocytopenia, hypertension, or hyperuricemia. Factors that are useful include complement levels, which are low in lupus flare and usually normal in preeclampsia; serum hepatic transferase levels, which are generally normal in a lupus flare but may be elevated in preeclampsia; the presence of RBC casts in the urine, which implies active lupus; and very gradual onset of proteinuria, which is characteristic of lupus flare. In preeclampsia, proteinuria appears abruptly or increases from baseline values rapidly.
E. Treatment
   1. **Corticosteroids** can be used during a lupus flare. The usual dose is 60 mg of prednisone daily for 2 to 3 weeks, which then is tapered to the lowest dose that controls symptoms. Patients should be monitored closely for the development of glucose intolerance, hypertension, and preeclampsia, which have been associated with corticosteroid therapy.
   2. Because of the fetal risks associated with **NSAID** use, pregnant women with SLE usually are switched from NSAID to aspirin. In the Hopkins Lupus Pregnancy Center, low-dose, or "baby," aspirin (81 mg) is administered to women with prior fetal loss and antiphospholipid antibodies, or who have a history of pregnancy-induced hypertension or preeclampsia (4).
   3. **Immunosuppressive agents** are used only for patients with significant organ involvement. When immunosuppressive agents are used, azathioprine is preferred. Cyclophosphamide should not be used if possible.
   4. **Antihypertensives** are used in many SLE patients before pregnancy or initiated during pregnancy when hypertension develops. Antihypertensive agents with good safety records in pregnancy include methyldopa, hydralazine, and labetalol (see Chap. 8, sec. **II.E.5**).

5. In pregnant women, **antiphospholipid antibodies** (lupus anticoagulant or anticardiolipin) are associated with fetal death, particularly in the second trimester. Studies have shown that low-dose aspirin and moderate-dose heparin improve fetal outcome. A regimen of aspirin, 81 mg/day, and 40 mg/day of prednisone for 10 weeks, tapered over 4 weeks to a maintenance dose of 5 mg/day, has shown good results (5). In addition, therapy with low-dose aspirin, heparin, or warfarin usually is recommended for approximately 3 months after delivery for women with a history of thromboembolic events.

F. **Neonatal lupus erythematosus** (NLE) consists of a transient rash in the newborn period, complete heart block, or both. NLE is a rare syndrome that occurs in a minority of infants delivered only to mothers who have antibodies to the Ro (SS-A) or La (SS-B) antigens, or both. Among infants at risk for NLE, fewer than 25% develop cutaneous NLE, while fewer than 3% develop congenital heart block. In subsequent pregnancies, the risk for recurrence of cutaneous NLE is about 25% and the risk for heart block is between 8% and 16%. Although no treatment has been proven to be effective in reversing fetal heart block *in utero*, the administration of dexamethasone to the mother may be beneficial in preventing extension of the fetal myocarditis (6).

References

1. Davison JM. The physiology of the renal tract in pregnancy. *Clin Obstet Gynecol* 1985;28(2):257–265.
2. Safari HR, Alsulyman OM, Gherman RB, Goodwin TM. Experience with oral methylprednisolone in the treatment of refractory hyperemesis gravidarum. *Am J Obstet Gynecol* 1998;178(5):1054–1058.
3. Baron TH, Richter JE. Gastroesophageal reflux disease in pregnancy. *Gastroenterol Clin North Am* 1992;21(4):777–791.
4. Petri M, Howard D, Repke J, Goldman DW. The Hopkins Lupus Pregnancy Center: 1987–1991 update. *Am J Reprod Immunol* 1992;28(3–4):188–191.
5. Silveira LH, Hubble CL, Jara LJ, et al. Prevention of anticardiolipin antibody-related pregnancy losses with predisone and aspirine. *Am J Med* 1992;93(4):403–411.
6. Rider LG, Buyon JP, Rutledge J, Sherry DD. Treatment of neonatal lupus: case report and review of the literature. *J Rheumatol* 1993;20(7):1208–1211.

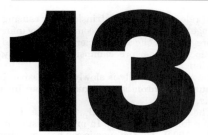

Hematologic Diseases of Pregnancy

Rebecca Kolp and
Karin Blakemore

I. **Anemia** is a decrease in hemoglobin to less than 11 g/dL. Anemias can be classified based on mean corpuscular volume (MCV). If the MCV is less than 80 fL, the anemia is microcytic; the two most common causes of microcytic anemia are iron deficiency and thalassemia. If the MCV is 80 to 100 fL, the anemia is normocytic; a relatively common cause of normocytic anemia is sickle cell disease. If the MCV is greater than 100 fL, the anemia is considered macrocytic; the most common causes of macrocytic anemia are vitamin B_{12} and folate deficiencies.

A. **Physiologic anemia of pregnancy.** During pregnancy, plasma volume increases 25% to 60%, starting at 6 weeks' gestation and continuing through delivery. The red blood cell (RBC) mass increases only 10% to 20% in pregnancy. The disproportionate increase in plasma volume compared with RBC mass results in blood dilution, and hematocrit falls 3% to 5%.

B. **Iron deficiency anemia**

1. **Diagnosis** is based on the slow onset of symptoms such as fatigue, headache, and malaise. In severe cases, pallor, glossitis, stomatitis, koilonychia (in which the outer surfaces of the nails are concave), pica, splenomegaly, shortness of breath, or advanced high-output heart failure can occur. Iron deficiency should be suspected when hemoglobin is less than 11 g/dL and MCV is less than 80 fL.

2. **Laboratory tests.** The basic workup for iron deficiency anemia includes a complete blood cell count (CBC), a peripheral blood smear (PBS), and a serum ferritin test. The diagnosis is confirmed if the PBS reveals small, hypochromic erythrocytes of various shapes and sizes; the MCV is less than 80 fL; the mean corpuscular hemoglobin concentration (MCHC) is less than 30 g/dL; and serum ferritin is less than 10 ng/mL. The serum ferritin level is more sensitive and specific than the serum transferrin level or serum iron studies.

3. **Treatment** consists of iron sulfate, 325 mg p.o. b.i.d. The hemoglobin level should increase within 6 to 8 weeks. For those patients who are unresponsive to or unable to tolerate oral therapy, i.v. administration of iron dextran is an alternative.

C. **Megaloblastic anemia** is characterized by macrocytosis (MCV greater than 100). Macrocytosis results from impaired DNA synthesis. Nuclear maturation is delayed, which affects erythrocytes, leukocytes, and thrombocytic cell lines, which in turn leads to anemia, leukopenia, hypersegmented polymorphonuclear leukocytes, and thrombocytopenia. Altered DNA synthesis stems from nutritional causes in 95% of cases. During pregnancy, folic acid requirements increase from 50 μg/day in the nonpregnant state to 800 to 1,000 μg/day. The etiology of folate deficiency is insufficient dietary intake of leafy green vegetables such as spinach. Women with sickle cell disease are at increased risk for folic acid deficiency. Phenytoin, nitrofurantoin, trimethoprim, and alcohol decrease absorption of folic acid. A less common cause of megaloblastic anemia is vitamin B_{12} deficiency, which often is a result of a long-term vegetarian diet or decreased intestinal absorption due to active tropical sprue, regional enteritis, or chronic giardiasis. Pernicious anemia, which results from decreased release of gastric intrinsic factor causing malabsorption of vitamin B_{12}, is age related and often accompanied by infertility, and thus it is rarely seen in pregnancy. Folic acid deficiency is associated with neural tube defects, abruptio placentae, preeclampsia, prematurity, and intrauterine growth retardation.

1. **Diagnosis.** Megaloblastic anemia usually is slowly progressive. It can manifest as bleeding caused by thrombocytopenia or as an infection resulting from leukopenia.

2. **Laboratory findings.** The basic workup for B_{12} or folate deficiency includes CBC, PBS, serum folate, serum B_{12}. In megaloblastic anemia, MCV usually is greater than 100 fL, but the anemia can be normochromic, with normal mean corpuscular hemoglobin (MCH) and MCHC findings. The PBS shows hypersegmented neutrophils and erythrocyte inclusions. The fasting serum folate level is less than 6 μg/L (normal is 6 to 12 μg/L). RBC folate is less than 165 μg/L. In severe disease, serum iron concentration and serum lactate dehydrogenase (LDH) increase. In vitamin B_{12} deficiency, the findings are all similar to those in folate deficiency. Serum B_{12} is less than 190 ng/L (normal is 190 to 950 ng/L), measured by radioimmunoassay. The Schilling test, which is used to assess causes of malabsorption of vitamin B_{12}, usually is postponed until postpartum.

3. **Treatment.** Folate deficiency anemia is treated with 1 mg t.i.d. of folic acid orally. Within 7 to 10 days, the white blood cell and platelet counts should return to normal. Hemoglobin will gradually increase to normal levels after several weeks of therapy. Vitamin B_{12} therapy entails 6 weekly injections of 1 mg of cyanocobalamin. Affected patients may require monthly injections for life. These women usually require treatment with iron and folate as well. Of note, replacement of folic acid can mask a vitamin B_{12} deficiency.

D. **Sickle cell disease** describes a group of hemoglobinopathies that may cause severe symptoms during pregnancy (Hb S, Hb SC, Hb SThal) or may be quiescent in an unaffected Hb AS carrier. Hb SS is the most common of these phenotypes, affecting 1 in 708 African-Americans. Affected patients may experience hemolytic anemia, recurrent pain crises, infection, and infarction of more than one organ system. A point mutation, which substitutes an amino acid at the sixth portion in the N-terminus of both beta chains of hemoglobin, causes sickling hemoglobinopathies. In Hb S, valine replaces glutamic acid. Hb S, when deoxygenated, forms insoluble tetramers inside RBCs. The tetramers cause the RBCs to become rigid and, consequently, trapped in the microvasculature, which in turn causes vascular obstruction, ischemia and infarction. This obstruction and infarction may lead to a vasoocclusive crisis, which may be associated with fever as well as skeletal, abdominal, and chest pain. Vasoocclusive crises may be initiated by an event such as hypoxia, acidosis, dehydration, infection, or psychologic stress. Patients with sickle cell disease are at increased risk during pregnancy because of its increased metabolic requirements, vascular stasis, and relatively hypercoagulable state.

1. **Diagnosis.** Episodes of pneumonia, pyelonephritis, cholecystitis, congestive heart failure, urinary tract infection, stroke, pulmonary embolism, retinal hemorrhage, preeclampsia, spontaneous abortion, preterm delivery, intrauterine growth retardation, and stillbirth are increased in patients with sickle cell disease. Most affected patients are diagnosed in childhood. Some present in pregnancy with previously undiagnosed symptoms such as a pain crisis or infection, splenic sequestration, or acute chest syndrome, which is associated with chest pain, pulmonary infiltrates, leukocytosis, and hypoxia. Jaundice may result from RBC destruction.

2. **Laboratory findings.** The anemia is normocytic, with a hemoglobin concentration of 5 to 8 g/dL and hematocrit less than 25%. An increased reticulocyte count is found. The peripheral blood smear may show sickle cells and target cells. Diagnosis is confirmed by hemoglobin electrophoresis. All African-American patients should be screened with a

hemoglobin electrophoresis to assess carrier status and offered genetic counseling that includes carrier state testing of the father of the baby. All patients at risk for offspring with hemoglobinopathies should receive counseling. Amniocentesis and chorionic villus sampling (CVS) allow in utero diagnosis by restriction fragment length polymorphism and polymerase chain reaction.

3. **Treatment.** Management consists of aggressive prenatal care. Folic acid supplements are administered to maintain erythropoiesis. Infections are treated aggressively with antibiotics. Severe anemia (hemoglobin less than 5 g/dL, hematocrit less than 15%, or reticulocyte count less than 3%) is treated with blood transfusion. Pain crises are managed with oxygen, hydration, and analgesia. Controversy surrounds prophylactic exchange transfusion. The advantages of transfusion are an increase in hemoglobin A, which improves oxygen-carrying capacity, and a decrease in hemoglobin S–carrying erythrocytes. Risks of transfusion are hepatitis, human immunodeficiency virus (HIV), transfusion reaction, and allosensitization. Treatment for acute chest syndrome is the same as for pain crises. Splenic sequestration is treated with blood transfusion. Medroxyprogesterone (Depo-Provera) injections have been found to decrease the number of pain crises.

4. **Pregnancy considerations.** An increase in prematurity, stillbirth, low-birth-weight babies, spontaneous abortion, and intrauterine growth retardation is associated with sickle cell disease. The degree of fetal assessment varies according to the clinical severity of the disease. In advanced cases, semiweekly nonstress tests and biophysical profiles should begin at 32 weeks' gestation, and serial obstetric ultrasound examinations used to help diagnose intrauterine growth retardation. After pregnancy, patients should practice early ambulation and wear pressure stockings to prevent thromboembolism. Intrauterine devices and combination oral contraceptives are contraindicated. Progestin-only pills, depomedroxyprogesterone, and subcutaneous implants or barrier devices are recommended for contraception.

5. **Heterozygous status** (Hb AS) is common (4% to 14%) in African-Americans. Women with sickle cell trait are at increased risk for renal infection, papillary necrosis, and, rarely, splenic infarction. There is no direct fetal compromise from maternal sickle cell trait. Patients should be screened for asymptomatic urinary tract infections, and the father of the baby should be assessed for carrier status. Genetic counseling should be offered to patients whose partners have Hb S, Hb C, Hb β-thal, and other potentially deleterious phenotypes.

E. **Thalassemias** are hematological disorders that result from limited synthesis of globin chains, which are the protein portions of hemoglobin. There are two types of thalassemias, α and β, which result from decreased production of structurally normal α- and β-globulin chains, respectively. Both diseases are transmitted as autosomal recessive traits. Table 13-1 shows the various types of α- and β-thalassemias and the degree of anemia they cause, based on the number of affected globin chains.

1. **Diagnosis.** Thalassemia is generally a microcytic hypochromic anemia, characterized by an MCV of less than 80 fL.

2. **Laboratory findings.** Quantitative hemoglobin electrophoresis is required for diagnosis. In homozygous β-thalassemia, Hb F is increased by 20% to 60% and may be as high as 90%. In heterozygous β-thalassemia, Hb A_2 is increased slightly more than 3.5%, and a slight increase in Hb F may be present. Low MCV and elevated Hb A_2 are the criteria for diagnosing carriers. Hb H has unique electrophoretic properties. Asymptomatic carriers of α-thalassemia often have normal amounts of Hb A_2 and Hb F, so pedigree studies are often helpful during workup of these patients. If a pregnant woman is found to be a carrier for thalassemia, her partner is offered testing. DNA-based prenatal testing using amnio-

Table 13-1. α- and β-Thalassemias and the degree of anemia they cause

	Number of α chains in α-thalassemia			
	0	1	2	3
Diagnosis	Hydrops fetalis	Hemoglobin H disease	Silent carrier	Silent carrier
Red blood cell morphology	Increased nucleated red blood cells	Microcytic Heinz bodies, targets	Microcytic slight hypochromia	Normal
Hemoglobin electrophonesis	Increased Barts hemoglobin	Increased hemoglobin H cells	Decreased hemoglobin A$_2$	Normal
Prognosis	Death	Moderate to severe anemia	Mild anemia	No symptoms

	Number of β chains in β-thalessemia	
	0	>0
Diagnosis	Cooley's anemia Homozygous	Heterozygous
Red blood cell morphology	Decreased mean corpuscular volume	Decreased mean corpuscular volume
	Target cells	Stippling
	Hypochromia	
	Nucleated red blood cells	
Hemoglobin electrophonesis	Increased hemoglobin F	Increased hemoglobin A$_2$
Prognosis	Death in childhood	Mild to moderate anemia

centesis or CVS is available if both members of the couple are found to be carriers.

3. **Treatment** varies depending on severity of disease. Asymptomatic α-thalassemia carriers and patients with heterozygous β-thalassemia require no special care other than counseling and information about the availability of prenatal diagnosis after assessment of the father. Homozygous disorders may necessitate multiple blood transfusions and splenectomy. All homozygous patients should receive supplemental folate to meet the requirements of accelerated erythropoiesis.

II. **Thrombocytopenia**
   A. **Maternal thrombocytopenia.** Thrombocytopenia is the most common hemostatic abnormality in pregnancy, occurring in 5% to 7% of all pregnancies, and defined as a maternal platelet count of less than 150,000/μL. The most common physical signs of thrombocytopenia are petechiae, easy bruising, epistaxis, gingival bleeding, menorrhagia, and hematuria. In general, the lower the platelet count, the higher the risk of bleeding. If the platelet count is more than 20,000/μL the obstetrician is usually anxious; the patient, however, seldom bleeds. The risk of spontaneous bleeding increases when the platelet count drops below 20,000/μL.

B. Fetal or neonatal thrombocytopenia. Normal fetal platelet counts range from 150,000 to 250,000/μL. The most serious complication of fetal thrombocytopenia is intracranial hemorrhage. In alloimmune thrombocytopenia, 20% of offspring suffer intracranial hemorrhages, half of which occur *in utero*. *In utero* intracranial hemorrhage does not appear to be a consequence of maternal idiopathic thrombocytopenic purpura (ITP), although intracranial hemorrhage can occur in the neonate. Neonatal thrombocytopenia is more common than fetal thrombocytopenia. Thrombocytopenia in neonates may be asymptomatic, or an affected neonate may present with petechiae or severe hemorrhage.

C. Causes of maternal thrombocytopenia in pregnancy. A prospective study of 15,471 healthy pregnant women who delivered during a 7-year period showed that 6.6% of the mothers had a platelet count of less than 150,000/μL. Of these patients, 73.6% had gestational or incidental thrombocytopenia. Twenty-one percent had thrombocytopenia associated with hypertensive disorders of pregnancy, and 3.8% had immunologic thrombocytopenia [systemic lupus erythematosus (SLE), ITP]. Other rare causes of maternal thrombocytopenia are disseminated intravascular coagulopathy, thrombotic thrombocytopenia purpura, hemolytic uremic syndrome, HIV, and drug-induced thrombocytopenia.

D. Gestational thrombocytopenia. Gestational thrombocytopenia is a benign condition in both the mother and the fetus. It occurs in 4% to 8% of normal pregnancies and accounts for 75% of maternal thrombocytopenia in pregnancy. Other names for the disorder include incidental, asymptomatic, and pregnancy-associated thrombocytopenia.

   1. Diagnosis. Gestational thrombocytopenia is usually a diagnosis of exclusion, for which the following three cardinal criteria are present: a mild degree of thrombocytopenia (70,000 to 150,000/μL); no prior history of thrombocytopenia; and no bleeding symptoms. The pathophysiology is unknown but may be related to increased physiological platelet turnover. Gestational thrombocytopenia usually resolves by 6 weeks postpartum and can recur in subsequent pregnancies.

   2. Management. A careful history to exclude other causes of thrombocytopenia is usually the first step. The history should be followed by a review of earlier platelet counts (at the time of first visit). In gestational thrombocytopenia, *no intervention is necessary*. About 2% of the offspring of mothers with gestational thrombocytopenia have mild thrombocytopenia (higher than 50,000/μL). None have severe thrombocytopenia.

E. Preeclampsia or HELLP (hemolysis, elevated liver enzymes, and low platelet) syndrome is the most common pathologic cause of maternal thrombocytopenia in obstetric practice (about 25%). HELLP syndrome results from increased platelet turnover related to either endothelial damage or consumptive coagulopathy. Symptoms spontaneously resolve by the fifth postpartum day. Around 0.4% of the offspring of mothers with HELLP syndrome will have mild thrombocytopenia, mainly as a consequence of prematurity.

F. Idiopathic thrombocytopenic purpura. ITP is the most common autoimmune disease in pregnancy, occurring in 1 to 2 per 1,000 pregnancies. ITP affects women of reproductive age more frequently than men (at a ratio of 3 to 1). Although it is idiopathic, the pathophysiology is reasonably well understood. Lymphocytes produce antiplatelet antibodies directed at platelet surface glycoproteins. The IgG-coated platelets are cleared by splenic macrophages, resulting in thrombocytopenia. The course of ITP is unaffected by pregnancy. Placental transfer of the IgG platelet antibodies can result in fetal or neonatal thrombocytopenia.

   1. Diagnosis. Isolated maternal thrombocytopenia should be present without splenomegaly or lymphadenopathy. Secondary causes of maternal thrombocytopenia should be ruled out (e.g., preeclampsia, HIV, SLE, drugs). Maternal bone marrow examination should reveal normal or increased megakaryocytes. Detection of platelet-associated antibodies is consistent with but not diagnostic of ITP. These antibodies are detected in 30% of patients with nonimmune thrombocytopenia. The absence of platelet-associated IgG makes the diagnosis less likely. Currently, no diagnostic test exists for ITP.

2. **Antenatal management.** Patients with ITP may experience greater morbidity from the therapeutic regimens used to treat the disease than from the disease itself. The goal of therapy is to raise the platelet count to a safe level (more than 20,000 to 30,000/μL) with the least amount of intervention possible; it is important to remember that a safe platelet count is not necessarily a normal platelet count.

   a. **Medical therapy.** When the maternal platelet count falls below 20,000 to 30,000/μL, corticosteroids are the treatment of choice. It is reasonable to begin with prednisone (1 to 2 mg/kg/day) and start tapering the dosage after the platelet count rises to a safe level. Steroids are thought to suppress antibody production, inhibit sequestration of antibody-coated platelets, and interfere with the interaction between platelets and antibody. Seventy percent to 90% of patients respond to therapy within 3 weeks. High doses of i.v. γ-globulin (0.4 g/kg/day for 5 days for 3 weeks or 1 g/kg/day for 1 week) are recommended for patients who do not respond to steroids. The proposed mechanism of action of γ-globulin is prolongation of the clearance time of IgG-coated platelets by the maternal reticuloendothelial system. Eighty percent of patients treated with γ-globulins respond within days, and remission lasts 3 weeks. The main drawback of γ-globulin treatment is its cost.

   b. **Splenectomy** rarely is indicated during pregnancy. Immunosuppressive therapy and danazol are contraindicated in pregnancy. Although the efficacy of these treatments in increasing maternal platelet count is well established, they are potentially harmful to the developing fetus.

G. **Idiopathic thrombocytopenic purpura and fetal or neonatal thrombocytopenia.** Ten percent to 15% of pregnancies complicated by ITP are associated with severe fetal or neonatal thrombocytopenia (fewer than 50,000/μL). It is now generally accepted that no correlation exists between fetal and maternal platelet counts. Unfortunately, no association between the presence or the level of maternal platelet antibodies and fetal platelet count exists either. This lack of association may be explained by the fact that fetal thrombocytopenia is related not only to the level of antiplatelet antibodies but also to the fetal reticuloendothelial system and the fetal capacity to produce platelets.

   1. **Incidence and complications.** The neonate platelet count declines after delivery, reaching a nadir at 48 to 72 hours of life. As many as 34% of neonates with severe thrombocytopenia experience hemorrhagic sequelae. The incidence of intracranial hemorrhage in one series was 1.5%, with a perinatal mortality of 0.5%. Unlike alloimmune thrombocytopenia, in which 50% of the intracranial hemorrhages occur *in utero*, no convincing evidence definitely attributes in utero intracranial hemorrhage to classic maternal ITP. Notification of a pediatrician for close monitoring of the neonatal platelet count is very important in preventing the devastating sequela of neonatal intracranial hemorrhage.

   2. **Intrapartum management.** For years, the assumption that a fetus with a platelet count lower than 50,000/μL is at significant risk for intrapartum hemorrhage, coupled with the belief that cesarean delivery is less traumatic than spontaneous vaginal delivery has led to the recommendation of cesarean delivery for severe fetal thrombocytopenia (less than 50,000/μL) in ITP patients. Traditionally, fetal scalp platelet counts were obtained after cervical dilatation. Although this technique is relatively simple, falsely low platelet counts (less than 50,000/μL), which can lead to inappropriate cesarean section, may be found in as many as 50% of cases. More recently, cordocentesis has been used to determine fetal platelet count before the onset of labor.

   3. **Is fetal thrombocytopenia secondary to chronic idiopathic thrombocytopenic purpura associated with intrapartum fetal hemorrhage?** A review of English-language publications on ITP in pregnancy between 1980 and 1990 found that all perinatal deaths and intracranial hemorrhages were reported in articles that did not specify either the timing of

the infant platelet count measurement or the timing of the hemorrhage. Therefore, the temporal relationship between these events and delivery was unclear. After reviewing more than 1,000 pregnancies complicated by ITP, a study found no documented cases of fetal hemorrhage, either before or during labor, and estimated that the risk of fetal hemorrhage intrapartum is less than 0.5%. The risk of fetal loss as a result of cordocentesis, however, is 1% to 2%, and prolonged fetal bradycardia leads to emergency cesarean delivery in a similar percentage of cases. The risk of the procedure and the morbidity associated with emergency cesarean delivery far outweigh the risk of intrapartum fetal hemorrhage; therefore, cordocentesis does not appear to be medically justified for fetal platelet determination in ITP.

4. **Delivery.** The assumed benefit of cesarean delivery for women with ITP has been refuted. In a retrospective study, the incidence of neonatal intracranial hemorrhage was lower with vaginal delivery than with cesarean (0.5% versus 2.0%). The investigators, however, did not subdivide the cesarean section group into elective surgeries and surgeries performed after the onset of labor. Other reviews found equal morbidity in thrombocytopenic neonates after cesarean or vaginal delivery. Without evidence that cesarean section provides fetal benefit, we believe that spontaneous vaginal delivery without antepartum or intrapartum fetal platelet determination to be the most reasonable method of delivery for pregnant patients with ITP.

5. **Surgery for patients with thrombocytopenia.** Excessive surgical bleeding when the platelet count is more than 50,000/μL. Platelet transfusions may be used to elevate the platelet count to this level before surgery. Platelet transfusions are available both as platelet concentrates and as platelet-enriched plasma. It is reasonable to expect an increase in platelet count of 1,000 to 10,000/μL for each unit of platelets transfused. In the presence of clotting abnormalities, epidural anesthesia can increase the risk of intraspinal epidermal hematoma. When the platelet count is more than 100,000/μL, the patient is a candidate for regional anesthesia. If the platelet count is between 50,000 to 100,000/μL, however, obtaining a bleeding time might help to determine whether the patient is at increased risk for an intraspinal bleed. If the bleeding time is prolonged, epidural anesthesia should be avoided.

B. **Alloimmune thrombocytopenia.** Alloimmune thrombocytopenia is the result of a platelet antigen incompatibility analogous to the incompatibility that causes Rh hemolytic disease. In alloimmune thrombocytopenia, the fetal platelets carry a specific paternal antigen that is not present on maternal platelets. These fetal platelets can traverse the placenta and isoimmunize the mother. The maternal antiplatelet antibodies cross to the fetal circulation and cause fetal thrombocytopenia. In contrast to ITP, the maternal platelet count is normal in alloimmune thrombocytopenia; it is only the fetus who becomes thrombocytopenic.

1. **Clinical implications.** Unlike Rh disease, 20% to 59% of diagnosed alloimmune thrombocytopenia occur in primiparous women. In about 80% of cases, the thrombocytopenia is a benign, self-limited condition of 1 to 16 weeks' duration postpartum. Twenty percent of offspring, however, can suffer intracranial hemorrhage, often *in utero*. Ninety percent of subsequent pregnancies are similarly or more severely affected. If alloimmune thrombocytopenia has complicated a previous pregnancy, appropriate prenatal management needs determination of fetal platelet genotype so that antenatal therapy can be initiated if the fetus is at risk.

Five known human platelet alloantigen systems have been described: PLA I, Bak, Br, Ko, and Pen (Table 13-2). The platelet antigens are localized to specific membrane glycoprotein complexes. All are implicated in alloimmune thrombocytopenia. These human antigen systems are biallelic and are inherited as autosomal codominant traits. Parental genotypes

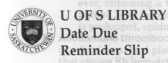

Table 13-2. Platelet-specific antigen systems

System	Antigens	Original name	Glycoprotein	Amino acid position	Gene frequency	Populations studied
HPA-1	HPA-1a	Zw a, Pl A1	III a	Leucine 33	0.8900	U.S. (W)
					0.9200	U.S. (AA)
					0.9950	Korean
					0.8460	Dutch
	HPA-1b	Zw b, Pl A2	III a	Proline 33	0.1100	U.S. (W)
					0.0800	U.S. (AA)
					0.0050	Korean
					0.1540	Dutch
HPA-2	HPA-2a	Ko b	I ba	Threonine 145	0.0900	U.S. (W)
					0.1800	U.S. (AA)
					0.1300	Korean
					0.0660	Dutch
	HPA-2b	Ko a, Sib a	I ba	Methionine 145	0.9200	U.S. (W)
					0.8200	U.S. (AA)
					0.8700	Korean
					0.0660	Dutch
HPA-3	HPA-3a	Bak a, Lek a	II b	Isoleucine 843	0.6700	U.S. (W)
					0.6300	U.S. (AA)
					0.6700	Korean
					0.5550	Dutch
	HPA-3b	Bak b, Lek b	II b	Serine 843	0.3300	U.S. (W)
					0.3700	U.S. (AA)
					0.3300	Korean
					0.4450	Dutch

HPA	Allele	Antigen	CD	Amino acid	Position	Frequency	Population
HPA-4	HPA-4a	Pen a, Yuk b	II b	Arginine	143	1.0000	U.S. (W)
						1.0000	U.S. (AA)
						1.0000	Korean
						0.9917	Japanese
						1.0000	Dutch
	HPA-4b	Pen b, Yuk a	III a	Glutamine	143	0.0000	U.S. (W)
						0.0000	U.S. (AA)
						0.0000	Korean
						0.0083	Japanese
						0.0000	Dutch
HPA-5	HPA-5a	Br b, Zav b	I a	Glutamic acid	505	0.1100	U.S. (W)
						0.2100	U.S. (AA)
						0.0300	Korean
						0.9800	Dutch
	HPA-5b	Br a, Zav a, Hc a	I a	Lysine	505	0.8900	U.S. (W)
						0.7900	U.S. (AA)
						0.9700	Korean
						0.0920	Dutch

AA, African-American; W, white.

determine whether the fetus is potentially at risk. When a father is homozygous for a platelet antigen allele lacking in the mother, all of the offspring will be at risk for alloimmune thrombocytopenia. When the father is heterozygous, however, only half of the fetuses will be at risk. When the father is heterozygous, amniocentesis can be performed to determine whether the fetus is at risk; the fetal platelet genotype is determined using the reverse dot blot technique.

3. **Management.** Optimal management of pregnant patients at risk for alloimmune thrombocytopenia is still evolving. Therapeutic options include maternal administration of steroids alone, maternal administration of i.v. γ-globulin with or without steroids, and fetal platelet transfusions using washed, irradiated maternal platelets. Fetal blood sampling is often performed at 20 to 22 weeks' gestation, after which a therapeutic protocol is initiated based on the initial fetal platelet count. If a previous offspring was severely affected, therapy is initiated as early as 12 weeks for subsequent pregnancies. More than one fetal blood sampling procedure may be necessary, particularly if failure of maternal therapy necessitates serial fetal platelet transfusions. At the time of labor, fetal blood sampling can be offered to the patient before allowing vaginal delivery. The patient also might choose an elective cesarean section near term.

III. **Leukemia.** Acute leukemia rarely complicates pregnancy. The incidence is less than 1 in 75,000 pregnant patients. When leukemia is present in pregnant patients, the need for chemotherapy, radiotherapy, and supportive care including blood products is important. Remission occurs in 50% to 80% of patients, but the median survival is 1 year.

A. **Diagnosis.** Signs of leukemia are sternal tenderness, skin pallor, petechiae, ecchymoses, and hepatosplenomegaly. Symptoms of leukemia include fatigue, severe infection, and easy bleeding.

B. **Laboratory findings.** In acute lymphocytic leukemia (ALL), acute myelogenous leukemia (AML), or monocytic leukemia, a normocytic and normochromic anemia and thrombocytopenia are found on CBC. Patients with ALL have a normal or increased white blood cell count. In acute nonlymphocytic leukemia (ANLL), most patients present with significantly increased white blood cell counts. The diagnosis is confirmed by bone marrow biopsy.

C. **Pregnancy effects.** No evidence exists that pregnancy has a deleterious course on leukemia. Exposure to single drugs or combination drug therapy during the second and third trimesters is not associated with gross fetal abnormalities in most cases. Regarding chemotherapy during the first trimester, studies are more inconclusive. Patients should be informed carefully about the chemotherapeutic agents that are to be used throughout the pregnancy and their possible effects on the fetus. In early pregnancy, it is important to consider the mother's disease state and her desires before recommending termination of the pregnancy. Patients with ALL should not consider future pregnancies for several years. Patients with ANLL should be advised against future pregnancy at any time because of the poor prognosis of this disease.

IV. **Thromboembolic disease** of some kind occurs in 7 in 10,000 women during pregnancy. The risk of thromboembolic disease is five times greater in pregnancy than in the nonpregnant state. Pregnancy is a hypercoagulable state. Eighty percent of antepartum deep venous thromboses (DVT) occur in the third trimester, when venous stasis is at its maximum. A significant number of embolic events occur after delivery. The risk of DVT after cesarean section increases three- to sixteenfold. DVT risk increases with age, multiparity, prior thrombotic event, and prior cesarean section.

A. A **superficial thrombus** is the most common type of thromboembolism in pregnancy. These clots rarely travel to the deep venous system. Superficial thromboses are treated with elevation of the affected body part and application of moist heat. No antiinflammatory agents or anticoagulants are administered for benign disease. Monitor patients carefully to be sure that the clot does not enter the deep venous system.

B. Deep venous thrombosis occurs in the lower extremities or in pelvic veins. Leg edema, calf pain, and Homan's sign are not particularly helpful in diagnosis because these effects can all be produced by many other causes, and DVT can be present without any of them.

    1. Diagnosis by Doppler ultrasound. In femoral veins, the interpretation of Doppler ultrasound may be difficult if the uterus is in the supine position, compressing the inferior vena cava especially after 20 weeks' gestation.

    2. Treatment. Intravenous heparin is the treatment for DVT. The appropriate dose is a 70 to 100 U/kg i.v. bolus of heparin, followed by infusion of 15 to 20 U/kg/hour, targeting a partial thromboplastin time (PTT) of 1.5 to 2.5 × control. After initial inpatient treatment, therapy should be continued with heparin injections, every 12 hours s.q., until 6 to 12 weeks postpartum, to maintain a PTT of 1.5 to 2.0 × control. Warfarin (Coumadin) is contraindicated in pregnancy because it has been found that one-third of fetuses exposed to Coumadin late in pregnancy developed central nervous system injuries or ophthalmologic abnormalities. Pregnant women exposed to Coumadin in the first trimester had a high incidence of teratogenicity and miscarriage. In studies of patients on long-term anticoagulation therapy with Coumadin, it has been shown when Coumadin was replaced with heparin at 6 weeks' gestation, none of the patients delivered children with warfarin embryopathy. Low-molecular-weight heparins have not been well studied in pregnancy and should be discontinued for at least 24 hours before placement of an epidural anesthetic.

C. Pulmonary embolism. The symptoms of dyspnea, pleuritic chest pain, tachypnea, and tachycardia typically used to diagnose pulmonary embolism (PE) are all common in pregnancy for other reasons. Normal arterial blood gas values also are altered in pregnancy, so these findings must be interpreted using pregnancy-adjusted normal valves.

    1. Diagnostic studies. The chest radiograph is important, because it helps rule out other disease processes and enhances interpretation of the ventilation-perfusion ($\dot{V}/\dot{Q}$) scan. A $\dot{V}/\dot{Q}$ scan is necessary for diagnosing pulmonary embolism. A normal scan finding is accurate in excluding PE. Most fetal exposure to radiation occurs when radioactive tracers are excreted in the maternal bladder. Therefore, fetal radiation exposure can be limited by prompt voiding after the $\dot{V}/\dot{Q}$ procedure. High-probability results on scans may be accepted as an indication for treatment because the reliability of $\dot{V}/\dot{Q}$ testing is 90%. Intermediate- or low-probability results require arteriography for further evaluation before a commitment to long-term anticoagulation is made. Pulmonary angiography poses fewer radiation risks to the fetus than might be expected. Spiral computed tomography of the chest may also be considered for the diagnosis of PE. This modality has not yet been used extensively in pregnancy.

    2. Treatment is the same as that for DVT. As with DVT, the most important time to provide prophylaxis for future pregnancies is during the 6-week postpartum period. No difference exists between the prophylaxis provided to a patient who experienced a DVT and that provided to a patient who experienced a PE. Prophylactic therapy consists of heparin, 5,000 units s.q. every 12 hours.

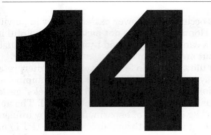

Perinatal Infections

Stephanie Cogan and
Karin Blakemore

I. **Human immunodeficiency virus**
   A. **Epidemiology**
      1. In the United States, approximately 89% of women with acquired immunodeficiency syndrome (AIDS) are of childbearing age. Among women of childbearing age, 1.7 in 1,000 were infected with the human immunodeficiency virus (HIV) in 1992. This prevalence is expected to increase as more HIV-infected women survive for longer periods of time and in a healthier state. During the 4 years between 1989 and 1992, between 1,000 and 2,000 infants per year were born with the HIV infection. Furthermore, during the years 1990 to 1994, the rate of progression of HIV to AIDS in women was three times that of men.
      2. The World Health Organization has predicted that by the year 2000, 3 million women worldwide will have died of AIDS, 10 million children will have acquired perinatal HIV infection, and 10 million children will have been orphaned because of HIV. Cases of AIDS will increase to 12 to 18 million worldwide, with as many as 30 to 40 million HIV-infected persons.
      3. The pregnancy rate in HIV-infected women is approximately 6%. More HIV-infected women now than in the past are choosing to continue unplanned pregnancies; others are choosing to conceive.
      4. Among patients at the gynecology and obstetrics clinic at Johns Hopkins Hospital who agree to be tested, the rate of HIV infection is approximately 5%. Of those patients whose test results indicated HIV infection, 3% had no known risk factors.
      5. Approximately 50% of women elect to continue an unplanned pregnancy despite a known HIV infection.
      6. It is impossible to predict accurately who is or is not infected. Of infected women screened in Baltimore, 44% had no identifiable risk factors except heterosexual intercourse, frequently with a partner not previously known to have had a risk factor.
   B. **Perinatal HIV transmission**
      1. The rate of **perinatal transmission** of HIV is approximately 25% to 30%. Studies have demonstrated that 20% to 30% of perinatal transmission is transplacental, or true vertical transmission. The remaining 70% to 80% of cases of perinatal infection occur intrapartum. Rarely in the United States does transmission occur postnatally.
      2. **Evidence of transplacental transmission** has been supported by research demonstrating placental cellular HIV growth *in vitro*, HIV isolation from amniotic fluid, and HIV isolation from fetal blood obtained at cordocentesis. Specimens for these research protocols were obtained at the time of pregnancy termination. Data showing the bimodal distribution of infection and identifying identical DNA serotypes in neonates and mothers support this hypothesis.
      3. **Intrapartum transmission** leads to later disease manifestation in infants than transplacental transmission, mimicking the pattern of hepatitis B virus (HBV) infection. Especially important to note is that infants infected

intrapartum who eventually show positive HIV test results initially had negative results on HIV polymerase chain reaction (PCR), p24 antigen, and HIV IgA and IgM tests, indicating an absence of established infection, at birth. Also, an increase in infection has been observed in presenting fetuses of twin pregnancies, compared with the second twins of the same pregnancies. This increase is postulated to result from the first twin's longer exposure to maternal genital secretions.

4. **Postnatal infection** is believed to result from breast-feeding. In areas where a stable supply of clean water is available, breast-feeding of infants by HIV-infected mothers is discouraged. If clean water is unavailable, consider that whereas breast-feeding is associated with a 14% risk of HIV transmission to infants, the risk of fatal diarrhea illness is higher than 14% in some areas.

5. Strategies for the **prevention** of vertical transmission include decreasing the viral load either chemically or immunologically.

C. **Diagnosis** of HIV infection is based on an initial screening test for specific antibodies using enzyme-linked immunosorbent assay (ELISA), usually against core (p24) or envelope (gp44) antigens. Positive results are confirmed by Western blot. The median time between infection with HIV and the development of AIDS is 10 years, with a range of a few months to 12 or more years. Clinical progression of the disease is monitored by evaluating the CD4 cell count. It is the absolute CD4 count that has been used as a criterion for therapeutic intervention.

1. **At CD4 counts of more than 500/mL,** patients usually do not demonstrate clinical evidence of immunosuppression.

2. **At CD4 counts of 200 to 500/mL,** patients are more likely to develop symptoms and require intervention than at higher counts.

3. **At CD4 counts of less than 200/mL,** or at higher CD4 counts accompanied by thrush or unexplained fever with temperatures higher than 37.8°C for 2 or more weeks, patients are at increased risk for developing complicated disease.

D. **Management.** HIV testing should be offered to all pregnant women as part of routine prenatal care. Patients with HIV are at increased risk for infections such as tuberculosis, bacterial pneumonia, and *Pneumocystis carinii* pneumonia (PCP). The care of the HIV-infected obstetric patient parallels that of the nonpregnant HIV-infected patient and entails monitoring of immune status, prophylaxis for opportunistic infections, and assessment for the presence of sexually transmitted diseases. Prophylaxis against PCP with aerosolized pentamidine appears to be safe in pregnancy. Trimethoprim-sulfamethoxazole double strength (TMP/SMX-DS, Bactrim) also appears to be safe.

1. **Strategies to prevent perinatal transmission**
   a. Decrease fetal viral exposure by preventing chorioamnionitis and decreasing the duration of labor. Decrease fetal contact with infected fluids by preventing ruptured membranes and mucosal inflammation.
   b. The AIDS Clinical Trial Group 076 trial results reveal a decrease in the perinatal HIV transmission rate from 25% to 8%. It is therefore vitally important to offer this regimen to all infected women. To successfully follow the regimen, women require knowledge of their HIV infection status, early access to prenatal care, and appropriate counseling about HIV and available treatment or prophylaxis. Counseling for patients who undergo HIV testing is now mandatory throughout the state of Maryland.

2. The decision to initiate **zidovudine (Retrovir, AZT) therapy** is based on gestational age and the woman's health. If maternal CD4 count is greater than 500 mL and the viral load by RNA PCR is less than 10,000 copies/mL, zidovudine is initiated at 14 to 16 weeks' gestation; the dosage is 600 mg/day in two or three divided doses.
   a. A large viral load with a low CD4 count mandates recommendation of maternally indicated triple-drug therapy, after a discussion of the known and postulated fetal effects of the therapy. Triple-drug therapy

is associated with the disappearance of detectable viral burden and an increase in CD4 count. The therapy consists of two nucleoside analogues and a protease inhibitor, usually zidovudine, 600 mg/day in two to three equal doses; lamivudine (3TC), 150 mg b.i.d.; and nelfinavir, 750 mg t.i.d.

b. As always in medicine, individualization of therapy is required. Patients who do not comply with multiple medication schedules need a simplified regimen. Patients who have been exposed to other combination therapies may need to continue the regimens they currently use. Cross-drug toxicity, drug resistance, and patient allergies also must be considered.

c. Patients who have demonstrated zidovudine failure are advised to take zidovudine for fetal indications because of a lack of data showing a decreased perinatal HIV transmission rate with other regimens.

3. **Other medications** recommended are TMP/SMX-DS, once daily, for prophylaxis against PCP when the CD4 count is less than 200/mL; and azithromycin, 1,200 mg once a week for *Mycobacterium avium-intracellulare* complex prophylaxis when the CD4 count is less than 100/mL. Routine vaccinations include the hepatitis B series, one-time pneumonia vaccine, and an annual influenza vaccine. Rubella vaccine may be administered as indicated. Severely immunocompromised patients may fail to mount an appropriate response to vaccines.

4. **Serum monitoring** of HIV-infected patients includes obtaining a baseline CD4 count, HIV RNA PCR quantification, complete blood cell count, and liver function tests, and assessing cytomegalovirus (CMV) and toxoplasmosis status.

a. If the CMV results are positive, an ophthalmologic evaluation is indicated. The risk of CMV retinitis is present in patients with a CD4 count of less than 50/mL; for these patients, consideration of oral ganciclovir, 1 g/day, is warranted. Toxoplasmosis in HIV-infected patients usually is caused by reactivation of latent disease (seroprevalence 10% to 30%). Toxoplasmosis risk is increased in patients with a CD4 count of less than 100/mL (75% cases occur with a CD4 count less than 50/mL); prophylaxis is provided by TMP/SMX-DS.

b. After a patient is started on antiretroviral therapy, a set of laboratory studies should be repeated on a monthly basis for 2 months, then every 2 or 3 months, depending on her response to therapy. An effective therapeutic regimen should result in an increase in the patient's CD4 count and a substantial decrease in her viral load; undetectable viral levels are to be expected on the triple-drug regimen. Failure to achieve such an effect warrants a reevaluation of the regimen. Keep in mind that a patient who demonstrates an increase in CD4 count or a decrease in viral load should nonetheless continue to receive prophylactic care consistent with her initial levels. Do not discontinue opportunistic infection prophylaxis; the risk of these illnesses remains high because, it is postulated, less effective CD4 cells form after HIV infection.

c. Patients requiring zidovudine only for fetal indications must be informed of the possibility that their risk of drug resistance will increase with one-drug therapy. Pregnancy is the only indication for such therapy at this point. Our practice is to administer zidovudine in combination with 3TC in an attempt to decrease the risk of resistant viral serotypes.

5. **Drug toxicity**

a. Nausea and vomiting can occur with any of the commonly prescribed medications, which is a significant problem when the patient is pregnant. Because of possible drug interactions, a careful review of all medications is indicated, especially when systemic antifungal agents are in use.

b. Indinavir (U.S. FDA Pregnancy Category C), a frequently prescribed protease inhibitor, carries the risk of nephrolithiasis and requires the consumption of an additional liter of fluid daily. The list of drugs that interact with indinavir is extensive. Because indinavir crosses the placenta, and because the fetus cannot voluntarily increase its oral intake, nelfinavir (U.S. FDA Pregnancy Category B) is the preferred protease inhibitor in pregnancy. The major additional side effect of nelfinavir is diarrhea. Nelfinavir also has an extensive drug interaction list.

    c. Lamivudine (U.S. FDA Pregnancy Category C) has minimal toxicity. TMP-SMX DS, however, has been shown to increase 3TC's serum levels; the therapeutic implications of this interaction are unclear.

    d. Zidovudine (U.S. FDA Pregnancy Category B) is associated with a high incidence of reversible gastrointestinal intolerance, insomnia, myalgias, asthenia, malaise, and headaches. Furthermore, bone marrow suppression resulting in anemia, neutropenia, or both can be quite severe, occasionally necessitating the use of erythropoietin (U.S. FDA Pregnancy Category C), blood transfusions, or a change in nucleoside analogues. Macrocytosis usually is observed during the first month of zidovudine therapy and has been used as a measure of patient compliance. A mild, reversible elevation of transaminases can be seen during zidovudine therapy. Fingernail discoloration usually appears at 2 to 6 weeks of therapy. Rarely, nucleoside analogue therapy is associated with severe effects of lactic acidosis or severe hepatomegaly with steatosis, either of which warrants discontinuation of therapy.

  6. Intrapartum therapy consists of the administration of zidovudine, 2 mg/kg i.v. during the first hour of labor, then 1 mg/kg/hour throughout the remainder of labor. Again, avoid artificial rupture of membranes, fetal scalp electrode, and intrauterine pressure catheter.

  7. Special management concerns include safe sex, postpartum contraception, premature rupture of membranes (PROM), patient compliance, and psychosocial issues.

  8. Fetal therapy. Maternal administration of AZT is associated with a decrease in the risk of vertical transmission by as much as two-thirds for mildly symptomatic pregnant women with HIV and CD4 of more than 200/mL who receive antepartum as well as intrapartum zidovudine therapy. Maternal zidovudine therapy is followed by 6 weeks of neonatal zidovudine therapy. No evidence of teratogenicity has been shown with zidovudine therapy. The regimen in most recent trials is as follows:

    a. Antepartum, 100 mg p.o. five times per day or 200 mg t.i.d.

    b. Intrapartum, 2 mg/kg body weight i.v. over 1 hour, then 1 mg/kg/hour until delivery

    c. Neonatal, 2 mg/kg p.o. every 6 hours for 6 weeks.

II. Cytomegalovirus

  A. Epidemiology. Cytomegalovirus is the most common congenital infection, affecting 0.4% to 2.3% of neonates. Cytomegalovirus is ubiquitous. The virus has been isolated from saliva, cervical secretions, semen, and urine; it can also be contracted by exposure to infected breast milk or blood products. Therefore, transmission can occur from mother to child both *in utero* and postpartum.

  B. Clinical manifestations

    1. Maternal infection. In immunocompetent adults, CMV infection is silent; symptoms appear in only 1% to 5% of cases. These symptoms include low-grade fever, malaise, arthralgias, and, occasionally, a pharyngitis with lymphadenopathy. Mothers determined to be seronegative for CMV before conception or early in gestation have a 1% risk of acquiring the infection during pregnancy, with a 30% to 40% rate of fetal transmission. Fewer than 15% of infected fetuses subsequently develop significant sequelae. A higher risk of sequelae is seen in fetuses infected earlier in gestation than in those infected later. Preterm neonates are at greatest risk of infection. Fetal infection also can result from recurrent or reactivation of maternal CMV infection. Previously acquired immunity, however, confers a decreased likelihood of clinically apparent disease, because partial protection to the fetus is provided by maternal antibodies. Of note, acquired immunity does not impede transmission, but evidently prevents the serious sequelae that develop with primary maternal infection.

2. **Fetal infection.** Manifestations of CMV in the neonate may include focal or generalized organ involvement. Common clinical findings in fetal infection include petechiae, hepatosplenomegaly, jaundice, microcephaly with periventricular calcifications, intrauterine growth retardation (IUGR), premature delivery, inguinal hernias in boys, and chorioretinitis. Nonimmune hydrops has also been reported.

3. **Morbidity and mortality.** Approximately one-third of neonates with symptomatic infection die from severe disease, generally with cerebral involvement. Infants who survive symptomatic CMV are at high risk for significant developmental and neurologic problems. Sixty percent to 70% of these survivors suffer hearing loss; visual disturbances, motor impairments, language and learning disabilities, and mental retardation are also common.

C. **Diagnosis**

1. **Maternal infection** currently can be detected reliably only by documenting maternal seroconversion using serial IgGs during pregnancy. If seropositivity is identified at least several months before conception, symptomatic fetal infection is unlikely. In practice, however, this testing does not occur. Most primary infections are clinically silent, so the majority are undiagnosed. Screening of asymptomatic pregnant women for seroconversion is not recommended because distinguishing primary from secondary CMV infection is frequently difficult using CMV serology. The CMV IgM test result is positive in only 75% of primary infections and in 10% of secondary infections.

2. **Fetal infection.** Antenatal ultrasonography may enable the detection of the fetal anomalies that characterize CMV infection: IUGR, intracranial calcifications, hepatic calcifications, and hydrops fetalis.

D. **Management.** Even if acute maternal infection can be demonstrated, effective *in utero* therapy for the fetus does not exist. Given the difficulty in distinguishing primary from secondary maternal CMV infection, counseling patients about pregnancy termination is problematic because most infected fetuses do not suffer serious sequelae and because only 10% of infected fetuses have a serious handicap. Women should be informed that their preterm infants may not have acquired sufficient transplacental maternal IgG to confer adequate immunity, so breast-feeding in women with active infection is discouraged.

III. **Varicella-zoster virus**

A. **Epidemiology.** The incidence of varicella in pregnancy is approximately 0.7 in 1,000 pregnancies. Of fetuses born to mothers who had active disease during the first 20 weeks of pregnancy, 20% to 40% are infected. The risk of congenital malformation after fetal exposure to primary maternal varicella before 20 weeks' gestation is estimated to be approximately 5%. Herpes zoster is also uncommon in women of childbearing age; the majority of infants delivered to affected women exhibit normal development with no adverse sequelae.

1. The major mode of **transmission** is respiratory, although direct contact with vesicular or pustular lesions also may result in disease. Nearly all persons are infected before adulthood, 90% before the age of 10.

2. Varicella outbreaks occur most frequently during the winter and spring. The incubation period is 13 to 17 days. Infectivity is greatest 24 to 48 hours before the onset of rash and lasts 3 to 4 days into the rash. The virus is rarely isolated from crusted lesions.

B. **Clinical manifestations**

1. **Maternal infection.** The risk of varicella pneumonia appears to increase in pregnancy starting several days after the onset of the characteristic rash. Early signs and symptoms of varicella pneumonia should be managed aggressively.

2. **Fetal infection** with varicella-zoster virus occasionally can lead to one of three major outcomes: intrauterine infection, which rarely causes congenital abnormalities; postnatal disease, ranging from typical varicella

with a benign course to fatal disseminated infection; and shingles, appearing months or years after birth. The sequelae of congenital varicella syndrome have been attributed to the occurrence of infection during the first and second trimesters. Those afflicted may exhibit a variety of abnormalities, including cutaneous scars, limb-reduction anomalies, malformed digits, muscle atrophy, IUGR, cataracts, chorioretinitis, microphthalmia, cortical atrophy, microcephaly, and psychomotor retardation. The precise risk of this syndrome is not known with certainty, although it is estimated to be quite small.

3. **Morbidity and mortality.** When varicella pneumonia occurs during pregnancy, maternal mortality may reach 40% in the absence of specific antiviral therapy. If maternal infection occurs within 5 days of delivery, hematogenous transplacental viral transfer may cause significant infant morbidity, incurring infant mortality rates between 10% and 30%. Sufficient antibody transfer to protect the fetus apparently requires at least 5 days after the onset of the maternal rash. Women who develop chickenpox, especially near term, should be observed for and educated about signs and symptoms of labor; they should receive tocolytic therapy if labor begins before day 5 of the maternal infection. Neonatal therapy is also important when a mother develops signs of chickenpox less than 3 days postpartum.

C. **Diagnosis**
1. **Clinical.** The diagnosis of acute varicella-zoster in the mother usually can be established by the characteristic clinical cutaneous manifestations.
2. **Laboratory studies.** Confirmation of the diagnosis may be obtained by examining scrapings of lesions, which may reveal multinucleated giant cells. For rapid diagnosis, varicella-zoster antigen may be demonstrated in exfoliated cells from lesions by immunofluorescent antibody staining.
3. **Ultrasonography.** Detailed ultrasound examination is probably the best means for assessing a fetus for major limb and growth disturbances. Other abnormalities that have been detected before 20 weeks' gestation include polyhydramnios, hydrops fetalis, multiple hyperechogenic foci within the liver, limb defects, and hydrocephaly. Although ultrasound can be offered in pregnancies with maternal varicella, it is less likely to be helpful in cases of zoster. Zoster (shingles) is extremely rare in pregnancy, and the majority of infants born to affected mothers have been found to be normal at delivery.

D. **Management**
1. **Exposure of a previously uninfected woman during pregnancy**
   a. Obtain an IgG titer within 24 to 48 hours of a patient's exposure to a person with noncrusted lesions. The presence of IgG within a few days of exposure reflects prior immunity. Absence of IgG indicates susceptibility.
   b. **Varicella-zoster immune globulin.** To prevent maternal infection in patients without IgG, some advocate administering varicella-zoster immune globulin (VZIG) within 96 to 144 hours of exposure, in a dosage of 125 U/10 kg up to a maximum of 625 units, or 5 vials, i.m. Because it is difficult to obtain serologic test results in a timely manner, and because no proven benefit results from administration of VZIG for the prevention of maternal-fetal transmission or the amelioration of maternal symptoms and sequelae, many experts do not currently recommend VZIG administration for pregnant women who have been exposed to varicella-zoster. If the mother becomes infected, a risk of fetal infection and the potential sequelae exists. Women with varicella early in gestation, however, may be advised to continue with the pregnancy because the risk of congenital varicella is very small.
2. **Maternal illness.** Generally, the disease in pregnant patients is similar to that in nonpregnant patients and requires no specific treatment. In the event that maternal clinical illness develops, the patient should receive

supportive care with fluids and analgesics. If evidence of pneumonia or disseminated disease appears, the patient should be admitted to the hospital for treatment with intravenous acyclovir. A decrease in maternal morbidity and mortality occurs in pregnant women afflicted with varicella pneumonia who are treated with acyclovir during the last two trimesters, and the drug is safe to use at this stage of gestation. The dosage of acyclovir is 10 to 15 mg/kg i.v. every 8 hours for 7 days, or 800 mg p.o. five times/day.

IV. **Parvovirus B19**
  A. **Epidemiology.** Thirty percent to 60% of adults have acquired immunity to human parvovirus B19. Most clinical infections, which are known as erythema infectiosum or fifth disease, occur in school-aged children. The virus is spread primarily by the respiratory route. Outbreaks usually occur in the midwinter to spring months.
  B. **Clinical manifestations**
    1. **Adult infection.** Sixty percent of infected adults have acute joint swelling, usually with symmetrical involvement of peripheral joints; the arthritis may be severe and chronic.
    2. **Fetal infection.** Maternal infection with human parvovirus B19 in pregnancy, whether symptomatic or asymptomatic, usually culminates in the delivery of an asymptomatic, normal infant. It is estimated that only one-third of maternal infections are associated with fetal infection. On transplacental transfer of the virus, however, fetal red blood cell (RBC) precursors may be infected. Infection of fetal RBC precursors can result in fetal anemia, which, if severe, leads to nonimmune hydrops fetalis. The likelihood of severe fetal disease is increased if maternal infection occurs during the first 18 weeks of pregnancy, but the risk of hydrops fetalis persists even when infection occurs in the late third trimester. Fetal IgM production after 18 weeks' gestation probably contributes to the resolution of infection in fetuses who survive. Fetal demise may occur at any stage of pregnancy.
    3. **Morbidity and mortality.** Although no direct evidence that parvovirus B19 causes congenital anomalies exists, there is some evidence that possible damage to the fetal myocardium results from infection. Studies suggest that the overall risk of fetal death after maternal parvovirus B19 infection is lower than 20%, and the risk is lower still in the second half of pregnancy.
  C. **Diagnosis** can be suspected on epidemiologic grounds in the event of an ongoing regional outbreak or if a family member is known to be affected. Children, the most common transmitters of parvovirus B19 infection, present with systemic symptoms such as fever, malaise, myalgia, and headaches as well as with a confluent, indurated facial rash that imparts the characteristic "slapped-cheek" appearance of fifth disease. The rash spreads over 1 to 2 days to other areas, especially exposed surfaces such as the arms and legs, and is usually macular and reticular in appearance. A pregnant woman who has been exposed to a child with fifth disease, presents with an unexplained morbilliform or purpuric rash, or has a known history of chronic hemolytic anemia and who presents with an aplastic crisis should be evaluated for parvovirus B19 virus by obtaining IgG and IgM titers. For patients who have had contact with an infected individual, titers should be drawn 10 days after exposure. Parvovirus B19 IgM appears 3 days after the onset of illness, peaks in 30 to 60 days, and may persist for 4 months. Parvovirus B19 IgG usually is detected by the seventh day of illness and persists for years; IgM therefore indicates a relatively recent infection.
  D. **Management.** No specific antiviral therapy exists for parvovirus B19.
    1. **Prophylaxis.** Empiric i.v. γ-globulin should be administered to immunocompromised patients with known exposure to parvovirus B19 and should be used for treatment of women in aplastic crisis with viremia.
    2. **Detection of fetal hydrops.** When maternal infection is identified, serial sonography should be performed. Although hydrops fetalis usually develops within 6 weeks of maternal infection, it can appear as late as 10

weeks after maternal infection. Weekly or biweekly ultrasound scans can be performed.

3. **Intrauterine blood transfusion** has been demonstrated to be a successful therapeutic measure for correcting the fetal anemia in fetal hydrops. Single or serial intrauterine transfusions may be undertaken.

V. Rubella

A. **Epidemiology.** Despite immunization programs in the United States, up to 20% of adults remain susceptible to rubella infections. The number of reported cases of congenital rubella syndrome, however, is now at an all-time low. **Transmission** results from direct contact with the nasopharyngeal secretions of an infected person. The most contagious period is the few days before the onset of a maculopapular rash. The disease is communicable, however, 1 week before and for 4 days after the onset of the rash. The incubation period ranges from 14 to 21 days.

B. **Clinical manifestations**
1. **Maternal infection.** Rubella is symptomatic in 50% to 70% of those who contract the virus. The illness is usually mild, with a maculopapular rash that generally persists for 3 days; generalized lymphadenopathy (especially postauricular and occipital), which may precede the rash; and transient arthritis.
2. **Fetal infection** after maternal viremia leads to a state of chronic infection. At least 50% of all fetuses are infected when primary maternal rubella infection occurs in the first trimester, which, as the period of organogenesis, is when the greatest risk of congenital anomalies exists. Multiple organ system involvement can occur. Permanent congenital defects include ocular defects such as cataracts, microphthalmia, and glaucoma; heart abnormalities, especially patent ductus arteriosus, pulmonary artery stenosis, and atrioventricular septal defects; sensorineural deafness; occasional microcephaly; and encephalopathy that culminates in mental retardation or profound motor impairment. The severely affected infant may also present with purpura, "blueberry muffin skin," "salt and pepper skin," retinopathy, IUGR, and hepatosplenomegaly. Late manifestations include diabetes mellitus, thyroid disorders, and precocious puberty.
3. **Morbidity and mortality.** Rubella in pregnancy is no more severe than in nonpregnant women; no association with an increased complication rate exists. Spontaneous abortion occurs in 4% to 9%, and stillbirths in 2% to 3% of pregnancies complicated by maternal rubella. The overall mortality for infants with congenital rubella syndrome (CRS) is 5% to 35%. As many as 50% to 70% of infants infected *in utero* may appear to be unaffected at birth but subsequently exhibit symptoms of CRS.

C. **Diagnosis**
1. **Serology.** Diagnosis is usually confirmed by serology because viral isolation is technically difficult; moreover, results from tissue culture may take up to 6 weeks to obtain. Many rubella antibody detection methods exist, including hemagglutination inhibition and radioimmunoassay, and latex agglutination. Specimens should be obtained as soon as possible after exposure, 2 weeks later, and, if necessary, 4 weeks after exposure. Serum specimens from both acute and convalescent phases should be tested; a fourfold or greater increase in titer or seroconversion indicates acute infection. If the patient is seropositive on the first titer, no risk to the fetus is apparent. Primary rubella confers lifelong immunity; protection, however, may be incomplete. Antirubella IgM can be found in both primary and reinfection rubella. Reinfection rubella usually is subclinical, rarely is associated with viremia, and infrequently results in a congenitally infected infant.
2. **Fetal infection.** Prenatal diagnosis is made by identification of IgM in fetal blood obtained by direct puncture under ultrasound guidance at 22 weeks' gestation or later. The presence of rubella-specific IgM antibody in blood obtained by cordocentesis indicates congenital rubella infection because IgM does not cross the placenta.

D. **Management.** Pregnant women should undergo rubella serum evaluation as part of routine prenatal care. A clinical history of rubella is unreliable. If the patient is nonimmune, she should receive rubella vaccine after delivery, and contraception should be used for a minimum of 3 months after vaccination. A woman who is inadvertently vaccinated in early pregnancy should be informed that the possibility of teratogenicity is theoretical and that the data do not support the assumption that the pregnancy should be terminated. If a pregnant woman is exposed to rubella, immediate serologic evaluation is mandatory. If primary rubella is diagnosed, the mother should be informed about the implications of the infection for the fetus. If acute infection is diagnosed during the first trimester, the option of therapeutic abortion should be considered. In women who decline this option, immune globulin may be given because it may modify clinical rubella. Immune globulin, however, does not prevent infection or viremia and affords no protection to the fetus.

VI. **Hepatitis B virus**

A. **Epidemiology.** Hepatitis B virus (HBV) transmission in North America occurs most commonly via parenteral exposure or sexual contact. Mother-to-infant transmission appears to be a significant mode of maintenance and transmission of infection throughout the world. Possible sources of mother-to-infant infection are infected amniotic fluid and blood. Transmission most frequently appears to occur during delivery.

B. **Clinical manifestations**

1. **Maternal infection.** The prodrome of HBV often is associated with non-hepatic symptoms such as rash, arthralgias, myalgias, and occasional frank arthritis. Jaundice occurs in a minority of patients.

2. **Fetal infection.** Whether infection occurs *in utero* or intrapartum, the presence of hepatitis Be antigen (HBeAg) in a fetus carries an 85% to 90% likelihood of developing chronic HBV and the associated hepatic sequelae.

3. **Morbidity and mortality.** In otherwise healthy women, no worsening of the course of the disease appears to occur during pregnancy. No increases in neonatal sequelae such as malformation, IUGR, spontaneous abortions, or stillbirths appear to exist.

C. **Diagnosis** is confirmed by serology.

1. **HBsAg** appears in the blood before clinical symptoms develop and implies carrier or infective status.

2. **HBeAg** is found with progression of the infection and implies high infectivity.

3. The disappearance of HBeAg and the appearance of **anti-HBeAg** signals a decrease in infectivity.

4. **Anti-HBcAg** indicates partial convalescence.

5. **Anti-HBsAg** indicates immunity or recovery.

6. If a patient is tested during the period in which results for HBsAg are negative but those for anti-HBsAg are not yet positive, HBV can be identified by anti-HBsAg, especially IgM, in high titers.

7. The risk of fetal transmission is highest in mothers who are HBeAg-positive at the time of delivery.

D. **Management.** If significant gastrointestinal symptoms develop, including hepatitis and an inability to tolerate oral feeding, patients may require hospitalization for parenteral hydration. The U.S. Centers for Disease Control and Prevention (CDC) recommend universal screening of pregnant women for HBV. The need for identification of HBV-infected pregnant women is compelled by the availability of hepatitis B immune globulin (HBIG) and HBV vaccines, which interrupt vertical transmission of the virus in nearly 90% of cases. HBIG, 5 mL, is administered to adults for prophylaxis as soon as possible after exposure. HBIG, 0.5 mL should be administered to neonates within 12 hours of birth to infected mothers. HBIG administration should be followed by the standard three-dose immunization series, with HBV vaccinations at the time of HBIG administration. At Johns Hopkins Hospital, recombinant hepatitis B vaccine is offered to all pregnant women deemed to be at high risk for contracting hepatitis B, such as those with histories of sexually transmitted diseases or i.v. drug use.

VII. Hepatitis C virus

A. Epidemiology. Transmission of the hepatitis C virus (HCV) appears to be similar to that of the hepatitis B virus, with an increased incidence among intravenous drug abusers, recipients of blood transfusions, and patients with multiple sex partners. Parenteral transmission occurs via blood and body fluids. Fewer transmissions from blood product transfusions occur now than in the past, however, as a result of blood bank screening.

B. Clinical manifestations. Persistent disease is common after hepatitis C virus infection.

1. **Maternal infection.** HCV causes acute hepatitis in pregnancy but may go undetected if liver function tests and HCV antibody tests are not obtained. As long as several months may elapse before positive results are detected on HCV antibody tests. Importantly, a high percentage of adults suffer chronic hepatitis after an acute infection; it is reasonable to assume that the same disease pattern is likely for infants infected *in utero.*

2. **Fetal infection.** If transmission occurs transplacentally, the neonate is at increased risk for acute hepatitis and for probable chronic hepatitis or carrier status. To date, however, no teratogenic syndromes associated with this virus have been defined. Unfortunately, the *in utero* transmission rate of HCV appears to be approximately 50% greater than that of HBV.

C. Diagnosis. Serum analysis is performed to detect antibody to HCV; because it takes up to 1 year after infection to become seropositive, however, many cases may be missed by serum analysis.

D. Management. No known method to prevent vertical transmission exists. Prevention of maternal infection by blood product screening has been the mainstay of management. According to a CDC report published in 1990, the results of studies to evaluate immune serum globulin for prophylaxis have been equivocal. Until such data are conclusive, it is reasonable to administer immune globulin in a 0.5 mL dose to infants at risk for HCV infection immediately after birth and 4 weeks later, to prevent neonatal HCV acquisition from an anti-HCV antibody–positive mother.

VIII. Rubeola

A. Epidemiology. Rubeola (measles) is extremely rare in pregnancy because of low susceptibility in adults. The highest incidence is in children; a shift in age-specific attack rates to adolescents and young adults, however, has been observed in the United States. Epidemics tend to occur during the winter and spring months. Transmission of the rubeola virus occurs via direct or indirect contact with respiratory droplets, which can remain infectious even when suspended in the air for several hours. The incubation period is 10 days.

B. Clinical manifestations. The prodrome, which consists of fever, cough, conjunctivitis, and coryza lasts 1 to 2 days; Koplik spots (pinpoint, gray-white spots surrounded by erythema) appear on the second or third day; a rash emerges on the fourth day. Patients remain contagious from the onset of symptoms until 2 to 4 days after the appearance of the maculopapular and characteristic semiconfluent rash. Measles may be complicated by pneumonia, encephalitis, or otitis media. Pneumonia occurs in 3.5% to 50.0% of adults who contract measles, and superinfection may occur. Superinfection should be suspected in patients who demonstrate clinical deterioration, an elevated white blood cell count with a leftward shift, and a chest radiograph with evidence of multilobar infiltrates. Pneumonia during pregnancy is associated with preterm labor and delivery.

1. **Fetal infection.** No definitive evidence of a teratogenic influence exists. Infants born to infected mothers are at the greatest risk for morbidity and neonatal death.

2. **Morbidity and mortality.** Maternal measles can lead to preterm delivery or spontaneous abortion. Measles in premature newborns may be associated with a high mortality rate.

C. Diagnosis. Clinical diagnosis is considered to be reliable. When the patient's presentation is atypical, laboratory confirmation of the diagnosis may be required. Serologic studies using complement fixation, hemagglutination inhibition, or indirect fluorescent antibodies are commonly employed. A pregnant woman with measles should be evaluated for preterm labor, volume depletion, hypoxemia, and secondary bacterial pneumonitis. An increase in liver function test results is observed, but liver dysfunction has been determined to be insignificant thus far.

D. Management. Susceptible (nonimmune) women should receive a vaccine postpartum and should be advised to use contraception for 3 months after vaccination because the vaccine is of the live, attenuated viral variety. Susceptible pregnant women who are exposed to measles should receive immune globulin, 0.25 mg/kg. Measles is not a contraindication for breast-feeding. No specific therapy is available for measles other than supportive measures and close observation for the development of complications.

IX. Mycoplasma

A. Epidemiology. *Mycoplasma* species are common inhabitants of genital mucosal membranes. Colonization rates are higher among patients from lower socioeconomic groups. Women who do not employ barrier methods of contraception are more likely to be colonized, and the rate of colonization increases with the number of sexual partners.

B. Clinical manifestations

   1. Maternal infection. *Mycoplasma hominis* and *Ureaplasma urealyticum* are both commonly identified in women with bacterial vaginosis. The exact role of these organisms in reproduction has yet to be elucidated; they have been implicated, however, in infertility, habitual abortion, and low birth weight. An association between chorioamnionitis and mycoplasmal infection has also been reported.

   2. Fetal infection. Studies have failed to demonstrate that adverse pregnancy outcomes are associated with maternal infection. In neonates with meningitis, however, *Mycoplasma* species were the organisms most frequently isolated from cerebrospinal fluid.

C. Diagnosis is confirmed by cervical culture.

D. Management. *M. hominis* infections respond to clindamycin. Infections by *Ureaplasma* species usually respond to tetracyclines and to erythromycin, which is the antibiotic employed during pregnancy. No immunizations to prevent colonization exist. Moreover, mycoplasmic organisms are so widespread that a large component of sexually active adults will eventually become colonized.

X. Toxoplasmosis

A. Epidemiology. In the United States, the incidence of acute toxoplasmosis infection during pregnancy has been estimated to be 0.2% to 1.0%. Congenital toxoplasmosis in the United States has an incidence estimated at 1 in 1,000 to 1 in 8,000 live births. Transmission occurs primarily via ingestion of undercooked or raw meat containing cysts or of water or food contaminated by the feces of infected cats. Transmission may also occur transplacentally when a woman acquires infection during pregnancy.

B. Clinical manifestations

   1. Maternal infection. Specific symptoms that signal acute toxoplasmosis infection are uncommon in pregnant women. Infection in pregnant women is often subclinical or may be mistaken for influenza. A mononucleosis-like syndrome, with fatigue, malaise, cervical lymphadenopathy, and atypical lymphocytosis, may occur. *Toxoplasma gondii* can infect virtually all cells and tissues. It is during the spreading phase of parasitemia that placental infection and subsequent fetal infection occur. The overall risk of fetal infection resulting from acute maternal infection is estimated to be 30% to 40%, and the rate of transmission increases with gestational age.

   2. Fetal infection. During the first trimester, the rate of toxoplasmosis transmission is approximately 15%. Although the transmission rate itself is lower earlier in gestation, fetal morbidity and mortality rates are higher with early transmission. The rate of second trimester transmission is approximately 30%, and the rate of third trimester transmission is 60%. The most severely affected neonates are those in whom

Table 14-1. Interpretation of *Toxoplasma* serologies

	IgM	IgG	Interpretation
(i)	+	–	Possible acute infection; IgG titers should be reassessed in several weeks
(ii)	+	+	Possible acute infection
(iii)	–	+	Remote infection
(iv)	–	–	Susceptible, uninfected

IgM titres may remain elevated for up to 1 year.

transmission occurred during the first trimester, and first trimester transmission is associated with possible intrauterine fetal demise and spontaneous abortion. Although infected neonates generally have mild or asymptomatic disease at birth, the infection does not follow a benign course. Sequelae such as visual loss as well as psychomotor and mental retardation develop. Hearing loss is demonstrated in 10% to 30% of affected infants and developmental delay in 20% to 75%.

   C. Diagnosis. Screening for toxoplasmosis is not routine in the United States. Because most pregnant women with acute toxoplasmosis are asymptomatic, the diagnosis is unsuspected until an affected fetus is born. For women who present with symptoms of acute toxoplasmosis, however, both IgM and IgG titers should be measured as soon as possible. Interpretation of *Toxoplasma* serology is shown in Table 14-1.

   1. A negative IgM finding rules out acute or recent infection, unless the serum is tested so early that an immune response has not yet been mounted. A positive test finding is more difficult to interpret because IgM may be elevated for more than a year after infection.

   2. Serologic tests that are generally employed include the Sabin-Feldman dye test, the indirect fluorescent antibody test, and ELISA.

   3. Prenatal diagnosis of fetal toxoplasmosis may be achieved by DNA PCR via amniocentesis. In cases of suspected prenatal infection, the placenta should be assessed pathologically for *Toxoplasma* cysts.

   D. Management. For women who elect to continue with their pregnancies after toxoplasmosis has been diagnosed, therapy must be initiated immediately and continued for a year or more in the infant to diminish the risk of the sequelae of congenital toxoplasmosis. Medical therapy is believed to confer a decrease in risk of damage of approximately 50%.

   1. **Spiramycin** is available to physicians in the United States through the FDA. Its effect is to decrease the risk of maternal-fetal transmission, and its use is recommended for treating acute maternal infections diagnosed before the third trimester, with continuation of the therapy for the duration of the pregnancy. If amniotic fluid PCR for *Toxoplasma* is negative, spiramycin is employed as a single agent. The dose is 500 mg p.o. five times per day, or 3 g/day in divided doses.

   2. **Pyrimethamine and sulfadiazine.** These two agents act synergistically against *T. gondii*. The dosage is pyrimethamine, 25 mg p.o. daily, and sulfadiazine, 1 g p.o. four times daily, for 28 days. Folinic acid, 6 mg i.m. or p.o., is administered three times a week to prevent toxicity. During the first trimester, pyrimethamine is not recommended because it could be a teratogen. Sulfadiazine is omitted from the regimen at term.

XI. Herpes simplex virus

   A. Epidemiology. Approximately 1 in 7,500 liveborn infants suffer perinatal transmission of herpes simplex virus (HSV). Whether pregnancy alters the rate of recurrence or frequency of cervical shedding is the subject of dispute. Surveys indicate that the incidence of asymptomatic shedding in pregnancy is 10% after a first episode and 0.5% after a recurrent episode.

1. **Primary maternal infection** with HSV type 2 is the result of direct contact, generally sexual contact, of the patient's mucous membranes or intact skin with the virus.
2. **Fetal infection** with the herpes simplex virus can occur via three different routes. *In utero* transplacental infection is one mechanism that can account for congenital HSV; ascending infection from the cervix can also occur. The most common route, however, is intrapartum, in which the infant makes direct contact with infectious maternal genital lesions during delivery.

B. **Clinical manifestations**
   1. **Maternal infection.** Primary infections of the genitals are often severe; they may, however, be mild or even asymptomatic. Vesicles appear 2 to 10 days after exposure on the cervix, vagina, or external genital area. Swelling, erythema, and pain are common, as is lymphadenopathy near the affected region. The lesions generally persist 1 to 3 weeks, with concomitant viral shedding. Upon resolution of the primary infection, the virus travels to and remains in the spinal sensory ganglia. Reactivation occurs in 50% of patients within 6 months of the initial outbreak, and subsequently at irregular intervals. Recurrent outbreaks are generally milder, and the usual duration of viral shedding in recurrent outbreaks is less than 1 week.
   2. **Fetal infection.** Congenital HSV infections, which produce fetal malformations, are exceedingly rare. Few, if any, neonatal infections are asymptomatic. The majority ultimately produce disseminated or central nervous system (CNS) disease or both. In infants who survive systemic infections, frequently no neurological or ophthalmic sequelae develop. Pneumonia may also occur in the infected neonate.
   3. **Morbidity and mortality.** The risk of transmission during a primary outbreak may approach 50%, with a much smaller risk during recurrent maternal HSV. Neonatal disseminated or CNS infection carries a 50% mortality rate.

C. **Diagnosis.** To exclude the possibility of an infection, 7 to 10 days must be allowed for isolation of the virus in tissue culture because low numbers of infective particles may require as long as 6 days to produce the characteristic cytopathic changes *in vitro*. With the use of an HSV-specific ELISA in tissue cultures, it is possible to provide preliminary evidence to support a diagnosis of active infection within 24 to 48 hours of culturing.
   1. Serology is of limited value in diagnosis because no single antibody titer is predictive of the presence or absence of genital shedding of the virus at any point in time.
   2. To reduce the likelihood of a misdiagnosis, the patient should point out where her lesions are, as well as any sites of previous infection. A sample from the endocervical canal and exfoliated cells from all suspicious areas should be obtained for viral culture.
   3. Smears of scrapings from the base of vesicles may be stained using Tzanck or Papanicolaou techniques, which reveal multinucleated giant cells that implicate HSV infection in 60% to 80% of cases.

D. **Management.** Patients with a history of genital herpes should undergo a careful perineal examination at the time of delivery. Active genital HSV in patients in labor or with ruptured membranes warrants cesarean section, regardless of the duration of membrane rupture. Vaginal delivery is indicated if no signs or symptoms of HSV are present. The use of acyclovir to treat HSV infection currently is not recommended during pregnancy because its effects on the fetus are unknown. Symptomatic treatment measures such as sitz baths can be advised; topical ointments, however, should be discouraged because they may cause dissemination of the infection and delay the healing process.

XII. **Group B streptococcus**
   A. **Epidemiology.** Group B streptococcus (GBS), primarily *S. agalactiae,* can be isolated from the vagina, rectum, or both of approximately 15% to 40% of obstetric patients. Vaginal colonization presumably results from contamination by rectal flora rather than sexual transmission. Colonization is more

prevalent among diabetic patients than in other populations, and infection rates in gestational diabetes are similar to those in pregestational diabetes. Although maternal colonization is common, invasive disease in term neonates is rare. Maternal-fetal transmission can occur via an ascending route *in utero* or during passage of the fetus through the vagina. The vertical transmission rate varies from 42% to 72%. No more than 1% to 2% of full-term infants delivered to colonized females, however, develop the serious sequelae of sepsis, pneumonia, or meningitis. In preterm infants, invasive disease is more common, with significant morbidity and mortality.

B. Clinical manifestations
1. **Maternal infection** is occasionally a cause of asymptomatic bacteriuria and acute cystitis. Several complications occur with increased frequency in GBS-infected women, including the following:
   a. Premature, prelabor rupture of membranes (PPROM)
   b. Preterm labor
   c. Chorioamnionitis
   d. Puerperal endometritis, especially after cesarean section
   e. Increased risk of bacteremia in patients with endometritis
   f. Increased risk of preterm delivery in patients with GBS bacteriuria, but decreased risk after antibiotic therapy
2. **Fetal infection.** GBS is acquired in the immediate perinatal period as a result of contamination of the infant with the microorganism from the mother's genital tract. GBS is a leading cause of pneumonia, sepsis, and meningitis during the first 2 months of life.
3. **Neonatal morbidity and mortality.** The overall neonatal mortality rate is currently approximately 15%, although low-birth-weight infants continue to be at high risk. Early-onset GBS disease has an incidence of 1.3 to 3.7 cases per 1,000 live births. Late-onset GBS infection, which occurs approximately 24 days after birth, affects 0.5 to 1.8 in 100 live births and carries a mortality rate of approximately 10%. Most affected infants are full term. Meningitis occurs in 85%, but infants may also present with bacteremia without localizing symptoms. Neurologic sequelae develop in approximately 50%.

C. Diagnosis. Definitive diagnosis is made by culture, and the highest yield is found when samples are obtained from both the lower vagina and the rectum. These samples must be inoculated immediately into Todd-Hewitt broth or onto selective blood agar.

D. Management. When GBS is suspected, broad-spectrum antibiotic coverage should be initiated until culture results are known. In cases of lower urinary tract infection, the treatment is ampicillin or penicillin, 250 mg p.o. four times per day for 3 to 7 days. For pyelonephritis, hospitalization is required, and ampicillin, 1 to 2 g i.v. every 6 hours, is administered. When the patient has been afebrile and asymptomatic for 24 to 48 hours, she may be discharged, and an oral regimen of ampicillin or penicillin should be followed to complete a total of 7 to 10 days of therapy. Only some obstetric patients with genital colonization require treatment, including patients with PPROM, preterm labor, rupture of membranes of longer than 18 hours' duration, multiple gestations, and overt chorioamnionitis. The drug of choice for intrapartum treatment of GBS infection is penicillin, 5 million units i.v. loading dose, followed by 2.5 million units i.v. every 4 hours.. For patients with an allergy to beta-lactam antibiotics, clindamycin, 600 mg i.v.; erythromycin, 1 to 2 g i.v.; or vancomycin, 500 mg i.v., is administered every 6 hours.

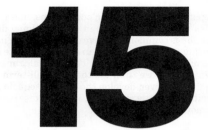

Surgical Disease and Trauma in Pregnancy

Anne Hardart and
Michael Lantz

General Considerations for the Pregnant Surgical Patient

The diagnosis and management of surgical disease during pregnancy is a challenge for both the obstetrician and surgeon, who must strive to maintain the pregnancy and provide definitive therapy as promptly as possible. Surgical disease in pregnancy is complicated by many factors that may result in a delay in diagnosis or treatment and consequently a less favorable outcome.

I. **Physiologic and anatomic changes in pregnancy**
   A. The enlarging uterus displaces abdominal organs and brings adnexal structures into the abdomen.
   B. Compression of inferior vena cava by the uterus decreases venous return and may cause supine hypotension syndrome.
   C. The patient's hyperadrenocortical state masks inflammatory symptoms.
   D. Relative leukocytosis may make determination of infection difficult, especially when leukocytosis is a key variable in determining infective pathology.
   E. Increased plasma volume and decreased hematocrit, as well as relatively decreased blood pressures, make evaluation of acute blood loss difficult.
   F. The ability of the omentum to contain peritonitis is reduced during pregnancy.
   G. The patient's hypoalbuminemic state predisposes to edema.

II. **Consequences of pregnancy for the diagnosis of surgical problems**
   A. Symptoms are masked by normal anatomic and physiologic changes.
   B. The differential diagnosis is expanded to include obstetric pathology.
   C. The potential harm to the fetus of diagnostic and therapeutic intervention must be considered.
   D. Delay in diagnosis is common, given the complexities of the clinical picture and the desire to protect the fetus. Prompt diagnosis and initiation of definitive therapy, however, are essential in minimizing maternal and fetal morbidity and mortality.

III. **Complications of nonobstetric surgery in the pregnant patient** include preterm labor, preterm delivery, and fetal loss. Recent abdominal surgery, however, does not complicate vaginal delivery, nor has incisional dehiscence been associated with vaginal delivery.

IV. **Diagnostic radiology in the pregnant patient.** Teratogenic and oncogenic risks of ionizing radiation are highest between 8 and 15 weeks' gestation. Exposure of the fetus to less than 10 rads is believed to pose little risk (1).

V. **Management of the pregnant surgical patient**
   A. **Optimal timing** of surgery is during the second trimester. Surgery during the first trimester carries an increased risk of spontaneous abortion because of possible disruption of the corpus luteum. Preterm labor and inadequate operative exposure complicate third trimester surgery.
   B. **Intraoperative management** should include left lateral uterine displacement, avoidance of uterine manipulation, optimal maternal oxygenation, and external fetal monitoring if gestational age is in the viable range.

C. **Perioperative care.** Current data do not support the use of intraoperative tocolytics (2).

Acute Abdomen in Pregnancy

I. **Acute appendicitis** is the most common surgical complication of pregnancy, affecting approximately 1 in 1,500 pregnancies.
   A. **Clinical presentation** includes anorexia, nausea, vomiting, fever, abdominal pain (the location of which depends on gestational age), abdominal tenderness, rebound tenderness, and, less commonly, leukocytosis.
   B. **Diagnosis.** Clinical suspicion is essential in making the diagnosis. Unfortunately, the classic signs of appendicitis, including right quadrant pain preceded by periumbilical pain, rebound tenderness, and obturator, psoas or Rovsing's signs, are often absent in the pregnant patient. The leukocyte count may or may not be elevated, although a shift to the left is a significant finding. Ultrasonography may be useful in ruling out other diagnoses.
   C. **Therapy**
      1. **Laparoscopy** may be useful if the diagnosis is uncertain (e.g., in the presence of a history of pelvic inflammatory disease). After 12 to 14 weeks' gestation, however, laparoscopy carries an increased risk of uterine perforation; open laparoscopy is therefore advisable if labaroscopy is considered after 12 to 14 weeks.
      2. **Laparotomy** is indicated if clinical suspicion of appendicitis is high, regardless of the stage of gestation. The location of the incision depends on gestational age. The acceptable negative laparotomy rate is 20% to 35%.
      3. **Antibiotics** should be administered postoperatively in cases of perforation, peritonitis, or periappendiceal abscess.
   D. **Complications** of appendicitis include preterm labor (10% to 15%), spontaneous abortion (3% to 5%), maternal morbidity and mortality, and perforation. If the delay in diagnosis is longer than 24 hours, morbidity is increased, with significant rates of perforation and fetal loss. Furthermore, maternal mortality may approach 5%, largely because of surgical delay.
   E. **Differential diagnosis** includes ectopic pregnancy, pyelonephritis, acute cholecystitis, pelvic inflammatory disease, preterm labor, abruption, degenerating myoma, adnexal torsion, and chorioamnionitis. Pyelonephritis is the most common misdiagnosis.

II. **Acute cholecystitis** is the second most common surgical complication of pregnancy. Pregnant patients are predisposed to cholelithiasis because of their decreased intestinal motility and delayed emptying of the gallbladder; 3.5% of pregnant women have asymptomatic gallstones (3).
   A. The **clinical presentation** is similar to that for nonpregnant patients, consisting of an abrupt onset of right upper quadrant pain, nausea, vomiting, anorexia, fever, dyspepsia, intolerance to fatty foods, and abdominal tenderness. Symptoms may be localized to the flank, right scapula, or shoulder.
   B. **Diagnostic evaluation** should consist of blood work, including leukocyte count, serum amylase, and total bilirubin, and ultrasound of the right upper quadrant to visualize calculi, wall thickness, and presence or absence of pericholecystic fluid. Experience with endoscopic retrograde cholangiopancreatography (ERCP) during pregnancy is limited, but the procedure may be considered if common bile duct stones are present. If ERCP is warranted, the amount of fluoroscopy may be kept to a minimum.
   C. **Differential diagnosis** includes acute fatty liver, abruptio placentae, pancreatitis, acute appendicitis, HELLP syndrome (hemolysis, elevated liver enzymes, and low platelets), and pneumonia.
   D. **Therapy**
      1. **Nonoperative management** may be sufficient and includes bowel rest, intravenous hydration, nasogastric suction, antibiotics, analgesics, and fetal monitoring. Cholecystectomy can be performed safely postpartum.

2. Successful use of **ERCP with sphincterotomy and percutaneous chole-cystotomy** has been reported.
3. **Surgical management** is required in approximately 25% of cases and is indicated in cases of failure of conservative therapy, recurrence in the same trimester, suspected perforation, sepsis, or peritonitis.
   a. Surgery is safest during the second trimester. The physician should consider delaying first trimester cases until the second trimester, and delaying third trimester cases until postpartum.
   b. **Laparoscopy versus laparotomy.** The safety of laparoscopy during pregnancy remains unproved. Many cases of successful laparoscopic procedures in pregnancy, however, have been reported in the literature. In one survey, 134 cases were performed in the first trimester, 224 in the second trimester, and 54 in the third. Carbon dioxide was used in all cases; in most cases, an insufflator pressure of 11 to 15 mm Hg was used. Because of the theoretical complication of puncturing the uterus with the Veress needle, open laparoscopy may be preferable. Laparoscopy is contraindicated late in the third trimester because of the increased risks of uterine perforation and poor exposure. Near term, open cholecystectomy remains the preferred technique. Intraoperative cholangiography should be avoided unless gallstone pancreatitis is suspected.

III. **Ovarian torsion and ruptured corpus luteum.** Adnexal torsion is an uncommon complication of pregnancy and occurs when an enlarged ovary twists on its pedicle. The most common causes of adnexal torsion are corpus luteum cysts, followed by dermoids and other neoplasms.
   A. The clinical presentation is characterized by mild to severe distress associated with acute, usually unilateral, pain, with or without diaphoresis; nausea; and vomiting. An adnexal mass may be palpable. The patient may have a history of induction of ovulation.
   B. Diagnostic evaluation includes ultrasound with Doppler flow studies to visualize cysts, rule out ectopic pregnancy, and evaluate blood flow to the ovaries.
   C. **Therapy**
      1. If intrauterine pregnancy has been confirmed by ultrasound, conservative management is indicated for ruptured corpus luteum cysts, which usually regress by 16 weeks' gestation.
      2. Operative management is indicated for an acute abdomen and cases of suspected torsion or infarction. Whether to remove the ovary or untwist it will depend on the assessment of viability of the ovary that has undergone torsion. Persistent cysts, cysts larger than 6 cm, or cysts with solid elements may also require surgery. Depending on gestational age, laparoscopy may be considered when the diagnosis is uncertain.
      3. Progestins should be administered postoperatively to prevent spontaneous abortion during the first 10 weeks of pregnancy, especially when the ovary containing the corpus luteum of pregnancy is involved.
   D. **Differential diagnosis** includes acute appendicitis, ectopic pregnancy, diverticulitis, small bowel obstruction, pelvic inflammatory disease, and pancreatitis.
   E. **Complications** of torsion include adnexal infarction, chemical peritonitis, and preterm labor.

Trauma in Pregnancy

I. **Incidence and etiology.** One in 12 pregnancies is complicated by trauma (1). Motor vehicle accidents are the most common cause, followed by falls and direct assaults. Physicians should be aware of the increasing incidence of domestic assaults on pregnant women. Maternal outcome is similar to that in trauma to nonpregnant women.

II. Assessment of the pregnant trauma patient

A. Stabilize the mother first

B. Conduct a primary survey

1. **Airway** should be established and maintained as for nonpregnant patients.

2. **Breathing.** Administer oxygen (O_2) by nasal cannula, face mask, or endotracheal tube to maintain saturation at 95% or greater. Intubation should be performed early. Maternal O_2 saturation of 91% correlates with a fetal partial oxygen pressure of approximately 60 mm Hg.

3. **Circulation**

   a. Place the patient in the left lateral decubitus position, or manually deflect the uterus to the left with a wedge under right hip, if gestational age is greater than 20 weeks.

   b. Two large-bore i.v. catheters should be placed.

   c. Crystalloid in form of lactated Ringer's solution or normal saline should be administered in a 3:1 ratio to the estimated blood loss. The volume should be adjusted upward to compensate for the normal hypervolemic state of pregnancy.

   d. Transfusion is indicated if the estimated blood loss is greater than 1 L. Because of increased blood volume during pregnancy, patients may lose up to 1,500 mL of blood before clinical instability becomes apparent.

   e. Vasopressors should be avoided if possible because they depress uteroplacental perfusion, but vasopressors should not be withheld if they are indicated, such as in cases of cardiogenic or neurogenic shock.

C. Conduct a secondary survey

1. Examination of entire body, with particular attention to abdomen and uterus, should be performed after the patient is stabilized.

2. Fetal surveillance to assess well-being and estimate gestational age is also included in the secondary survey.

D. Perform diagnostic tests

1. Diagnostic peritoneal lavage is riskier in pregnant than in nonpregnant patients but still has a morbidity rate of less than 1% (4). It may be indicated in cases of blunt trauma or stab wounds if the patient has altered sensorium, unexplained shock, major thoracic injury, or multiple orthopedic injuries.

2. **Computed tomographic** (CT) scan should be performed if patient is stable.

3. **Ultrasound** is less useful for assessing injury than other modalities; it may be used, however, for screening or for obstetric indications.

4. **Other laboratory tests** include Rh status, complete blood cell count (CBC), Kleihauer-Betke test, and toxicology screen.

E. Cesarean section for fetal distress may be considered if the mother is stable, depending on gestational age, condition of fetus, and the extent of injury to the uterus.

F. The use of **tocolytics** in cases of trauma is controversial but not contraindicated. Standard tocolytic agents produce symptoms such as tachycardia, hypotension, and altered sensorium that may complicate management of the trauma patient in preterm labor.

III. Blunt trauma most commonly is caused by motor vehicle accidents. Pregnant women should be instructed to wear seat belts with three-point restraints and with the lap belt secured over the bony pelvis and not across the fundus.

A. Complications include retroperitoneal hemorrhage (which is more common in the pregnant than the nonpregnant patient), abruptio placentae, preterm labor, placental laceration, uterine rupture, and direct fetal injury. These complications are more likely in the presence of pelvic fractures. Splenic rupture is the most common cause of intraperitoneal hemorrhage. Bowel injuries, in contrast, are less common during pregnancy than at other times. Fetal death is caused most commonly by maternal death, and correlates with severe injuries, expulsion from the vehicle, and maternal head injury.

B. Evaluation

1. Laboratory tests, as listed in sec. **II.D.4,** should be performed, including hematocrit, blood type and screen, and Kleihauer-Betke.

   2. Nitrazine and fern tests of vaginal secretions should be performed to rule out rupture of membranes.
   3. X-ray studies with abdominal shielding should be performed as indicated.
 C. **Abruptio placentae** in the trauma patient (see Chap. 9, sec. I) occurs in up to 38% of cases of blunt trauma with major maternal injury and in up to 2.4% of cases of blunt trauma with minor maternal injury (4).
   1. **Clinical evaluation.** Abruptio placentae is likely in the presence of hypertonic contractions, vaginal bleeding, fetal tachycardia, late decelerations, uterine tenderness, rupture of membranes, or serious maternal injury.
   2. **Diagnostic evaluation**
      a. Electronic monitoring is considered to be the most sensitive method for diagnosing abruptio placentae. If contractions occur less frequently than every 10 minutes, abruptio placentae is an unlikely diagnosis. Twenty percent of patients with contractions more frequent than every 10 minutes have abruptio placentae.
      b. A CBC should be obtained to assess for thrombocytopenia or acute anemia. Fibrinogen determination and prothrombin and partial thromboplastin times may be useful; disseminated intravascular coagulation, however, typically occurs only after abruptio placentae is clinically evident.
      c. A Kleihauer-Betke test should be performed to identify any degree of fetomaternal hemorrhage. Rh-negative, unsensitized women require 300 μg of $Rh_o(D)$ immune globulin (RhoGAM) for every 30 mL of whole fetal blood in the maternal blood. The usefulness of routinely performing a Kleihauer-Betke test, however, remains uncertain.
      d. Ultrasound is less useful in diagnosing abruptio placentae than fetal monitoring, but should be used to estimate gestational age, locate the placenta, and assess the amniotic fluid index.
   3. **Management** consists of observation, although the period required is the subject of controversy. Two to 6 hours may be sufficient if the patient is not having contractions and exhibits no signs of abruptio placentae; some obstetricians, however, advocate observation for 24 hours from the time of trauma.
IV. **Penetrating trauma.** Management of pregnant patients with penetrating trauma is the same as that of nonpregnant women. Tetanus toxoid should be administered if indicated.
 A. **Gunshot wounds.** The incidence of fetal mortality from gunshot wounds is 40% to 70%, whereas maternal mortality occurs in 5% of patients (1). As with blunt injuries, the incidence of bowel injuries is decreased in pregnant patients.
   1. **Evaluation** includes thorough examination of all entrance and exit wounds. Radiographs may help localize the bullet, and CT may also be helpful.
   2. **Management.** Surgical exploration is mandatory in gunshot wounds to the abdomen or flank.
 B. **Stab wounds** carry a more favorable prognosis than gunshot wounds.
   1. **Evaluation** consists of local exploration of the wound. Diagnostic peritoneal lavage may be considered if the fascia has been penetrated. CT may be helpful in assessing the extent of the injury.
   2. **Laparotomy** is indicated if intraperitoneal bleeding is suspected.
V. **Cardiopulmonary resuscitation in pregnancy.** Because cardiac arrest in a pregnant patient is usually the result of an acute insult rather than a chronic illness, maternal survival is more common than in the general population. The chance of fetal survival is also improved by the generally healthy state of the pregnant patients who arrest.
 A. **Causes** of cardiac arrest in the pregnant patient, other than trauma, include pulmonary embolism, amniotic fluid embolism, stroke, maternal cardiac disease, and complications of tocolytic therapy such as pulmonary edema (seen with beta agonists).
 B. **Standard resuscitative protocols** should be followed without modification. Compression of abdominal and pelvic vessels by the gravid uterus can be minimized by manually deflecting the uterus to the left during chest compression.

    C. Pharmacologic agents should be administered as indicated; pressors, however, should be avoided, if possible, because they decrease uteroplacental perfusion.

VI. Postmortem cesarean section, or emergency cesarean section to save the fetus may be considered after severe maternal injury. Although, by definition, postmortem cesarean section is performed only after maternal death has occurred, delivery of the fetus may relieve aortocaval compression and allow for improved venous return and subsequent maternal survival (5). Cesarean section, however, is contraindicated in unstable patients because blood loss from surgery can precipitate death.

    A. The following criteria should be met before postmortem cesarean section is performed:

        1. Cardiac arrest and nonresponse to cardiopulmonary resuscitation have occurred.

        2. Estimated gestational age is greater than 26 weeks; estimated fetal weight is greater than 1,000 g.

        3. Unfavorable maternal outcome is anticipated.

        4. Neonatal support is available.

    B. Technique

        1. A sterile field is unnecessary and time-consuming to establish.

        2. The procedure should be performed immediately at bedside.

        3. Cardiopulmonary resuscitation should be continued.

        4. If it is believed that maternal survival is possible, broad-spectrum antibiotic prophylaxis should be administered.

        5. Careful documentation in the medical record after the procedure is essential because legal issues often arise in the aftermath of maternal death. Physicians performing postmortem cesarean sections under indicated circumstances, however, are at minimal legal risk.

    C. Timing of postmortem cesarean section is critical to its success. The decision to perform the procedure should be made within 4 minutes of cardiac arrest, with delivery within 5 minutes. Chances of fetal survival are excellent if delivery occurs within 5 minutes and poor if delivery occurs after 15 minutes. Nevertheless, infant survival after more than 20 minutes postarrest has been reported; therefore, if any signs of fetal life are present at any time after maternal death, an attempt at delivery should be made. In cases of maternal brain death, however, delivery is not emergent if the fetus is mature, a normal fetal heart rate is present, and signs of fetal distress are absent; in such cases, the patient's family should be consulted before surgery is performed.

References

1. The American College of Obstetricians and Gynecologists. *Trauma during pregnancy. ACOG technical bulletin no. 161.* Washington, DC: American College of Obstetricians and Gynecologists, 1991;165–170.
2. Kort B, Katz VL, Watson WJ. The effect of nonobstetric operation during pregnancy. *Surg Gynecol Obstet* 1993;177(4):371–376.
3. Nathan L, Huddleston JF. Acute abdominal pain in pregnancy. *Obstet Gynecol Clin North Am* 1995;22(1):55–68.
4. Lavery JP, Staten-McCormick M. Management of moderate to severe trauma in pregnancy. *Obstet Gynecol Clin North Am* 1995;22(1):69–90.
5. The American Heart Association. Guidelines for cardiopulmonary and emergency cardiac care, part IV: special resusitation situations. *JAMA* 1992;268(16):2242–2250.

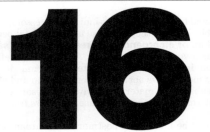

Ectopic Pregnancy

Mona Sadek and
Jean Anderson

Ectopic pregnancy (EP) is defined as implantation of the blastocyst anywhere other than in the endometrial cavity (from Greek "out of place").

I. **Incidence.** Approximately 2% of pregnancies are ectopic. The incidence more than quadrupled between 1970 and 1987 (from 1 in 200 live births to 1 in 43). EPs account for 10% of all maternal mortality. Seventy-five percent of pregnancies occurring after failure of tubal sterilization procedures are likely to be EPs (1).

The implications of EP for future fertility are significant: The overall conception rate after an EP is 60%. In pregnancies occurring after the initial ectopic pregnancy, spontaneous abortion accurs in one-sixth and approximately one-third are recurrent EPs. Only one-third of women with a history of EP eventually deliver a liveborn infant. The incidence of heterotopic pregnancy (combined intrauterine and extrauterine gestation) is an uncommon event: 1 in 4,000 to 1 in 30,000 to 40,000 pregnancies. The incidence rises significantly when ovulation-inducing agents are used.

The incidence of EP is higher in nonwhite women than in white women. The highest age-specific incidence rates per 100,000 women are observed in women 25 to 34 years of age.

II. **Etiology.** The increase in incidence of EPs has been correlated with (a) the improved treatment of pelvic inflammatory disease (PID), which, in the past, would have rendered the patient infertile, as well as an increase in the incidence of PID; (b) the use of intrauterine devices (IUDs), especially those that contain progesterone; (c) the increase in surgical procedures for the treatment of fallopian tube disease; (d) the greater number of elective sterilizations; (e) improved diagnostic techniques; and (f) other contributing factors, including diethylstilbestrol exposure, endometriosis, and the use of ovulation-induction agents.

The vast majority of EPs are tubal. Most tubal pregnancies are found in the distal two-thirds of the tube. The ampulla is the most common site of implantation, accounting for 78% of EPs; 12% are located in the isthmus, 5% are in the fimbriae, and 2% are cornual or interstitial. The remainder are abdominal, cervical, or ovarian.

III. **Diagnosis.** EP may represent a surgical emergency, and therefore timely diagnosis is essential (Fig. 16-1).

A. **Clinical manifestations** are diverse and depend on whether rupture has occurred. The patient typically presents with complaints of spotting, followed by severe lower abdominal pain, occasionally accompanied by syncope, dizziness, or neck or shoulder pain.

1. The **classic triad of signs and symptoms** of EP includes (a) history of a missed menstrual period followed by abnormal vaginal bleeding, (b) abdominal or pelvic pain, and (c) a tender adnexal mass. This triad is seen in less than 50% of patients.

2. The most frequently experienced symptoms of EP are **pelvic and abdominal pain** (95%) and **amenorrhea with vaginal spotting or bleeding** (60% to 80%).

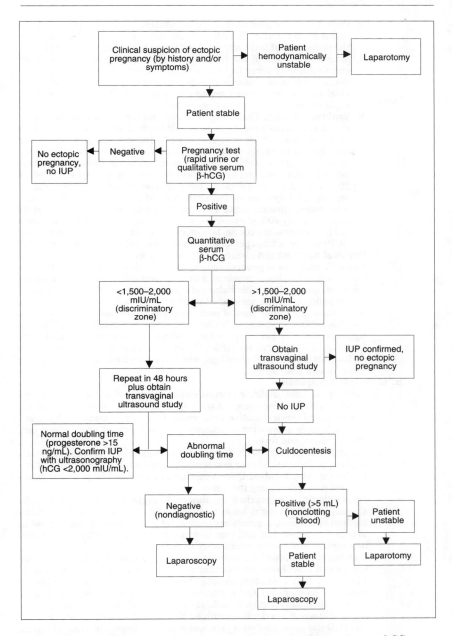

Figure 16-1. Algorithm for ectopic pregnancy diagnosis and management. hCG, human chorionic gonadotropin; IUP, intrauterine pregnancy.

a. **Pain.** The early pain from an EP is usually colicky and is believed to result from tubular distention. Pain may be perceived anywhere in the abdomen but is usually confined to the lower abdomen and is more severe on the side of the EP. With a large hemoperitoneum, pleuritic chest pain may occur from diaphragmatic irritation. Exquisite tenderness occurs on abdominal palpation and vaginal examination; cervical motion tenderness, especially, is seen in 75% of women with ruptured or rupturing tubal pregnancies.

b. **Vaginal spotting.** That the patient has no history of a missed menstrual period does not exclude an EP. Vaginal spotting occurs when endocrine support for the endometrium declines, resulting in scanty, dark brown bleeding, either intermittent or continuous. The uterus grows during the first 3 months of tubal gestation because of stimulation by placental and ovarian hormones and is slightly enlarged in 25% of cases. Uterine decidual casts are passed in 5% to 10% of cases, accompanied by cramps similar to those of a spontaneous abortion.

c. A **palpable adnexal mass or mass in the cul-de-sac** is reported in approximately 40% of cases; however, absence of a mass does not rule out EP. Conversely, a corpus luteum cyst with an intrauterine pregnancy (IUP) may result in a palpable adnexal mass and be mistaken for an EP.

3. **Physical examination** elicits abdominal or pelvic tenderness in 97% of cases. Tenderness is generalized in 45% of patients with EP, is located bilaterally in the lower quadrants in 25%, and is located unilaterally in the lower quadrant in 30%. Rebound tenderness may or may not be present, depending on the amount of peritoneal irritation. Cervical motion tenderness is another sign of peritoneal irritation that also suggests a possible EP in the absence of infection or ovarian torsion (2). Additional signs are shoulder pain, believed to be secondary to peritoneal irritation from the hemoperitoneum (15%); Cullen's sign (periumbilical ecchymosis from intraperitoneal bleeding), which is a rare finding; and low-grade fever (in less than 10%).

B. **Differential diagnosis**

1. **Salpingitis.** This condition is most commonly mistaken for a tubal pregnancy because it also presents with abdominal pain, abnormal vaginal bleeding, and cervical motion tenderness. However, patients with salpingitis will have a negative pregnancy test, an elevated white blood cell (WBC) count, and fever.

2. **Threatened abortion.** With threatened abortion, bleeding is usually more profuse, pain is in the lower midline abdominal area, and cervical motion tenderness may be absent. A corpus luteum cyst may be palpated as an adnexal mass, confusing the issue.

3. **Appendicitis.** Amenorrhea or abnormal vaginal bleeding is usually absent. Persistent right lower quadrant pain, with fever and gastrointestinal symptoms, suggests appendicitis. Cervical motion tenderness is usually less severe but still may be present. A pregnancy test would also be negative (unless coexistent with an IUP).

4. **Ovarian torsion.** Initially, pain from ovarian torsion usually waxes and wanes and later becomes constant as vascular supply is compromised. There may be a coexistent elevated WBC count and a palpable adnexal mass, but a pregnancy test is negative (unless coexistent with an IUP).

5. Other differential diagnoses include dysfunctional uterine bleeding (usually painless and heavier than with an EP), persistent corpus luteum cyst, and IUD use associated with pain and severe dysmenorrhea (pain is often midline and pregnancy test negative). Gastroenteritis or urinary tract infection or calculus early in pregnancy may also mimic an EP (2).

C. **Laboratory tests**

1. **Pregnancy tests**

a. **Urine.** Urinary pregnancy tests for human chorionic gonadotropin (hCG) are most often latex agglutination inhibition slide tests, which have a sensitivity in the range of 50 to 80 mIU/mL. Although simple and rapid, these tests are positive in only 50% to 60% of EPs.

They are qualitative and thus can be either positive or negative, but they are useful because of the rapidity in obtaining results. They can be positive at levels of 25 mIU/mL or greater.

   b. **Serum.** For distinguishing EP or other abnormal pregnancies from normal IUPs, the most sensitive test is the serum β-hCG radioimmunoassay, a quantitative test that is positive at levels of 5 mIU/mL [International Reference Preparation (IRP)]. Serial values allow comparison with normal doubling times: 1.4 to 1.5 days in early IUPs to 3.3 to 3.5 days in 6- to 7-week gestations. Approximately 85% of normal pregnancies fall within these limits; EPs are generally associated with lower β-hCG levels than normal IUPs. Pregnancies near 6 weeks demonstrating a less than 66% increase in hCG within a 48-hour period are either EPs or nonviable IUPs that are likely to abort.

2. **Hemoglobin and hematocrit.** Baseline levels are obtained, and serial levels are useful if the diagnosis is uncertain. An acute drop over the first few hours of observation is more important than the initial reading. After acute hemorrhage, initial readings may at first be unchanged or only slightly decreased; subsequent decline represents restoration of depleted blood volume by hemodilution.

3. **Leukocyte count** varies considerably in ruptured EPs. It is normal in 50% of EPs but has been reported to rise as high as 30,000.

4. **Progesterone.** Although a single level cannot predict whether a patient has an EP, levels can often be used to establish that there is an abnormal pregnancy (either incomplete abortion or EP). The serum progesterone level will be less than 15 ng/mL in 81% of EPs and in 93% of abnormal IUPs, but in only 11% of normal IUPs. Conversely, less than 2% of EPs and not more than 4% of abnormal IUPs have progesterone levels of more than 25 ng/mL. Thus, a single serum progesterone level of more than 25 ng/mL strongly indicates a normal IUP, and a level of less than 15 ng/mL suggests an abnormal pregnancy. It has been suggested that serum progesterone be used as a screening test; however, this measuring of serum progesterone has not always been found to be useful, given the time needed to obtain the results of serum determinations at most institutions.

D. **Ultrasound (US)** allows the clinician to rule out an IUP when an EP is suspected. A positive US diagnosis can be made by identifying an extrauterine fetus, but this is an uncommon finding. In practice, an IUP sac or fetus seen on US essentially excludes the presence of an EP.

   1. **Abdominal US.** An IUP is usually not recognized using abdominal US until 5 to 6 weeks' gestation or 28 days after timed ovulation. An adnexal mass seen on US is suggestive of EP; fetal heart motion outside the uterus is diagnostic, however. With a range of serum hCG concentrations of 6,000 to 6,500 mIU/mL (IRP) a normal IUP can be visualized by transabdominal sonograms 94% of the time. The absence of an intrauterine sac when the hCG level is more than 6,000 mIU/mL is diagnostic of an EP in 86% of cases. At the time of initial evaluation, however, less than 25% of patients with EPs have hCG levels of more than 6,000.

   US findings suggestive of early IUPs may be apparent in some cases of EP. The appearance of a small sac or collapsed sac may actually be a blood clot or decidual cast.

   2. **Vaginal US** is more sensitive and specific; however, 10% of EPs are still missed by this procedure. Earlier and more specific diagnoses are made with the following diagnostic criteria: (a) identification of a gestational sac of more than 1 to 3 mm eccentrically placed in the uterus and surrounded by a decidual-chorionic reaction, and (b) a fetal pole within the sac, especially when accompanied by fetal heart motion. A point of differentiation between false and genuine sacs is the presence of a yolk sac. Using vaginal US, a gestational sac can usually be seen when serum hcG concentrations are as low as 1,000 mIU/mL.

E. **US and β-hCG levels.** In hemodynamically stable patients, evaluation of suspected EP involves serial determinations of serum β-hCG levels and vaginal or abdominal US.

1. If the β-hCG level is more than 6,000 mIU/mL and an intrauterine sac is seen by abdominal US, an EP is ruled out, except for rare cases of heterotopic pregnancy. The critical or discriminatory zone for vaginal US is between 1,500 and 2,500 mIU/mL (IRP).

2. If the β-hCG level is more than 6,000 mIU/mL and no intrauterine sac is seen on abdominal US, or if the β-hCG level is above 1,500 to 2,500 mIU/mL and no intrauterine sac is seen on a vaginal US, an EP is very likely.

3. If the β-hCG level is less than 6,000 mIU/mL and a definite intrauterine gestantional sac is visualized on abdominal US (1,500 to 2,500 mIU/mL and a definite intrauterine gestantional sac on vaginal US), a spontaneous abortion is likely, but an EP must be ruled out. A serum progesterone level determination may be useful.

4. With β-hCG levels of less than 6,000 mIU/mL and an empty uterus on abdominal US (greater than 1,500 to 2,500 mIU/mL and an empty uterus on vaginal US), no diagnosis can be made. A serum β-hCG level determination can confirm a pregnancy 8 days after fertilization. An intrauterine gestational sac cannot be identified even with vaginal US until 28 days after conception; the time between 8 and 28 days results in the "20-day window." A progesterone level determination may again be useful, but it is not always rapidly available in most institutions. Serial β-HCG levels and follow-up ultrasonography are used to resolve the diagnosis.

F. **Culdocentesis** is a simple technique for identifying hemoperitoneum. The cervix is pulled toward the symphysis with a tenaculum, and a 20-gauge spinal needle is inserted through the posterior vaginal fornix into the cul-de-sac. The presence of old clots or bloody fluid that does not clot suggests hemoperitoneum secondary to a ruptured EP. Clotting, if it occurs, suggests aspiration from an adjacent blood vessel or brisk bleeding from a ruptured EP. Culdocentesis may be unsatisfactory with a history of previous salpingitis and pelvic peritonitis because of an obliterated cul-de-sac. Purulent fluid points to a diagnosis of salpingitis. Contraindications include a deeply retroverted uterus or a mass in the cul-de-sac.

G. **Curettage** is useful in differentiating between threatened or incomplete abortions and tubal pregnancies. Stovall et al. recommend that curettage be carried out in cases in which the progesterone level is less than 5 ng/mL, β-hCG titers are rising abnormally and are less than 2,000 mIU/mL, and no IUP has been visualized by transvaginal US (3). If curettings yield placental or fetal tissue, a simultaneous EP is unlikely. If curettings yield decidual tissue but no villi, follow-up is needed with serial hCG determinations and US. The presence of decidua alone on pathologic examination implies extrauterine pregnancy, although it may be seen in a complete abortion.

IV. **Treatment.** The initial management decision is based on the patient's stability. Patients in shock, with a surgical abdomen, should be taken to the operating room as soon as possible, resuscitated with intravenous fluids using two large-bore intravenous cannulas and a Foley catheter in place (maintaining urine output at more than 33 mL/hour). Blood tests that should be undertaken at once, including a type and cross-match for four units of packed red blood cells, complete blood count, prothrombin time, partial thromboplastin time, and renal panel.

A. **Surgical management.** The operative procedure is selected based on the rate of bleeding, patient stability, the extent of damage to the fallopian tube, and the desire for future fertility. There are two primary approaches:

1. **Laparoscopy.** Advantages include definitive diagnosis, concurrent route to remove the mass, direct route to inject chemotherapeutic agents into the mass, and quicker recovery period. Disadvantages include possible difficulty in identification of an early unruptured tubal pregnancy, and control of profuse hemorrhage is difficult to impossible.

2. **Laparotomy** is the last resort, but one should not delay with a patient with obvious hemorrhage and hemodynamic compromise. In this case, after hemostasis is obtained, the treatment of choice is complete or partial salpingectomy. With a ruptured interstitial or cornual pregnancy, hysterectomy may be required in rare circumstances. Laparotomy is also indicated when adhesive disease precludes adequate visualization through the laparoscope.

B. **Conservative surgical approaches** are preferred whenever possible, unless the patient does not wish to preserve childbearing potential. **Salpingectomy** is not conservative, as it involves the removal of the entire fallopian tube. This is done when the size and extent of the EP are such that salvage of the tube is not possible. Briefly, conservative options include the following:

1. **Salpingostomy** involves incision of the fallopian tube, creating a new opening (stoma). It is used to remove a small pregnancy less than 2 cm long in the distal third of the tube. A linear incision 2 cm or shorter is made on the antimesenteric border over the pregnancy, which usually extrudes from the incision and may be removed. Any bleeding sites are cauterized with laser or needle-point cautery, and the incision is left to heal by secondary intention. Sherman et al. (4) and Timonen and Nieminen (5) showed higher subsequent pregnancy rates with salpingostomy over salpingectomy, making it the preferred method. Salpingostomy can also be done laparoscopically.

2. **Salpingotomy** involves incision of the fallopian tube, with reapproximation of the cut edges. It is performed as described for salpingostomy, except that a one-layer closure with 7-0 interrupted absorbable, nonreactive [e.g., polyglactin (Vicryl), polyglycolic acid (Dexon)] sutures is used to reapproximate the cut edges. This can also be done laparoscopically. Salpingostomy may be preferred to salpingotomy because it is simpler and has equivalent success rates for future pregnancy.

3. **Segmental resection (partial salpingectomy) and anastomosis (immediate versus delayed)** involves excising the involved portion of fallopian tube and reapproximating the remaining ends. It is recommended for unruptured ectopics in the isthmus because salpingotomy or salpingostomy in this narrow region might result in scarring and further narrowing. Segmental resection may also be done with ruptured ampullary ectopics in an unstable patient, when hemostasis needs to be rapidly obtained and childbearing potential preserved. The mesosalpinx is incised, the EP is excised, the mesosalpinx is sutured, thus reapproximating tubal stumps, and the cut ends of the tubes are anastomosed to each other in layers with interrupted 7-0 Vicryl sutures.

4. **Fimbrial evacuation** involves squeezing the EP out of the fimbriated end. The so-called milking, or suctioning, of the ectopic mass from distally implanted tubal pregnancies is not recommended because of a doubling in recurrence rates of EPs over those treated with salpingotomy and a high rate of surgical reexploration for recurrent bleeding secondary to persistent trophoblastic tissue.

5. **Cornual resection,** which involves excision of the cornu, is reserved for the very rare occurrence of a cornual EP. In this procedure, a wedge of the outer one-third of the interstitial portion of fallopian tube, together with the EP, is removed to avoid recurrence of EP in the tubal stump without creating a defect in the uterus, where rupture would be a concern. Laparotomy is required.

V. **Complications**

A. **Persistent trophoblastic tissue.** With conservative approaches, there is a significant risk that not all trophoblastic tissue is evacuated, necessitating close follow-up postoperatively. With persistent or increasing hCG values, reexploration or chemotherapy with methotrexate (MTX) may be chosen based on the patient's stability and hCG level.

B. **Persistent EP** is the most common complication and the major reason for secondary intervention after initial conservative surgical therapy of an EP. There is little information concerning reproductive outcome after treatment of this complication. Salpingectomy appears to be the most dependable treatment, offering the greatest assurance for complete resolution of persistent EP. Issues regarding further fertility often influence the decision of deferring salpingectomy and opting for repeat salpingostomy or MTX.

Conservative surgery should be followed with weekly β-hCG determinations until they reach nonpregnant levels. An hCG clearance occurs in two

Table 16-1. Single-dose methotrexate protocol for ectopic pregnancy treatment

Day	Therapy
0^a	hCG, D&C, CBC, AST, BUN, creatinine, blood type (including Rh)
1	MTX, hCG
4^b	hCG
7^c	hCG

AST, aspartate aminotransferase; BUN, blood urea nitrogen; CBC, complete blood cell count; D&C, dilation of the cervix and curettage of the uterus; hCG, quantitative beta-human chorionic gonadotropin (mIU/mL); MTX, intramuscular methotrexate, 50 mg/m²; Rh, rhesus factor.
[a]In patients not requiring D&C before MTX initiation (hCG of 2,000 mIU/mL and no gestational sac on transvaginal ultrasound), day 0 and day 1 are combined.
[b]The hCG titer on day 4 is usually higher than the hCG titer on day 1.
[c]If there is a <15% decline in titer between days 4 and 7, give second dose of methotrexate, 50 mg/m² on day 7. If ≥15% decline in hCG titer between days 4 and 7, follow weekly until hCG is <10 mIU/mL.
From ref. 3, adapted with permission.

phases: an initial phase, with a half-life of 5 to 9 hours, and a second, longer phase, with a half-life of 22 to 32 hours. When removal of tissue is fairly complete, serum hCG levels will be 20% or less of intraoperative or preoperative levels within 72 hours after surgery. If hCG levels continue to fall, expectant management with serial hCG determinations is sufficient. If they plateau or rise, further treatment options (salpingectomy, partial salpingectomy, or MTX) should be considered.

C. **Chronic EP** is often an enigma and not diagnosed until exploratory laparotomy. Patients are stable, display intermittent symptoms, and have a high incidence of false-negative pregnancy tests and culdocentesis, distinguishing them from patients with acute EP. Approximately 6% of EPs are chronic (range, 3% to 20%). Dense adhesions and occasional abscess formations are surgical features that characterize chronic EP. Patients may have fever, adnexal mass, and vaginal bleeding for a longer period of time secondary to death of the embryo and degeneraton of the trophoblast.

VI. **Medical management**

A. **Systemic MTX.** MTX, a folic acid analogue, inhibits dehydrofolate reductase and DNA synthesis and has been used in the treatment of unruptured EP. MTX targets rapidly dividing cells, including fetal cells, trophoblast, bone marrow cells, and cells of the buccal and intestinal mucosa. Its repeated use is limited by dose- and duration-dependent side effects: severe leukopenia, bone marrow aplasia, thrombocytopenia, ulcerative stomatitis, diarrhea, liver cell necrosis, hemorrhagic enteritis, and even death from intestinal perforation. The current single-dose MTX protocol, developed by Stovall et al. for treatment of an unruptured EP, is summarized in Table 16-1. Stovall recommends that patients with subnormally rising hCG titers of less than 2,000 mIU/mL undergo dilation of the cervix and curettage of the uterus (D&C). The hCG titer is repeated the following day, and if rising, MTX (50 mg/m²) is given i.m. For patients with rising hCG titers of more than 2,000 mIU/mL, a D&C is not required, and MTX can be administered on day 0.

Before treatment, all patients should have a normal platelet and WBC count, normal liver function tests, and normal renal function. A blood type/Rhesus test should be done to assess the need for Rh_o (D) immune globulin (RhoGAM). An hCG titer is drawn on days 4 and 7, although the level will usually be higher on day 4 than day 1. If the titer on day 7 is less than that on day 4, weekly hCG levels are followed until negative. If not, or if it is not declining, a second dose of MTX (same dosage) is given, and the titers are followed days 4 and 7, as above.

Table 16-2. Criteria for methotrexate therapy

Stovall and Ling, 1993[a]

Hemodynamically stable

hCG titers increased after curettage

Transvaginal ultrasonography showed an unruptured ectopic pregnancy of <3.5 cm in greatest diameter

Desire for future fertility

American College of Obstetricians and Gynecologists, 1990[b]

Ectopic size of 3 cm or less

Desire for future fertility

Stable or rising hCG levels with peak values of <15,000 mIU/mL

Tubal serosa intact

No active bleeding

Ectopic pregnancy fully viable at laparoscopy

Selected cases of cervical and cornual pregnancy

---

hCG, human chorionic gonadotropin.
[a]From ref. 3, adapted with permission.
[b]From American College of Obstetricians and Gynecologists. *Ectopic pregnancy. ACOG technical bulletin #150.* Washington, DC: American College of Obstetricians and Gynecologists, 1990.

Patients should be informed that the failure rate with EP of less than 3.5 cm is 5% and that the majority of patients have an increase in abdominal/pelvic pain during treatment. This pain is often difficult to distinguish from pain due to rupture of the EP. Patients should be followed with transvaginal US and hemoglobin determinations and surgically managed if there is evidence of rupture.

1. **Strict criteria** are required for MTX therapy (Table 16-2). The most important selection criterion for medical management involves patient stability. Fetal cardiac activity is a relative contraindication because it is associated with a significantly higher failure rate (14%) than in the absence of cardiac activity (5%).
2. **Contraindications** to MTX therapy are listed in Table 16-3.
3. **Disadvantages** of single-dose systemic MTX include prolonged time for the hCG titers to decline and the EP to resolve (70 to 120 days) and the need for close monitoring of outpatients for rupture and MTX side effects, making compliance an important consideration in patient selection.

B. **Local (transvaginal/laparoscopic) treatment**

1. Transvaginal intratubal MTX has been undertaken but has a significant failure rate (30%.) Laparoscopic intratubal MTX has not been found to be successful in a randomized trial and so has been abandoned because of the need for surgery for persistence of EP.
2. Laparoscopic intratubal **prostaglandin and hyperosmolar glucose** injections have been tried, but not found to be more effective than salpingostomy; therefore, they are not recommended.
3. **Cervical EPs.** MTX, as well as other substances such as actinomycin-D, have also been used in the treatment of cervical EPs. Direct injection of various agents has been reported using laparoscopy or transvaginally with the aid of US. Injection of MTX under US guidance is associated with a less than 80% success rate. Although MTX injection with US avoids surgery, it has a lower success rate than systemic MTX (92%).
4. RU-486, a progesterone receptor–blocker, has not shown effectiveness in limited reports of EP.

Table 16-3. Contraindications to methotrexate therapy

Stovall and Ling, 1993[a]

Hepatic dysfunction: aspartate aminotransferase level >2 times normal

Renal disease: serum creatinine level >130 mmol/L (1.5 mg/dL)

Active peptic ulcer disease

Blood dyscrasia: leukocyte count <3,000 cells/μl or platelet count 100,000/μl

American College of Obstetricians and Gynecologists, 1990[b]

Contraindications listed above, plus:

Poor patient compliance

History of active hepatic or renal disease

Presence of fetal cardiac activity

[a]From ref. 3, adapted with permission.
[b]From American College of Obstetricians and Gynecologists. *Ectopic pregnancy. ACOG technical bulletin #150.* Washington, DC: American College of Obstetricians and Gynecologists, 1990.

VII. **Fertility after EP.** The choice of surgical procedure in the management of an EP is not a significant determinant of fertility outcome in women with EPs. A history of previous infertility is the single most important factor influencing future fertility. It is recommended that conservative surgery be performed in women desiring subsequent pregnancy. Women with a single remaining fallopian tube have a 58% chance of an IUP after conservative therapy.

   A. The overall cumulative clinical pregnancy rate of 59% at 36 months compares favorably with the reported cumulative clinical pregnancy rates after salpingotomy for unruptured EP.

   B. **MTX** is consistent with subsequent fertility: as high as 80% in one population, with a mean interval of 32 ± 1.1 months, and 87% of these intrauterine, 13% EPs.

   C. Conservative surgery for small unruptured EP yields tubal patency in more than 80% of patients. In small, uncontrolled studies, a 40% to 60% IUP rate with a 10% to 20% risk of recurrent EP after linear salpingostomy has been reported. It is noteworthy that a recurrent EP occurs in the contralateral tube as often as in the operated oviduct. Women with a history of infertility have a lower rate of IUP (41%) compared with those with a normal reproductive history (85%).

   D. When comparing outcome after conservative surgery with that after salpingectomy, a similar subsequent fertility and EP recurrence are found. Fertility is improved, however, in patients with contralateral adhesive disease or history of infertility (76% vs. 44%) when conservative management is chosen instead of salpingectomy. Future pregnancy data following salpingotomy in patients with a tubal pregnancy in a sole patent oviduct (20% ectopic recurrence) suggest that a conserved tube is at similar risk for repeat EP as is a diseased contralateral tube that was not operated on.

   E. The risk of recurrence increases in patients who have had two or more EPs. Only one out of three will conceive, and 20% to 57% of these will result in EPs.

VIII. **Follow-up.** Patients should be advised to take birth control pills or use other reliable contraception until initial inflammation resolves (6–12 weeks). Contraception will avoid the confusion between rising hCG levels from a new pregnancy and those of a persistent EP, should conception occur in the immediate postoperative period. They should undergo extensive counseling regarding their recurrence risk for an EP and the absolute necessity for early medical care. It is important to give RhoGAM (300 μg) postoperatively in an Rh-negative woman to prevent Rh isoimmunization in a future pregnancy.

References

1. Gabbe SG, Niebyl JR, Simpson JL (eds). *Obstetrics: normal and problem pregnancies*, 2nd ed. New York: Churchill Livingstone, 1991.
2. Niswander KR, Evans AT (eds). *Manual of obstetrics: diagnosis and therapy*, 4th ed. Boston: Little, Brown, 1991.
3. Stovall TG, Ling FW. Single-dose methotrexate: an expanded clinical trial. *Am J Obstet Gynecol* 1993;168:1759–1762.
4. Sherman D, Langer R, Sadovsky G, et al. Improved fertility following ectopic pregnancy. *Fertil Steril* 1982;37:497–502.
5. Timonen S, Nieminen U. Tubal pregnancy, choice of operative method of treatment. *Acta Obstet Gynecol Scand* 1967;46(3):327–329.

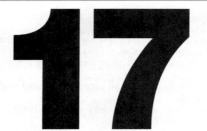

Acute and Chronic Pelvic Pain

Vanna Zanagnolo and
Vanessa Cullins

I. **General principles.** When presented with a female patient with abdominopelvic pain, the most important initial determination is whether the patient exhibits an acute surgical abdomen. The next two most important considerations are (a) whether she is pregnant and (b) whether she requires immediate hospitalization. If the patient is pregnant, ectopic pregnancy must be considered, as untreated ectopic pregnancy may lead to death from intraperitoneal hemorrhage. Immediate hospitalization is required for any patient for whom an outpatient evaluation or treatment is likely to delay management or lead to further complications.

II. **Acute abdomen**

A. **Clinical presentation and general approach.** Findings associated with acute abdomen include pain, usually of sudden onset, tenderness to palpation, rebound tenderness, and diminished or absent bowel sounds. Rapid assessment to identify patients requiring urgent intervention must be performed. This assessment should include history, if obtainable, and physical examination, including pelvic examination. Signs of distress (including confusion, obtundation, diaphoresis, and hypotension) indicate need for prompt intervention.

1. **Intravascular volume and hemodynamic status should be assessed immediately and frequently reassessed.** A sudden increase in pulse rate or change in postural blood pressure (BP) is often the only early indication of internal bleeding. Postural hypotension (supine to upright fall in systolic BP of more than 10 mm Hg or increase in heart rate of more than 20 beats/minute) indicates moderate blood loss (10% to 20% of circulatory volume); supine hypotension suggests severe blood loss of more than 20% of circulatory volume. Further blood loss results in shock, with peripheral vasoconstriction, diaphoresis, and ischemic organ damage.

2. **Shock** requires rapid restoration of circulatory volume and admission to an intensive care unit. **Septic shock,** usually manifested by fever, hypotension, tachycardia, peripheral vasodilatation, and diaphoresis, requires rapid initiation of both antibiotic and intravascular volume support.

B. **Differential diagnoses** vary depending on the age of the patient.

1. **Torsion of an adnexa and mesenteric lymphadenitis** may be more prevalent in preadolescent and adolescent girls.

2. **Salpingitis, tubo-ovarian abscess, ectopic pregnancy, severe uterine atony postabortion (postabortal syndrome) or postpartum, postabortion uterine perforation, and ruptured ovarian cyst** must be considered in women of reproductive age; **Crohn's disease, acute cholecystitis, perforated peptic ulcer, acute pyelitis, renal calculi, or splenic rupture** are rare but may be in the differential diagnosis.

3. In older women, acute abdomen suggests **torsion, acute cholecystitis, perforated ulcer, or acute diverticulitis.**

4. **Acute appendicitis** is part of the differential diagnosis in all age groups.

C. **Laboratory evaluation.** In addition to a sensitive pregnancy test, a type and crossmatch, complete blood cell count (CBC), and platelet count should be obtained. Hemoglobin and hematocrit are inaccurate indicators of the degree of acute blood loss; they may be normal initially despite considerable blood loss.

D. Therapy should be instituted as soon as hemodynamic compromise is identified. Begin restoration of intravascular volume immediately.

1. Two large-bore intravenous lines should be established with 14- to 18-gauge catheters in large peripheral veins. Isotonic saline, lactated Ringer's solution, or 5% hetastarch (Hespan) can be used until blood products are available. The rate of volume infusion should be guided by the patient's condition and degree of suspected volume loss. Six units of packed red blood cells should be available at all times until the patient's condition has stabilized.

2. After hemodynamic stabilization, surgical exploration (laparotomy or laparoscopy) is the next step if acute intraabdominal bleeding or acute appendicitis is suspected.

3. If sepsis is the working diagnosis, the patient should be hospitalized and treated with broad-spectrum, intravenous antibiotic therapy; continued blood pressure support; and intravascular volume support.

4. For the patient who is hemodynamically stable upon presentation, indications for surgical exploration rather than observation should be based on the most likely diagnosis.

III. Acute pelvic pain

A. General approach. Acute pelvic pain presents as both pelvic and lower abdominal pain. This pain may be caused by dysfunction of genitourinary, gastrointestinal, or musculoskeletal system. A detailed history, selective use of diagnostic tests, and a well-considered differential diagnosis are necessary for accurate diagnosis and appropriate therapy.

1. **History.** The onset, character, location, and radiation pattern of the pain must be determined and correlated with changes with micturition, bowel movements, intercourse, activity, and stress. Menstrual, sexual, contraceptive, and past medical and surgical histories may provide important details for accurate diagnosis. Diagnosis and treatment at the time of a previous, similar episode of pain can be important information; temper this information with recognition that the diagnosis could have been incorrect if not confirmed by laparoscopic or tissue diagnosis.

2. **Physical examination.** Complete physical examination, including pelvic and rectovaginal examination, should be performed. Evaluate pain locations and change in pain characteristics during examination maneuvers. Attempt to distinguish between changes associated with the palpating abdominal versus vaginal hand.

3. **Laboratory tests** include a pregnancy test for patients of reproductive age, CBC, and routine urine analysis. Determination of erythrocyte sedimentation rate (ESR) and electrolyte and chemistry panels may be helpful.

4. **Culdocentesis** should be considered infrequently, given the availability of ultrasonography and diagnostic laparoscopy.

5. **Ultrasonography** should be considered when faced with the following circumstances:
   a. **Inadequate pelvic examination** because of pain or obesity,
   b. **Suspected ectopic pregnancy,** or
   c. **Adnexal mass suspected,** yet not confirmed by examination. Ultrasonography can also localize an intrauterine device or confirm fluid in the cul-de-sac.

6. **Diagnostic laparoscopy** should be considered if the diagnosis remains unclear despite noninvasive testing or attempted treatment. Laparoscopy should be considered if it might preclude laparotomy or if the patient's condition fails to improve with conservative measures.

B. Early pregnancy-related causes of acute pelvic pain. Complications of early pregnancy that may cause acute pelvic pain include abortion (threatened, inevitable, incomplete, complete, or septic); incomplete involution of the uterus postabortion, with subsequent bleeding and intrauterine massive clot formation; and ectopic pregnancy.

1. **Spontaneous abortion** is generally accompanied by vaginal bleeding and crampy, midline, intermittent, lower abdominopelvic pain.

2. **Septic abortion** is associated with additional findings of malaise, elevated temperature, and elevated white blood cell (WBC) count. Dilation of the cervix and curettage of the uterus (D&C) is the treatment of choice for incomplete, inevitable, missed spontaneous abortion, or incomplete postabortal involution of the uterus; septic abortion requires intravenous antibiotic therapy in addition to D&C. D&C should be performed immediately after the first dose of antibiotic has been given.

3. **Ectopic pregnancies** are usually associated with intermittent or continuous, crampy pain with vaginal bleeding. Before rupture of an ectopic pregnancy (and development of an acute abdomen), **physical examination** usually reveals unilateral adnexal tenderness and may reveal a tender adnexal mass (see Chap. 16).

C. **Pelvic infection or pelvic inflammatory disease (PID)** includes acute cervicitis, endometritis, and acute salpingitis, with infectious complications of pyosalpingitis, tuboovarian abscess, and perihepatitis. Patients usually present with bilateral lower quadrant abdominopelvic pain. Fever may be present.

1. **Pelvic examination** may reveal purulent or mucopurulent cervical discharge, cervical motion tenderness, uterine tenderness, and bilateral adnexal tenderness.

2. **Laboratory tests.** An elevated WBC count and ESR may be present. Classic gonococcal salpingitis occurs near the time of the menses and is often associated with fever and peritoneal signs. Nongonococcal salpingitis (usually associated with *Chlamydia trachomatis* infection) is less likely to be associated with acute peritonitis or fever, regardless of inciting cervical pathogen(s). Most upper gynecologic tract infections are polymicrobial.

3. **Management.** Complications of pelvic infection, such as infertility, chronic pelvic pain (CPP), and ectopic pregnancy can be minimized with early, aggressive, broad-spectrum, antibiotic treatment. Mildly symptomatic individuals who can tolerate oral antibiotic therapy may be candidates for outpatient treatment. This approach requires frequent clinical follow-up (e.g., at 48 to 72 hours, at 1 to 2 weeks, and at 1 month after initiation of therapy).

D. **Disorders of uterus and adnexa**

1. **Degenerating myoma**

a. **Clinical presentation** includes acute, usually constant, sharp pain in the region of the myoma, often in association with pregnancy.

b. **Pelvic examination.** The uterus is irregular, usually enlarged, and tender to palpation.

c. **Laboratory findings.** Mild leukocytosis may be present.

d. **Imaging studies.** Pelvic examination may be supplemented by **ultrasonography,** which can provide objective information regarding the size and location of individual myomas.

e. **Treatment**

(1) **Therapeutic alternatives** include conservative therapy [e.g., heating pad, bed rest and a nonsteroidal antiinflammatory drug (NSAID) such as ibuprofen, 600 mg p.o. q6h (not p.r.n.)] with serial examinations; i.v. or i.m. ketorolac (30 to 66 mg), which can give dramatic relief, if not pregnant; and hormonal therapy, if not pregnant [e.g., leuprolide, 3.75 mg i.m.; nafarelin acetate (Synarel Spray), intranasally b.i.d.; or other gonadotropin-releasing hormone (GnRH) agonist].

(2) If not pregnant, **operative treatment** includes myomectomy or hysterectomy. GnRH agonist therapy is generally used as an interim management tool to reduce myoma volume prior to operative treatment. Severity of symptoms, reproductive plans, patient age, and patient desires should guide therapeutic decisions.

2. **Pelvic pain of adnexal origin (ovarian torsion, intracapsular or extracapsular ovarian hemorrhage, or rupture of an ovarian cyst or endometrioma)**

a. **Clinical presentation.** Severe colicky, unilateral pain and low-grade temperature is associated with ovarian torsion. Sudden onset of bilateral pain localized to a predominant side is more likely associated with ovarian cyst rupture or capsular hemorrhage.

  b. **Examination,** depending on whether the process is unilateral or bilateral, reveals localized or diffuse abdominopelvic tenderness with worsening of pain on bimanual examination; rebound tenderness and abdominal guarding may be present.

  c. **Laboratory findings.** Although leukocytosis and an elevated ESR can be associated with torsion, these findings are usually not present with ovarian hemorrhage or rupture. Obtain **abdominal and transvaginal sonographic evaluation if the pelvic examination is unrevealing.** If diagnosis remains unclear, **diagnostic laparoscopy** is necessary.

  d. **Treatment.** Analgesia with close observation is the management option of choice in the hemodynamically stable patient whose diagnosis is rupture of an ovarian cyst or ovarian hemorrhage. Conservative management should continue as long as the patient remains hemodynamically stable and clinically improves. Operative laparoscopy or laparotomy may be necessary for ovarian torsion, significant intracapsular or extracapsular ovarian hemorrhage, or insufficient clinical improvement during conservative management.

E. Nongynecologic disorders that cause acute pelvic pain are most commonly gastrointestinal in origin and include acute appendicitis, diverticulitis, viral gastroenteritis, and mesenteric lymphadenitis.

  1. Acute appendicitis

  a. **Clinical presentation.** Typical initial pain of acute appendicitis is diffuse, mild, and located in the epigastrium and periumbilical region. As inflammation progresses, the pain becomes more severe and localizes in the right lower quadrant. Anorexia, nausea, and vomiting are present in 50% of patients. Because elderly patients may have less severe pain and delayed localization in the right lower quadrant, the incidence of appendiceal perforation, morbidity, and mortality rates are higher.

  b. **Physical examination.** Patients with acute appendicitis classically have tenderness to direct palpation, rebound tenderness, and guarding in the right lower quadrant over the point where the inflamed appendiceal serosa is in contact with the parietal peritoneum. As the disease progresses, tenderness and muscle rigidity become more pronounced. If the infection fails to localize, generalized peritonitis ensues, with diffuse tenderness, guarding, distension, ileus, dehydration, tachycardia, and spiking fever.

  c. **Laboratory findings.** The WBC count is usually elevated, with a predominance of juvenile forms (shift to the left); ESR is elevated. Occasionally, pyuria without bacteriuria may be seen, which confuses the differentiation between pyelonephritis and appendicitis.

  d. **Ultrasonographic and radiographic findings.** In advanced disease, abdominal x-ray may show an indistinct right psoas muscle shadow, a "sentinel loop" ileus, or a soft-tissue mass with or without gas bubbles. Ultrasonographic findings of appendicitis consist of an incompressible, tender tubular structure with a diameter of 7 mm or greater. Identification of an appendicolith within the lumen of the tender, tubular structure is diagnostic of appendicitis. Appendiceal abscess may be evident on computed tomographic (CT) scan as well. In early appendicitis, diagnostic accuracy is improved by laparoscopy.

  e. **Management.** If unruptured, appendectomy is performed as soon as preoperative preparation is completed. Very ill patients who are dehydrated, have abnormal serum electrolytes, marked gastric and intestinal distension, or circulatory collapse from gram-negative sepsis must be stabilized prior to appendectomy (see sec. II). (See Chap. 15 for a discussion of surgery during pregnancy.)

  2. Mesenteric lymphadenitis, diverticulitis, and inflammatory bowel disease

  a. **Clinical presentation.** Mesenteric lymphadenitis generally presents as right lower quadrant or right pelvic pain; however, the pain of diverticulitis is usually left-sided. Inflammatory bowel disease commonly presents as episodic, subacute, or chronic abdominopelvic pain and may have associated bloody diarrhea.

b. **Diagnosis.** Imaging studies of the gastrointestinal tract, sigmoidoscopy, and stool examination for the presence of blood, leukocytes, and bacteria may provide useful information.

c. Consult a **gastroenterologist for evaluation and management.**

3. **Cystitis and trigonitis**

a. **Clinical presentation.** Cystitis and trigonitis may cause lower abdominal and pelvic pain that is generally midline in nature and accompanied by dysuria, urgency, frequency, or hematuria. Acute cystitis can result in significant tenderness on pelvic examination, especially with movement of the cervix or uterus.

b. **Diagnosis** can be confirmed with urinalysis and urine cultures; **cystoscopy** may be necessary if diagnosis is uncertain or symptoms persist after antibiotic therapy.

4. **Renal colic**

a. **Clinical presentation.** Renal colic because of renal or ureteral stone may present with severe, intermittent flank pain that may radiate to the lower abdomen, groin, labia, or vagina.

b. **Diagnosis.** Hematuria and passage of a stone or gravel add useful information.

c. **Intravenous pyelography, ultrasonography, or both** are usually necessary to confirm the diagnosis.

d. **Management.** Obtain a **urologic consultation to determine whether antibiotics and operative intervention are required.**

IV. **Chronic pelvic pain (CPP)**

A. **General principles.** Chronic and recurrent pelvic pain are common problems seen by the gynecologist. Chronic pain syndrome is a complex condition that involves the patient's social relationships and physical well-being. The initial search for a cause should concentrate on distinguishing between episodic CPP and continuous CPP.

B. **Episodic CPP** is cyclic, recurrent pain that has been present for at least 6 months and is associated with pain-free intervals. Dyspareunia, mittelschmerz (midcycle pelvic pain), and dysmenorrhea are examples of episodic pelvic pain.

1. **Dyspareunia, or pain with intercourse,** may be superficial or deep.

a. **Superficial dyspareunia** is usually caused by vulvitis, bartholinitis, atrophic dystrophy, infected urethral diverticulum, vulvar vestibulitis, tender episiotomy scar, or overly corrected posterior colporrhaphy. Vaginal dyspareunia caused by vaginismus (involuntary, vaginal introital, muscle spasm), chronic vaginal infection, or inadequate lubrication may be superficial or deep.

b. **Deep dyspareunia** is commonly caused by chronic, abdominopelvic processes such as endometriosis, levator ani syndrome, chronic PID, or severe pelvic adhesions. When dyspareunia develops after hysterectomy without salpingo-oophorectomy, it may be a result of a chronically infected vaginal cuff or to adhesions of one or both ovaries to the vaginal apex.

c. **Treatment** of dyspareunia requires correction of the underlying abnormality. Treat signs of infection with broad-spectrum aerobic and anaerobic antimicrobials; inadequate lubrication may be corrected through change in sexual practices and use of a water-based commercial lubricant (e.g., K-Y Jelly, Surgilube, Replens, Astroglide) or topical estrogen therapy, if the patient is estrogen deficient. Patients with vaginismus may require dilator, lubricant, and psychiatric therapy, depending on the underlying etiology. Patients undergoing dilator therapy usually require detailed instruction and psychological support. Consult a practitioner or a sex therapist before instructing your first patient with this disorder. Surgical misadventures that result in dyspareunia usually require surgical correction.

2. **Mittelschmerz, or midcycle pelvic pain,** is usually the result of peritoneal irritation caused by release of blood or follicular fluid from the ovary at ovu-

lation. The pain is generally unilateral and lasts a few hours, but in some patients can be intense and prolonged. Immediate treatment with NSAIDs and long-term prophylactic treatment of ovarian suppression with depot medroxyprogesterone acetate or oral contraceptives (OCPs) (formulations containing at least 5 μg of ethinyl estradiol) can be used to manage this pain.

3. **Dysmenorrhea** is severe cramping in the lower abdomen with possible extension to inner thighs that may be accompanied by sweating, tachycardia, headaches, nausea, vomiting, or diarrhea. This pain is usually midline, without an adnexal component. These symptoms typically occur during the first 1 to 3 days of menses. Dysmenorrhea is defined as primary when no pathologic condition is found. Secondary dysmenorrhea is associated with pelvic pathology.

   a. **Primary dysmenorrhea** is more common in patients younger than age 20. It has a tendency to occur with menarche and usually dissipates with time. It is more commonly associated with the systemic symptoms listed above than is secondary amenorrhea. Primary dysmenorrhea rarely lasts more than 3 to 5 days. Dyspareunia is usually absent.

      (1) **Etiology.** Primary dysmenorrhea arises from myometrial contractions caused by prostaglandin $F_{2\alpha}$ originating in secretary endometrium. The majority of prostaglandin release and the greatest intensity of symptoms occur in the first 48 hours of menses. Associated systemic symptoms are explained by entry of prostaglandins and prostaglandin metabolites into the systemic circulation.

      (2) **Diagnosis** is based on characteristics of pain, timing in relation to the menstrual cycle, absence of pathology, and response to treatment. Pelvic examination in nonmenstruating patients with primary dysmenorrhea does not demonstrate any tenderness or pathologic changes.

      (3) **Management.** Mainstay treatment options are NSAIDs, OCPs, or both. NSAIDs inhibit prostaglandin synthetase.

         i. **Propionic acid derivatives** (ibuprofen, 600 to 800 mg p.o. t.i.d. or q.i.d.; naproxen, 250 to 500 mg p.o. t.i.d.; ketoprofen, 50 to 75 mg p.o. t.i.d.) and **fenamates** (mefenamic acid, 250 mg p.o. q.i.d.; meclofenamate, 50 to 100 mg p.o. q.i.d.) are very effective for treatment of dysmenorrhea. Treatment is begun at the first sign of the impeding menses or at the sign of first bleeding and is continued q6–8h for 3 to 5 days (not p.r.n.). Absolute contraindications are gastrointestinal ulcers and hypersensitivity to NSAIDs. Approximately 80% of dysmenorrheic women improve with NSAIDs. A 3- to 6-month trial with at least two different agents and strict adherence to timing is recommended before abandoning this therapy.

         ii. **Alternative treatment is OCPs,** which cause a reduction in prostaglandins by inducing an atrophic, decidualized endometrium. **Any low-dose OCP (less than 50 µg ethinyl estradiol with progestin)** is acceptable. A 70% to 80% reduction in dysmenorrhea has been found after treatment with OCPs. A trial of at least 3 months of OCPs is necessary. Advantages to OCPs include contraception and menstrual regularity. If a woman has no contraindications to NSAIDs or low-dose OCPs and does not desire pregnancy, combination therapy is suggested. Advantages of a combination of a NSAID and OCPs include (a) greater efficacy because of the two different mechanisms of action, and (b) potential for faster relief because NSAIDs should provide relief during the very first cycle.

         If the patient fails a trial of either or both therapies, further investigation should determine the cause of pain. Consider diagnostic laparoscopy and hysteroscopy. If the investigation reveals no pathology, nonroutine therapies such as GnRH agonists, calcium channel blockers, or laparoscopic uterosacral or presacral nerve transection may be considered.

b. **Secondary dysmenorrhea** is more common in women older than 20 years of age. The pain may begin just before menses and continue during and after. Dyspareunia, if present, generally is worse during menses. Women with secondary dysmenorrhea tend to experience both midline and bilateral lower quadrant abdominal pain.

   (1) **Etiology.** Causes of secondary dysmenorrhea include fibroids, endometriosis, adenomyosis, chronic pelvic infection, adhesions, pelvic venous congestion, functional ovarian cysts, intrauterine device, and venous congenital or acquired outflow tract obstruction (e.g., cervical stenosis). The pain is a direct consequence of the specific condition or pathologic process.

   (2) **Diagnosis.** The most sensitive **diagnostic study** for the diagnosis of secondary dysmenorrhea is a careful **history and physical and pelvic examination.** It is important to observe the patient's movements while carefully examining the pelvis and upper and lower abdomen. Special attention should be paid to the urethra, adnexa, uterosacral ligaments, and posterior cul-de-sac. The role of **laboratory evaluation** is very limited. Blood counts help to evaluate ongoing, excessive blood loss that might be present in patients with fibroids or adenomyosis; determination of ESR may help to identify chronic inflammation. Blood chemistries, urine analysis, and urine cultures may help identify nongynecologic causes of secondary dysmenorrhea. Although seldom necessary for diagnosis, **ultrasonography** can document significant growth of myomas or the presence of ovarian cysts. **CT scan and magnetic resonance imaging (MRI)** are seldom of assistance. **Diagnostic laparoscopy** may be required to establish a diagnosis if noninvasive diagnostic measures and trial therapies have been ineffective.

   (3) **Treatment** is directed toward correcting the identified pathologic cause.

4. **Endometriosis.** Pain is the most common single symptom of endometriosis. The incidence of endometriosis at laparoscopy for pelvic pain varies from 3.6% to 52.0%. The pain of endometriosis is usually diffuse, intermittent lower quadrant abdominal pain associated with dysmenorrhea and dyspareunia.

   a. **Diagnosis** should suspected when there is a history of chronic pain that becomes more severe with menses. Pelvic examination may reveal uterine tenderness, adnexal tenderness, or both; lack of uterine mobility; uterosacral ligament nodularity and tenderness; or evidence of endometriosis in the vagina and the cervix. The specific diagnosis of endometriosis is made by direct biopsy at the time of laparoscopy or laparotomy or by direct biopsy of vaginal or cervical lesions.

   b. **Therapy** is medical or surgical, either definitive or conservative, depending on the severity of the disease and patient's reproductive plans.

5. **Adenomyosis**

   a. **Clinical presentation.** Adenomyosis is more common in parous, reproductive-age women. Cyclical or continuous pelvic pain, dysmenorrhea, and dyspareunia are classically associated with a mildly enlarged, boggy, and tender uterus. The pain may radiate to the anterior thigh.

   b. **Pelvic examination.** The uterus is symmetrically enlarged and tender to palpation. Adenomyosis is a histological diagnosis; it is usually a diagnosis of exclusion until the patient undergoes a hysterectomy, at which time tissue is provided for diagnostic confirmation.

   c. **Treatment.** Temporary relief of pelvic pain with uterosacral and paracervical block has been proposed as a diagnostic aid. Cyclic hormonal therapy has not been shown to be of value; NSAIDs provide little relief. GnRH agonist therapy has been inadequately assessed. Definitive treatment is hysterectomy.

6. **Cervical stenosis** is severe narrowing of the cervical canal. This narrowing impedes menstrual flow, thereby causing pain from an increase in intrauter-

ine pressure. The etiology of cervical stenosis may be congenital or secondary to cervical injury (e.g., electrocautery, cryosurgery, or conization with the formation of scar tissue). Patients usually give a history of severe cramping throughout the menstrual period and scant menstrual flow. Cerebral stenosis may occur from atrophy in postmenopausal patients, but is rarely symptomatic.

    a. **Diagnosis** is documented by the inability to pass a thin, silver wire probe through the internal os.

    b. **Treatment** consists of dilating the cervix with progressive metal dilators or osmotic dilators (e.g., *Laminaria*, Dilapan). Cervical stenosis often recurs, necessitating repeat procedure.

C. Continuous CPP is noncyclic, recurrent pelvic pain that has been present for 6 months or longer. Endometriosis and adenomyosis may also cause CPP (see sec. **IV.B.4–5**). Other gynecologic causes of CPP are loss of pelvic support, chronic pelvic inflammation with presence of dense pelvic adhesions, pelvic congestion syndrome, ovarian remnant syndrome, retained ovary syndrome, and nerve entrapment .

  1. Overview

    a. **Epidemiology.** The prevalence rate of CPP is approximately 12%; the lifetime incidence rate is 33%. This syndrome has been estimated to account for approximately 10% of outpatient gynecologic consultation and is responsible for approximately one-third of laparoscopies performed. CPP is the indication for 12% to 16% of hysterectomies performed in the United States.

    b. **Diagnosis.** A thorough, complete physical examination, including specific attempts to elicit trigonal or urethral tenderness and discover abdominal wall trigger points, should be performed.

    c. **Screening laboratory tests** include a CBC, stool guaiac, urine analysis and urine culture, endocervical testing for gonorrhea and chlamydia, and cervical cytology.

    d. **Special studies,** including gastrointestinal or genitourinary endoscopy and radiographic studies and nerve blocks conducted by an anesthesiologist, are obtained as indicated.

    e. **Laparoscopy** is recommended if initial evaluation and management fail to provide significant resolution of symptoms.

  2. Chronic pelvic inflammation, pelvic adhesions, and chronic salpingitis. Chronic infection, neurovascular damage, or anatomic distortion because of adhesion formation may lead to CPP.

    a. **Pelvic examination** can reveal any combination of adnexal, cervical motion, or uterine tenderness.

    b. **Endometrial biopsy** can confirm the diagnosis of chronic endometritis. Diagnostic laparoscopy is often necessary to establish a diagnosis of pelvic adhesions or chronic infection.

    c. Although **pelvic adhesions** are the only findings in 10% to 25% (1) of **diagnostic laparoscopies** for CPP, it is unclear as to whether the adhesions are the true cause of the pain or are an incidental finding (2).

    d. **Treatment.** Medical treatment of chronic infection consists of long courses (2 to 6 weeks) of broad-spectrum oral or parenteral antibiotics, or both. Operative laparoscopy with lysis of adhesions is a reasonable initial approach for the patient with adhesions and no evidence of infection. For patients who have become debilitated secondary to pelvic pain from chronic pelvic infection or adhesions, definitive surgery (total abdominal hysterectomy and bilateral salpingo-oophorectomy) may be the only therapeutic option when laparoscopic approaches fail. If the pain recurs, repeat adhesiolysis is usually not successful; consider consultation with a multidisciplinary CPP team.

  3. Pelvic congestion syndrome is characterized by continuous, bilateral abdominopelvic pain that worsens at day's end. The pain may be accompanied by deep dyspareunia and intensified upon standing or jumping. The pain is usually described as burning or throbbing, with radiation to the sacral area and back of legs.

    a. **Physical examination** may reveal tenderness of both adnexa, uterine tenderness, uterine enlargement, and posterior fornix tenderness, without induration or masses.

    b. **Diagnostic laparoscopy** may reveal prominent, enlarged, broad ligament veins.

    c. **Treatment.** Severe cases that do not respond to counseling and NSAID therapy for pain management may respond to hysterectomy or GnRH agonists.

4. **Ovarian remnant syndrome** occurs in a patient who previously underwent bilateral oophorectomy with or without total abdominal hysterectomy. In most cases, endometriosis or PID was present at the time of initial surgery and complete adnexectomy was difficult.

    a. **Clinical presentation.** Many patients experience cyclic pelvic pain, ranging from a pressure sensation or dull aching to severe stabbing pain.

    b. **Laboratory findings.** A finding of postmenopausal levels of follicle-stimulating hormone in a reproductive-aged woman helps eliminate the diagnosis.

    c. **Imaging studies**

        (1) **Vaginal ultrasonography** after hormone stimulation may show an ovarian cyst.

        (2) **CT scan or MRI** may be useful in defining the relation of the ovarian remnant to surrounding structures.

    d. **Treatment** is adequate excision of the ovarian remnant, with removal of contiguous adherent tissue such as pelvic peritoneum, underlying infundibulopelvic ligament, and vascular tissue.

5. **Retained ovary syndrome** is pelvic pain from posthysterectomy adherence of one or both ovaries to the vaginal apex.

    a. **Diagnostic laparoscopy** may show pelvic adhesions, follicular cysts, or hemorrhagic corpus lutea involving the retained ovaries.

    b. **Treatment.** Medical treatment can be attempted with ovarian suppression (using OCP formulations containing at least 35 μg of ethinyl estradiol). Usually, reoperation is indicated for oophorectomy or ovarian suspension.

6. **Gastroenterologic causes** of CPP include irritable bowel syndrome (IBS), inflammatory bowel disease, enterocolitis, diverticulitis, intestinal obstruction, intestinal neoplasms, hernias, abdominal angina, and intestinal endometriosis. Depending on the population, these diagnoses may account for 7% to 60% of office visits for CPP (3).

    a. **Gynecologic physical examination** should evaluate the abdomen for scars, hernias, and distension. Palpation of the abdomen can demonstrate diffuse or localized tenderness, with peritoneal signs or intraabdominal masses. A comprehensive rectal examination should evaluate the perineal region, function and tenderness of internal and external anal sphincter, and the puborectalis muscles. If gastrointestinal pathology is suspected, consult a gastroenterologist.

    b. **IBS** is a common gastrointestinal disorder that can present as pelvic pain (4). The pain is crampy and usually localized to the lower abdomen. It is often improved after bowel movements and typically is of greatest severity a few hours after meals. Complaints of constipation and intermittent diarrhea are common in patients with IBS. Patients also complain of abdominal distension and a sensation of incomplete evacuation after bowel movements. Associated psychiatric symptoms are often seen.

        (1) On **physical examination** tenderness is localized over the sigmoid colon. Discomfort and finding hard feces during rectal examination are suggestive of IBS. In young women, diagnosis is usually based on the patient's history and physical examination. Older individuals or patients who have not responded to initial treatment require CBC, WBC and occult blood counts from stool, proctosigmoidoscopy, and colonoscopy or barium enema; all these test results are normal in IBS patients.

(2) Treatment of IBS consists of reassurance, education, stress reduction, and bulk-forming agents. Bulk-forming agents (e.g., Citrucel, Metamucil, or daily bran intake of 20 g) are the single most effective components of therapy. Tincture of belladonna (5 to 10 drops p.o. t.i.d. q.a.c.), hyoscyamine (0.125 mg s.l. q.p.m. or 0.375 mg p.o. b.i.d.), and dicyclomine (20 mg p.o. q.i.d.) may be helpful in controlling the loose-stool component of this disorder. Low-dose tricyclic antidepressants such as amitriptyline (10 to 50 mg p.o. q.h.s.), doxepin (10 to 50 mg p.o. q.h.s.), or desipramine (50 mg p.o. q.h.s.) (5) are helpful in patients unresponsive to the previously mentioned treatments.

c. Inflammatory bowel disease

    (1) Clinical presentation. In both Crohn's disease and ulcerative colitis, visceral pain can originate from a nonobstructed and inflamed bowel, from obstruction, or from an extension of the disease process beyond the bowel wall (perforation, fistulas, or abscess formation). Pain is associated with bloating, abdominal distension, and the sensation of incomplete evacuation after a bowel movement. Approximately 80% of patients with Crohn's disease and 50% of patients with ulcerative colitis complain of mild to moderate abdominopelvic pain. The pain may be associated with diarrhea and fever among Crohn's sufferers; patients with ulcerative colitis usually experience bloody diarrhea.

    (2) Physical examination should evaluate for perineal disease such as fistulas or abscess.

    (3) Laboratory tests. WBC and ESR are usually elevated in Crohn's disease; iron deficiency or macrocytic anemia may be present in both diseases.

    (4) Small bowel follow through to view the ileum and **colonoscopy or sigmoidoscopy** to visualize edematous mucosa and ulcers are the most important diagnostic tests for Crohn's disease.

    (5) Management. Consult a gastroenterologist.

d. Diverticulitis

    (1) Clinical presentation. Diverticulitis most commonly presents with pain in the left lower abdominal quadrant that lasts hours or days, increases with eating, and decreases with bowel movements. Crampy diarrhea, constipation, dyspepsia, and fever may also be present.

    (2) Laboratory tests. The WBC count and ESR may be elevated. The diagnosis is confirmed with an abdominal **CT scan.**

    (3) Management. Consult a gastroenterologist.

e. Carcinoma of the colon and rectum

    (1) Clinical presentation. The most common symptoms are a change in bowel habits (75%) or abdominal pain (65%).

    (2) Diagnosis. Positive stool guaiac may be present with associated anemia. The diagnosis is made with **colonoscopy,** which is approximately 12% more accurate than barium enema.

    (3) Management. Consult a gastroenterologist and a surgeon.

f. Ischemic bowel disease

    (1) Clinical presentation. The typical patient is an older woman who complains of intermittent, dull, crampy abdominal pain that occurs 15 to 30 minutes after meals and lasts up to a few hours.

    (2) Diagnosis is confirmed with angiographic study.

    (3) Management. Consult a gastroenterologist.

g. Intestinal endometriosis. Twelve percent to 37% of patients with endometriosis have colonic involvement.

    (1) Clinical presentation. Symptoms of rectal and sigmoid involvement include abdominal pain, dyspareunia, tenesmus, constipation or diarrhea, and low back pain. Symptoms do not always fluctuate with the menstrual cycle.

    (2) **Diagnosis** is made via laparoscopy.

    (3) **Treatment.** A trial of medical treatment with a GnRH agonist can be attempted, but surgical extirpation may be necessary.

  h. **Lactose intolerance** should be ruled out in younger patients through a therapeutic trial of withholding milk products.

7. **Urogynecologic causes of CPP**

  a. **General approach.** Questions regarding urinary complaints should be part of **history** taking when evaluating pelvic pain.

    (1) **Clinical presentation.** Symptoms of urinary urgency, frequency, and dysuria correlate with a chronic lower urinary tract condition. Dyspareunia may be an associated symptom.

    (2) **Physical examination** should begin with neurologic examination of the lower extremities and perineal area. A pelvic examination should begin with gentle palpation of the pelvic floor musculature to assess its tone and tenderness, followed by gentle one-hand palpation of the urethra, trigone, and bladder. A bimanual examination is performed to palpate the bladder and reproductive organs. The vagina should be examined with a Sims-type speculum or the lower half of a bivalve speculum, looking for evidence of relaxation. In postmenopausal women, the urethral meatus should be examined for its caliber and evidence of hypoestrogenism.

    (3) **Laboratory tests.** A urine analysis with culture and sensitivity should be obtained. Infections among CPP sufferers should be treated according to bacterial sensitivities. If the patient continues to experience pain, proceed with further investigation after infection has resolved. Measurement of postvoid residuals may be helpful if the patient has a history consistent with incomplete bladder emptying or incontinence. Consult a urogynecologist or urologist before further evaluation.

    (4) **Cystourethroscopy** should be performed on all patients who have irritative lower urinary tract symptoms and no evidence of infection; evidence of chronic infection and presence of diverticula or tumors may be revealed. Two of the most common but poorly understood sources of CPP of urinary origin are **chronic urethral syndrome** and **interstitial cystitis.**

  b. **Chronic urethral syndrome** (6) is a set of irritative lower urinary tract symptoms, the causes of which are still controversial (urethral infection, urethral spasm, or urethral instability).

    (1) **Clinical presentation.** Patients may present complaining of urinary urgency, frequency, dysuria, postvoid fullness, urge or stress incontinence, vulvar irritation, dyspareunia, and pelvic or vaginal pain. A history of postcoital voiding dysfunction and dyspareunia is suggestive of the syndrome.

    (2) **Pelvic examination** reveals tenderness over the urethra and bladder base and suprapubic and sometimes pubococcygeal muscle tenderness.

    (3) **Laboratory tests.** Urine should be sent for culture and sensitivity; urethral culture for chlamydia should be performed if the patient fails to respond to initial therapy.

    (4) **Cystourethroscopy.** Findings of erythema and exudate, with or without cystic glandular dilatation, are fairly consistent with chronic urethral syndrome.

    (5) **Uroflowmetry.** Prolonged flow times and intermittent flow patterns can be consistent with urethral spasm and an inability to relax the urethra.

    (6) **Treatment** consists of bladder reeducation and antimicrobials. Suppression with trimethoprim (800 mg p.o. q.d.), sulfamethoxazole (160 mg p.o. q.d.), or nitrofurantoin (100 mg p.o. q.d.) can be given for 3 to 6 months. Doxycycline (100 mg p.o. b.i.d.) may be given for 10 days if chlamydia is suspected as a source of pain. Bladder reed-

ucation is indicated when **urethral muscular spasm** is implicated as a major cause of discomfort. Skeletal muscle relaxants, such as diazepam (2 to 10 mg p.o. t.i.d. to q.i.d.) or cyclobenzaprine (10 mg p.o. t.i.d.), may be tried. Smooth muscle relaxants, such as prazosin (1 mg p.o. b.i.d. to t.i.d.) or dibenzyline (10 mg p.o. b.i.d.), can also be used (7). Vaginal estrogen cream should be used on long-term basis in postmenopausal women with evidence of hypoestrogenism.

   c. **Interstitial cystitis** is a chronic inflammatory condition of the bladder wall that results in decreased bladder capacity and compliance.

      (1) **Clinical presentation.** Patients present with diurnal *and* nocturnal urinary frequency. Patients may also experience dyspareunia.

      (2) **Laboratory tests.** Urine analysis may reveal hematuria. Infection must be ruled out with a urine culture. Urine cytology is also obtained to rule out neoplasm.

      (3) **Pelvic examination** can reveal a tender bladder base.

      (4) **Diagnosis** is based on a triad of clinical findings typically associated with interstitial cystitis:

         i. **Irritative voiding** symptoms (frequency, urgency, nocturia, suprapubic pain) that are usually relieved by voiding

         ii. **The absence of objective evidence for another disease process**

         iii. **A characteristic** cystoscopic appearance

      (5) **Cystoscopy** shows submucosal hemorrhage and petechiae, often referred to as *glomerulations*.

      (6) **Bladder biopsy** typically shows nonspecific inflammation of the submucosa and muscularis.

      (7) **Treatment.** Hydrodistention as well as behavioral modification using increased voiding intervals may provide short-term relief for some patients. Intravesical instillation of dimethyl sulfoxide provides relief through antiinflammatory and analgesic properties. Amitriptyline (25 mg p.o. b.i.d. to q.i.d.) has been shown to provide relief. Pentosanpolysulfate (Elmiron) has been approved for the treatment of interstitial cystitis. Typical dosage is 100 mg p.o. three times daily. Surgical therapies (augmentation cystoplasty, cystectomy) are a last resort.

  8. Musculoskeletal causes of CPP. The character of pain from musculoskeletal dysfunction is similar to that of gynecologic pain and is often altered by hormonal influences of menstruation and pregnancy. Treatment depends on the underlying nongynecologic disorders. Consult a neurologist or orthopedic surgeon if musculoskeletal pain does not resolve after a trial of NSAIDs, rest, and heat.

D. Chronic pain syndrome (CPS). Women with CPS often experience increased anxiety and depression for which a psychiatrist, psychologist, or social worker are often needed. CPS should be approached from the standpoint of both physical and lifestyle case management.

  1. Diagnosis is usually determined only after multiple organic causes have been evaluated and possibly treated. In general, the pain these patients experience is disproportional to any organic pathology that is found, and the intensity of the pain increases even though the patients' ongoing pathology remains constant or improves. The patient usually has multisystem symptoms. Common signs and symptoms that suggest CPS, when they occur sequentially or together, include the following:

    a. Increasing tenderness during subsequent pelvic examinations

    b. IBS

    c. Decreased libido with or without dyspareunia

    d. Chronic musculoskeletal problems without organic pathology

    e. Diminishing physical activity

    f. Signs of depression

    g. Altered family and social roles

Many women with CPS have one or all of the following:

       h. Current physical or psychological abuse
       i. History of childhood sexual, psychological, or physical abuse
       j. Genetic predisposition to depression
   2. Special management considerations. Most of these patients "doctor shop" because a "cure" is not easily found. Many of these patients develop addictions to narcotics and/or anxiolytics prescribed by unknowing physicians. Medication that is not helping the patient must be discontinued. Any controlled medications that are prescribed should be monitored closely for physical effect on the patient and patient usage (or abuse).

     These patients generally require **frequent visits** initially. Gradually taper visits as improvement occurs. It is important that the patient is regularly reminded of improvement, if improvement is occurring. This can be achieved through comparing serial pain scores and symptom questionnaires.

References

1. Stoval TG, Elder RF, Ling FW. Predictors of pelvic adhesions. *J Reprod Med* 1989;34(5):345–348.
2. Porpora MG, Gomel V. The role of laparoscopy in the management of pelvic pain in women of reproductive age. *Fertil Steril* 1997;68(5):765–779.
3. Reiter RC. A profile of women with chronic pelvic pain. *Clin Obstet Gynecol* 1990;33(1):130–136.
4. Longstretch GF. Irritable bowel syndrome: diagnosis in the managed care era. *Dig Dis Sci* 1997;42(6):1105–1111.
5. Greenbaum DS, Mayle JE, Vanegeren LE, et al. Effects of desipramine on irritable bowel syndrome compared with atropine and placebo. *Dig Dis Sci* 1987;32(3): 257–266.
6. Schmidt RA. The urethral syndrome. *Urol Clin North Am* 1985;12(2):349–354.
7. Barbaslias GA, Meares EM Jr. Female urethral syndrome: clinical and urodynamic perspectives. *Urology* 1984;23(2):208–212.

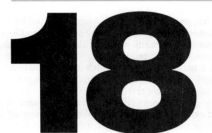

Infections of the Genital Tract

Mimi Yum and
Jeffrey Smith

I. Infections of the lower genital tract. Symptoms caused by infections of the lower genital tract are among the most common presenting complaints of gynecologic patients.

   A. Vulvar infections. Normal vulva is composed of the following: skin, with stratified squamous epithelium containing sebaceous, sweat, and apocrine glands, and underlying subcutaneous tissue, including Bartholin's glands. Vulvar itching or burning accounts for approximately 10% of gynecologic office visits.

      1. Parasites

         a. Pediculosis pubis (the "crab louse") is among the most contagious sexually transmitted diseases and is transmitted through close contact (sexual or nonsexual) or sharing of towels or sheets. It is usually restricted to vulvar areas but may infect eyelids and other body parts. The parasite deposits eggs at base of the hair follicle. The adult feeds on human blood and moves slowly.

           (1) Symptoms of infection include intense, constant itching in the pubic area caused by an allergic reaction, accompanied by macular-papular lesions on the vulva.

           (2) Diagnosis is made by gross visualization of eggs or lice in the pubic hair or microscopic identification of crab-like louse under oil.

         b. Scabies (the "itch mite") is transmitted via close contact (sexual or nonsexual) and may infect any part of the body, especially flexural surfaces of the elbows and wrists and external genitalia. The adult female burrows beneath the skin, where she lays eggs, and travels quickly across the skin.

           (1) Symptoms of infection include severe but intermittent itching. The itching may be more severe at night. It may present as papules, vesicles, or burrows. The hands, wrists, breasts, vulva, and buttocks are most commonly affected.

           (2) Diagnosis is made by microscopic examination of skin scrapings under oil.

         c. Treatment for pediculosis pubis and scabies requires an agent that kills adults and eggs.

           (1) Permethrin cream, 5% (Nix cream)

              i. Pediculosis pubis. Two applications are made 10 days apart in order to kill newly hatched eggs.

              ii. Scabies. Ten-minute applications b.i.d. for 2 days.

           (2) Gamma-benzene hexachloride, 1%, (Kwell) lotion, cream, shampoo

              i. Pediculosis pubis. Apply after showering to affected areas for 12 hours on 2 successive days.

              ii. Scabies. In adults, apply 30 mL of lotion over the entire skin surface, leaving the lotion on for 12 hours. Pruritus may persist for a couple of days and may be treated with antihistamines.

           (3) These treatments are **contraindicated** in pregnant or breast-feeding patients.

(4) Clothes and linens should be laundered in hot water and heat-dried.
2. **Molluscum contagiosum** is a benign infection by poxvirus and is spread by close sexual or nonsexual contact and autoinoculation. The incubation period ranges from several weeks to months.
   a. **Signs and symptoms** include domed papules with central umbilication, ranging from 1 to 5 mm in diameter. Up to 20 lesions may appear at one time.
   b. **Diagnosis** is made by gross inspection or microscopic examination of white, waxy material expressed from nodule. Wright or Giemsa staining for intracytoplasmic molluscum bodies confirms diagnosis.
   c. **Treatment** consists of evacuation of the white material, excision of the nodule with a dermal curet, and treatment of the base with ferric subsulfate (Monsel's solution) or 85% trichloroacetic acid. Cryotherapy with liquid nitrogen can also be used.
3. **Condyloma acuminatum (genital or venereal warts)** is an infection of the vulva, vagina, or cervix with human papillomavirus (HPV). HPV infection is the most common sexually transmitted disease and is associated with cervical, vaginal, and vulvar intraepithelial lesions, as well as squamous carcinoma and adenocarcinoma. The subtypes that cause exophytic condylomata are usually not associated with the development of carcinoma.
   a. Peak **incidence** is among 15- to 25-year-olds. Pregnant, immunosuppressed, and diabetic patients are at increased risk.
   b. **Signs and symptoms** include soft, pedunculated lesions on any mucosal or dermal surfaces that range in size and formation. Lesions are usually asymptomatic unless they are traumatized or secondarily infected, causing bleeding, pain, or both.
   c. **Diagnosis** is made primarily via gross inspection. Colposcopic examination may aid in identification of cervical or vaginal lesions. Microscopic recognition of HPV changes in biopsy specimens or Pap smears can confirm diagnosis. DNA typing may also be performed.
   d. **Treatment** consists of removing lesions if they are symptomatic or for cosmesis. There is no therapy for complete eradication of the virus.
      (1) **Podophyllin.** Paint the lesion each week for 4 to 6 weeks. Podophyllin should be washed off in 6 hours. This treatment is contraindicated in pregnant patients.
      (2) **Trichloroacetic acid,** apply every 1 to 2 weeks until lesions slough off.
      (3) **Topical 5-fluorouracil,** daily application for 7 to 10 days.
      (4) **Imiquimod cream 5%,** apply three times per week, up to 16 weeks.
      (5) **Cryotherapy, electrocautery, or laser treatment** may be used for larger lesions.
B. **Genital ulcers**
   1. **Genital herpes** is a recurrent, sexually transmitted infection by herpes simplex virus (HSV) (80% are type II) that results in genital ulcers. Infection with genital herpes has reached epidemic proportions, with an incidence in the United States of 500,000 to 2 million cases per year. The prevalence is 10 to 30 million cases per year. The incubation period is 3 to 7 days.
      a. **Signs and symptoms**
         (1) **Primary infection** may result in systemic as well as local manifestations. The patient may experience a virus-like syndrome with malaise and fever, then paresthesias of the vulva that are followed by vesicle formation. These are often multiple, resulting in shallow, painful ulcers that may coalesce. Multiple crops of vesicles and ulcers can occur in a 2- to 6-week period. The symptoms last for approximately 14 days, peaking at approximately day 7. The outbreak is self-limited, and lesions heal without scar formation. Viral shedding can continue for 2 to 3 weeks after the appearance of lesions.
         (2) **Recurrent herpetic outbreaks** are usually shorter in duration (averaging 7 days), with less severe symptoms. They are often preceded by a prodrome of itching or burning in the affected area. Systemic symptoms are usually absent. Fifty percent of infected

women experience their first recurrence within 6 months and have an average of four recurrences in the first year. Thereafter, the rate of recurrence is quite variable. Latent herpes virus resides in the dorsal root ganglia of S2, S3, and S4. Its reactivation can be triggered by some defect in the immune response—for example, pregnancy or an immunocompromised state.

   b. Complications include herpes encephalitis (rare) and infection of the urinary tract resulting in retention, severe pain, or both.

   c. Diagnosis is usually by inspection alone; however, if a definitive diagnosis is needed, a viral culture can be obtained. The vesicle should be opened, then vigorously swabbed. Sensitivity of a viral culture is approximately 90%. Immunologic or cytologic tests are not as sensitive.

   d. Treatment

   (1) **Goals** of treatment include shortening the clinical course, preventing complications, preventing recurrence, and decreasing transmission.

   (2) The virus cannot be completely eradicated.

   (3) In severe cases or immunosuppressed patients, acyclovir, i.v. 5 mg/kg q8h for 5 days, should be administered.

   (4) For primary outbreaks in outpatients, acyclovir, 200 mg p.o., is administered five times a day for five days. Treatment reduces the duration of symptoms but does not affect the latency of the virus. Topical acyclovir administered to affected areas three to four times a day can also speed healing and provide symptomatic relief. It is less effective than the oral form. For recurrences, acyclovir, 200 mg p.o., is administered five times a day for 5 days. For prophylaxis, acyclovir, 200 mg p.o. two to five times a day *or* 400 mg p.o. b.i.d., is administered.

   e. Counseling. Patients should be advised to remain abstinent from the onset of prodromal symptoms until complete reepithelialization of lesions. HSV infection may facilitate human immunodeficiency virus (HIV) infection. There is probably no association with the development of squamous intraepithelial lesion.

2. **Granuloma inguinale (donovanosis)** is a chronic, ulcerative infection of the vulva caused by *Calymmatobacterium granulomatis*, a gram-negative rod. It is extremely rare in the United States, but common in tropical countries. Granuloma inguinale is not highly contagious, usually requiring chronic exposure, but it can be transmitted via sexual contact or close nonsexual contact. The incubation period ranges from 1 to 12 weeks.

   a. Signs and symptoms begin with an asymptomatic nodule that then ulcerates, forming multiple beef-red, painless ulcers that coalesce. Destruction of the vulvar architecture is common. Minimal adenopathy may occur.

   b. Diagnosis. Microscopic examination of smears and biopsy specimens reveal pathognomonic intracytoplasmic Donovan's bodies, clusters of bacteria with a bipolar (safety pin) appearance.

   c. Treatment

   (1) **Tetracycline,** 500 mg p.o. q6h for 2 to 3 weeks or until complete clinical response seen.

   (2) **Chloramphenicol,** 500 mg p.o. t.i.d. for 21 days.

   (3) **Surgical excision** may be required if medical treatment fails.

3. **Lymphogranuloma venereum** is a chronic infection of lymphatic tissue by *Chlamydia trachomatis* (serotypes L1, L2, and L3). It is rare in the United States, with fewer than 500 cases per year, and is seen more commonly in the tropics. It infects males five times more frequently than females. The vulva is the most common site of infection in females, but the rectum, urethra, or cervix may be involved. The incubation period is 4 to 21 days.

   a. Signs and symptoms

   (1) **Primary infection** is a small (2 to 3 mm), shallow, painless ulcer that heals rapidly and spontaneously.

    (2) **The secondary phase** begins 1 to 4 weeks later and is marked by painful adenopathy in inguinal and perirectal areas that can coalesce and enlarge forming buboes. Systemic symptoms may also develop.

    (3) **The tertiary phase** is marked by the rupture and drainage of the buboes, forming sinuses. Extensive tissue damage may occur.

  b. Diagnosis is made by culture of pus or lymph node aspirate. A *Chlamydia* antibody titer of greater than 1:64 is also considered diagnostic.

  c. Centers for Disease Control and Prevention (CDC) treatment recommendation

    (1) **Doxycycline,** 100 mg p.o. b.i.d. for 21 days (at least)

    (2) **Tetracycline or erythromycin,** 500 mg p.o. q6h for 3 to 6 weeks

    (3) **Aspiration of fluctuant nodes** (*not* incision and drainage)

4. Chancroid is an acute, sexually transmitted infection caused by *Haemophilus ducreyi*. It is common in developing countries but rare in the United States. It infects males five to ten times as often as females and may facilitate transmission of HIV. Chancroids are highly contagious, but infection requires broken skin or traumatized tissue. The incubation period is 3 to 6 days.

  a. Signs and symptoms

    (1) Infection initially presents as a **small papule** that develops into a **pustule,** then ulcerates. Multiple lesions at different stages can be seen at one time. The ulcers are shallow, with ragged borders, and painful.

    (2) **Inguinal adenopathy** (usually unilateral) is seen in 50% of cases.

    (3) The recurrence rate at the same site is approximately 10%.

  b. Diagnosis is made by culture and Gram's stain (demonstrating extracellular "school of fish") of purulent exudate or lymph node aspiration.

  c. CDC recommended regimen

    (1) **Azithromycin,** 1 g p.o. (one dose)

    (2) **Erythromycin,** 500 mg p.o. q6h for 7 days

    (3) **Alternatives:** ceftriaxone, 250 mg i.m. (one dose); or trimethoprim and sulfamethoxazole (Bactrim DS), p.o. b.i.d. for 7 days; or ciprofloxacin, 500 mg p.o. b.i.d. for 3 days

5. Syphilis is a chronic disease caused by *Treponema pallidum* considered to be the great imitator of medicine (particularly before the advent of acquired immunodeficiency syndrome) because of its multitude of clinical manifestations. It is a moderately contagious disease, with 10% infectivity rate for a single sexual encounter with an infected partner. Individuals are contagious during primary and secondary stages and through the first year of the latent stage. There has been a recent increase in incidence, with as many as 40,000 persons per year becoming infected in the United States. Syphilis has a multitude of nongynecologic manifestations. The organism can penetrate skin or mucous membranes, and the incubation period is 10 to 90 days.

  Primary syphilis is characterized by a hard, painless chancre that is usually solitary and that may appear on the vulva, vagina, or cervix. Extragenital lesions may occur. The chancres heal spontaneously. Nontender regional adenopathy occurs. Lesions of the vagina or cervix resolve without recognition.

  Secondary syphilis is a systemic disease that occurs after hematogenous spread of the organism, from 6 weeks to 6 months after primary chancre. There are multiple manifestations, including the classic maculopapular rash on the palms and soles. Mucous patches and condyloma latum, large, raised gray-white lesions, may develop on the vulva. They are usually painless and may also be associated with painless adenopathy. These symptoms can resolve in 2 to 6 weeks.

  Latent-stage syphilis follows an untreated secondary stage and can last 2 to 20 years. Symptoms of secondary syphilis may recur.

  Tertiary syphilis develops in up to one-third of untreated or inadequately treated patients. The disease can affect the cardiovascular, central nervous, and musculoskeletal systems, resulting in varied disorders, such as aortic aneurysms, tabes dorsalis, generalized paresis, change in mental status, optic atrophy, gummata of skin and bones, and endarteritis.

   a. **Diagnosis** is made by screening with nonspecific serologic tests such as the VDRL and the rapid plasma reagin tests. False-positive results may be seen in 1% of patients. Biologic false-positive results, usually of low titers, may be caused by pregnancy, autoimmune disorders, chronic active hepatitis, intravenous drug use, febrile illness, immunization. Serologic tests become positive 4 to 6 weeks after exposure, usually 1 to 2 weeks after appearance of the primary chancres.

   If the nonspecific test is positive, a more specific antitreponemal test is performed such as fluorescent-labeled *Treponema* antibody absorption (FTA-ABS) or microhemagglutination assay for antibodies to *T. pallidum*.

   Dark-field microscopy of clear serum expressed from a primary or secondary syphilitic lesion is required to identify the spirochete, a very thin, elongated, spiral-shaped organism.

   b. **Treatment** recommended by the CDC is outlined in Table 18-1.

   c. **Follow-up.** After treatment of early syphilis, VDRL or rapid plasma reagent titers should be obtained every 3 months for 1 year (the tests should be run by the same laboratory). Titers should decrease by fourfold in 1 year. If not, retreatment is required. If the patient has been infected for longer than 1 year, titers should be followed for 2 years. The specific FTA-ABS test will remain positive indefinitely.

   Neurosyphilis must be ruled out in those with more than 1-year duration of disease. Cerebrospinal fluid should be tested for FTA-ABS reactivity.

C. Vaginitis is characterized by pruritus, discharge, dyspareunia, and dysuria. Odor is one of the most common complaints encountered by the gynecologist in office practice.

   The vagina is normally colonized by a number of organisms, including *Lactobacillus acidophilus*, diphtheroids, *Candida*, and other flora. Its physiologic pH is approximately 4.0, which inhibits overgrowth of pathogenic bacteria. There is also a physiologic discharge composed of bacterial flora, water, electrolytes, and vaginal and cervical epithelium. It is typically white, floccular, odorless, and seen in dependent areas of the vagina.

   Diagnosis of vaginitis usually requires microscopic examination of vaginal discharge. There are three major types, as follows:

   1. **Bacterial vaginosis (BV) (nonspecific vaginitis)** is the most common cause of vaginitis. It is generally not considered to be a sexually transmitted disease, as it has been reported in young girls and nuns who have not been sexually active. There is no single infectious agent, rather a shift in the composition of normal vaginal flora with an up to tenfold increase in anaerobic bacteria and increase in the concentration of *Gardnerella vaginalis*. There is also an associated decrease in the concentration of lactobacilli.

      a. **Signs and symptoms.** The characteristic discharge of BV is thin, homogeneous, and gray-white and has a fishy odor. The discharge can be copious and is adherent to vaginal walls on speculum examination. Vulvar or vaginal pruritus or irritation is rare.

      b. **Diagnosis** is made by the following methods:

         (1) **Microscopic identification of clue cells** (constituting more than 20%) on a wet smear. Clue cells are vaginal epithelial cells with clusters of bacteria adhering to the cell membrane, creating a stippled appearance. Few inflammatory cells or lactobacilli should be noted.

         (2) **The pH of the discharge** should be equal to or greater than 4.5.

         (3) **Positive "whiff" test,** which means that an aminelike (or fishy) odor is released with the addition of potassium hydroxide (KOH) solution (10% to 20%) to the discharge.

         (4) **Erythema of the vagina** is rare.

Table 18-1. Centers for Disease Control 1993 recommended treatment of syphilis

1. Primary and secondary syphilis
   Recommended regimen
   > Benzathine penicillin G, 2.4 million units i.m. in a single dose

   Penicillin allergy (nonpregnant)
   > Doxycycline, 100 mg p.o. two times/day for 2 wk
   > *or*
   > Tetracycline, 500 mg p.o. four times/day for 2 wk
   > *or*
   > Erythromycin, 500 mg p.o. four times/day for 2 wk

2. Latent syphilis
   Recommended regimens
   > Early latent syphilis (<1 yr)
   > > Benzathine penicillin G, 2.4 million units i.m. in a single dose
   > Late latent syphilis (>1 yr)
   > > Benzathine penicillin G, 7.2 million units total, administered as three doses of 2.4 million units i.m. each, at 1-wk intervals

   Penicillin allergy (nonpregnant)
   > Doxycycline, 100 mg p.o. two times/day
   > *or*
   > Tetracycline, 500 mg p.o. four times/day

   Both drugs administered for 2 wk in duration <1 yr, otherwise 4 wk

3. Late syphilis
   Recommended regimen (without neurosyphilis)
   > Benzathine penicillin G, 7.2 million units total, administered as three doses of 2.4 million units i.m., at 1-wk intervals

   Penicillin allergy
   > Same as for late latent syphilis

4. Neurosyphilis
   Recommended regimen
   > 12–24 million units aqueous crystalline penicillin G daily, administered as 2–4 million units i.v. every 4 hr, for 10–14 days

   Alternate regimen (if compliance assured)
   > 2.4 million units procaine penicillin i.m. daily, plus probenecid, 500 mg p.o. four times/day, both for 10–14 days

5. Syphilis during pregnancy
   Recommended regimens
   > Penicillin regimen appropriate for the pregnant woman's stage of syphilis. Some experts recommend additional therapy (e.g., a second dose of benzathine penicillin, 2.4 million units i.m.) 1 week after the initial dose, particularly for women in the third trimester and for those who have secondary syphilis during pregnancy

   Penicillin allergy
   > A pregnant woman with a history of penicillin allergy should be treated with penicillin after desensitization.

6. Syphilis among human immunodeficiency virus–infected patients
   Primary and secondary syphilis
   > Recommended benzathine penicillin 2.4 million units i.m. Some experts recommend additional treatments such as multiple doses of benzathine penicillin G,

(continued)

Table 18-1. (continued)

as in late syphilis. Penicillin-allergic patients should be desensitized and treated with penicillin

Latent syphilis (normal cerebrospinal fluid examination)

Benzathine penicillin G, 7.2 million units as three weekly doses of 2.4 million units each

From Centers for Disease Control. 1993 sexually transmitted diseases treatment guidelines. *MMWR Morb Mortal Wkly Rep* 1993;42:27–46. Reprinted with permission.

   c. Treatment
      (1) Metronidazole (Flagyl), 500 mg p.o. b.i.d. for 7 days
      (2) Metronidazole (Metrogel), per vagina b.i.d. for 5 days
      (3) Clindamycin 2% cream, per vagina once a day for 7 days
2. *Trichomonas* **infection** is sexually transmitted infection by protozoa *Trichomonas vaginalis.* It accounts for approximately 25% of infectious vaginitis. *Trichomonas* is a hardy organism, able to survive on wet towels and other surfaces. Its incubation period ranges from 4 to 28 days.
   a. Signs and symptoms may vary greatly. The classic discharge is frothy, thin, malodorous, and copious. It may be gray, white, or yellow-green. There may be erythema or edema of the vulva and vagina. The cervix may also appear erythematous and friable.
   b. Diagnosis
      (1) A wet-slide preparation reveals the unicellular fusiform protozoon, which is slightly larger than a white blood cell. It is flagellated, and motion can be observed in the specimen. Many inflammatory cells are usually present.
      (2) The vaginal discharge should have a pH of 5.0 to 7.0.
      (3) Asymptomatic patients who are infected may first be recognized with detection of *Trichomonas* on a Pap smear.
   c. Treatment consists of metronidazole, 2 g p.o. (one dose). The patient's sex partner should be treated as well.
3. **Candidal vaginitis** is not a sexually transmitted infection, as *Candida* is a normal vaginal inhabitant in up to 25% of women and is found in the rectum and oral cavity at an even greater percentage. *Candida albicans* is the pathogen in 80% to 95% of cases of vulvovaginal candidiasis, with *C. glabrata* and *C. tropicalis* accounting for the remainder. Risk factors for infection include immunosuppression, diabetes mellitus, hormonal changes (e.g., pregnancy), broad-spectrum antibiotic therapy, and obesity.
   a. Signs and symptoms. The severity of symptoms does not correlate with the number of organisms. The predominant symptom is pruritus, which is often accompanied by vaginal irritation, dysuria, or both. The classic vaginal discharge is white, curdlike, and without an odor. Speculum examination often reveals erythema of the vulva and vaginal walls, sometimes with adherent plaques.
   b. Diagnosis is made when a KOH preparation of the vaginal discharge reveals hyphae and buds (a 10% to 20% solution of KOH causes lysis of red and white blood cells, facilitating identification of the fungus). The clinician may need to view many fields in order to find the pathogen. A negative KOH preparation does not necessarily rule out the infection. The patient can be treated based on the clinical picture. A culture can be obtained with results made available within 24 to 72 hours.
   c. Treatment consists of topical application of an imidazole or triazole, such as miconazole, clotrimazole, butoconazole, or terconazole. These drugs can be prescribed as a cream, suppository, or both. Duration of therapy varies with the medication selected. A single dose of fluconazole (Diflucan), 150 mg p.o. (one dose), has a high efficacy rate.

D. **Cervicitis** is characterized by a severe inflammation of the mucosa and submucosa of the cervix. Histologically, one may see infiltration by acute inflammatory cells as well as occasional necrosis of the epithelial cells. The primary pathogens of mucopurulent cervicitis are *C. trachomatis* and *Neisseria gonorrhoeae*, both of which are transmitted sexually. Mucopurulent cervicitis can be diagnosed by gross inspection. A Gram's stain can be used to confirm the diagnosis.

1. *C. trachomatis* is the most common sexually transmitted organism in the United States.
   a. **Demographics.** There are approximately 4 million new infections per year. The prevalence of chlamydial cervicitis is approximately 3% to 5%, but may be as high as 15% to 30% in some populations. Approximately 20% to 40% of sexually active women have positive microimmunofluorescent *Chlamydia* antibody titers. Risk factors include age younger than 24 years, low socioeconomic status, multiple sex partners, and unmarried status.
   b. **Microbiology.** *C. trachomatis* is an obligatory intracellular organism that preferentially infects the squamocolumnar cells, thus the transition zone of the cervix.
   c. **Signs and symptoms.** Chlamydial infection is asymptomatic in 30% to 50% of cases and may persist for several years. Patients with cervicitis may complain of vaginal discharge or spotting or postcoital bleeding. On examination, the cervix may appear eroded and friable. A yellow-green mucopurulent discharge may be present. A Gram's stain should reveal more than 10 polymorphonuclear leukocytes per oil immersion field.
   d. **Diagnosis** by culture is the optimal test. Culture should be obtained by swabbing the endocervix. The synthetic swab should be rotated for 15 to 20 seconds to ensure obtaining epithelial cells. Sensitivity is approximately 75%.

   A rapid slide test (monoclonal antibody test) provides quicker, cheaper results. This test has a sensitivity of 86% to 93% and a specificity of 93% to 99%.

   DNA probe tests are currently being developed.
   e. **CDC treatment recommendations**
      (1) **Doxycycline,** 100 mg p.o. b.i.d. for 7 days
      (2) **Azithromycin,** 1 g p.o. (one dose)
         Alternative regimen
      (3) **Ofloxacin,** 300 mg p.o. b.i.d. for 7 days
      (4) **Erythromycin base,** 500 mg p.o. q.i.d. for 7 days
      (5) **Erythromycin ethylsuccinate,** 800 mg q.i.d. for 7 days
      (6) **Sulfisoxazole,** 500 mg p.o. q.i.d. for 10 days

   Sex partners should be referred to a clinic or physician for treatment. A test of cure is necessary only in pregnant patients or if symptoms persist.

2. Gonorrhea
   a. **Microbiology.** *N. gonorrhoeae* is a gram-negative diplococcus that infects columnar or pseudostratified epithelium; thus, the urogenital tract is a common site of infection. Pharyngeal and disseminated gonorrhea are other manifestations of this infection. The incubation period is 3 to 5 days.
   b. **Demographics.** The number of reported infections dropped as of 1975, but have since risen again to epidemic levels. The age group most affected is 15- to 19-year-olds, constituting 80% of infections. Prevalence ranges from 1% to 2% to as high as 25% in some populations. Risk factors are essentially the same as those for *Chlamydia* cervicitis. Although the incidence of gonorrhea in the total population is higher in males by a ratio of 1.5 to 1, the risk of transmission from male to female is 80% to 90%, whereas the risk of transmission from female to male is approximately 25%.
   c. **Signs and symptoms.** As with chlamydial infections, patients are often asymptomatic; however, they may present with vaginal discharge, dysuria, or abnormal uterine bleeding.

    d. Diagnosis. Culture with selective medium is the best test for gonorrhea. A sterile cotton swab is inserted into the endocervical canal for 15 to 30 seconds; the specimen is then plated on the medium. Culturettes may also be used but may be associated with decreased sensitivity. A Gram's stain demonstrating intracellular diplococci is diagnostic, but sensitivity is only about 60%.

    e. CDC treatment recommendations

        (1) **Ceftriaxone,** 125 mg i.m. (one dose)

        (2) **Cefixime,** 400 mg p.o. (one dose)

        (3) **Ciprofloxacin,** 500 mg p.o. (one dose)

        (4) **Ofloxacin,** 400 mg p.o. (one dose)

        Because coinfection with chlamydia is common, the patient should also be treated for chlamydia, and sex partners should be referred for treatment.

E. Urinary tract infection (UTI). Infections of the lower urinary tract (urethra and bladder) are experienced by 10% to 20% of adult women per year. Females are more susceptible because of the shorter urethral tract and the colonization of distal urethra by bacteria from the vulvar vestibule. UTIs are characterized by dysuria, urinary frequency, and urinary urgency and possible suprapubic tenderness. Findings include acute bacterial cystitis of more than 10^5 organisms per mL. The most common pathogens are *Escherichia coli* and *Staphylococcus saprophyticus.*

    1. Diagnosis. A clean-catch, midstream urine specimen should be obtained for microscopic examination, culture, and sensitivities (culture or refrigerate within 2 hours of obtaining specimen). The gold standard for diagnosis is more than 10^5 organisms per mL; however, as few as 10^2 organisms per mL can confirm cystitis. A pelvic examination should be performed to rule out vulvovaginitis, cervicitis, and other causes.

    2. Treatment

        a. Single-dose regimen: Bactrim DS

        b. Three-day regimen: Bactrim DS, b.i.d.; nitrofurantoin, 100 mg q6h; ciprofloxacin, 250 mg b.i.d.

        c. Seven- to 14-day regimen is used with the above antibiotics in patients who are pregnant, who are immunosuppressed, who are diabetic, who have anatomic abnormalities, or who have failed previous therapy.

    3. Prevention. For women with recurrent postcoital UTI, postcoital prophylactic antibiotics and voiding immediately after intercourse may be recommended. Drinking cranberry juice has been shown to decrease the incidence of recurrent UTIs.

II. Infections of the upper genital tract

A. Endometritis (nonpuerperal)

    1. Pathophysiology. This disease is caused by the ascension of pathogens from the cervix to the endometrium. Pathogens include *C. trachomatis, N. gonorrhoeae, Streptococcus agalactiae,* cytomegalovirus, HSV, and *Mycoplasma hominis.* Organisms that produce bacterial vaginosis may also produce histologic endometritis, even in women without symptoms. Endometritis is also an important component of pelvic inflammatory disease (PID) and may be an intermediate stage in the spread of infection to the fallopian tubes.

    2. Signs and symptoms

        a. Chronic endometritis. Many women with chronic endometritis are **asymptomatic.** The classic symptom of chronic endometritis is **intermenstrual vaginal bleeding.** Postcoital bleeding and menorrhagia may also be present. Other women may complain of a dull, constant lower abdominal pain. Chronic endometritis is a rare cause of infertility.

        b. Acute endometritis. When endometritis coexists with acute PID, **uterine tenderness** is common. It is difficult to determine whether inflammation of the oviducts or of the endometrium produces the pelvic discomfort.

    3. Diagnosis. The diagnosis of chronic endometritis is established by endometrial biopsy and culture. The classic histologic findings of chronic endometritis are an inflammatory reaction of monocytes and plasma cells in the endometrial stroma (five plasma cells per high-power field). There is no correlation between the presence of small numbers of polymorphonuclear leukocytes and chronic endometritis. A diffuse pattern of inflammatory infiltrates of lymphocytes and plasma cells throughout the endometrial stroma is associated with severe cases of endometritis. This may even be associated with stromal necrosis.

4. **Treatment.** The treatment of choice for chronic endometritis is doxycycline, 100 mg p.o. twice daily for 10 days. Broader coverage of anaerobic organisms may be considered, especially in the presence of bacterial vaginosis. When associated with acute PID, treatment should focus on the major etiologic organisms including *N. gonorrhoeae* and *C. trachomatis* as well as broader polymicrobial coverage.

B. **Pelvic inflammatory disease** is an infection of the upper genital tract. The disease process may include the endometrium, fallopian tubes, ovaries, myometrium, parametria, and pelvic peritoneum. It is the most significant and one of the most common complications of sexually transmitted infection.

1. **Demographics.** Approximately 1 million patients are treated for PID annually, of which 250,000 to 300,000 are hospitalized and 150,000 undergo a surgical procedure for a complication of PID. PID is the most common serious infection of women aged 16 to 25.

There has been a rise in the incidence of PID in the past 2 to 3 decades resulting from a number of factors, including more liberal social mores, increasing incidences of sexually transmitted pathogens such as *C. trachomatis*, and more widespread use of nonbarrier contraceptive methods such as the intrauterine device (IUD).

Approximately 15% of cases of PID occur following procedures such as endometrial biopsy, curettage, hysteroscopy, and IUD insertion. Eighty-five percent of cases occur as spontaneous infections in reproductive age women who are sexually active.

2. **Pathophysiology and microbiology.** Like endometritis, PID is caused by the spread of infection via the cervix. Although PID is associated with sexually transmitted infections of the lower tract, it is a polymicrobial process.

One theory of the pathophysiology is that a sexually transmitted organism such as *N. gonorrhoeae* or *C. trachomatis* initiates an acute inflammatory process that causes tissue damage, thereby allowing access by other organisms from the vagina or cervix to the upper genital tract.

Menstrual flow may facilitate infection of the upper tract by causing loss of cervical mucous plug, causing loss of the endometrial lining with its possible protective effects, and providing a good culture medium (menstrual blood) for bacteria.

A positive endocervical culture for a particular pathogen does not necessarily correlate with positive intraabdominal cultures.

Isolates obtained directly from the upper genital tract include a variety of bacteria, including *C. trachomatis, N.gonorrhoeae*, and multiple other aerobic and anaerobic bacteria (Table 18-2).

3. **Prevention.** Emphasis must be placed on aggressive treatment for lower genital tract infection and early aggressive treatment of upper genital tract infection. This will help reduce the incidence of long-term sequelae. Treatment of sexual partners and education are important in reducing the rate of recurrent infections.

Both clinical and laboratory studies have shown that the use of contraceptives changes the relative risk of developing PID.

Barrier methods of contraception provide both a mechanical obstruction and a chemical barrier. Nonoxynol 9, the chemical used in spermicidal preparations, is lethal to both bacteria and viruses.

Oral contraceptive use is associated with a lower incidence of PID and with a milder course of infection when it does occur. The protective effect is unclear but may be related to change in cervical mucus consistency, shorter menses, or atrophy of the endometrium.

4. **Risk factors**
   a. **Previous history of PID**

Table 18-2. Microorganisms isolated from the fallopian tubes of patients with pelvic inflammatory disease

Type of agent	Organism
Sexually transmitted disease	*Chlamydia trachomatis*
	Neisseria gonorrhoeae
	Mycoplasma hominis
Endogenous agent, aerobic or facultative	*Streptococcus* species
	Staphylococcus species
	Haemophilus species
	Escherichia coli
Anaerobic	*Bacteroides* species
	Peptococcus species
	Peptostreptococcus species
	Clostridium species
	Actinomyces species

From Weström L. Introductory address: treatment of pelvic inflammatory disease in view of etiology and risk factors. *Sex Transm Dis* 1984;11(4 suppl):437–440. Reprinted with permission.

    b. Multiple sex partners, defined as more than two partners in 30 days (Increased risk is not seen with serial monogamy.)

    c. Infection by a sexually transmitted organism. Fifteen percent of patients with uncomplicated anogenital gonorrhea will develop PID at the end of or just after menses.

    d. Use of an IUD can increase the risk of PID three to five times. The greatest risk for PID occurs at the time of insertion of the IUD and in the first 3 weeks after placement.

  5. Signs and symptoms. The most common presenting symptom is abdominopelvic pain. Other complaints are variable, including vaginal discharge or bleeding, fever and chills, nausea, and dysuria. Fever is seen in 60% to 80% of patients.

  6. Diagnosis of PID is difficult because the presenting signs and symptoms vary widely. In patients with cervical, uterine, and adnexal tenderness, PID is accurately diagnosed only about 65% of the time. Because of the sequelae of PID, especially infertility and chronic pelvic pain, PID should be suspected in at-risk women and treated aggressively. Diagnostic criteria outlined by the CDC help improve the accuracy of the diagnosis and the appropriateness of treatment.

    a. Minimum criteria for clinical diagnosis (all three should be present) are as follows:

      (1) Lower abdominal tenderness

      (2) Cervical motion tenderness

      (3) Adnexal tenderness

    b. Additional criteria for a diagnosis. Routine criteria are simple procedures that support and/or confirm the presence of an acute inflammatory process. Elaborate criteria should be reserved for clinical situations where the patient presents with more severe clinical findings and where other serious diagnoses must be ruled out.

      (1) Routine

        i. Oral temperature >38.3°C

        ii. Abnormal cervical or vaginal discharge

        iii. Elevated erythrocyte sedimentation rate, C-reactive protein, or both

        iv. Laboratory documentation of cervical infection with *N. gonorrheae* or *C. trachomatis*

(2) Elaborate
  i. Histopathologic evidence of endometritis
  ii. Tubo-ovarian abscess on sonography or other imaging study
  iii. Laparoscopy
7. Treatment for PID should have as its goal prevention of tubal damage that leads to infertility and ectopic pregnancy and prevention of chronic infection. Many patients can be successfully treated as outpatients and early ambulatory treatment should be the initial therapeutic approach. Antibiotic choice should target the major etiologic organisms (*N. gonorrheae* and *C. trachomatis*), but should also address the polymicrobial nature of the disease. The CDC recommendations for outpatient management of the disease include the following two regimens:
  a. Regimen A. Cefoxitin, 2 g i.m., plus probenecid, 1 g p.o. in a single dose concurrently; or ceftriaxone, 250 mg i.m., or other parenteral third-generation cephalosporin (e.g., ceftizoxime or cefotaxime), plus doxycycline, 100 mg p.o. two times a day for 14 days.
  b. Regimen B. Ofloxacin, 400 mg p.o. two times a day for 14 days, plus either clindamycin, 450 mg p.o. four times a day, or metronidazole, 500 mg p.o. two times a day for 14 days.
  Patients treated with an outpatient regimen should be reevaluated in 48 hours to assess the success of treatment.
  c. Criteria for hospitalization of patients with acute pelvic inflammatory disease include:
    (1) Suspected pelvic or tuboovarian abscess
    (2) Pregnancy
    (3) Temperature >38°C
    (4) Uncertain diagnosis
    (5) Nausea and vomiting precluding oral medications
    (6) Upper peritoneal signs
    (7) Failure to respond to oral antibiotics within 48 hours
    (8) Adolescents
    Conservative practitioners may consider hospital admission for all cases of acute PID, especially in nulligravidas or patients thought to be unable to adhere to the outpatient regimen.
  d. The CDC recommended **treatment schedules for inpatient treatment** are as follows:
    (1) Cefoxitin, 2 g i.v. every 6 hours, or cefotetan, 2 g i.v. every 12 hours, plus doxycycline, 100 mg every 12 hours p.o. or i.v. After discharge from the hospital, continue doxycycline, 100 mg p.o. twice a day for a total of 14 days.
    (2) Clindamycin, 900 mg i.v. every 8 hours, plus gentamicin, loading dose i.v. or i.m. (2 mg/kg) followed by maintenance dose (1.5 mg/kg) every 8 hours. After discharge from the hospital, continue doxycycline, 100 mg p.o. twice a day for 14 days total, or clindamycin, 450 mg p.o. five times daily for 10 to 14 days. The regimen should be continued for at least 48 hours after the patient improves. Patients should be discharged on an oral regimen and followed up as outpatients after approximately 7 days.
8. Sequelae. Approximately 25% of PID patients experience long-term sequelae. Infertility affects up to 20%. Women with a history of PID have a six to ten times higher risk for ectopic pregnancy. Chronic pelvic pain and dyspareunia have been reported.
  Fitz-Hugh–Curtis syndrome is the development of fibrous perihepatic adhesions resulting from the inflammatory process of PID. This can cause acute right upper quadrant pain and tenderness.

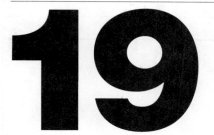

Fertility Control

Carolyn Donovan,
Pamela Cailliau,
Paul Blumenthal, and
Vanessa Cullins

I. Contraception

A. Natural method (the rhythm method). With this method, a couple voluntarily avoids or interrupts sexual intercourse during the fertile phase of the woman's cycle. This method is appropriate for women who are unable to use other methods, those with regular menstrual cycles, or those with religious or philosophical beliefs that prevent them from using other contraception methods.

1. **The menstrual cycle** is divided into three phases for purposes of assessing the likelihood of conception.
   a. **Phase I (relatively infertile phase)** lasts from onset of menstruation until the time of preovulation.
   b. **Phase II (fertile phase)** lasts from several days preovulation to 48 hours postovulation.
   c. **Phase III (absolutely infertile phase)** lasts from 48 hours after ovulation until the onset of menstrual bleeding, about 10 to 16 days.
2. **Methods for determining the phase of the cycle**
   a. **Testing cervical mucus.** During phases I and III, the mucus is scant, thick, and tacky, and breaks quickly when stretched. During phase II, the mucus is more abundant, thick, and clear, and stretches easily.
   b. **Measuring basal body temperature.** Basal body temperature should be measured in the morning. A sustained temperature rise of 0.2° to 0.6°C indicates that ovulation has occurred. The postovulatory infertile period begins the morning of the third sustained temperature rise until the onset of menstrual bleeding.
3. **Advantages.** There are no physical side effects. The method is economical, there is an immediate return to fertility on cessation of the method, and there are no method-related health risks.
4. **Disadvantages.** There is a high failure rate (pregnancy rate of 10 to 30 per 100 women per year). The method offers no protection against sexually transmitted diseases (STDs), including hepatitis B virus (HBV) and human immunodeficiency virus (HIV), and it inhibits spontaneity.

B. Barrier methods and their usage are shown in Fig. 19-1.

1. **Condoms**
   a. **Types** of condoms include latex (plain or treated with spermicide), vinyl, and natural. The spermicide will immobilize or kill sperm, providing added protection if breakage or leakage occurs.
   b. **Directions for use.** The condom should be applied before vaginal penetration and should cover the entire length of the erect penis. It should not be applied tightly (a reservoir should be left to retain the ejaculate). Adequate lubrication should be used, and the condom should be removed immediately after ejaculation and disposed of properly.
   c. **Condom use is appropriate** for all women especially those with more than one sex partner, even if using another method, and for those at risk for STDs.

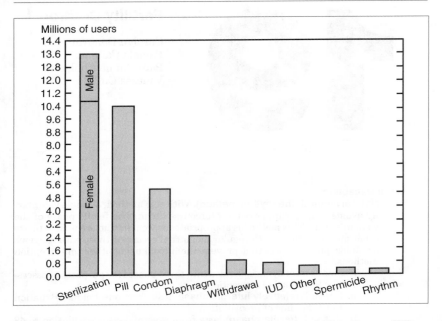

Figure 19-1. Contraceptive methods used in 1989 by women aged 15 to 44 years. IUD, intrauterine device. (From Cunningham GF, MacDonald PC, Gant NF, Leveno KJ, Gilstrap LC. *Williams obstetrics,* 19th ed. Norwalk, CT: Appleton & Lange, 1993. Reproduced with permission.)

    d. Advantages. There are no method-related health risks. Condoms are fairly effective in preventing pregnancy if used properly, and they are the only contraceptive method that provides protection against STDs.

    e. Disadvantages. Condoms have a high failure rate (pregnancy rate of 3 to 15 per 100 women per year), and only synthetic condoms protect against HBV and HIV. If either partner has a latex allergy, a nonlatex (e.g., natural, vinyl) product should be used.

  2. A diaphragm is a dome-shaped rubber cup attached to a flexible ring that is inserted into the vagina (spermicide is applied to the inside of the rubber cup) and prevents sperm from entering the upper reproductive tract. Diaphragms are most appropriate for women who want a user-controlled method, cannot or do not want to use a hormonal method, are at risk for STDs, and who have infrequent sex. Diaphragms may be used by breast-feeding mothers.

    a. Types of diaphragms include flat spring, coil spring, and arching spring.

    b. Fitting. The diaphragm should lie just posterior to the symphysis pubis and deep into the cul-de-sac so that the cervix is completely covered and behind the center of the membrane (Fig. 19-2). The largest diaphragm that fills this space comfortably should be selected. If the diaphragm is too small, there is an increased possibility of pregnancy. A diaphragm that is too large may produce vaginal pain, ulceration, and urinary tract infections.

    c. Instructions for use. Spermicide should be applied before each coital act; each application of spermicide is effective for only 1 to 2 hours. The diaphragm should be left in place for a minimum of 8 hours after the last coital act.

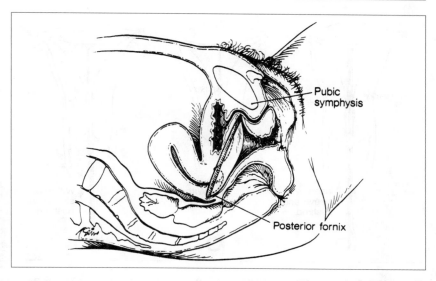

Figure 19-2. A diaphragm in place creates a physical barrier between the vagina and cervix and importantly provides for intimate contact between the contraceptive jelly or cream and the cervix. (From Cunningham GF, MacDonald PC, Gant NF, Leveno KJ, Gilstrap LC. *Williams obstetrics*, 19th ed. Norwalk, CT: Appleton & Lange, 1993. Reproduced with permission.)

      d. Advantages. There are no method-related health risks. A diaphragm is effective in preventing pregnancy if used properly and provides some protection against STDs (additional protection is provided if used in combination with spermicide). There is also a decreased risk of cervical cancer, compared with women not using any contraceptive method.

      e. Disadvantages. There is high failure rate (pregnancy rate of 5 to 20 per 100 women per year). There is a slight risk of toxic shock syndrome (when the diaphragm is used properly, the risk is very low) and an increased risk of urinary tract infections (caused by the mechanical obstruction of the egress of urine). The diaphragm requires initial fitting.

      f. Precautions. Women with uterine prolapse, cystocele, rectocele, or structural abnormalities of the reproductive tract (uterine malposition) must ensure that the diaphragm remains properly positioned during use. It may not be an appropriate method if the anatomical defect is such that the device will not remain in position.

   3. A cervical cap is also a dome-shaped cap that fits over the cervix.

      a. Conditions requiring caution. A cervical cap cannot be left on the cervix for longer than 48 hours. Only women with a normal Pap smear are candidates for use. It is recommended that women who use cervical caps have a repeat Pap smear 3 months after initiating use.

      b. Failure rates with the cervical cap are 8 to 20 per 100 women per year.

   4. Spermicides are agents that cause destruction of the sperm cell membrane, thereby affecting mobility.

      a. Types of spermicides include aerosol foams, creams, vaginal suppositories, jellies, films, and sponges. All contain a spermicidal agent, usually nonoxynol 9.

      b. Advantages. There are no method-related health risks or systemic side effects. Spermicide serves as a lubricant and also provides some pro-

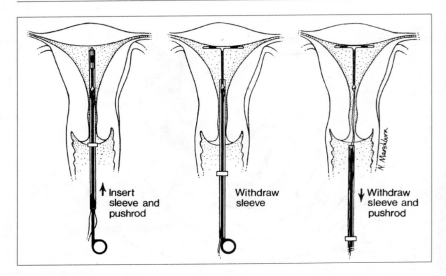

Figure 19-3. Insertion of Copper T380A using the withdrawal technique. (From Cunningham GF, MacDonald PC, Gant NF, Leveno KJ, Gilstrap LC. *Williams obstetrics,* 19th ed. Norwalk, CT: Appleton & Lange, 1993. Reproduced with permission.)

tection against STDs. The risk for cervical neoplasia is decreased compared with nonusers (as a result of the antiviral activity of spermicide).

   c. Disadvantages of spermicides include a high failure rate (first-year pregnancy rate of 10 to 25 per 100 women per year) and effectiveness for only 1 to 2 hours.

C. Intrauterine devices (IUDs) are flexible plastic devices sometimes medicated with metal or a slowly released hormone. Copper-releasing devices interfere with the ability of the sperm to pass through the uterine cavity; progestin-releasing devices thicken the cervical mucus and thin the endometrial lining. In general, modern IUDs work by preventing fertilization or conception.

   1. Types include copper-containing (Copper T380A, Nova T, Multiload 375) and hormone-releasing (Progestasert and LevoNova/Mirena) IUDs.

   2. Insertion. Figure 19-3 shows insertion of a Copper T380A IUD. Insertion and removal of an IUD is safe and easy when properly performed by a trained provider.

   3. Advantages. IUDs are highly effective at preventing pregnancy (pregnancy rate of 0.3 to 1.0 per 100 women per year) and immediately effective after insertion. Long-term protection is provided with copper IUDs (up to 8 years). IUDs can be used for emergency postcoital contraception (the inflammatory response of the endometrium probably prevents implantation), and they do not affect breast-feeding.

   4. Disadvantages. Among properly counselled and selected users, the risk of pelvic inflammatory disease (PID) is minimally increased compared with risk for non-IUD users. Most of the slight observed increased risk is associated with insertion or removal. The IUD string must be checked after every period. Dysmenorrhea and menorrhagia frequently occur within the first few months after device insertion. IUDs offer no protection against STDs.

   5. Conditions requiring caution. The IUD should not be used if pregnancy is suspected, if there is current pelvic infection or a recent history of PID or purulent cervicitis. IUDs should also not be used if there is unexplained vaginal bleeding or suspicion of pelvic malignancy. Women with more than one sex partner, or immunocompromised women should consider another method because of the increased risk of infection.

6. **Side effects** include cramping and abnormal menstrual bleeding (irregular or heavy).

7. **Complications** include uterine and pelvic infection (PID, actinomycosis), expulsion, uterine perforation, and ectopic pregnancy.

D. **Hormonal contraceptives**

1. **Combined oral contraceptives (COCs)** consist of synthetic estrogen and progestin preparations and cause suppressed ovulation, thickening of cervical mucus, and alteration of endometrium (Table 19-1). COCs are appropriate for most women, especially those with a history of anemia, dysmenorrhea, menorrhagia, metrorrhagia, or ectopic pregnancy, and for breast-feeding mothers after 6 months postpartum.

   a. **Advantages.** COCs are highly effective (first-year pregnancy rate of 1 to 3 per 100 women per year) and offer protection against ovarian and endometrial cancer and some causes of PID. Periods are lighter, shorter, and regular, with fewer menstrual cramps. Benign breast disease, ectopic pregnancy, and iron-deficiency anemia are also reduced.

   b. **Disadvantages.** COCs have rare but serious side effects in some women and offer no protection against HBV, HIV, or other STDs. Contraceptive effectiveness is decreased when COCs are taken with certain medications (rifampin, carbamazepine, phenytoin, barbiturates). They must be taken every day.

   c. **Conditions requiring caution.** Women with the following conditions should not use COCs: known pregnancy, heavy smoker older than 35 years [increased risk of myocardial infarct (MI) and cerebrovascular accident (CVA), and acute thrombophlebitis], history of thromboembolic or vascular disorders, deep vein thrombophlebitis, pulmonary embolus, coronary artery disease, angina, congestive heart failure, MI, history of breast cancer, jaundice, active liver disease, or benign or malignant liver tumors.

   d. **Risk factors.** If any two of the following are present, avoid this method of contraception: age older than 35 years, smoker, hypertension (blood pressure of more than 160/90 mm Hg), diabetes mellitus, first-degree relative with a history of MI or CVA at younger than 50 years.

   e. **Side effects and how to treat them**

      (1) **Amenorrhea.** Rule out pregnancy. If the patient is not pregnant and taking the pills correctly, reassure the patient and consider raising the estrogen dose and/or decreasing the progestin dose.

      (2) **Breast fullness or tenderness.** Confirm the absence of breast disease by examination and mammography if necessary. If not resolved after 3 months on COCs, consider switching to lower dose formulation or another method of contraception.

      (3) **Depression, severe vascular headache, or migraine (frequently associated with nausea).** Discontinue the pills and use another method.

      (4) **Hypertension.** If hypertension is a result of COC use, consider switching the patient to progestin-only pills or nonhormonal contraception. Check the patient's blood pressure on visits. If the systolic pressure is more than 160 mm Hg on two visits, discontinue the pills. If the diastolic pressure is more than 110 mm Hg on one visit or more than 90 mm Hg on three visits, discontinue the pills. Have the patient eliminate caffeine from the diet. If hypertension persists, change contraceptive method.

      (5) **Spotting or intermenstrual bleeding.** Reassure the patient that spotting or intermenstrual bleeding usually decreases by the fourth month of use. Consider increasing the estrogen dose (to 50 μg ethinyl estradiol) for several cycles until spotting resolves, then return to lower dose. If spotting returns, continue with a higher estrogen dose. Alternatively, consider lowering progestin dose and observe effect on cycle control.

Table 19-1. Composition of some oral contraceptives marketed in the United States

Product	Type	Progestin	Estrogen
Mead Johnson Co.			
Ovcon-50	Combination	1.0 mg norethindrone	50 μg ethinyl estradiol
Ovcon-35	Combination	0.4 mg norethindrone	35 μg ethinyl estradiol
Organon, Inc.			
Desogen	Combination	0.15 mg desogestrel	30 μg ethinyl estradiol
Mircette	Combination	0.15 mg desogestrel	20 μg ethinyl estradiol and 10 μg ethinyl estradiol (5 days)
Ortho Pharmaceutical, Inc.			
Modicon	Combination	0.5 mg norethindrone	35 μg ethinyl estradiol
Ortho-Novum 1 + 35	Combination	1.0 mg norethindrone	35 μg ethinyl estradiol
Ortho-Novum 1 + 50	Combination	1.0 mg norethindrone	50 μg mestranol
Ortho-Novum 10/	Combination-biphasic	0.5 mg norethindrone	35 μg ethinyl estradiol
Ortho-Novum 11/	Combination-biphasic	1.0 mg norethindrone	35 μg ethinyl estradiol
Micronor	Progestin	0.35 mg norethindrone	
Ortho-Novum 7/	Combination-triphasic	0.5 mg norethindrone	35 μg ethinyl estradiol
Ortho-Novum 7/	Combination-triphasic	0.75 mg norethindrone	35 μg ethinyl estradiol
Ortho-Novum 7/	Combination-triphasic	1.0 mg norethindrone	35 μg ethinyl estradiol
Parke-Davis			
Loestrin 1 + 20	Combination	1.0 mg norethindrone acetate	20 μg ethinyl estradiol
Loestrin 1.5 + 30	Combination	1.5 mg norethindrone acetate	30 μg ethinyl estradiol
Estrostep 5/	Combination-triphasic	1.0 mg norethindrone acetate	20 μg ethinyl estradiol
Estrostep 7/	Combination-triphasic	1.0 mg norethindrone acetate	30 μg ethinyl estradiol
Estrostep 9/	Combination-triphasic	1.0 mg norethindrone acetate	35 μg ethinyl estradiol
Searle Laboratories			
Demulen 1 + 35	Combination	1.0 mg ethynodiol diacetate	35 μg ethinyl estradiol
Demulen 1 + 50	Combination	1.0 mg ethynodiol diacetate	50 μg ethinyl estradiol
Syntex Laboratories			
Brevicon	Combination	0.5 mg norethindrone	35 μg ethinyl estradiol
Norinyl 1 + 35	Combination	1.0 mg norethindrone	35 μg ethinyl estradiol

(continued)

Table 19-1. (continued)

Product	Type	Progestin	Estrogen
Norinyl 1 + 50	Combination	1.0 mg norethindrone	50 μg mestranol
NOR QD	Progestin only	0.35 mg norethindrone	
Tri-Norinyl 2/	Combination-triphasic	0.5 mg norethindrone	35 μg ethinyl estradiol
Tri-Norinyl 9/	Combination-triphasic	1.0 mg norethindrone	35 μg ethinyl estradiol
Tri-Norinyl 5/	Combination-triphasic	0.5 mg norethindrone	35 μg ethinyl estradiol
Wyeth Laboratories			
Allesse	Combination	0.1 mg levonorgestresl	20 μg ethinyl estradiol
Lo Ovral	Combination	0.3 mg norgestrel	30 μg ethinyl estradiol
Nordette	Combination	0.15 mg levonorgestrel	30 μg ethinyl estradiol
Ovral	Combination	0.5 mg norgestrel	50 μg ethinyl estradiol
Ovrette	Progestin only	75 μg norgestrel	
Triphasil 6/	Combination-triphasic	50 μg levonorgestrel	30 μg ethinyl estradiol
Triphasil 5/	Combination-triphasic	75 μg levonorgestrel	40 μg ethinyl estradiol
Triphasil 10/	Combination-triphasic	125 μg levonorgestrel	30 μg ethinyl estradiol

    f. Missed pills. If one pill is missed, instruct the patient to take two pills at the next scheduled time and complete the pack as usual. If two or more consecutive pills are missed, instruct the patient to finish the package of pills and use an alternative contraceptive method for the remainder of the cycle.

  2. Progestin-only pill (Table 19-2) causes suppression of ovulation, thickening of cervical mucus, and alteration of the endometrium.

    a. Types include levonorgestrel, norgestrel, norethindrone, and ethynodiol diacetate.

    b. The progestin-only pill is indicated for breast-feeding women after 6 weeks postpartum, women who cannot or do not want to use estrogen, and women with anemia.

    c. Advantages. The first-year pregnancy rate is 3 to 6 per 100 women per year. The pill is rapidly effective (within 24 hours of initiation of

Table 19-2. Composition of progestin-only oral contraceptives

Progestin	Dose (μg)	Brand names
Norethindrone	350	Micronor, Nor-QD, Noriday
Norethindrone	75	Micro-Novum
Norgestrel	75	Ovrette, Neogest
Levonorgestrel	30	Microlut, Microval
Ethynodiol diacetate	500	Femulen

From Cunningham GF, MacDonald PC, Gant NF, Leveno KJ, Gilstrap LC. *Williams obstetrics*, 19th ed. Norwalk, CT: Appleton & Lange, 1993. Reprinted with permission.

use), and fertility returns immediately when the pill is discontinued. Its use does not affect breast-feeding and may improve anemia. Menstrual flow is decreased. The use of the pill offers some protection against endometrial cancer and protects against some causes of PID, and there is decreased benign breast disease.

   d. Disadvantages of the progestin-only pill include amenorrhea and intermenstrual bleeding. It must be taken every day

   e. Advantages over COCs. Low-dose progestin-only pills have not been associated with breast cancer. Women with a past history of thromboembolic disorders can use progestin-only pills, and there is no evidence that the progestin-only pill causes liver tumors.

3. **Progestin-only injectable contraceptives** cause suppression of ovulation, thickening of cervical mucus, alteration of endometrium (atrophy), and a change in tubal motility.

   a. Types of progestin-only injectable contraceptives include medroxyprogesterone acetate (Depo Provera), 150 mg i.m. every 3 months, and norethindrone (Noristerat), 200 mg i.m. every 2 months.

   b. Advantages. Progestin-only injectable contraceptives are very effective (first-year pregnancy rate of 0.3 to 0.9 per 100 women per year); they are also rapidly effective (less than 24 hours after injection) and long-acting. They can be used by women older than age 35 years.

   c. Disadvantages. Return to fertility is delayed up to 5 to 7 months, and some patients experience weight gain, irregular bleeding, amenorrhea (roughly 50% of users), excessive bleeding (rare), and serum lipid changes.

4. **Implants (Norplant System, Jadelle, Implanon)** consist of thin, flexible capsules filled with levonorgestrel or desogestrel that are inserted under the skin of a woman's arm. They cause suppression of ovulation, thickening of cervical mucus, alteration of the endometrium (atrophy), and a change in tubal motility.

   a. Advantages. Implants are highly effective (pregnancy rate of 0.2 to 0.5 per 100 women per year) and effective within 24 hours of placement. This method of contraception provides long-term protection (3 to 5 years) and immediate return of fertility on removal of the capsules.

   b. Disadvantages. This method of contraception requires a minor surgical procedure to insert and remove the capsules and provides no protection against STDs.

   c. Side effects include mastalgia, breast tenderness, weight gain or loss, irregular bleeding or spotting, amenorrhea, hirsutism, and hair loss.

   d. Complications include capsule expulsion, inadequate insertion of capsules, and capsules being inadvertently inserted too deeply in subcutaneous tissue (can be detected by x-ray or sonography to assist removal).

E. **Voluntary sterilization** is appropriate for couples who desire permanent sterilization and for women with medical problems that might subject them to high-risk pregnancy.

1. **Tubal ligation** is the one of the most frequently used method of fertility control (second to oral contraceptives).

   a. Types

   (1) **Postpartum tubal ligation (bilateral partial salpingectomy)**
      (a) **Pomeroy** (Fig. 19-4); variations include Parkland (tube transected separately); Uchida (tube buried in the mesosalpinx); Irving (tube buried in the myometrium).
      (b) **Filshie clip.** A spring-loaded titanium clip is applied to the tube, occluding it.

   (2) **Interval tubal ligation**
      (a) **Minilaparotomy.** The Pomeroy procedure (see Fig. 19-4) performed using a 3- to 4-cm suprapubic incision under local anesthesia with sedation or under general anesthesia.
      (b) **Laparoscopic**
         i. **Silastic rings** are placed around loop of tube, resulting in necrosis and occlusion.

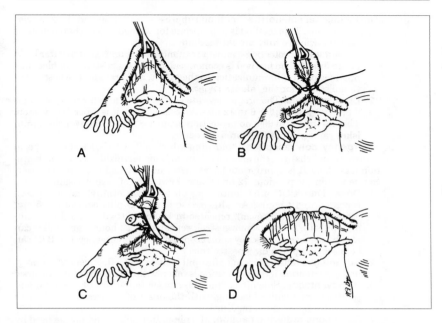

Figure 19-4. Modified Pomeroy technique of female sterilization. (From Sciarra JJ. Surgical procedures for tubal sterilization. In: Sciarra JJ, Zatuchni GI, Daly MJ, eds. *Gynecology and obstetrics.* Vol 6. Philadelphia: JB Lippincott Co., 1990:2. Reproduced with permission.)

        ii. Clips (Filshie, Hulka). Spring-loaded clips are placed across diameter of tube, producing occlusion.

        iii. Cautery (bipolar, unipolar). An electric current is passed through a portion of the tube, resulting in necrosis and occlusion.

    (c) Advantages. The procedure is highly effective and has no long-term side effects. The first-year pregnancy rate is 0.1 to 0.5 per 100 women per year (laparoscopy) versus 0.4 to 1.0 per 100 women per year (minilaparectomy). All procedures can be performed under either local or general anesthesia. All interval procedures are provided on an outpatient basis.

    (d) Disadvantages. The procedure is permanent and offers no protection against STDs. Surgical risks accompany the procedure. There is a risk of ectopic pregnancy, should pregnancy occur after the procedure.

2. Vasectomy

    a. Advantages over female sterilization

        (1) Outpatient procedure under local anesthesia

        (2) Failure rate of 3 to 4 per 1,000 procedures (can be detected by postoperative semen analysis)

        (3) Less expensive and fewer complications

        (4) No change in sexual function and no long-term side effects

    b. Disadvantages. The procedure is permanent, offers no protection against STDs, and is not effective immediately, requiring up to 20 ejaculations before becoming effective. Surgical risks also accompany the procedure.

F. **The lactational amenorrhea method** suppresses ovulation and thickens cervical secretions. This method is appropriate for women at less than 6 months postpartum who are **fully breast-feeding.**
   1. **Advantages.** Protection against pregnancy starts immediately after birth of the infant. The method is economical, decreases postpartum bleeding, provides passive immunization to the infant, and provides the best nutritional source for the infant.
   2. **Disadvantages.** The pregnancy rate for the first 6 months postpartum is 2 per 100 women; for 6 to 12 months postpartum, it is 6 per 100 women. This method provides no protection against STDs. Effectiveness diminishes rapidly if not fully breast-feeding.
G. **Emergency contraception** ["morning-after" pill (COCs)] reduces sperm transport and changes the endometrium, making fertilization and implantation less likely. It is appropriate for women who have had unprotected intercourse within the previous 72 hours and for victims of sexual assault.
   1. **Dose.** Four COC pills containing 30 to 35 μg ethinyl estradiol p.o., repeated in 12 hours. An alternative is 2 COC pills containing 50 μg ethinyl estradiol (Préven), repeated in 12 hours, (two doses). Progestin-only pills (0.75 mg levonorgestrel, repeated in 12 hours) and IUDs can also be used as emergency contraception. In an emergency, the IUD can be inserted up to 5 days postcoitus.
   2. **Advantages** of the morning-after pill include 98% effectiveness for pregnancy prevention if the medication is taken within 72 hours of intercourse.
   3. **Disadvantages.** Side effects include nausea (one-third of patients) and spotting or irregular bleeding, with the onset of menses within 7 to 10 days after ingestion of medication.
   4. **Conditions requiring caution.** Morning-after pill should not be used by women in whom pregnancy is suspected or with active thromboemblic process.
II. **Elective abortion**
A. **Epidemiology (United States).** In the United States, more than one-half of all pregnancies are unintended; slightly less than half of these unintended pregnancies end in abortion. The abortion rate in 1992 was 27.5 for every 100 recognized pregnancies. This rate has been fairly constant since 1980.

   In 1990, approximately 83% of pregnancy terminations were performed on patients 18 to 34 years old. Eighty-two percent of the patients were unmarried, and for 50% it was a first pregnancy. Ninety percent of abortions took place in the first 12 weeks after the last menstrual period. Ninety-nine percent were performed using suction and/or instrumental evacuation.
B. **Indications.** The debate over abortion policy in this country is one of the most divisive and complex issues of our time. It will not be addressed here except to briefly outline the legal foundation for current abortion practices in this country.

   In 1973, the U.S. Supreme court in *Roe v Wade* legalized elective pregnancy termination during the first trimester of pregnancy. Individual states were given the latitude to regulate second trimester procedures in "ways that are reasonably related to maternal health." In *Doe v Bolton*, the court specified that the concept of "health" was based on the judgment of the attending physician and included psychological, emotional, and familial factors.

   States may prohibit abortion after the fetus reaches viability unless the life or health of the mother is threatened. Termination of pregnancies when the fetus is not expected to survive for a meaningful period after birth because of genetic or congenital abnormalities (e.g., anencephaly or trisomy 13) is generally considered acceptable at any gestational age.
C. **Procedures**
   1. **Methods of cervical dilation.** Dilation before surgical or medical abortion may be indicated for a nulliparous patient or for a patient with an undilated and uneffaced cervix. The agents that cause dilation may be inserted before suction curettage.
      a. **Osmotic agents** include *Laminaria* (genus of seaweed), Lamicel (magnesium sulfate sponge), and Dilapan (tents of polyacrylonitrile). When inserted in the cervix, these devices slowly absorb water and expand,

allowing the cervix to soften and dilate. They also cause the release of prostaglandin, which ultimately disrupts the stroma of the cervix. This results in a soft, flaccid cervix that is easy to dilate. **Medical agents** include misoprostol (50 to 200 μg). When taken 12 to 24 hours (orally) or 4 to 6 hours (vaginally) before the procedure, it softens and dilates the cervix. Mifepristone, 100 mg taken orally 24 to 36 hours before the procedure, is also effective.

    b. **Technique.** The cleansed cervix is grasped with a tenaculum. The cervical canal is carefully sounded, without rupturing the membranes, to identify the length of the canal, its diameter, and the resistance of the internal os. A device of appropriate size is then inserted, using a uterine-packing forceps so the tip passes just beyond the internal os. After about 6 hours, the device will have swollen and thereby dilated the cervix, allowing easier mechanical dilation and curettage.

    c. **Warnings.** Do not use aspirin for pain from abortions for two reasons:

        (1) Aspirin is an antipyretic and could obscure the early signs of uterine infection.

        (2) Aspirin is a prostaglandin synthase inhibitor that might prevent local production of prostaglandins, which aid in cervical effacement and uterine contractions.

2. **First trimester termination**

    a. **Surgical**

        (1) Menstrual extraction

            (a) The technique includes aspiration of the endometrial cavity using a 5- to 7-mm cannula and a syringe within 1 to 3 weeks after failure to menstruate and a negative pregnancy test.

            (b) Complications include an implanted zygote missed by the curet, failure to recognize an ectopic pregnancy, and uterine perforation.

        (2) Vacuum aspiration (manual vacuum aspiration, suction curettage)

            (a) Technique

                i. Perform a pelvic examination to determine the shape and position of the uterus.

                ii. Insert a sterile speculum and remove the osmotic dilators if any were placed before the procedure.

                iii. Instill 1 to 3 mL of 1% lidocaine at the site where the tenaculum is to be placed. **Grasp the anterior or posterior lip of the cervix,** with tenaculum.

                iv. Instill 5 to 10 mL of 1% lidocaine at 4 and 8 o'clock paracervically to produce a paracervical block.

                v. Dilate the cervical canal by serial insertion of tapered rods that increase progressively in size (Pratt, Hegar, or Denniston dilators may be used).

                vi. Use a canulla size approximately the same diameter (mm) as the weeks of gestation (weeks since last menstrual period) ± 1 week.

                vii. Insert a suction curet, activate the vacuum, and remove the products of conception.

                viii. Remove the suction curet after aspiration is complete, and, if there is doubt that all of the products of conception have been removed, gently insert a sharp curet to ensure that the uterine cavity is empty.

                ix. Reintroduce the suction curet for a few seconds to remove any remaining tissue, if a sharp curet was used.

                x. Examine the tissue to verify that products of conception consistent with the gestational age are present. If the pregnancy is in the later stages, count fetal parts.

                xi. Remove all instruments from the vagina.

            (b) Complications include uterine perforation, retention of the products of conception, bleeding, and infection.

(3) **The manual vacuum aspirator** (Karman cannula) is a plastic, syringe-powered, reusable aspirator. It is especially useful in less developed countries as a low-cost, low-tech alternative to the traditional electric pump–powered aspiration method. It is used in some centers in the United States for pregnancy termination, usually up to 10 or 11 completed weeks, and for management of incomplete abortion.

(4) **Hysterotomy.** Laparotomy and uterine incision for pregnancy termination is almost never indicated. Data collected for 1990 show that it represented less than 0.01% of all elective terminations that year.

b. **Medical. Mifepristone (RU-486) and methotrexate with misoprostol** have been used independently to induce first trimester abortion with a success rate (complete abortion, no suction curettage) approximately 93% when the gestation is less than 7 weeks from last menstrual period. Several different protocols have been published in the literature. For mifepristone, most protocols involve the oral administration of 200 to 600 mg, followed 36 hours later by oral or vaginal administration of 400 to 800 μg of misoprostol. For methotrexate, the protocol requires 50 mg/m^2 i.m., followed in 5 to 7 days by 800 μg of misoprostol by vagina. Medical abortion procedures require accurate dating, as success rates are inversely related to gestational age.

3. **Second trimester termination**
   a. **Surgical**
      (1) **Vacuum aspiration (instrumental removal of fetal tissue, or D&E).** The procedure for surgical abortion between 14 and 22 weeks is identical to the first trimester procedure, with the following caveats:
         (a) **Ultrasonographic confirmation** of gestational age is essential.
         (b) **Preoperative cervical preparation** is mandatory and is often carried out over the 1 to 2 days before the procedure to maximize adequate cervical dilation and minimize the chances of cervical laceration and uterine injury. Sequential insertion of osmotic dilators is most frequently used.
         (c) **Dilation** to 1.5 to 2.0 cm is usually necessary to allow for passage of instruments into the uterine cavity.
         (d) **Some practitioners recommend amniotomy** before beginning vacuum aspiration, because amniotomy allows the uterus to contract, reducing blood loss and bringing the products of conception closer to the cervical os.
         (e) **In addition to application of the vacuum aspirator,** instrumental removal of the products of conception is usually required. At gestations greater than 15 weeks, the fetal calvarium frequently requires crushing and removal with special forceps.
         (f) **Intraoperative ultrasound** is frequently employed and is used routinely by some practitioners.
         (g) **It is essential to examine and account for** all fetal parts and a volume of placental tissue consistent with the gestational age.
         (h) **As gestational age increases,** the skill required of the operator increases dramatically, especially after 16 weeks of gestation. Complications such as cervical trauma, uterine perforation, hemorrhage, and retained products are more common after 18 weeks and may result in significant morbidity.
      (2) **Hysterotomy.** Laparotomy and uterine incision for pregnancy termination is rarely indicated. It represented less than 0.01% of all elective terminations in data collected for 1990.
   b. **Medical**
      (1) **Medical second trimester abortion,** also referred to as induction abortion, comprises a number of methods for inducing fetal death and/or uterine contractions that lead to expulsion of the products of conception, include the following:

      (a) **I.v., high-dose oxytocin**
      (b) **Intraamniotic 20% saline or 30% urea**
      (c) **Intraamniotic prostaglandin**
         i. **PGE_2**
         ii. **$PGF_{2\alpha}$**
      (d) **Vaginal or rectal prostaglandin**
         i. **PGE_2**
         ii. **$PGF_{2\alpha}$**
         iii. **Misoprostol**
   (2) Medical abortions offer several advantages over D&E:
      (a) **Procedures do not require anesthesia,** although analgesia is usually necessary.
      (b) **A skilled operator** is not required for administration of vaginal or rectal suppositories or high-dose oxytocin.
   (3) Disadvantages, compared with D&E:
      (a) **Procedure can take 24 hours or more.**
      (b) **Major complications and mortality** appear to be two to three times higher in induced procedures.
      (c) **Fever and severe gastrointestinal side effects** are common with the use of some prostaglandins.
  4. Prophylactic antibiotics (e.g., doxycycline, 100 mg p.o. b.i.d. for 3 days) should be administered to all patients, starting immediately after any aspiration procedure, to reduce the incidence of significant uterine and pelvic infections.
  5. Complications are similar for all gestational ages and methods. In general, the later the gestational age, the higher the risk of complications.
    a. Anesthesia can cause complications including drug reaction, circulatory collapse, seizures, cardiac damage, and cerebrovascular accident. The risk of death from termination performed under general anesthetic is two to four times higher than for procedures performed under local anesthetic. Lidocaine for paracervical blocks should be limited to no more than 2 mg/kg of body weight. The use of lidocaine with epinephrine may reduce systemic absorption. Small amounts of vasopressin can be used with lidocaine to reduce bleeding.
    b. Cervical dilation can result in cervical laceration with resultant hemorrhage and possible infertility or cervical incompetence. Occasionally a cervical laceration can tear into the uterine artery, necessitating hysterectomy. Prevention primarily involves avoiding the tear by using osmotic dilators and using metal dilators carefully and only as necessary. Once a laceration has occurred, it can be sutured with interrupted Vicryl or chromic sutures.
    c. Incomplete evacuation usually presents during the first 7 postoperative days with persistant heavy bleeding (heavier than a normal menstrual flow), cramping, fever, and uterine tenderness. If left untreated, it can eventually lead to sepsis with its attendant potentially severe organ system damage and death. Reaspiration is the treatment of choice and should not be delayed in favor of antibiotic treatment.
    d. Sustained fever of 101.5°F or higher that appears within 7 days of termination of the pregnancy should be considered evidence that products of reproduction have been retained, causing sepsis, until proven otherwise. Treatment includes reaspiration and administration of appropriate broad-spectrum antibiotics [e.g., gentamicin and clindamycin (Ampicillin)] and careful monitoring for signs of septic shock.
    e. Low-grade fevers without signs of sepsis can be treated with reaspiration and oral antibiotics (e.g., doxycycline, 100 mg p.o. for 10 days).
    f. Uterine perforation is the most common major complication of surgical abortion. Treatment depends on gestational age, the extent of the tear, and the amount of bleeding. Recognition is obviously crucial. Typical signs of uterine perforation include
      (1) Onset of diffuse abdominal pain during a procedure

      (2) Onset of brisk, bright red bleeding

      (3) Observation of mesenteric fat or small bowel in the cannula or forceps

  g. Once the suspicion of perforation arises, laparoscopy is almost always indicated to assess the extent of the damage, rule out any parametrial hematomas, and prepare for completion of the abortion procedure under direct vision. If damage is minimal (e.g., fundal perforation without bleeding), treatment should consist of overnight observation and introduction of a uterotonic agent such as oxytocin, misoprostol, or methylergonovine maleate (Methergine). Significant damage requires immediate laparotomy or laparoscopic repair.

  h. Uterine atony should be treated by uterine massage and the administration of methylergonovine or other uterotonic agents. The presence of retained products of conception should be ruled out, or they should be evacuated; they are the most common cause of hemorrhage due to atony.

  i. Postabortal hematometra typically develops 1 to 12 hours after a suction abortion. It typically presents with uterine pain and an enlarged, boggy uterus with or without moderate bleeding. Bimanual uterine massage will sometimes expel a moderate-sized clot, giving immediate relief of symptoms and firming of the uterus. Reaspiration is often required.

  j. Other rare complications include

      (1) Molar pregnancy

      (2) Disseminated intravascular coagulation

      (3) Amniotic fluid embolism

      (4) Undiagnosed twin pregnancy

      (5) Postabortal psychosis

6. Long-term complications. Although many studies are open to methodologic criticism, there is no credible evidence to suggest that a history of pregnancy termination increases a woman's risk of infertility, spontaneous abortion, psychological illness, or sexual dysfunction.

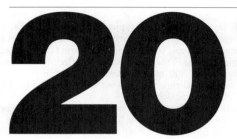

Benign Vulvar Lesions

Cornelia Liu Trimble
and Edward Trimble

I. **Infections.** Many benign lesions of the vulva are infectious. A number of these infections can involve squamous epithelium elsewhere. The vulva and perineum have estrogen and progesterone receptors and thus are subject to stronger hormonal influences than skin elsewhere. Furthermore, as the vulva and perineum are often sequestered by clothing, they are prone to chronic dampness from perspiration.

   A. **Bacterial infections and sexually transmitted diseases (STDs).** Common bacterial infections include those that cause folliculitis (*Staphylococcus*), furuncles (*Staphylococcus*), and Bartholin's gland abscesses (polymicrobial). **Treatment** strategies should focus on hygiene measures, with sitz baths and antibiotics if necessary.

     The Bartholin's gland may become occluded and superinfected, manifesting as an abscess. These lesions are usually polymicrobial in origin, although approximately 10% may be caused by *Neisseria gonorrhoeae*. Of note, attempts at incision and evacuation are therapeutic only when the lesion has become fluctuant. The incision should be made proximal to the hymeneal ring, and a Word catheter may be inserted. To bring a firm lesion to fluctuance, sitz baths are recommended. Recurrences are common. Surgical marsupialization may be required.

   B. **STDs** that may involve the vulva include gonorrhea and syphilis, as well as human papillomaviruses (HPVs). Gonorrhea will often present as an acute inflammatory reaction in the region of the urethra, or at Bartholin's or Skene's glands. Diagnosis is made by culture. Assessment for other STDs, such as chlamydia, as well as a Papanicolaou's (Pap) smear, should be performed.

     1. **Syphilis**

       a. **Primary syphilis** has an incubation period of 3 weeks. The primary lesion is a painless, indurated papule that can be as large as 2 cm in diameter. This lesion will progress to an ulcer, which then resolves in up to 8 weeks. Inguinal lymph nodes may be shotty. The chancres may be multiple and, on the vulva, may be superinfected. The diagnosis can be made by darkfield microscopic examination. The VDRL is positive in 70% of patients with primary syphilis. If the test is negative, and the disease is suspected clinically, it should be repeated weekly for 4 weeks with negative results before the patient is considered to be free of the disease.

       b. Vulvar manifestations of **secondary syphilis** include soft, nontender papules that may be larger than the primary lesions. The VDRL will be positive at this stage of the disease.

       c. The pathognomonic lesion of **tertiary syphilis** is the condyloma latum.

       d. The recommended Centers for Disease Control and Prevention **therapy** for primary syphilis is a single i.m. dose of 2.4 million units of benzathine penicillin G. Treatment schedules for later stages of this disease are covered Chap. 18. As with all STDs, assessment for other STDs should ensue.

     2. **Chancroid** represents another STD that, although more common in men than in women, also may present as a vulvar ulcer. The incubation period

ranges from 3 to 10 days. These lesions typically are quite painful. Bilateral inguinal adenopathy is common. Because the causative organism, *Haemophilus ducreyi*, is difficult to culture, biopsy and Gram's stain are often necessary for diagnosis. **Treatment** consists of trimethoprim, 160 mg, and sulfamethoxazole, 800 mg, p.o. twice a day for 10 days. For patients allergic to sulfa, erythromycin, 500 mg, every 6 hours for 10 days is the treatment of choice.

3. **Granuloma inguinale** is a contagious, chronic STD. The causative organism is *Calymmatobacterium granulomatis*. The lesions are granulomatous and locally destructive; however, they are rarely painful. The diagnosis may be made by histologic or cytologic demonstration of the Donovan body, which is highlighted with Wright's or Giemsa stain. Although the acute lesion responds to tetracycline, surgery may be indicated in later, chronic stages to remove areas of chronic infection and distortion.

4. **Lymphogranuloma venereum** is a chronic STD, caused by three serotypes of *Chlamydia trachomatis*, L1, L2, and L3. The primary lesion may present as a papule, a shallow ulcer, or a small, herpetiform lesion. This arises after an incubation period of 3 to 12 days. The inguinal lymph nodes may become involved in the second stage of the disease. This generally occurs 10 to 30 days after initial infection but may occur 4 to 6 months later. An enlarged inguinal lymph node is sometimes called a *bubo*. Chronic, untreated infection can lead to proctocolitis and bowel strictures, progressive vulvar induration and fibrosis, and in some cases, stenosis of the urethra and vagina. The diagnosis of lymphogranuloma venereum is based on a positive serologic test result, isolation of the organism, or histologic identification of the bacterium. Effective antibiotics include tetracycline, sulfadiazine, chloramphenicol, erythromycin, and rifampin. The recommended tetracycline dosage is 1 g loading dose, then 500 mg four times a day for 14 days. If surgery is indicated for repair of strictures or fistulas, patients should receive antibiotics for several months before time of operation.

C. **Viral infections.** Viral infections of the lower genital tract are common. The most common include condyloma acuminatum, molluscum contagiosum, and herpes simplex.

1. **Condyloma acuminatum,** or venereal warts, are caused by HPV infection. HPV types 6 and 11 are the most common types producing exophytic lesions on the lower genital tract. These lesions are frequently multifocal. Malignant transformation is uncommon. The exophytic lesions may be pruritic and may become superinfected. Although they may regress spontaneously during pregnancy or other immunocompromised states, they may instead flourish. **Treatment** consists of local destruction, either by topical 5-fluorouracil or podophyllin or by surgical excision. Systemic and intralesional interferon has also been used. A Pap smear of the cervix should be obtained. Infection with HPV (types 16, 18, 31, 33) typically does not manifest as exophytic lesions, but rather as vulvar intraepithelial neoplasia and is covered in more detail in the section on squamous carcinomas.

2. **Molluscum contagiosum** is a poxvirus that is spread by close contact. The lesions are multiple, small, umbilicated papules filled with white, waxy material. Most patients are entirely asymptomatic. Although the diagnosis is most often made clinically, histologic demonstration of intracytoplasmic molluscum bodies is pathognomonic. **Therapy** consists of curettage and excision of the lesions under local anesthesia.

3. **Herpes simplex virus (HSV)** infection is the most common cause of vulvar ulcers. HSV-1 is typically associated with oral infections, although it can produce genital lesions. HSV-2 is more often the cause of lesions of the lower genital tract. The infection is highly contagious. It may be preceded by malaise, fever, or a prodromal tingling sensation at the site of the eventual lesion. Recurrent ulcers are often in the same location. They are frequently painful. Of note, viral shedding may persist for several weeks after the ulcers have resolved, although this is much more likely

with a primary infection. Recurrences are usually milder than primary lesions. **Treatment** for both the initial lesions and recurrences consists of acyclovir, 200 mg, five times a day for 10 days.

II. **Inflammatory lesions.** Two rare causes of ulcerative lesions of the vulva are Crohn's disease and Behçet's disease.

A. In **Crohn's disease,** vulvar ulcers may precede gastrointestinal symptoms by months or even years. Crohn's ulcers are typically linear and may result in draining fistulas.

B. **Behçet's disease** comprises a constellation of relapsing oral and genital ulcers associated with ocular inflammation. Any one or all three of these components may be present, but uveitis is less frequent than ulcerations. The patient with ocular manifestations is at risk for meningoencephalitis, which may be fatal. These ulcers may not produce symptoms. Systemic corticosteroid treatment is the most widely used and effective treatment.

III. **Benign neoplastic lesions of the vulva.** Not all pedunculated or exophytic lesions of the vulva are warts. In addition to the ones discussed previously, other exophytic lesions include squamous hyperplasia, keratoacanthomas, fibroepithelial polyps, seborrheic keratoses, and lipomas, as well as other, very rare entities. Ectopic tissue, such as papillary hidradenomas or endometriosis, may also present as a mass lesion.

A. In **squamous hyperplasia,** there are variable increases in the thickness of the horny layer of skin (hyperkeratosis), as well as in the basal layer (acanthosis). These may be red or white, well-delineated or poorly defined. Evaluation should include colposcopy and full-thickness biopsy. There is no proved association between hyperplasia and squamous carcinoma. Topical corticosteroids are the treatment of choice for squamous hyperplasia of the vulva. An isolated, heaped-up lesion consistent with squamous hyperplasia is called a *keratoacanthoma*.

B. **Acrochordons,** or skin tags, are frequently pedunculated but may be sessile and have a rubbery consistency. These do not need to be removed unless they are symptomatic. On histologic examination, these are fibroepithelial polyps.

C. **Seborrheic keratoses** are flat, raised pigmented lesions common elsewhere on the body. Although these lesions are benign, all pigmented vulvar lesions should be evaluated carefully. Both melanomas and squamous carcinoma of the vulva may be similar in appearance.

D. **Lipomas** are benign tumors composed of adipose tissue. They are soft and sometimes pedunculated.

E. On occasion, **ectopic tissue** can cause symptoms on the vulva. **Papillary hidradenomas** occur on the milk line and present as a firm, encapsulated nodule that can measure up to 2 cm in greatest dimension. These occur predominantly in postpubertal white women. The most frequent location is on the labia majora or in the interlabial folds. Most commonly, these nodules are asymptomatic.

Endometriotic foci on the vulva are relatively uncommon. They may occur in a site of previous surgery, such as an episiotomy site. These lesions appear bluish-red and undergo cyclic enlargement.

Other benign lesions that may occur on the vulva include granular cell tumors, syringomas, hemangiomas, and pyogenic granulomas. These are all rare lesions.

IV. **Benign pigmented and hypopigmented lesions**

A. **Nevi** of the intradermal, junctional, and compound varieties are common on the external genitalia. These lesions should be excised carefully, as the differential diagnosis includes melanoma and squamous carcinoma. Nevi are either pigmented or white (hypopigmented or amelanotic).

Both seborrheic keratoses and vulvar intraepithelial lesions may be pigmented.

B. **Lichen sclerosus** is characterized by itching, with low, flat-topped white maculopapules on the vulva and perineum. These can grow together to form well-defined plaques. Often, the labia minora may disappear from atrophy. Multiple punch biopsies should be taken to confirm the diagnosis. Topical testosterone appears to be the most successful agent to decrease pruritus, edema, and scarring associated with lichen sclerosus.

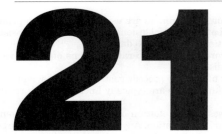

Urogynecology and Pelvic Relaxation

R. Bradley Lucas and
René Genadry

I. Urogynecology
A. Etiology of urinary incontinence

1. **Genuine stress incontinence** is the most common form of urinary incontinence and results from abnormal transmission of abdominal pressure to the bladder. Normally, intraabdominal pressure is transmitted equally to the proximal urethra and bladder, allowing urinary continence. Changes in anatomy and support cause an unequal pressure-transmission ratio. Higher pressures transmitted to the bladder than to the urethra lead to urinary incontinence.

2. **Detrusor instability** is uninhibited bladder contractions that lead to urinary incontinence; it can arise from a number of causes. **Local bladder irritation** can lead to instability; one of the more common origins of this irritation is urinary tract infection. Upper central nervous system lesions cause a type of detrusor instability termed **detrusor hyperreflexia.** These lesions may arise from cerebral vascular accidents, multiple sclerosis, or trauma. Spinal cord lesions lead to incontinence through abnormal reflex activity. This is commonly called **reflex incontinence.** Spinovascular disease can result from diabetes mellitus, atherosclerosis, and meningomyelocele. Between 5% and 27% of patients will develop *de novo* **detrusor instability** within 6 months of surgery for stress incontinence (1). New obstruction of urine outflow can possibly cause autonomic nerve damage and resultant detrusor instability.

   Idiopathic detrusor instability is, however, the most common form of this problem. Idiopathic detrusor instability results from a loss of the previously learned inhibition of detrusor muscle contractions.

3. **Acquired urinary incontinence through fistulas** leads to persistent wetness for the patient. Ureterovesical, urethrovesical, and vaginovesical fistulas may result from disease or previous obstetric or gynecologic surgery.

4. Several **congenital defects** lead to urinary incontinence. **Ectopic ureter** and **bladder extrophy** lead to continuous urine loss. **Hypospadias** may cause the absence of part or all of the urethra and lead to urinary incontinence because of intrinsic urethral deficiency (see sec. **I.C.3**).

5. **Urethral diverticulum** may allow urine to pool after voiding and cause troublesome postvoid dribbling.

6. **Urinary retention with overflow incontinence** is found in patients with neurologic disease in which lower motor neurons are affected, such as diabetic peripheral neuropathy. This distal sensory or sensorimotor polyneuropathy is characterized by segmental demyelination and axonal degeneration. The pathogenesis is still uncertain but thought to be metabolic in origin. Uremia and hypothyroidism can cause similar problems with peripheral innervation of the detrusor muscle.

7. **Functional incontinence (impaired mobility)** should be considered in patients who may have difficulty with ambulation.

8. **Medications, delirium, and urinary tract infections** can all lead to transient episodes of incontinence.

B. Investigation of urinary incontinence
  1. Patient history
   a. A **general medical history** should include the patient's health status, list of medications, questions regarding any chronic disease and recent medical problems, and a review of systems. Question the patient about any pharmacologic therapies and previous surgeries.
   b. A **classification of symptoms** should include the nature of the urine loss, the onset, the duration of the problem, and the precipitating causes. This should include a careful history of the evolution of the problem, as well as previous medical or surgical attempts at therapy. It is important to establish early on how compromising the problem is to the patient's lifestyle. If a treatment plan is formed based on history alone, the physician may be wrong as much as 40% of the time (2).

   The physician should decide whether a conservative plan might be helpful or whether a complete evaluation is warranted. For instance, Kegel exercises can be initiated if there is a typical history of stress incontinence with no further problems.
   c. Begin a **voiding log** after the patient's first visit. The patient should record episodes of voiding and leakage of urine, as well as any accompanying urge. Estimates of the amount of leakage and measurements of input and output are important. Encourage the patient to record these events during several "normal" 24-hour periods.
  2. Physical examination
   a. A **general physical examination** should establish the severity of any chronic diseases such as diabetes mellitus or chronic obstructive pulmonary disease.
   b. A skilled **neurologic examination** should localize any lesions in the cerebrum, brain stem, cerebellum, spinal cord, or peripheral nervous system. A mental status evaluation will help rule out dementia, brain tumors, and normal-pressure hydrocephalus. It will also help determine which treatment plan would be most accepted by the patient. Test cranial nerves to isolate central nervous system lesions or to diagnose early multiple sclerosis. Evaluate muscle strength and look for muscle atrophy and spasticity. Measure deep tendon reflexes to assess spinal cord structure. Hyperreflexia reveals supranuclear lesions.

   Finally, sacral cord integrity is evaluated with three tests: (a) stroking the skin lateral to the anus to elicit the anal reflex; (b) tapping or squeezing the clitoris to elicit the bulbocavernous reflex; and (c) stimulating the urethral or vesical mucosa to do the same. Proper reflexes with these tests demonstrate an intact spinal cord from L5 to S5. Ask the patient to cough and watch for contraction of the periurethral striated sphincter. This demonstrates an intact spinal cord from T6 to L1. This screening examination should tell the physician whether to refer the incontinent patient to a neurologist.
   c. A thorough **pelvic examination** will identify any areas of pelvic relaxation as well as their severity. Note any further atrophic changes at the vulva or vagina, which may result from estrogen deficiency. Furthermore, fistulas or a urethral diverticula may be discovered with a careful examination. Use the fixed blade of a Graves speculum to hold aside vaginal walls during inspection.
  3. Laboratory
   a. **Urinalysis and culture** is needed before any further workup of the incontinent patient. Stress and urgency incontinence may both result from urinary tract infection. A normal urinalysis helps exclude metabolic, neoplastic, and other intrinsic problems of the upper urinary tract and bladder.
   b. **Blood glucose and calcium tests** are necessary to rule out diabetes mellitus and hyperparathyroidism. Kidney function should be evaluated with a blood urea nitrogen/creatinine test.

4. **Office cystometrics** can provide some useful information. These tests should be performed in a logical and sequential manner. Consider antibiotic prophylaxis after instrumentation.

   a. A **bladder capacity test** consists of slowly filling the bladder with sterile saline. Document when the patient first feels an urge to urinate. An urge to void at less than 150 mL indicates small bladder capacity or an irritable bladder. Continue filling until the patient states she can no longer continue without voiding. Normal maximum capacity is between 300 and 600 mL.

   b. A **cough stress test** should be performed with a full bladder. Watch for descent of the bladder neck and proximal urethra into the pelvis. Look for loss of urine with cough. Small amounts of urine loss with cough suggest stress urinary incontinence. Delayed leaking or sudden, large amounts of urine loss suggest detrusor instability. A positive cough stress test in the supine position in which there is a relatively empty bladder and little Valsalva raises the possibility of intrinsic sphincter deficiency.

   c. A **cotton swab test** will evaluate bladder neck mobility. A cotton swab with lidocaine gel is placed in the urethral meatus. Ask the patient to strain. A greater than 45-degree change from the horizontal indicates hypermobility.

   d. The **Marshall test** and **Bonney test** are tests commonly performed in the office. Both require the patient to cough with a full bladder. Support the urethrovesical angle with placement of Allis clamps at the anterior vaginal wall for the Marshall test. For the Bonney test, insert fingers into the lateral fornices of the vagina. In both tests, take care to stay lateral to the angle avoiding compression of the urethra. No leakage of urine when the urethrovesical angle is returned to its proper anatomic location may indicate genuine stress urinary incontinence. As there will likely be some degree of urethral compression, these tests should not be used as a substitute for urodynamic testing.

   e. Measure **residual urine** by placing a catheter in the bladder after the patient voids. More than 50 mL of residual urine may indicate a large cystocele or a motor problem with the bladder, which leads to overflow incontinence.

5. **Urodynamic laboratory studies** are useful in the evaluation of urinary incontinence. They should definitely be considered when no pure genuine stress incontinence is present according to the history, when recurrent incontinence is present, and when severe stress incontinence is present.

   a. **Cystometry** is the most helpful of urodynamic laboratory studies. Its purpose is to check bladder compliance and rule out detrusor instability by determining whether the bladder fills to a reasonable capacity without a rise in pressure. In this study, an attempt is made to reproduce the filling and voiding functions of the bladder, with the cystometrogram demonstrating the relationship of volume and pressure (compliance = volume/pressure).

      Multichannel cystometry measures intraabdominal pressure and intravesical pressure. A probe is placed in the rectum or vagina to duplicate intraabdominal pressure. The bladder is instilled with normal saline at a rate of 50 to 100 mL per minute for filling cystometry. The **bladder capacity testing** should be performed as outlined in sec. **I.B.4.a.**

      Detrusor pressure is equal to the vesical pressure minus the abdominal pressure and should remain stable. During and after filling, provocative tests should be performed. Have the patient stand, cough, and bounce. Turn on running water. Uninhibited detrusor contractions indicate detrusor instability. Urine leakage with a stable detrusor indicates stress urinary incontinence.

   b. A **urethral closure pressure profile** goes even further in evaluating stress urinary incontinence. Multichannel cystometry also allows for measurements of intraurethral pressure. As the transducer is withdrawn from the urethra, pressures are measured. Continent patients will always have an intraurethral pressure greater than or equal to the intravesical pressure. Urinary incontinent patients, however, will have an intraurethral pressure that is less than the intravesical pressure during stress incontinence. The functional length of the urethra correlates with the length of urethra that exhibits positive pressure above bladder pressure.

A **leak point pressure** can be identified. This is the minimum abdominal pressure that leads to urinary incontinence. Patients with severe incontinence caused by an intrinsic sphincter defect are not able to generate intraurethral pressure higher than intravesical pressure. In these patients, minimal increases in intraabdominal pressure lead to intravesical pressure higher than intraurethral pressure. The leak point pressure helps identify these patients with intrinsic sphincter deficiency. Leak pressures of less than 60 cm H_2O with 200 mL in the bladder indicate intrinsic sphincter deficiency.

   c. Uroflowmetry is used to identify detrusor weakness or outlet obstruction. The volume of urine voided is measured in mL per second. Volumes of more than 200 mL should have peak flow rates between 20 and 30 mL per second.

   d. Urethrocystoscopy is best performed after cystometry because irritation from the media or the scope might cause detrusor contractions and create a false-positive recording during cystometry. The urethra should be examined closely on entering, as erythema will develop during the procedure. Look for exudates or orifices from diverticula. Also, look for any ectopic ureter, which would cause persistent leaking. Visualize the anatomy of the urethrovesical junction. After studying the urethra, look for any intrinsic lesions in the bladder and identify the ureteral orifices.

C. Treatment

   1. Detrusor instability is generally more responsive to nonsurgical therapy.

      a. Behavioral therapy such as changing the amount of fluid intake or types of food can have dramatic effects. Increasing water intake with meals can dilute any irritants that are causing detrusor contractions. Have the patient decrease caffeine, alcohol, and citrus fruit intake. The patient can also benefit from limiting cigarettes and artificial sweeteners.

        Bladder training is the most effective means of correcting urge incontinence. Ninety percent of patients with detrusor instability have no definable irritant (3). Bladder training introduces the patient again to the discipline of toilet training. With encouragement from the physician and staff and motivation from the patient, remarkable results can take place. Have the patient sit on the toilet every 15 minutes during the waking day. She must attempt to urinate. If she has an urge to urinate before the next scheduled time, have her attempt to "hold it." After 3 days, the interval is increased to 30 minutes. The intervals increase (15 minutes to 30 minutes to 45 minutes to 1 hour to 1.5 hours to 2 hours and to 3 hours) every 3 days until the patient is voiding every 3 hours.

      b. Medication for the treatment of urge incontinence is used to affect neurotransmitter activity at the neuromuscular unit. Therefore, most of these drugs have anticholinergic properties. Most common are **propantheline** at doses of 7.5 to 30.0 mg two to four times a day or the **tricyclic antidepressant imipramine,** at doses of 12.5 to 25.0 mg two to three times a day. These drugs are usually safe if they are titrated to avoid the bothersome anticholinergic side effects of constipation, drowsiness, and blurry vision. Tell the patient to expect some dry mouth. Vagal blockade from antimuscarinic effects can increase the heart rate. Avoid using them in patients with cardiac arrhythmias and narrow-angle glaucoma.

        Oxybutynin is an **antispasmodic agent** that can alleviate detrusor irritability. It also has some anticholinergic properties. Use a dose of 2.5 to 5.0 mg two to four times a day.

Calcium channel blockers is a class of drugs being used more often for urge incontinence. Tolterodine, a drug with anticholinergic properties, is dosed as 1 to 2 mg two times a day.

c. **Functional electrical stimulation** can be successful in both stress urinary incontinence and detrusor instability. Proper stimulation results in contraction of pelvic floor muscles and relaxation of bladder muscle. Before functional electrical stimulation is undertaken, an electromyogram (EMG) is necessary to confirm an intact reflex loop from the afferent pathways of the pudendal nerve to the sacral nerve roots to the efferent pathways to the pelvic floor muscles. The physician can confirm whether functional electrical stimulation will be beneficial by performing urodynamic studies at the same time. Loss of detrusor muscle spasms during stimulation can predict successful therapy. If the above criteria are met, the patient can be fitted with either a vaginal or rectal stimulator. A stimulator that generates a biphasic impulse is used.

Treatment of urge incontinence requires an electrical current from 65 to 100 mA at a duration of 1 msec and a frequency of 20 Hz. The patient may stimulate herself at home for 20 minutes a day for 5 days. The inhibition of bladder spasms lasts much longer for idiopathic detrusor instability than for neurogenic detrusor instability (e.g., after spinal cord trauma).

d. **Psychological counseling** can be used to augment any of the above treatments. Psychosocial problems in an individual's life may disrupt any attempts at correction of urinary incontinence. For example, the patient may have some motivation for or secondary gains from having urinary incontinence.

2. **Genuine stress incontinence**

a. **Nonsurgical therapy** also has an important place in treatment of urinary stress incontinence.

(1) **Behavioral therapy** includes **dietary changes,** bladder training, and optimization of overall health. Have the patient measure her voids and then decrease fluid intake until her urine output is only 1,000 mL per day. Tell the patient to decrease caffeine and alcohol intake, as both have diuretic effects.

Bladder training (see sec. I.C.1.a) has been found to decrease the frequency of incontinence episodes by 50% (4).

Lifestyle changes such as decreased tobacco use, weight loss, and improved care for chronic disease states will decrease abdominal and pelvic floor pressure, which can decrease the severity and the number of episodes of stress urinary incontinence.

(2) **Pelvic floor rehabilitation** with **Kegel exercises** is an effective but seldom used modality. Strengthening the levator ani and urogenital sphincter muscles through exercise will help restore the anatomy of the proximal urethra and pelvic floor. Also, improved muscle tone will help the patient constrict her urethral lumen. The resting tone will be increased and the strengthened muscles will increase the intraluminal pressure at times of stress. To perform Kegel exercises, the patient identifies the muscles by stopping her urine in midstream. She then contracts these muscles ten to 20 times for 5 seconds. Have the patient do this three times a day. This type of pelvic muscle rehabilitation is successful only with an intense program lasting several months and requires support and enthusiasm from the physician and staff. Some form of biofeedback will greatly increase the chance of success.

(3) **Biofeedback** through auditory or visual stimuli allows the patient to recognize physiologic events in her body. The patient can learn to influence these signals and subsequently control the events. EMG recordings are most often used for stress urinary

incontinence. The patient learns to contract her perineal muscles and not her abdominal muscles.

The use of vaginal cones might also be considered a form of biofeedback. The patient is asked to hold progressively heavier cones in her vagina. The muscles used to prevent the cone from slipping out are the pelvic floor muscles that need to be strengthened. One month of therapy has been shown to be successful in 70% of patients (5).

(4) **Medical therapy** for genuine stress urinary incontinence is generally aimed at increasing urogenital sphincter tone. Alpha agonists such as pseudoephedrine, ephedrine, and norepinephrine can be used. Imipramine also has alpha agonist activity. These medications should be used with caution in elderly patients with hypertension or heart disease.

Unless there is a contraindication, postmenopausal patients with stress urinary incontinence should be placed on **estrogen replacement.** Estrogen will thicken urethral mucosa as well as improve periurethral muscle tone. Commonly employed oral therapies or conjugated equine estrogen vaginally at a dose of 1 g/day should be used. The dose and frequency should be decreased after some initial improvement is seen.

(5) **Mechanical devices,** most notably the Smith-Hodge vaginal pessary, can be used to correct genuine stress urinary incontinence by helping predict which patients would benefit from surgical procedures for stress incontinence. Continence is restored surgically by anatomic corrections that improve urethral closure pressure, increase functional urethral length, and support the urethrovesical junction (6). Placement of a Smith-Hodge pessary may uncover the weak sphincter and identify patients who should have a surgical sling procedure. Placement of a Smith-Hodge pessary may also identify patients at risk for incontinence after cystocele repair (some women develop incontinence after a cystocele repair because of a weak urethral sphincter).

b. There are a number of prerequisites for **surgical treatment** of genuine stress urinary incontinence. The degree of incontinence must be such that it is debilitating to the patient's lifestyle. A complete evaluation should rule out other possibilities of incontinence. The patient should understand the goal of the surgery and any failure risk. The patient must also have a strong desire to have surgery.

Patients with a mixed disorder should be identified before surgery. Detrusor instability should be treated with bladder training before the surgery.

Concurrent repair of rectocele and relaxed vaginal outlets, when present, will give further support to the bladder and ameliorate symptoms.

(1) **Anterior colporrhaphy with Kelly plication** is a procedure well-tolerated by patients and can be done under local anesthesia. The anterior repair, however, does not go very far in restoring the anatomy. The bladder neck is rarely restored to a retropubic position. Commonly quoted success rates are 85%, with a reduction to 70% after 2 years.

(2) **Retropubic urethropexy** elevates the urethrovesical angle to restore continence. An incision that allows for good exposure is needed. Before the urethropexy, consideration should be given to closing the posterior cul-de-sac with 2-0 polydioxanone sutures. This is especially important in patients with existing enteroceles.

Next, the space of Retzius is opened through gentle, blunt dissection (sharply, if the patient has had previous surgery); 2-0 sutures are passed on both sides through paravaginal fascia alongside the urethrovesical junction. The first is placed at the level of the junction 2 cm from the midline; the second is placed just distal. The urethrovesical junction is then elevated as the sutures are passed through Cooper's ligament. Opinions differ as to whether a permanent or absorbable suture is better for long-term cure.

The procedure just described is also commonly known as a **Burch colpourethropexy**. A **Marshall-Marchetti-Krantz** operation differs in that the sutures are passed through the symphysis pubis instead of Cooper's ligament. Studies give these procedures an 85% to 90% success rate after 2 years.

(3) Common **needle urethropexy procedures** are the modified Pereyra, the Stamey, and the Gittes. These procedures should be considered if the patient does not need abdominal surgery for another reason. The recovery time may be quicker and less painful, at the expense of less optimal long-term results.

With a **modified Pereyra**, anterior colporrhaphy dissection is continued past the urethrovesical junction. Blunt dissection opens the space of Retzius from below. Permanent suture is passed in a helical fashion through the pubourethral ligaments and musculofascial tissues. Continue laterally and then repeat on the other side. A suprapubic incision is then carried down to the fascia. Needle ligature carriers are passed through the fascia and behind the symphysis pubis until the vaginal finger is met. The suture can then be withdrawn and the pubourethral support elevated as the suture is tied.

A **Stamey procedure** uses endoscopy to visualize the urethrovesical junction while sutures are placed. Stamey also introduced the idea of polyethylene terephthalate fiber (Dacron) graft for urethral support instead of the patient's tissue.

The **Gittes technique** uses no incisions. The same ligature carriers are passed through small scalpel punctures to a finger elevating the anterior vaginal wall lateral to the urethrovesical junction.

3. **Intrinsic sphincter deficiency (or low-pressure urethra)**, although technically a form of stress urinary incontinence, is considered separately because its treatment options are more limited. These patients have a low urethral closure pressure (lower than 20 cm H_2O) and a low leak point pressure (lower than 60 cm H_2O). Postoperative scarring can immobilize the urethra and decrease urethral outflow resistance; therefore, procedures that increase outflow resistance are needed.

a. **Suburethral sling procedures** provide the suburethral support necessary to increase outflow resistance. The **Goebel-Stoeckel procedure** harvests fascia from the fascia lata. An **Aldridge procedure** harvests fascia from the rectus muscle. Inorganic or synthetic materials have been used but are associated with a higher rate of infection.

After incising the vaginal mucosa 1 cm posterior to the external urethral meatus, the tissues of the posterior urethra and bladder neck are laterally dissected. An abdominal incision is carried down to rectus fascia, and two incisions are made in this fascia. Blunt dissection from above and below open space behind the pubic bone and lateral to the urethra. The urogenital diaphragm is pierced with a Kelly clamp from above. The sling can be loosely passed under the urethra and drawn up for support. Ridley quoted an 88% success rate (7).

Another procedure, the vaginal **mucosa sling** or **suburethral patch,** can provide similar results. Vaginal mucosa is dissected off the paravesical fascia, similar to an anterior repair. A small 1 cm × 1 cm patch of vaginal mucosa below the urethra is left, however. Permanent suture is attached to the four corners of the patch and passed up behind the symphysis pubis with Pereyra needles. The suture is then tied above the abdominal fascia.

Urinary retention and voiding dysfunction can result from tight slings. Patients should expect a catheter to be used postoperatively in order to rest the bladder. Patients should be counseled preoperatively that a week of postoperative urinary retention is not uncommon. Rarely, patients can have dysfunction as long as 4 to 6 weeks postoperatively, requiring an indwelling catheter or intermittent self-catheterization.

    b. Periurethral bulking agents such as fat or collagen injections have received increased support among urogynecologists for the treatment of intrinsic urethral deficiencies. The procedure is well-tolerated by patients and very effective. Determine that leak point pressure is less than 60 cm H_2O. Under cystoscopic guidance, the surgeon injects the bulking agent either transurethrally or periurethrally. The injection is located at the bladder neck at the 4 and 8 o'clock positions. The patient is skin tested at a date before the procedure to identify potential problems of hypersensitivity. The greatest drawback of this procedure is that the agents are eventually resorbed and the effects lost. This is balanced, however, by the fact that it is an outpatient procedure. The effectiveness of the periurethral bulking agents is indirectly proportional to the amount of urethral hypermobility experienced by the patient.

  D. Urethral diverticula classically present with dribbling after voiding and expression of pus from the urethra. The patient may present, however, with complaints of recurrent infection, dyspareunia, or vaginal pressure and pain. It is important to include urethral palpation in the examination whenever a patient has genitourinary complaints. Asymptomatic urethral diverticulae should not be removed.

    Urodynamic assessment is necessary before any surgery for urethral diverticula (see sec. **I.B.5.a**). After the diverticular orifice is identified, the urethral closure pressure profile should be checked. If the opening is distal to the peak urethral closure pressure, a Spence procedure is the operation of choice. If the orifice is on the proximal side, an excision through vaginal mucosa followed by layered closure is preferred. The Spence procedure was designed to marsupialize the diverticulum. A urethrotomy is performed by cutting the floor of the urethra all the way to the orifice of the diverticulum. The sac is then excised. A running, locking suture around the opening completes the marsupialization.

II. Pelvic relaxation

  A. Pelvic floor support is composed of a layer of striated muscle (the levator ani and the coccygeus muscle) and its fascial covering. The levator ani is divided into the pubococcygeal and the iliococcygeal muscles and is the most important component of pelvic support, followed by the endopelvic fascia. Also important to pelvic support is the urogenital diaphragm and perineal membrane.

    This support system is a dynamic system, requiring that the levator ani have a constant resting tone to maintain closure of the pelvic floor. The muscular floor can then support the pelvic organs in their proper position.

  B. Risk factors for pelvic organ prolapse are similar in that they cause damage or atrophy to the musculofascial floor. **Nerve damage** causes the muscles to atrophy. When the muscles become too weak or damaged, the endopelvic fascia becomes the primary support. Fascia, however, does not stretch or attenuate—it breaks. **Obstetric trauma** from a prolonged second stage of labor or pudendal nerve injury from forceps delivery, **chronic increases in intraabdominal pressure, aging,** and **estrogen deficiency** are all well-recognized risk factors for pelvic relaxation.

  C. Discussion of the **types of pelvic organ prolapse** focuses on the organs that are herniating and their location. Examples of types include **relaxed vaginal outlet, rectocele, enterocele, cystocele, uterine prolapse, and vaginal prolapse.** These defects are further defined by descriptions of mild, moderate, severe, or first-, second-, and third-degree prolapse, allowing for clear documentation and communication between physicians. The surgeon should decide if the problems are related to a global defect or a focal defect.

    Investigation of pelvic organ prolapse should begin with a careful medical history. The patient should be carefully questioned about any problems with urinary or fecal incontinence. Does the patient need to "splint" her vagina with her fingers to evacuate stool? The patient should be asked about fecal incontinence, as she may not volunteer this information.

1. **Clinical evaluation** should be comprehensive, with the patient in supine and standing positions to give a better chance of reproducing the problems. Quantify any descent of the bladder, urethra, vagina, uterus, and rectum. Repeat this with a Valsalva maneuver. Check for enterocele with rectovaginal exam while the patient stands.

   Stroking the vaginal mucosa or cervix with a cotton swab often identifies fragile epithelium resulting from estrogen deficiency. A cotton swab test should also be performed to evaluate the bladder neck support (see sec. I.B.4.c).

2. **Diagnostic tests** may help unmask urinary incontinence. Severe uterine prolapse can cause anatomic distortions that conceal urinary incontinence, which patients with severe uterine prolapse are prone to have. Diagnostic tests also help separate focal from global defects.

   a. **Urodynamics studies** should be performed to rule out any problems with urge incontinence before surgical correction of stress urinary incontinence is undertaken (see sec. I.B.5).

   b. **Dynamic fluoroscopic imaging** can be a useful adjunct to the physical examination. This study should be reserved for patients who are having repeat surgery for prolapse. It can precisely identify fascial tears and confirm an enterocele (8).

   c. Similarly, **dynamic magnetic resonance imaging** can provide more objective information on the location and severity of hernias (9).

   d. **Anal manometry** and ultrasound studies should be considered to evaluate fecal incontinence.

D. **Preventing pelvic organ prolapse** should be a goal during vaginal deliveries and hysterectomies. The obstetrician should be aware of the damaging effect that a prolonged second stage of labor or improperly placed forceps can have on the pudendal nerve and the pelvic floor. The gynecologist's patient can benefit greatly from proper support of the vaginal vault after hysterectomy.

   The contributing factors to pelvic relaxation rarely go away and, in fact, usually progress. Abdominal forces directed to the pelvis distribute the pelvic pressure to the areas of weakest support. Correction of defects at one site but not another can be a great disservice to the patient. Traction of the vaginal axis in more posterior or anterior directions, as in vaginal vault fixations or colpourethropexy, will allow these forces to cause problems. The former places the patient at risk for cystocele and anterior enterocele; the latter places the patient at risk for rectocele and posterior enterocele.

E. **Management of pelvic organ prolapse** should be aimed at improving the patient's symptoms for the present and the long-term. It is not recommended to attempt to surgically improve an asymptomatic patient's pelvic relaxation.

1. **Nonsurgical therapy** is always part of the treatment plan and can be especially useful for patients who are poor surgical candidates.

   a. **Encouraging behavioral alterations** such as decreased tobacco use and weight loss should not be overlooked. Constipation problems can usually be addressed successfully. Behaviors helpful in improving stress urinary incontinence will usually improve pelvic relaxation [see sec. I.C.2.a.(1)].

   b. **Hormone replacement** is effective as a primary treatment for mild pelvic relaxation and as a preoperative adjunctive therapy. Estrogen improves elasticity, thickens the vaginal mucosa, and improves local blood supply. These effects increase muscle tone in the pelvis and make the fascia more resistant to breaking.

      Preoperative estrogen supplementation thickens the vaginal mucosa and decreases its fragility. As a result, dissection of mucosa off the fascia during surgery is much more efficient.

   c. **Pelvic training, biofeedback, and Kegel exercises** should be made part of the therapeutic plan for every patient with mild to moderate problems [see sec. I.C.2.a.(2)–(3)].

    d. Vaginal pessaries will support prolapsed organs and improve many symptoms when sized correctly. Sometimes, as in the severely ill patient, they are the only treatment option.

        (1) Proper care for the pessaries includes regular and frequent cleaning of the device. Patients who use these devices should be seen in the office frequently so the vaginal mucosa can be examined for infection and abrasion. Oral or vaginal estrogen therapy will help protect the mucosa. The commonly employed oral therapies or conjugated equine estrogen vaginally at a dose of 1 g/day should be used.

        (2) Pessary types in use today include the Smith-Hodge, Gellhorn, Gehrung, cube, donut, and ring. The Smith-Hodge should be used for patients with stress urinary incontinence [see **sec. I.C.2.a.(5)**]. The Gellhorn is a rigid acrylic pessary that can be used for third-degree uterine prolapse and procidentia. The Gehrung pessary, which is made of flexible plastic and arch-shaped, is the only pessary that will allow coitus when placed properly. Generally, it is used in patients with third-degree prolapse and cystocele or rectocele, and insertion can be difficult. The cube is also designed to correct third-degree prolapse and is sometimes the only pessary that will support a procidentia. This device, with a string, is squeezed before insertion, creating a vacuum that sucks the vaginal walls toward it. Difficulties often arise in removing the cube because of the suction. The donut pessary is made of silicone and used for third-degree uterine prolapse. The ring is used for patients with lesser degrees of prolapse.

2. Surgical therapy

    a. Anterior colporrhaphy is used to restore the fascia and muscular support of the urethra and bladder. This anterior repair is used in patients with a large posterior cystocele who need digital support to fully empty the bladder. Patients will usually require other concurrent procedures to repair further fascial defects. A small cystocele may also be corrected abdominally.

    b. Posterior colporrhaphy is used to repair those fascial defects that allow herniation of rectocele. Lateral dissection is extended far enough to mobilize pararectal fascia and levator ani muscles. No. 0 delayed-absorbable vertical mattress sutures are used to plicate the pararectal fascia. Several sutures can be used to approximate the levator ani at the midline. Complete dissection of the rectovaginal wall over its entire length will expose a high rectocele and enterocele when present.

    c. Perineorrhaphy for a relaxed vaginal outlet often accompanies a posterior repair. The muscles of the perineum are identified by making a transverse incision at the mucocutaneous junction and a V-shaped incision over the perineal body. No. 0 delayed-absorbable suture is used to plicate the pararectal fascia and levator ani.

    d. Enterocele repair requires either preoperative or intraoperative diagnosis of the enterocele by the astute surgeon. The entire posterior wall of the vagina must be dissected to its apex. After thorough dissection, the surgeon can often visualize the protruding hernia sac. Small bowel may or may not fill the enterocele sac. A rectal exam or a probe placed in the bladder, or both, will aid in identification of an enterocele sac. The sac is mobilized and entered sharply, intestinal contents are identified and displaced, and several high purse-string sutures are applied around the neck of the sac. The remaining peritoneum is excised. The uterosacral ligaments are then plicated (10).

    e. Transvaginal sacrospinous colpopexy is used to affix the vagina to the sacrospinous ligament when vaginal vault prolapse is identified. An Allis clamp is placed on the vaginal vault, and the area of the vault that could be held to the ligament with the least amount of tension is identified. The vault can be attached to one or both sacrospinous ligaments.

Alternatively, the vagina can be affixed to the sacrotuberous ligament. A perineal incision is made, and blunt dissection is used to enter the rectovaginal space. Rectal pillars formed from fibers of the cardinal/uterosacral ligament complex extend from vagina to rectum and sacrum. Lateral to these pillars are the pararectal spaces and the sacrospinous ligaments. Adequate exposure with Breisky-Navratil refractors and a notched speculum will reveal the sacrospinous ligament. A Miya hook ligature carrier, Shutt suture punch, or Deschamps ligature carrier is used to place permanent suture through the ligament. A thorough understanding of the surrounding anatomy is necessary.

The sacrospinous ligament lies within the inferior aspect of the coccygeus muscle. The coccygeal muscle originates at the ischial spine and inserts at the coccyx. Pudendal vessels run below the ischial spine. The inferior gluteal vessels lie behind the ligament. The sciatic nerve originates at the sacral plexus above the coccygeal muscle then travels lateral to the ischial spine. A free needle is used to place the sutures subepithelially through the vagina. An anterior colporrhaphy and the upper part of a posterior colporrhaphy are performed at this point if needed. Afterwards, the sutures can be tied. This procedure has good long-term success, often above 90% (11).

f. **Abdominal sacrocolpopexy** is an excellent procedure for vaginal prolapse. In this procedure, the vaginal vault is fixed to the sacral promontory with autologous or synthetic material. The surgeon should make sure to attach the lateral vaginal corners and 3 to 4 cm of posterior vaginal vault to the graft. The peritoneum is opened over the sacral promontory, and one end of the graft is attached with permanent suture. There should be no tension in the graft. The graft is then covered with peritoneum. Because presacral venous bleeding can be troublesome, the surgeon should be prepared to control it with steel tacks. Success rates of long-term results of more than 93% are typical (12).

References

1. Vierhout ME, Mulder AFP. De novo detrusor instability after Burch colposus pension. *Acta Obstet Gynecol Scand* 1992;71:414–416.
2. Stanton SL, Ozsoy C, Hilton P. Voiding difficulties in the female: prevalence, clinical, and urodynamic review. *Obstet Gynecol* 1983;61:144–147.
3. Fantl JA, Hurt WG, Dunn LJ. Dysfunctional detrusor control. *Am J Obstet Gynecol* 1977;129:299–303.
4. Fantl JA, et al. Bladder training in the management of lower urinary tract dysfunction in women. *J Am Geriatric Soc* 1990;38:329–332.
5. Peattie AB, Plevnik S, Staunton SL. Vaginal cones: a conservative method of treating genuine stress incontinence. *Br J Obstet Gynaecol* 1988;95:1049–1053.
6. Bhatia NN, Bergman A, Gunning JE. Urogynamic effect of vaginal pessary in women with stress urinary incontinence. *Am J Obstet Gynecol* 1983;147:876–884.
7. Ridley JH. Appraisal of the Goebel-Stoeckel Sling procedure. *Am J Obstet Gynecol* 1966;95:714–721.
8. Brubaker L, et al. Pelvic floor evaluation with dynamic fluoroscopy. *Obstet Gynecol* 1993;82:863–868.
9. Goodrich MA, et al. Magnetic resonance imaging of pelvic floor relaxation: dynamic analysis and evaluation of patients before and after surgical repair. *Obstet Gynecol* 1993;82:883–891.
10. Nichols DH, Genadry RR. Pelvic relaxation of the posterior compartment. *Curr Opin Obstet Gynecol* 1993;5:458–464.
11. Morley GW, Delancey JOL. Sacrospinous ligament fixation for eversion of the vagina. *Am J Obstet Gynecol* 1988;158:872–881.
12. Addison WA, et al. Abdominal sacral colpopexy with Mersiline mesh in the retroperitoneal position in the management of posthysterectomy vaginal vault prolapse and enterocele. *Am J Obstet Gynecol* 1995;153:140–146.

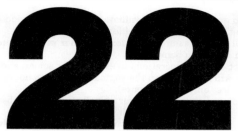

Sexual Assault and Domestic Violence

Ginger J. Gardner and
J. Courtland Robinson

I. **Epidemiology.** Violence against women is a diverse and disturbing problem affecting many women. The violence may be domestic or stranger abuse, may be physical or sexual, and may occur at any stage of life. Overall, domestic violence is the single most common cause of injury to women. Nearly 25% of women in the United States (more than 12 million) will be abused by a current or former partner sometime during their lives.

Violence against women often results in acute as well as long-standing physical and emotional pain. Women may present to gynecologists or be referred for chronic pelvic pain. During pregnancy, battering may begin or escalate and can result in poor pregnancy outcomes, including miscarriage, preterm labor, and low birth weight. Violence occurs in up to 20% of pregnancies, more prevalent than common disorders such as preeclampsia, gestational diabetes, and placenta previa.

As health care providers, we are often the first and sometimes the only professionals whom victims of violence may encounter. It is therefore our responsibility to identify patients with a history of abuse, to understand the possible physical and emotional consequences, and to provide appropriate treatments and resources.

II. **Rape crisis evaluation and treatment.** Rape crisis typically involves an acute attack, often by a stranger, leading the patient to present immediately to the emergency department. The evaluation and treatment approach is as follows:

A. **Report patient statement.**
1. Make sure a chaperon who is the same sex as the patient is present at all times for the history and examination.
2. Ask about the patient's injuries.
   a. What was the nature of the sexual violation?
   b. What has the patient done since the event—for example, has she showered, changed clothes, and so forth?
3. Do not impose interpretation on the description—document the patient's exact description of the event.
4. Document medically relevant information only. Do not include the time and place of the event, as such descriptions will be covered in the police report. Any description of such events by the physician may only increase the possibility of a discrepancy in the patient's report of attack when reviewed later.
5. Do not use legal terms such as "sexual assault" or "rape." It is acceptable to comment on findings "consistent with the use of force."
6. Take a thorough sexual and gynecologic history, including history of infections, pregnancy, use of contraception, and last consensual intercourse.

B. **Examine the patient and collect evidence.**
1. Be sensitive and gentle.
2. Document the patient's emotional condition.
3. Be thorough and systematic and record all evidence of injury; use drawings and photographs as needed.
4. Collect appropriate clothing from the patient (if she has not yet changed) and give it to the proper personnel.

5. Perform a full skin examination and evaluate all orifices for evidence of laceration, bruising, bite marks, or use of foreign objects.
6. Perform an overall general examination for any other injuries, such as abdominal trauma or broken bones.
7. Collect dry and wet swabs of secretions to evaluate for semen and hair (evidence of coitus will be present in the vagina for up to 48 hours after attack, in other orifices only up to 6 hours).
8. Collect oral, cervical, and rectal cultures for sexually transmitted diseases (STDs).
9. Perform irrigation of the vaginal vault; examine samples immediately and send to the crime laboratory to evaluate for sperm.
10. Take samples of and perform combings of the patient's genital hair.
11. Obtain fingernail scrapings.
12. Obtain a baseline syphilis serology.
13. Perform serologic tests for herpes simplex virus, hepatitis B virus, human immunodeficiency virus (HIV), and cytomegalovirus.
14. Maintain the chain of collecting evidence—give samples directly to rape crisis personnel.

C. Treat the patient.
1. Suture lacerations as needed.
2. Treat presumptively for STDs. Approximately 43% of sexual assault victims have at least one preexisting STD. The actual risk of acquiring an STD from sexual assaults is unclear; however, Chlamydia appears to be the most common pathogen. Following are treatment options.
    a. Ceftriaxone, 250 mg i.m., and doxycycline, 100 mg p.o. b.i.d. for 7 days.
    b. Spectinomycin, 2 g i.m., and doxycycline, 100 mg p.o. b.i.d. for 7 days.
    c. Erythromycin may be used as a substitute for doxycycline if the patient is known to be pregnant.
    d. Azithromycin, 1 g p.o. (one dose), may be substituted for doxycycline to enhance patient compliance and for ease of administration.
    e. Floxin, 200 mg b.i.d., for gonococcal and Chlamydia infection.
3. Provide immediate contraception. The chance of pregnancy after an assault is reported to be 2% to 4% in victims not protected by some form of contraception at the time of attack. The available options include the following:
    a. Oral contraceptive tablets containing ethinyl estradiol, 50 μg, two pills p.o. immediately; repeat in 12 hours (This method is approximately 75% effective.)
    b. Ethinyl estradiol, 5 mg q.d. for 5 days
    c. Conjugated equine estrogen, 20 to 30 mg q.d. for 5 days
    d. Intrauterine device placement
4. Provide follow-up.
    a. Follow up at 1 to 2 weeks for psychological evaluation.
    b. Follow up at 3 to 4 weeks for repeat hepatitis B testing, cultures for test of cure, and a pregnancy test.
    c. Follow up at 3 to 6 months for repeat HIV testing.
    d. Provide 24-hour hotline numbers and social work resources.

III. Domestic violence evaluation and treatment. Although some women are victims of an acute attack or rape, others find themselves in long-standing abusive or destructive relationships that include domestic violence. Women are more likely to be injured, raped, or killed by a current or former male partner than by all other types of assailants combined. Women who are injured as a result of domestic violence are more likely to suffer serious injury or loss of consciousness than are victims of stranger violence. The approach to evaluation and treatment should involve screening, assessment, and patient empowerment, as described below.
A. Screening
1. Ask about domestic violence as part of a routine patient evaluation. Abuse crosses all ethnic, religious, and socioeconomic divides—ask as frequently as possible.

2. **Ask periodically.** Studies show that women asked about violence more than once during detailed in-person interviews or asked more than once during pregnancy report higher prevalence rates.
3. **Interview the patient in private** without her partner, children, or other relatives present. Be aware that the batterer often accompanies the woman to the appointment and wants to stay close at hand to monitor what she says to the physician. Find a way for him to be excused from the room to allow for a private patient-physician interview.
4. **Assure patient confidentiality.** Never ask what she did wrong or why she has not left her partner—avoid being judgmental. Avoid value-laden terms such as "abused" and "battered." Instead ask questions such as the following:
   a. Have you been hit, slapped, kicked, or otherwise physically hurt by someone?
   b. Are you in a relationship with a person who threatens or physically hurts you?
   c. Has anyone forced you to have sexual activities that made you uncomfortable?
   d. Does your partner treat you well?
   e. Does your partner criticize you or your children a lot?
   f. Has your partner ever hurt or threatened you or your children?
   g. Has your partner ever hurt pets or destroyed objects in your home or something you especially cared about?
   h. When you argue or fight with your partner, what happens?
   i. Does your partner throw or break objects during arguments?
   j. Is your partner jealous?
   k. Has your partner ever tried to keep you from taking medication you needed or from seeking medical help?
   l. Does your partner make it difficult for you to find or keep a job or go to school?
   m. Does your partner ever withhold money when you need it?
   n. Has your partner ever forced you to do something you did not want to do?
   o. Does your partner abuse drugs or alcohol? What happens?
5. Ask about a history of **previous trauma, chronic pain, or psychological distress.**
6. Most important, regardless of the method, **make time to screen.** According to Dr. Richard Jones at the University of Connecticut, "If you ask about domestic violence early on, it probably takes less time than the multiple visits for PMS or pelvic pain you face with many patients. Long range, in fact, it's probably a very good use of your time and the patient's."

B. **Assessment.** Typically, a battered woman has numerous emergency room visits for injury. Her injuries usually involve multiple sites (such as three or more body parts), affect the head and torso (accidental injuries are more likely to be peripheral), and are in various stages of healing. The patient may say she is accident prone or have a vague or inconsistent description of the mechanism of injury in relation to the bodily damage.

   In contrast, the patient may report a variety of somatic complaints. Patients may have headaches, insomnia, choking sensations, hyperventilation, or back and chest pain. Victims may have gastrointestinal disturbance and they are twice as likely to report a history of functional bowel disorder. Rather than use descriptors of or show evidence of physical pain, some patients may present with mood changes, anxiety, eating disorders, drug use and abuse, or suicidal thoughts. Battered women actually account for 25% of women who attempt suicide, and a suicide threat on the part of the batterer or the victim may be a warning that homicide may actually occur. Such complaints certainly warrant a full assessment for underlying disease; they should also serve as a possible indicator of domestic violence (Fig. 22-1).

General presentations
Statement "I've been beaten."
Vague description of cause
Inconsistent description of cause
Time delay from occurrence
Multiple injuries
Various stages of healing
Depression and attempted
  suicide
Anxiety and panic disorders
Repetitive somatoform symptoms
Substance and alcohol abuse
Eating disorders
Hostile, uncooperative behaviors

Gynecologic presentations
Sexually transmitted diseases,
  including human immunodefi-
  ciency virus
Unintended pregnancy
Chronic pelvic pain
Sexual dysfunction
Recurrent vaginal infections
Premenstrual stress syndrome

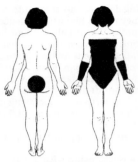

Obstetric presentations
Late prenatal care, missed
  appointments
Substance use and abuse
Multiple, repeated complaints
Poor weight gain and nutrition
Preterm labor
Low birth weight
Fetal injury and death
Maternal injury

Indirect clues
Accident prone
Immature personality
Hysteric
Psychosomatic complaints
Diffuse anxiety disorder
Help-rejecting behaviors
Masochistic

Physical examination demeanor
Flat affect
Embarrassed
Hesitant
Eye contact avoided
Frightened
Evasive
Hostile
Disassociation or zoning out
  during examination

Figure 22-1. Indicators of domestic violence. (From ACOG Family Violence Work Group. *Domestic violence: the role of the physician in identification, intervention, and prevention.* ACOG slide lecture presentation, 1995. Reprinted with permission.)

1. **Findings and signs specifically seen by obstetricians and gynecologists**
   a. Gynecologists
      (1) Chronic pelvic pain (Victims are more likely to have had pelvic surgery than nonabused patients.)
      (2) Premenstrual syndrome
      (3) Multiple or recurrent STDs
   b. Obstetricians
      (1) Unintended pregnancy
      (2) Late registration for prenatal care, no prenatal care, missed appointments
      (3) Fetal or maternal injury (Violence is often directed toward the woman's abdomen during pregnancy.)
      (4) Spontaneous abortion or stillbirth
      (5) Preterm labor
      (6) Low-birth-weight infants
2. The mechanism of injury during pregnancy may be direct or indirect. Partial abruption or premature rupture of membranes secondary to the mechanical force of trauma and infection or exacerbation of chronic illnesses such as asthma are examples of the direct effect of abuse on poor pregnancy outcome. Indirectly, elevated physical and psychological stress from abuse can be associated with resultant poor nutritional intake and cigarette, alcohol, or illegal drug abuse, leading to poor pregnancy outcomes.
3. Alternatively, the patient may directly reveal that she has been battered. If the patient reports she is a victim, or if you suspect battering without her disclosure, ask the following to assess the degree of the risk to the patient:
   a. How were you hurt?
   b. Has this happened before?
   c. When did it first happen?

The following exit plan has been proposed for a woman who feels that she or her children are in danger from her male partner:

1. Have a change of clothes packed for herself and her children, including toilet articles, necessary medications, and an extra set of house and car keys. These can be placed in a suitcase and stored with a friend or neighbor.
2. Cash, a checkbook, and a savings account book may also be kept with the individual chosen.
3. Identification papers, such as birth certificates, social security cards, voter registration card, utility bills, and a driver's license should be kept available because children will need to be enrolled in school and financial assistance may be sought. If available, financial records such as mortgage papers, rent receipts, or an automobile title should be taken.
4. Something of special interest to each child, such as a book or toy, should be taken.
5. A plan of exactly where to go, regardless of the time of day or night, should be decided upon. This may be a friend or relative's home or a shelter for battered women and children.

Figure 22-2. Exit plan for abused women. (From Helton A. Battering during pregnancy. *Am J Nurs* 1986;86:910–913. Modified with permission.)

    d. How badly have you been hurt in the past?
    e. Have you needed to go to the emergency room for treatment?
    f. Have you ever been threatened with a weapon, or has a weapon ever been used on you?
    g. Have you ever tried to get a restraining order against a partner?
    h. Have your children ever seen or heard you being threatened or hurt?
    i. Do you know how you can get help for yourself if you were hurt or afraid?
 C. Empowering the patient
    1. Discuss the seriousness of the situation.
    2. Treat patient injuries and assess emotional status for suicidal tendencies, depression, and substance abuse.
    3. Empower the woman to better protect herself and her children. Most women feel unable to leave an abusive relationship because of lack of financial resources or fear that the batterer will follow them.
    4. Discuss court restraining orders and laws against stalking.
    5. Provide the patient with phone numbers of resource agencies in the event of an acute outbreak of violence.
    6. Review an exit plan or exit drill (Fig. 22-2).
IV. Pediatric and geriatric abuse
 A. Childhood physical abuse. While screening women for current abusive encounters, it is important to recognize their risk factors include prior childhood sexual or physical abuse. The following is a review of the most common manifestations of childhood physical abuse. The victim and her children may have a history of or be at risk for such injuries.
    The most common injury sustained during physical child abuse is soft-tissue injury. Circumferential injuries may represent choking or forced restraint. Scars or bruises in various stages of healing may indicate repetitive abuse and, in contrast to accidental injuries, typically do not involve the bony prominences. The injury may represent the shape of the object used to inflict

the injury such as a belt buckle or a rope. Documented intraabdominal injuries in the absence of a previous high-impact injury are also suggestive of abuse, and the patient may present with nausea, vomiting, hematuria, hematemesis, melena, abdominal distention, or abdominal bruising.

The second most common injury in childhood physical abuse is multiple or complex fractures, which usually represent the late manifestations of abuse. Accidental fractures are uncommon in children younger than 1 year of age, and Salter-Harris fractures in infancy are virtually diagnostic of child abuse based on the large amount of force required to dislodge the tight attachment of the periosteum to the underlying bony cortex. Such fractures can be sustained when a child is violently swung by the arms or legs. Lateral or posterior rib fractures may indicate violent squeezing of the rib cage and can be seen most easily on roentgenograms as callus formation well after the abusive episode.

The third most common result of childhood physical abuse is intracranial injury. This type of injury usually occurs in shaken baby syndrome. It may be difficult to diagnose because of the absence of visible physical skull injury and because the nonspecific presentation can mimic infection, intoxication, metabolic disease, or electrolyte imbalance. Shaken baby syndrome can result in blindness or mental deficiency.

Burn injuries should also alert the clinician to the possibility of childhood abuse. Scald burns are the most common type of inflicted burn injury, usually inflicted after the child fails to be toilet trained or after periods of enuresis. The burn pattern may be in a stocking-and-glove dunking appearance, an oval appearance over the buttocks or genitalia, or a pour or splash appearance with a distribution that is difficult to attribute to childhood activity. A child's accidental scalding usually occurs when a child looks up and pulls a hot liquid on himself or herself. The burn is present on the face, arms, and upper trunk and usually involves the underside of the chin and axilla. Other types of splash burns should be considered suspicious for abuse. Branding injuries may also occur, such as cigarette or cigar burns, seen as multiple, deep, circular burns on the soles, palms, and genitalia. Accidental contact burns usually involve a smaller portion of the skin, are poorly marginated, and are more superficial than burns from abuse.

B. **Childhood sexual abuse.** The majority of childhood sexual abuse occurs between the ages of 6 and 14, especially between ages 12 and 14. The victim is typically a girl who sustains vaginal, anal, or oral penetration, and the perpetrator is usually a relative or an acquaintance. In contrast to physical abuse, there are rarely physical or laboratory findings of the trauma. It is the child's word that is the indicator of the abuse.

Some signs, however, can be used as diagnostic clues for childhood sexual abuse, especially if the abuse is recent or repetitive and leaves physical stigmata, as follows:

1. Genital findings
   a. Thickening or hyperpigmentation of labia majora, labia minora, or introitus
   b. Irregular or enlarged hymenal orifice
   c. Bruises, bleeding, and abrasions in the vulvovaginal area
   d. Vaginal discharge and pruritus
   e. Laxity of the anal sphincter, anal fissures or lacerations, or perianal scarring
   f. Positive acid phosphatase on the body or in the clothes; sperm in the child's urine

2. Childhood STDs. Although only 2% to 10% of abused children become infected, the findings of childhood syphilis, gonorrhea, condylomata acumata, and chlamydia should alert the clinician to evaluate for sexual abuse.

3. Behavioral problems. Abused children may demonstrate anxiety, sleep disturbances, withdrawal, somatic complaints, increased sex play, inappropriate sexual behavior, school problems, acting-out behaviors, self-destructive behaviors, depression, or low self-esteem.

    4. Adolescent pregnancy. Former victims of childhood sexual abuse may be at increased risk for conception during adolescence.

    5. Child's parent is in an abusive relationship. Forty-five percent to 59% of mothers of abused children have been abused or raped.

    Unlike partner violence, evidence of child abuse must be reported to the police or specified social agencies in all 50 states.

  C. Elder abuse. Elder abuse is a variant of domestic violence that affects as many as 2 million Americans, typically at the hands of adult family members or caregivers. Physicians should apply the same criteria in assessing the older individual as they would a younger woman for domestic violence.

V. Lesbian, gay, and bisexual relationships. Less is known about medical issues in the gay, lesbian, and bisexual community; however, domestic violence in same-sex relationships appears to be as common as in heterosexual relationships. The victims encounter the same spectrum of abusive behavior as their heterosexual counterparts, and they may face additional obstacles to disclosure, accessing care, and achieving safety. Physicians should approach screening, diagnosis, and treatment with special sensitivity.

Resource Information

National Domestic Violence Hotline (1-800-799-SAFE). This hotline provides a listing of local shelters and crisis centers. This number can be used as a resource for both clinicians and as a hotline for victims of abuse.

Call local government officials for state laws regarding stalking and restraining orders, for child abuse reporting agencies and child protective services, and for rape crisis centers and hotlines in the local area.

Call hospital departments, such as the psychiatry department, to find staff specializing in the area of physical and sexual abuse and specializing in social work.

Other national hotlines

National Resource Center on Domestic Violence and Department of Justice Information Center (800-537-2238)

National Assault Prevention Center (908-369-8972)

National Coalition Against Domestic Violence (303-839-1852)

National Institute for Violence Prevention (508-833-0731)

Selected Reading

American College of Obstetricians and Gynecologists. *Technical bulletin: domestic violence,* Washington, DC: American College of Obstetricians and Gynecologists, 1995.

American College of Obstetricians and Gynecologists. *Technical bulletin: sexual assault,* Washington, DC: American College of Obstetricians and Gynecologists, 1992.

Chambliss L, Bay R, Jones R. Domestic violence: an educational imperative? *Am J Obstet Gynecol* 1994;172:1035–1038.

Chez R, Jones R, Stark E, Warshaw C. Dialogues on domestic abuse. *Contemp OB/GYN* 1992;42:78–110.

Gazmararian J, Lazorick S, Apitz A, Ballard T, Saltzman L, Marks J. Prevalence of violence against pregnant women. *JAMA* 1996;275:1915–1920.

Gonzalez-Ibrahim E. Diagnostic points in child abuse. *Resident and Staff Physician* 1996;42:12–16.

Massachusetts Medical Society Committee on Violence. *Partner violence: how to recognize and treat victims of abuse,* 2nd ed. Waltham, MA: Massachusetts Medical Society, 1996.

Muram D. Child sexual abuse. *Obstet Gynecol Clin North Am* 1997;19:193–206.

Newberger E, Barkan S, Lieberman E, et al. Abuse of pregnant women and adverse birth outcome. *JAMA* 1992;267:2370–2372.

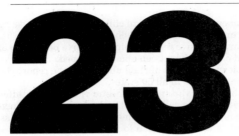

23

Breast Diseases

Cecilia Lyons and
Michael Choti

Breast cancer is the most common malignancy in women. The incidence of breast cancer has been increasing at an annual rate of 1.2% since 1940, and there are approximately 180,000 new cases diagnosed each year. It is the leading cause of death in women aged 40 to 55 years, and an estimated 45,000 women die yearly from this disease. One in nine women will develop breast cancer in her lifetime. Many women only see a gynecologist on a regular basis for checkup, and it is therefore crucial that the gynecologist is able to adequately detect and work up breast disease.

I. **Anatomy.** The adult breast lies between the second and sixth ribs in the cervical axis and between the sternal edge and midaxillary line in the horizontal axis. Breast tissue also projects into the axilla as the axillary tail of Spence. The breast is comprised of three major tissues: skin, subcutaneous tissue, and breast tissue consisting of both parenchyma and stroma. The parenchyma is divided into 15 to 20 segments that converge at the nipple in a radial arrangement. Between five to ten major collecting ducts open into the nipple. Each duct drains a lobe made up of 20 to 40 lobules. Each lobule consists of ten to 100 alveoli. Fascial tissues surround the breast. The major blood supply to the breast is from the internal mammary and thoracic arteries. The lymphatic drainage is unidirectional from the superficial to deep lymph plexuses. Flow moves toward the axillary (97%) and internal mammary nodes (3%).

II. **Methods for screening and diagnosis of breast cancer**

A. A complete **physician breast examination** should be performed once a year in the average-risk patient.

1. **Inspection** should first be performed with the patient sitting with her arms relaxed at her sides. The contour and symmetry of the breasts as well as skin changes or scars, position of the nipples, or appearance of a mass should be noted. Erythema or edema should be noted. Skin dimpling and nipple retraction sometimes can be seen when the patient is asked to lift her hands above her head and then press her hands on her hips thereby contracting the pectoralis muscles. Distortion of Cooper's ligaments may lead to skin dimpling.

2. **Palpation** is best performed with the flat portion of the fingers. The patient's breast should be palpated in a methodical fashion either in concentric circles or by quadrant until the entire breast is palpated. The entire axilla and supraclavicular areas should be palpated to detect adenopathy. If the nodes are suspicious, assessment of their consistency and number is important. The entire breast from the clavicle to the costal margin should be examined in both the upright and supine positions to best evaluate for any palpable dominant mass, nodularity, or tenderness. Any dominant mass should be evaluated and biopsied in most cases, regardless of the mammographic appearance, to rule out other synchronous cancers or multifocal disease. Many patients have a normally nodular breast parenchyma that can make the detection of a dominant mass difficult. Breast cancer that presents as a mass is often nontender and firm

with indistinct borders. It may be fixed to the skin or underlying fascia. The optimal time for breast examination is during the first 10 to 14 days after menses when the hormonal influence is the least. The nipple should also be checked for nipple discharge, as well as examined for skin changes, including retraction, erythema, and scaling. All positive findings should be well documented in writing and preferably with a drawing.

B. **Breast self-examination (BSE).** BSE is recommended for all women after age 20 years on a monthly basis. This skill should be demonstrated and taught to the patient. The patient should begin the examination with inspection in front of a mirror in a well-lit room. She should inspect her breasts with her hands along her sides and then raised above her head. She should look for abnormalities in her breast contour, asymmetry, skin changes, nipple alterations, or discharge. The patient should be instructed to palpate supraclavicular and axillary locations looking for masses or nodes. Then she should lie in the supine position with a pillow beneath her back on the side of the breast being examined to rotate her chest so that the breast being examined is symmetrically flattened against the chest wall. The patient should then systematically palpate each quadrant of her breast, including the area beneath the nipple. The nipples should be compressed for evidence of discharge. The patient should feel for masses or other changes from previous examination. If there are any findings of concern, she should immediately contact her physician.

C. **Screening mammography.** Mammography has been credited with reducing the mortality from breast cancer by up to 30%. It is important that the mammographic study is done adequately, looking at all breast tissue. It should include at least two views of both breasts: a mediolateral side view and a cranio-caudal view. Mammography is an essential part of the examination of women with a palpable mass even when cancer is obvious. The mammogram in such a situation is most useful in evaluating other areas of the breast. Mammographic abnormalities characteristic of breast cancer include spiculated, soft-tissue densities; microcalcifications; and architectural distortion of the breast without obvious mass. Microcalcifications can occur with or without an associated mass lesion. Suspicious calcifications occur in clusters and are often pleomorphic and small compared to benign calcifications. Approximately *15% of cancers are not apparent on mammogram.* This is true for both small and large lesions and especially true in younger patients. If a lesion is palpable on physical examination but not apparent on a mammogram, a biopsy should be done.

The following are guidelines for mammography screening to be undertaken with a broader program of monthly breast self-examination as well as yearly physician examination.

- A screening mammogram should be performed in all women between the ages of 35 and 40 years; in high-risk patients, this age should be lowered to 30 years.
- Mammography should be performed every 1 to 2 years in women between the ages of 40 and 50 years.
- Annual mammogram should be performed in patients 50 years of age and older.

D. **Diagnostic mammography.** Diagnostic mammography is used when the presence of a lesion has already been detected either as a result of physical examination or screening mammography. There is an overlap in radiographic characteristics between benign and malignant lesions. Mammography can be diagnostic if a lesion has very typical characteristics for cancer (i.e., spiculated or ill-defined margins). Diagnostic mammography includes further radiologic work up, including spot compression views, magnification images, and often, special studies that characterize findings more clearly. It is always important to compare mammograms with previous screening or diagnostic studies.

E. **Ultrasonography.** Ultrasound is a valuable supplement to, but never a substitute for, mammogram. Ultrasound is particularly useful in distinguishing cystic from solid lesions. Ultrasound may be used in patients with indeterminate mammographic abnormalities or in patients with dense breasts on mammography. Ultrasonographic features suspicious for cancer include solid masses with ill-defined borders or complex cystic lesions.

F. Other imaging techniques. Newer imaging modalities are under investigation to improve early detection screening and accuracy of breast cancer diagnosis, including magnetic resonance imaging, positron emission tomography scan, and digital mammography.

G. Biopsy techniques

1. **Fine-needle aspiration biopsy (FNAB)** is used to obtain cellular material from a breast abnormality for cytologic evaluation. This method is quick and less invasive than other methods. It involves introduction of a narrow-gauge (22 G) needle into a lesion under suction with multiple passes to obtain cellular material. It is important to be aware that this procedure is not 100% accurate and often cannot distinguish between invasive and non-invasive carcinomas. Typically, FNAB is used for palpable masses and can be done in the office. It can also be performed under ultrasonographic or stereotactic mammographic guidance.

2. **Stereotactic and ultrasound-guided core biopsy.** In this diagnostic method, a large-bore needle (14 G) is used to obtain the specimen, which consists of slender cylindric fragments or cores of tissue that are sent for histologic evaluation. Both frozen and permanent sections can be made. Multiple cores are often taken, often four to five. This procedure is commonly performed under stereotactic mammographic guidance on a mammographic abnormality, although it can also be performed under ultrasound guidance or directly on a palpable mass. Image-guided biopsy techniques are becoming more common, including larger core suction-assisted biopsy devices.

3. **Excisional biopsy** is typically performed under local anesthesia. With this approach, the abnormality is completely removed. It can be performed for both palpable and nonpalpable lesions. With a nonpalpable mammographic abnormality, needle localization and wire is used, which is called *needle localization breast biopsy*. With this technique, a needle or wire (or both) is first placed in the area of the lesion under mammographic guidance. The patient is then brought to the operating room where an excisional biopsy of the area of the tip of the needle is performed. Specimen radiograph during surgery should always be performed to confirm complete removal.

4. **Incisional biopsy.** With this method, only a portion of the mass is excised, usually under local anesthesia. Incisional biopsy is mostly used if the mass is too large for complete excision, the result of which would compromise definitive therapy, or in patients with inoperable disease to plan future systemic therapy. This type of biopsy is rarely performed except in unusual circumstances.

H. Workup of palpable breast mass. Evaluating a palpable mass requires a thorough history, physical, and mammography. In the majority of cases, the important presenting symptom is a painless mass. The presence of pain, however, should not lead to a false reassurance because as many as 10% of patients with cancer may present with breast pain. Less common symptoms include nipple discharge, nipple rash or ulceration, diffuse erythema of the breast, adenopathy, and symptoms associated with distant metastasis. Enlargement of the breast with or without a distinct mass, erythema, and peau d'orange are the hallmarks of locally advanced breast cancer and can sometimes be confused with mastitis. Early breast cancer can also be associated with a breast abscess or mastitis. Any non-lactating woman with an infection of the breast should be observed and biopsy should be considered if a residual abnormality is present after resolution of the infection. Ultrasound with needle aspiration is useful in distinguishing between cystic and solid lesions. Any mass that does not disappear on aspiration or does not completely resolve on ultrasound is an indication for FNAB with cytologic examination. Core or excisional breast biopsy should be considered for any persistent solid breast mass.

I. **Workup of mammographic abnormality.** There are multiple radiologic findings that usually require surgical consultation and consideration of breast biopsy even when the physical examination is unremarkable. Listed below are examples of such findings:

- Soft tissue density, especially if the borders are not well defined radiographically
- Clustered microcalcifications in one area of the breast
- Calcifications within or closely associated with a soft tissue density
- Asymmetric density or parenchymal distortion
- New abnormality compared with previous mammogram

When a woman's screening mammogram is ambiguous, diagnostic mammographic workup with special views should be performed and a decision made whether to perform a diagnostic biopsy. If a patient is being followed with mammography, typically a short-term follow-up study is recommended within 6 to 9 months. Biopsies of mammographic lesions include needle localization excision biopsy and stereotactic core biopsy.

III. **Common benign breast problems**

A. **Breast pain** is the most common breast symptom causing women to consult a physician. As previously discussed (see sec. **II.H**), although the vast majority of patients with pain have a benign etiology, up to 10% of patients with cancer have associated pain, often with an associated mass. Benign breast pain can be either cyclic or noncyclic. Cyclic pain usually is maximal premenstrually and relieved with the onset of menses and can be either unilateral or bilateral. Cyclic breast pain frequently radiates to the ipsilateral axilla and arm. Noncyclic breast pain can have various causes, including hormonal fluctuations, firm adenomas, duct ectasia, and macrocysts. Noncyclic pain may also arise from musculoskeletal structures such as soreness in the pectoral muscles from exertion or trauma. Painful costochondritis is another common cause of breast pain. With most noncyclic breast pain, however, no definite cause is determined. Although breast cancer can present only as pain, this is uncommon. The evaluation in such a patient should include a complete history and physical examination as well as mammography in women older than 35 years of age to exclude a suspicious density as the source of pain. Patients that do not have a dominant mass can be reassured; 85% to 90% require no further therapy. If further therapy is needed, the pattern should be characterized. Approximately 80% of women with cyclic pain and 40% of women with noncyclic pain will respond to medical therapy, including caffeine withdrawal, vitamin E, or danazol.

B. **Nipple discharge** is a common presenting complaint. All nipple discharge is not pathologic, and an attempt should be made to classify the discharge as physiologic, pathologic, or galactorrhea based on history, physical examination, and guiaic testing.

1. **Physiologic discharge** is nonspontaneous and usually bilateral. It arises from multiple ducts and is usually serous in character. It may be caused by exogenous estrogens, some tranquilizers, or nipple stimulation. This type of discharge is not associated with underlying breast disease and requires no further treatment. Reassurance is sufficient treatment.

2. **Galactorrhea** is also a typically bilateral, multiduct discharge with a milky character. If the nature of the nipple discharge is uncertain, staining can be performed for fat globules. Galactorrhea may have a variety of causes, including chest wall trauma, administration of oral contraceptives, phenothiazines, antihypertensives, and tranquilizing drugs. Several endocrine abnormalities will give rise to galactorrhea, including amenorrhea syndromes, pituitary adenomas, and hypothyroidism. An evaluation for endocrine abnormality should be performed with a prolactin level and thyroid function tests. Hyperprolactinemia should be evaluated with computed tomography scan and visual field testing.

3. **Pathologic discharge** can frequently be localized to a single duct. It is usually a spontaneous discharge that is intermittent. It may be greenish-gray, serosanguinous, serous, or bloody. The most common cause of pathologic

discharge is benign breast disease even if it contains blood. The quadrant of the breast where pressure results in discharge should be noted to localize the duct. Testing the fluid for occult blood is useful to identify subtle bloody discharge. The role of cytology in the evaluation of nipple discharge is controversial and should not be used to rule out carcinoma. A mammogram should be part of the evaluation of patients with a pathologic discharge. Any patient with an associated mammographic abnormality or palpable mass should be biopsied. Also, any persistent pathologic discharge or those that are bloody should be biopsied using a surgical terminal duct excision. Benign causes for pathologic nipple discharge include papilloma, duct ectasia, and fibrocystic changes. Carcinoma accounts for only 5% of pathologic discharge, and 3% to 11% of women with cancer have an associated nipple discharge.

C. Breast infections

1. **Puerperal mastitis** is an acute cellulitis of the breast in a lactating woman. If treatment is not begun promptly, puerperal mastitis could progress to abscess formation. Mastitis usually occurs during the early weeks of nursing. On inspection, there is often a cellulitis in a wedge-shaped pattern over a portion of breast skin. The affected tissue is red, warm, and very tender. Usually, there is no purulent drainage from the nipple because the infection is around rather than within the duct system. High fevers and chills as well as flulike body ache is common. *Staphylococcus aureus* is the most common organism, and antibiotic therapy should cover this organism. Antibiotic therapy recommended is dicloxacillin, 230 to 500 mg every 6 hours, or nafcillin or oxacillin, 2 g i.v. every 4 hours for 10 days. The patient should be encouraged to continue to breast-feed or pump milk to promote drainage from the affected segments. Warmth and manual pressure to engorged areas is also beneficial.

   If puerperal mastitis is not treated promptly or fails to respond to therapy, an abscess may form. Fluctuance may be absent, and it could be difficult to detect because of the numerous fibrous septa within the breast. If the puerperal mastitis does not resolve quickly with treatment, incision and drainage with cultures is indicated.

2. **Nonpuerperal mastitis** is now the most common type of breast abscess encountered. This type of abscess is most commonly subareolar with an area of tenderness, erythema, and induration. The patient is generally not systemically ill. This is usually a polymicrobial infection including anaerobes. Empiric antibiotic coverage should be broad and include coverage for anaerobes. Aspiration or simple incision and drainage can be performed in the acute phase, but this procedure may carry a 50% to 75% recurrence and complication rate. Subsequent elective reoperation with major duct excision should be considered in these patients to reduce the risk of recurrent infection.

D. Fibrocystic condition is the most common benign breast complaint. It occurs in approximately 10% of women younger than age 21 years and is more common in the premenopausal period. Common complaints are bilateral pain and tenderness, most often localized in the subareolar or upper outer regions of the breast. These symptoms are noted most often during the 7 to 14 days before menses. The pain is likely due to stromal edema, ductal dilation, and some degree of inflammation, but the true etiology is unclear. This condition should be considered a normal variation and not a disease, although some women can be significantly debilitated by persistent symptoms. Management should include regular examinations and imaging if indicated. Oral contraceptives suppress symptoms in 70% to 90% of patients and can be considered. Analgesics, such as acetaminophen, aspirin, and nonsteroidal antiinflammatory drugs, are also helpful. It has been suggested that restricted intake of methylxanthines may produce improvement. These include elimination of coffee, tea, chocolate, and caffeinated soda. Selected patients may also benefit from diuretic therapy. Often, reassurance that the symptoms are not related to a disease or serious pathologic condition is enough for the patient.

E. **Benign lumps**
1. **Fibroadenomas** are the most common mass lesions found in women younger than 25 years. Growth is generally gradual, and there may be occasional cyclic tenderness. If the lesion is palpable, increasing in size, or psychologically disturbing, core or excisional biopsy should be considered. Conservative management may be appropriate for small lesions that are nonpalpable and have been identified as fibroadenomas by mammography, ultrasound, FNAB, or core biopsy. Careful follow-up is essential. Carcinoma within a fibroadenoma is a very rare occurrence. A rare malignant variation of fibroadenoma called *cystosarcoma phyllodes* is treated by wide resection.
2. **Breast cysts** can be found in pre- or postmenopausal women. Physical examination often cannot distinguish cysts from solid masses. Ultrasound and cyst aspiration can be diagnostic, and no further therapy is needed. If a cyst does not resolve with aspiration, recurs within 6 weeks, or is complex on ultrasound, surgical consultation should be obtained.
3. **Fat necrosis** is frequently associated with breast trauma. It has also been reported to occur after breast biopsy, infection, duct ectasia, and reduction mammoplasty as well as after lumpectomy and radiotherapy for breast carcinoma. Fat necrosis may occur anywhere, but it is most common in the subareolar region. This process can be difficult to distinguish from breast cancer on both physical examination and mammography. A painless mass in the breast that is ill-defined, firm, and poorly mobile with associated skin thickening and retraction is a common presentation. When obvious trauma has occurred with mass and associated ecchymosis, the patient can be observed. In the absence of clear-cut evidence of trauma or if the mass persists, excisional biopsy must be done to rule out malignancy.

IV. **Breast cancer**
A. **Risk factors**
1. **Genetic predisposition.** A family history of breast cancer in a first-degree relative is associated with an increased risk of developing breast cancer. Less commonly, hereditary conditions are seen in which breast cancer develops in multiple generations with high frequency. Familial and hereditary breast cancer is more commonly seen in the younger patient and is more likely bilateral. Significant advances in determining the molecular genetics of breast cancer have been made with the discovery of susceptibility genes, including *BRCA1* and *BRCA2*.
2. **Gynecologic history.** Early menarche and late natural menopause are associated with somewhat increased risk of developing breast cancer. Multiparity confers a somewhat decreased risk, and the age at first childbirth alters the incidence, the older primigravida being at increased risk of developing breast cancer.
3. **Diet.** The data available presently is insufficient to provide firm dietary advice for reduction in breast cancer risk. The influence on the prognosis of already-diagnosed breast cancer has not been well studied, and at this time there is no sound basis for giving advice regarding dietary changes. Many studies have been made regarding the influence of dietary fat on the risk of development of breast cancer, and the results are contradictory. The relationship between vitamins and other micronutrients and breast cancer has not been adequately studied to date. Some studies have shown that smoking may be associated with increased risk.
4. **Hormones.** An increased risk of breast cancer associated with oral contraceptives in premenopausal women or with hormone replacement therapy in postmenopausal women presently is considered small or nonexistent. Prolonged use of such preparations may increase the risk. Any association between oral contraceptive use and the ultimate development of breast cancer may be related to time and duration of administration. Even though metaanalysis has failed to demonstrate an increased risk of developing breast cancer from oral contraceptive use, prolonged use, especially before the first pregnancy, may be associated with a slightly increased risk of developing breast cancer. The effect of hormone replacement therapy on breast cancer is unknown.

B. Prevention and early detection. Early detection is the key to improved breast cancer survival. All women who are at average risk should have yearly physician examinations, perform monthly BSE, and have screening mammography. A baseline mammogram should be obtained at age 35 to 40 years in the average risk woman, and earlier in high-risk patients. Between age 40 to 50 years, mammograms should be obtained every 1 to 2 years, and annually after age 50. New discoveries in molecular genetics of breast cancer may open up new possibilities for identification and screening of high-risk women using genetic testing.

C. Premalignant conditions
  1. Atypia
  a. Mammary dysplasia refers to a spectrum of clinical signs, symptoms, and histologic changes and is not precise. The essential part of the evaluation of a woman with mammary dysplasia is to rule out malignancy.
  b. Atypical hyperplasias are proliferative lesions of the breast that possess some, but not all, of the features of carcinoma *in situ*. Atypical hyperplasias are categorized as either ductal or lobular in type.
    (1) Atypical ductal hyperplasia is a lesion that has features of ductal carcinoma *in situ*: nuclear monomorphism; regular cell placement; and round, regular spaces in at least part of the involved duct.
    (2) Similarly, features of **atypical lobular hyperplasia** are characterized by changes similar to those of lobular carcinoma *in situ* (LCIS) but lack the complete criteria for that diagnosis. Atypical hyperplasia, a premalignant finding, is associated with a four- to five-fold risk of breast cancer, usually in the ipsilateral breast. Women with proliferative breast disease but no atypical hyperplasia, such as sclerosing adenosis, ductal epithelium hyperplasia, and intraductal papillomas, have a breast cancer risk approximately twice that of women with no proliferative breast lesions.
  2. LCIS is a proliferative premalignant condition associated with increased risk of developing breast cancer. It is usually an incidental finding not resulting in a palpable mass or mammographic abnormality, although it can be seen in association with or adjacent to a palpable or visible cancer. It is usually multicentric and is associated with a bilateral increased risk of breast cancer. Associated palpable or mammographic abnormality must be fully evaluated to rule out associated intraductal or invasive carcinoma. Patients with evidence of LCIS are considered high risk and should be followed carefully. Prophylactic bilateral mastectomy is rarely indicated.

D. Histologic subtypes of breast cancer
  1. Ductal carcinoma *in situ* (DCIS) refers to a proliferation of cancer cells within the ducts without invasion through the basement membrane into the surrounding stroma. Histologically, DCIS can be divided into multiple histologic subtypes: solid, micropapillary, cribriform, and comedo. DCIS can also be graded as low, intermediate, or high (Elston grade I, II, or III). DCIS is the early, noninfiltrating form of breast cancer with minimal risk of metastasis and an excellent prognosis with local therapy alone.
  2. Infiltrating ductal carcinoma (IDC) is the most common histologic type of invasive carcinoma, accounting for 60% to 75% of all tumors. These tumors can be associated with varying degrees of carcinoma *in situ*.
    a. Mucinous and tubular cancers are well-differentiated variants of IDC. These cancers account for approximately 5% of breast cancers, are often more circumscribed, have a lower risk of lymph node involvement, and have a better prognosis.
    b. Medullary carcinoma, which also accounts for approximately 5% of all breast cancers, can present as a grossly well-defined lesion that is microscopically poorly differentiated with intense infiltration of lymphocytes or plasma cells.
  3. Infiltrating lobular carcinoma is a variant of invasive cancer associated with microscopic lobular architecture. These cancers account for 5% to 10% of breast cancer and are more often multifocal and less evident on mammography. In reality, a spectrum of histologic appearance of infil-

Table 23-1. Staging of breast cancer

TX	Primary tumor cannot be assessed
T0	No evidence of primary tumor
Tis	Carcinoma *in situ*: intraductal carcinoma, lobular carcinoma *in situ*, or Paget disease of the nipple with no tumor
T1	Tumor ≤2 cm in greatest dimension
T1a	Tumor ≤0.5 cm in greatest dimension
T1b	Tumor >0.5 cm but ≤1 cm in greatest dimension
T1c	Tumor >1 cm but ≤2 cm in greatest dimension
T2	Tumor >2 cm but ≤5 cm in greatest dimension
T3	Tumor >5 cm in greatest dimension
T4	Tumor of any size with direct extension to chest wall or skin
T4a	Extension to chest wall
T4b	Edema (including peau d'orange) or ulceration of the skin of the breast or satellite skin nodules confined to the same breast
T4c	Both T4a and T4b
T4d	Inflammatory carcinoma
NX	Regional lymph nodes cannot be assessed (e.g., previously removed)
N0	No regional lymph node metastasis
N1	Metastasis to movable ipsilateral axillary lymph node(s)
N2	Metastasis to ipsilateral axillary lymph node(s), fixed to one another or other structures
N3	Metastasis to ipsilateral internal mammary lymph node(s)
M	Presence of distant metastasis cannot be assessed
M0	No distant metastasis
M1	Distant metastasis (including metastasis to ipsilateral supraclavicular lymph node(s))

Stage	Tumor size	Lymph node metastases	Distant metastases
0	Tis	N0	M0
I	T1	N0	M0
IIa	T0	N1	M0
	T1	N1	M0
	T2	N0	M0
IIb	T2	N1	M0
	T3	N0	M0
IIIa	T0	N2	M0
	T1	N2	M0
	T2	N2	M0
	T3	N1, N2	M0
IIIb	T4	Any N	M0
	Any T	N3	M0
IV	Any T	Any N	M1

From American Joint Committee on Cancer. Beahrs OH, Henson DE, Hutter RVP, Kennedy BJ, eds. *Manual for staging of cancer*, 4th ed. Philadelphia: JB Lippincott Co, 1992. Reprinted with permission.

trating cancer can exist, varying from ductal to lobular features. Carcinoma with mixed features is often called *infiltrating mammary carcinoma*.

E. Staging and prognostic factors. The most common staging system for breast cancer uses the tumor, node, metastasis classification based on the size of the tumor, involvement of regional lymph nodes, and presence or absence of distant metastasis (Table 23-1). Prognosis is most strongly correlated with tumor size and the status of the axillary lymph nodes. Other factors that correlate with improved prognosis include positive staining for estrogen (ER) and progesterone (PR) receptors, low tumor grade, low S-phase, and diploid DNA. Hormone status, in addition to providing prognostic information, can predict response to hormone therapy.

F. **Local treatment of primary breast cancer**

1. **Infiltrating cancer.** The principles of local treatment of infiltrating breast cancer involve treatment of the entire ipsilateral breast tissue as well as histologic determination of axillary lymph nodes for prognostic and therapeutic indications. Therapeutic options include breast conservation therapy and modified radical mastectomy.

   a. **Mastectomy.** Decades ago, mastectomy, complete surgical removal of the breast, was the only standard therapy for the treatment of breast cancer. For infiltrating cancer, complete removal of the breast tissue, in addition to sampling the axillary contents, is performed. With **modified radical mastectomy,** pectoralis muscles are preserved. With **radical mastectomy,** pectoralis muscles are removed with the mastectomy. Radical mastectomy is rarely performed today, and only when the tumor directly involves the chest wall. **Total mastectomy,** is removal of the entire breast tissue without axillary dissection. This operation is typically reserved for those with DCIS or if prophylactic mastectomy is being performed.

   Chest wall radiation therapy is sometimes indicated after mastectomy. It is administered in patients with large, locally advanced cancers or large numbers of lymph nodes involved. A patient undergoing mastectomy can also undergo reconstruction, either performed immediately at the time of the mastectomy or in a delayed fashion. Options for reconstruction include autologous muscle transfer (transverse abdominis muscle or latissimus muscle) or the placement of an expander and implant.

   b. **Breast conservation therapy (BCT).** BCT for infiltrating cancer requires complete resection of the tumor, axillary lymph node sampling, and radiation treatment to the remaining breast tissue. Complete surgical excision, also called *lumpectomy* or *partial mastectomy*, requires complete resection with negative margins. If disease is multifocal, or large, and negative margins cannot be achieved, BCT should not be recommended. Axillary sampling or dissection is often performed through a separate, small incision in the axillary region, where a portion of the axillary contents are removed and histologically analyzed for lymph node involvement. Radiation therapy is performed postoperatively on the entire breast and may include the supraclavicular and axillary regions. This form of therapy, in appropriate patients, results in survival comparable to that of mastectomy. Recurrence within the breast typically ranges from 0.5% to 1.0% per year.

   c. **Role of axillary node dissection.** Although sampling of the axillary nodes is considered standard treatment for IDC, there is an increasing trend in its selective use. In some cases, patients with very small cancers may be offered no axillary dissection. In addition, the use of lymphatic mapping and sentinel lymph node biopsy is being investigated. With this technique, a specific, or "sentinel," lymph node(s) is identified using a radioactive tracer injected into the region of the cancer, and only this node is biopsied, sparing the need for more radical node dissection.

2. **Treatment of intraductal cancer.** Patients who have only DCIS can be similarly offered options of mastectomy or BCT. In intraductal cancer, in which the risk of nodal involvement is less than 1%, lymph node sampling is not recommended. The patient may elect mastectomy or undergo lumpectomy followed by radiation therapy. In some cases of microscopic DCIS, lumpectomy alone can be considered.

3. **Adjuvant systemic therapy.** Patients with a higher risk of a systemic recurrence often undergo additional adjuvant systemic therapy. This therapy is often recommended in patients who are lymph node–positive or when the

tumor size is large. Systemic therapy consists of either **chemotherapy** or **hormonal therapy.** Adjuvant chemotherapy has been shown to reduce the odds of death by 25% in selected patients. Chemotherapy is typically administered postoperatively, can range from 3 to 6 months, and includes multiple drug combinations [doxorubicin (Adriamycin)-cyclophosphamide, cyclophosphamide-methotrexate-fluorouracil, and others]. If a patient is undergoing BCT, chemotherapy can be administered either before or after radiation therapy. In rare cases, including **inflammatory breast carcinoma,** or locally advanced disease, chemotherapy can be administered before surgical therapy. **Hormonal therapy** is the most common adjuvant systemic therapy recommended, most commonly using tamoxifen. This medication, administered at 20 mg/day, has been shown to be more effective in patients who are ER/PR-positive. Typically, tamoxifen therapy is administered for a duration of 5 years. This treatment is well tolerated. Side effects are rare and include thromboembolism and retinopathy.

4. **Treatment of metastatic disease.** Although breast cancer is rarely stage IV at the time of presentation, approximately one-third of patients will go on to subsequently develop distant metastatic disease. This cancer is rarely curable when advanced. Patients can be offered systemic therapy, either with chemotherapy or hormonal therapy. Patients who are ER/PR-positive are more likely to respond to hormone therapy. In addition to tamoxifen, other hormonal agents include progestins, including megestrol acetate (Megace) or aminoglutethimide. Various chemotherapeutic agents can be used in this situation, including high-dose chemotherapy with marrow or stem cell rescue.

G. **Pregnancy and breast cancer.** Breast cancer is especially difficult to diagnose during pregnancy and lactation. Pregnant patients do as well as their nonpregnant counterparts at a similar stage. Treatment during pregnancy is basically the same. The tumor can usually be fully excised or mastectomy can be performed if needed during pregnancy. There is no evidence that aborting the fetus or interrupting the pregnancy will lead to improved outcome. Radiotherapy should be avoided until after delivery. Even though there are no teratogenic effects of chemotherapy in the third trimester, most physicians delay treatment until after delivery because there is little evidence that this delay will have any significant impact on prognosis.

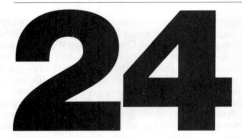

Perioperative Care and Complications of Gynecologic Surgery

Ralph Zipper,
Diljeet Singh,
Jeffrey Smith, and
J. Courtland Robinson

I. Intraoperative and postoperative hemorrhage

A. **Acquired and congenital bleeding abnormalities** that predispose a patient to intraoperative and postoperative bleeding can sometimes be discovered during preoperative evaluation from history, physical, and laboratory studies.

   1. **Coagulopathies** are more often acquired than congenital.

   2. **A history of bruising, bleeding, or postoperative bleeding, a family history of bleeding disorder, and the presence of liver disease** should all be followed up with appropriate laboratory studies to assess for bleeding potential.

   3. **Infection or sepsis** can predispose to disseminated intravascular coagulopathy.

   4. **Anemia, unusual bruising, or petechiae** evident on physical examination should be evaluated.

   5. **Recent use of medications that can affect coagulation** should be ascertained.

      a. **Aspirin, nonsteroidal antiinflammatory drugs**

      b. **Antibiotics**

         (1) **General use** with decreased oral intake can lead to vitamin K deficiency.

         (2) **Trimethoprim-sulfamethoxazole** can lead to thrombocytopenia, especially in the geriatric population.

         (3) **Moxalactam, cefoperazone, cefotetan, and cefamandole** can cause hypoprothrombinemia.

B. **Surgical causes** must be distinguished from **nonsurgical causes** in the management of intraoperative and postoperative bleeding.

   1. **Nonsurgical bleeding.** Coagulation abnormalities may arise during and after a procedure.

      a. **Transfusion** may give rise to dilutional abnormalities. For every 6 to 8 units of packed red blood cells (PRBC) administered, 2 units of fresh frozen plasma is recommended; for every 10 units of PRBC, 10 units of platelets should be given.

      b. **Infection or sepsis** may lead to the development of a disseminated intravascular coagulopathy.

   2. **Surgical bleeding.** The most conservative and least invasive approaches to surgical bleeding should be considered first to avoid complications. Aggressive supportive therapy with fluids and blood products is essential. Unnecessary delay must be avoided; with intraoperative bleeding, initial tamponade of bleeding vessels can allow time to communicate with the anesthesiologist, clear the surgical field of blood, and maximize exposure.

      a. **Arterial bleeding** is usually easy to identify. The thickness of arterial walls allows them to be grasped and clipped or ligated as appropriate.

         (1) **Arterial punctures** may be handled by placement of a figure-of-eight stitch with fine, permanent suture (e.g., 5-0 prolene).

         (2) **Large arteries that have been lacerated** can be repaired using a fine, permanent suture (e.g., 5-0 prolene). If needed, arterial

clamps can be placed above and below the site to reduce tension and interrupted stitches used to control bleeding.

(3) For the rare case of massive arterial bleeding, pressure on the distal abdominal aorta can be used to slow the bleeding while the vessel is identified and repaired. The length of time during which pressure is placed on the aorta must be carefully monitored to avoid compromising circulation to the lower extremities.

b. **Venous bleeding** can be more problematic to repair, because veins are thin-walled and easily torn.

(1) A venous puncture may be handled by placing a local hemostatic agent at the breach and applying pressure for 5 to 15 minutes.

(2) The vessel may need to be freed of surrounding tissues to be precisely ligated or clipped. **Major veins** that cannot be ligated but must be repaired if lacerated include the common and external iliacs. Continuous side-to-side closure with 5-0 prolene is the repair of choice.

(3) Postoperative intraperitoneal bleeding may cause only subtle changes in vital signs and urine output. A high index of suspicion must be maintained.

(a) Vital signs may remain stable for 12 to 18 hours before reflecting significant blood loss in a healthy patient.

(b) Abdominal distention does not always follow significant intraperitoneal bleeding (3 L or more).

(c) Delay in reexploration can be fatal.

(4) Postoperative bleeding from the vaginal vault is most often from the vaginal artery in the lateral vaginal fornix.

(a) The patient's return to the operating room should not be excessively delayed.

(b) In repairing bleeding, care should be taken to avoid bladder, ureter, and rectum.

(c) If bleeding cannot be visualized or controlled vaginally, an abdominal approach may be necessary.

II. Injury to adjacent organs

A. Ureteral injury is uncommon during gynecologic surgery, occurring in 0.3% to 0.5% of cases.

1. **Etiology and prevention.** Knowledge of ureteral anatomy, assessment of the potential for distortion of normal anatomy, and adequate exposure during the procedure are all essential in the prevention of injury.

a. **Conditions such as pregnancy, the presence of benign or malignant tumors, endometriosis, infection, uterine procidentia, and pelvic hematomas and lymphocysts** place the ureter at risk of involvement, distortion, or compression. In certain conditions, preoperative i.v. pyelography or the placement of ureteral catheters may be helpful in preventing injuries.

b. **Almost all major vaginal and abdominal operations** have been implicated in ureteral injury. The rarity of ureteral injury during subtotal hysterectomy suggests that it is the removal of the cervix that places the ureter at greatest risk. The lowest 3 cm of the ureter may therefore be the most vulnerable.

c. **The risk of ureteral injury is greater in some areas,** such as the pelvic brim (in the vicinity of the infundibulopelvic ligament), the ovarian fossa, the paracervical area (near the uterine artery), and the area between the vagina and the bladder (ureterovesical junction) (Fig. 24-1).

d. **Hazardous maneuvers** that lead to ureteral injury are clamping and oversewing to stop bleeding associated with loss of the uterine artery or ovarian pedicle, kinking or obstructing the ureter at the pelvic brim when reperitonealizing the pelvis, obstructing during procedure to obliterate the cul-de-sac, and clamping or suturing the vaginal cuff, which is associated with injury or obstruction at or near the uterovaginal junction.

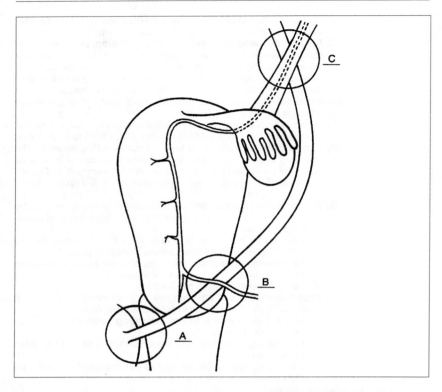

Figure 24-1. Common sites of ureteral injury associated with hysterectomy are ureterovesical junction (*A*); junction of uterine artery and ureter (*B*); and infundibulopelvic ligament (*C*). (From Shingleton HM. Repairing injuries to the urinary tract. *Contemp Obstet Gynecol* 1984;March:76. Adapted with permission.)

        e. Ureters may be kinked by nearby sutures, partially or completely **ligated** by sutures, **crushed** with a clamp, **cut,** partially or completely **resected, or subject to ischemic injury and necrosis.**

    2. Diagnosis

        a. In a minor injury, spontaneous healing may occur. **More serious injuries** not recognized during the procedure may produce symptoms postoperatively (Table 24-1).

        b. Ureteral ligation can lead to superimposed infection. An ischemic area at the point of ligation may rupture, leading to urinoma; fever, sepsis, flank pain, tenderness, ileus, and abdominal distention may be present.

        c. Radiologic evaluation, such as an i.v. pyelogram or a computed tomographic (CT) scan, that can confirm the diagnosis and help locate the injury is the response demanded by a proper index of suspicion.

    3. Repair and treatment

        a. Management depends on the patient's condition, the extent and location of the injury, the underlying diagnosis leading to surgery, and the local pathology and condition of periureteral tissues (Table 24-2).

        b. Management differs for injuries identified intraoperatively and postoperatively.

Table 24-1. Symptoms and signs of postoperative ureteral injury

Symptoms	Signs
Flank pain, tenderness	Urinoma
Fever, sepsis	Abnormal pyelogram
	Urine leak
	Obstruction
Ileus, abdominal distention	Anuria
	Silent loss of kidney
Urinary leak	
Vaginal	
Cutaneous	

From Shingleton HM. Repairing injuries to the urinary tract. *Contemp Obstet Gynecol* 1984;March:76. Adapted with permission.

(1) **If an injury is recognized intraoperatively,** the mobility of the ureter and bladder and the time required to repair the damage should be considered.

    (a) **If suture is found around the ureter,** it should be removed. Ureteral defect may be uncovered.

    (b) **For some injuries to the sheath and clamping and suturing injuries,** stenting the ureter and placing a drain at the site of injury may be sufficient therapy.

    (c) **When managing clamping injuries,** the extent to which the ureter is devitalized should be assessed; i.v. indigo carmine may show an unperceived leak. If there is no obvious severe damage or leakage, the ureteral sheath may be approximated with several 5-0 chromic sutures. Placement of a stent with drainage of the injury site further supports adequate healing.

    (d) **More extensive injuries to the lower ureter** may require additional surgery. Reimplantation into the bladder (ureteroneocystostomy) is the procedure of choice and is usually possible if the injury is within 6 cm of the bladder. The anastomosis must be tension free; mobilization of the bladder and psoas-muscle hitching can be used to bridge the gap when the ureter is short.

Table 24-2. Factors to consider in managing ureteral injury

If recognized intraoperatively	If recognized postoperatively
Mobility of ureter and bladder	Time interval to diagnosis
Time required to repair damage	Degree of impairment of renal function

Common to both

Age and general condition of patient
Underlying condition leading to original surgery
Level of and extent of injury
Associated pathology in area of injury

From Shingleton HM. Repairing injuries to the urinary tract. *Contemp Obstet Gynecol* 1984;March:76. Adapted with permission.

    (e) **Ureteroureterostomy** is the procedure of choice when a ureter is injured in the upper pelvis (approximately 7 cm or more from the bladder). **Anastomosis** is performed over a stent, and the site of injury is drained.

    (f) **Transureteroureterostomy** is potentially hazardous to both renal units and should be considered a last resort.

    (g) **Percutaneous nephrostomy** is rarely needed when an injury is discovered intraoperatively. However, if the patient's condition will not tolerate additional operative time, and there is significant risk of poor healing because of underlying conditions such as infection, malignancy, or past or planned radiation, delayed repair may be necessary.

  (2) An **injury may be uncovered postoperatively.** The time necessary for diagnosis and the degree of renal impairment should be considered when planning management.

    (a) Efforts should be made to **stent the ureter and allow healing without surgery.**

    (b) **Retrograde pyelography with cystoscopy and stent placement** should be attempted.

    (c) **Percutaneous nephrostomy with antegrade stent placement** can be performed if necessary. It may also be necessary to perform **percutaneous nephrostomy with delayed antegrade stent placement** to preserve renal function.

    (d) **Surgical repair** should be planned if circumstances prevent stent placement or if healing over the stent does not occur. The type of repair needed depends on the location of the injury and the extent of the ureteral damage and on underlying factors individual to each patient.

    (e) **The recovery potential of the kidney postobstruction** depends on the duration of the obstruction, the degree of obstruction, the degree of backflow, the presence or absence of infection, and the extent to which each kidney was functional before the injury.

B. Bladder injuries

  1. Etiology and prevention

    a. **Injuries to the bladder may occur** while incising the lower abdominal wall, during abdominal or vaginal hysterectomy, or during operations to correct stress-based urinary incontinence.

    b. **Damage occurs most frequently** while grasping the vaginal vault with clamps or suturing the cut edges of the vagina.

    c. **The risk of intraoperative damage** is reduced by adequate exposure of the wound, emptying of the bladder before incision, the use of sharp dissection during development of the bladder flap, and a good familiarity with bladder anatomy.

    d. **Bladder dissections** can be complicated, predisposing the patient to injury, by previous cesarean sections, pelvic infections, endometriosis, and distortion and obliteration of planes by benign and malignant tumors.

    e. **Methylene blue or indigo carmine** may be placed in the bladder if difficulty is anticipated, or an instrument may be placed in the urethra to help identify the proper planes. Methylene blue, indigo carmine, or sterile milk in the bladder can also help disclose a suspected injury.

    f. **An omental pedicle graft** may be placed at the base of the bladder during postirradiation hysterectomy to improve vascular supply.

  2. Repair and treatment

    a. **To avoid a potential nidus for stone formation,** absorbable suture should be used in repair.

    b. **Minor serosal or superficial seromuscular injuries** can be repaired with continuous or interrupted 3-0 absorbable suture.

    c. **Small lacerations** penetrating the bladder mucosa should be closed in two layers.

    d. Major lacerations may require mobilization of the bladder for tension-free repair.

    e. Injury to the bladder dome requires a double-layered closure of continuous 3-0 delayed absorbable suture.

    f. An injury to the bladder base should be assessed for extent and proximity to trigone and ureteral orifices. Continuous horizontal mattress sutures of 3-0 delayed absorbable suture may be used to close the first layer, approximating and inverting the bladder mucosa. Closure should go beyond the limits of the defect, and the security of this layer should be assessed by placing sterile milk or methylene blue in the bladder. One to two additional layers of vertical mattress sutures without tension should be used to approximate the relaxed bladder muscle. Cystoscopy with i.v. indigo carmine may be used if there is uncertainty about ureteral integrity.

    g. Postoperative bladder drainage should be employed, its duration depending on the extent and the location of the defect, the security of closure, the condition of the tissues, and patient comorbidities.

C. Genitourinary fistulas

    1. Most genitourinary fistulas are the result of pelvic surgery. The majority follow an abdominal hysterectomy performed for benign rather than malignant conditions. In developing countries, most fistulas are due to obstetric trauma.

    2. When intraoperative injury to the urinary tract is recognized and repaired, fistulas rarely result.

    3. Diagnosis

        a. A watery vaginal discharge that smells like urine suggests the presence of a fistula.

        b. Inspection alone can sometimes reveal the site of fistula.

        c. Placing a tampon or sequential cotton balls in the vagina after instilling methylene blue or indigo carmine into the bladder should help localize a fistula.

            (1) Blue dye on the most distal cotton ball suggests urethral urinary loss.

            (2) Dye on cotton balls in the upper vagina suggests vesicovaginal fistula.

            (3) Wet but undyed cotton balls in the upper vagina suggest a ureterovaginal fistula; i.v. administration of indigo carmine can substantiate the diagnosis.

        d. I.v. urography may help to evaluate renal function, detect ureteral obstruction, and rule out complex fistulas. **Cystoscopy** may be used to locate vesicovaginal fistulas, determine their relationship to ureteral orifices and the trigone, and evaluate the tissue around the fistula.

    4. Repair and treatment

        a. Virtually all posthysterectomy bladder fistulas are small and occur just anterior to the vaginal cuff in the bladder base. Once the cuff is healed, the **Latzo technique**—simple repair without excision of the fistula—can be performed relatively early in the postoperative period.

        b. A layering technique requires a 2- to 4-month delay to allow resolution of fistula site edema.

        c. In nonirradiated patients, both techniques have high success rates (88% to 100%).

        d. For ureteral fistulas, see sec. II.A.

D. Small bowel injury

    1. Procedures permitting injuries and prevention of injury

        a. When surgery has previously been performed in the same area, care should be taken to avoid injuring the bowel when entering the abdominal cavity. The incision may be extended beyond the width of the earlier opening to allow entry into the abdominal cavity.

        b. In cases with extensive adhesions secondary to such causes as infection, malignancy, previous surgery, and endometriosis, the risk of injury is high. The use of blunt rather than sharp dissection to release adhesions increases the risk of bowel laceration.

2. **Repair and treatment**
   a. **If the serosa is sufficiently injured to expose the muscularis,** prompt repair using 3-0 delayed absorbable suture in an interrupted fashion should be undertaken. A single seromuscular layer of sutures should be placed transverse to the longitudinal axis of the lumen to avoid luminal constriction.
   b. **If the defect exposes the lumen,** the loop should be mobilized and inspected.
      (1) **To minimize contamination,** rubber- or linen-shod clamps should be placed proximal and distal to the defect, packs placed, and the area suctioned.
      (2) **The size and location of the defect, the presence of mesenteric damage, and the health and viability of the neighboring tissues** should be assessed.
      (3) A **small defect** may be closed transverse to the longitudinal axis of the bowel with the placement of full-thickness interrupted 3-0 delayed absorbable suture. Suture line is reinforced with a second layer of seromuscular embrocating interrupted 3-0 delayed absorbable stitches. Care should be taken to avoid injury to the mesenteric vessels during repair.
      (4) **Resection with anastomosis** is necessary when the bowel wall is more extensively damaged or ischemic because of compromise of blood supply. Anastomosis with stapling is preferred to manual suturing; the use of staples decreases tissue handling and shortens the operation and the interruption of blood supply, improving healing overall.
   c. **Crush injuries** should be carefully inspected and reinforced with longitudinally placed 3-0 delayed absorbable interrupted stitches.
3. **Unrecognized or inadequately repaired bowel injuries** may lead to fistulas.

E. **Large bowel injuries**
   1. **Etiology and prevention**
      a. **Injuries to the large bowel** may occur during abdominal, vaginal, and obstetric procedures.
      b. **Risk factors** include extensive adhesions, endometriosis, pelvic inflammatory disease, benign or malignant tumors, inflammatory bowel disease, history of irradiation, or surgery.
      c. **Mechanical and antibiotic bowel preparation** is recommended when extensive pelvic disease is present or dissection is anticipated.
      d. **Subtotal hysterectomy** may be a prudent alternative to some planned hysterectomies, so that injury to the rectosigmoid colon can be avoided.
   2. **Repair and treatment**
      a. **Injuries to the rectosigmoid colon** are closed in much the same way as injuries to the small intestine. If the defect is large, if there is significant fecal contamination and the bowel is unprepared, or if the bowel wall is unhealthy or previously irradiated, a diverting loop colostomy or ileostomy may be appropriate.
      b. **Injury to the rectum** may occur during vaginal procedures. The defect should be closed by placing a row of 3-0 delayed absorbable sutures through the rectal mucosa and then reinforcing this with a two-layered closure of overlying tissue. Colostomy is rarely necessary.
      c. **The lower rectum and perineum** may be injured during delivery of a large infant, during a difficult forceps delivery, or when an episiotomy is extended. Recognition and proper repair is essential. Continuous 3-0 delayed absorbable suture should be used to approximate rectal mucosa. This should be reinforced with several interrupted 3-0 delayed absorbable sutures. Repair must go beyond the superior apex of the defect in the mucosa. If the anal sphincter is involved, it should be approximated with several interrupted 2-0 delayed absorbable

sutures. Finally, vaginal mucosa, perineal muscles, fascia, and skin should be approximated.

F. Intestinal-vaginal fistulas

   1. **Intestinal-vaginal fistulas in the upper one-third of the vagina** may result from abdominal or pelvic surgery and can be caused by injury to the small or large intestine. Repair may require concomitant colostomy.

   2. **Rectovaginal fistulas in the lower one-third of the vagina** generally require delayed repair.

III. Postoperative infection. Infections are a major source of morbidity during the postoperative period.

A. Prevention

   1. **The risk of infection** can be lessened with minimal operative time, careful dissection, meticulous hemostasis, and adequate drainage.

   2. **Procedure-related factors**

      a. **Antibiotic prophylaxis** is necessary before bowel surgery, vaginal hysterectomy, radical surgery for gynecologic cancer, and cesarean section performed more than 6 hours after rupture of membranes during labor.

      b. **Antibiotic prophylaxis for abdominal hysterectomy** probably is only necessary in the setting of significant comorbid conditions or in the geriatric population.

      c. **Closed-suction drainage** may reduce the risk of infection in cases with a greater than usual potential for collection of blood or peritoneal fluid, or in spaces that have been contaminated by bacterial spill.

      d. **Antibiotic therapy** (rather than prophylaxis) should be introduced intraoperatively in cases involving frank abscess or infection.

   3. **Patient-related factors**

      a. **Patients in whom bowel surgery is anticipated** should undergo bowel preparation.

      b. **Patients with comorbid conditions** (i.e., obesity, malignancy, cardiovascular disease, diabetes, collagen vascular disease, or other chronic illness) should be considered for antibiotic prophylaxis.

      c. **In patients who have a preoperative infection,** elective procedures should be postponed.

   4. **Antibiotic prophylaxis**

      a. A **single dose of an antibiotic** active against gram-positive and gram-negative aerobes and anaerobes should be given before the procedure. Primary pelvic pathogens include the coliforms, streptococci, fusobacteria, and bacteroides.

      b. **The antibiotic should be present** in the tissues at the time of contamination.

      c. **The shortest possible course** of antibiotic prophylaxis should be given.

      d. **The risk of complications** from antibiotic prophylaxis should not outweigh the risk of infection.

      e. **Cephalosporins** are a good choice (e.g., cefazolin, cephalothin).

      f. Ninety percent of patients with a **history of a penicillin allergy** do not react to cephalosporins.

      g. **Combinations** should be used for a specific indication, such as prevention of endocarditis. *Streptococcus faecalis*, which is frequently involved in patients undergoing genitourinary procedure, requires the synergism of penicillin and an aminoglycoside. In penicillin-allergic patients, vancomycin and an aminoglycoside are adequate. If surgery is complicated or longer than 1 hour, or if estimated blood loss is more than 1,500 mL, three doses of each antibiotic should be given.

B. Evaluation

   1. **If postoperative infection** is a concern, the patient should be evaluated for risk factors. Lack of prophylactic antibiotics, contamination of the surgical field by infected tissues or from spillage of large bowel contents, immunocompromised host, poor nutrition, chronic and debilitating severe illness, poor surgical technique, and preexisting infection are all possible contributors to postoperative infection.

2. **Potential sites of postoperative infection** include the lungs, the urinary tract, and the sites of surgery (including pelvic sidewall and vaginal cuff), incisions, and i.v. catheters.

3. **Fever**

a. **Standard definitions vary.** A **common definition** requires a temperature at or above 38°C (100.4°F) that appears after the first 24 hours following surgery on two occasions divided by at least 4 hours.

b. **Febrile morbidity** within the first 48 hours of surgery has been estimated to occur in up to 50% of gynecologic surgery patients. It often resolves without therapy.

c. Fever should be considered a **sign of infection;** the **diagnosis** of infection requires clinical and laboratory evidence of a specific pathogen.

4. **Evaluation for infection** should include a review of the patient's history and a thorough examination with specific attention to sites at risk [e.g., pulmonary examination, palpation of kidneys and costovertebral angles (CVA), evaluation of incision and catheter sites, extremity examination evaluating for deep venous thrombosis (DVT) or thrombophlebitis, and possibly a pelvic examination to evaluate vaginal cuff for cellulitis, hematoma, or abscess].

5. **Laboratory and radiologic assessment** should be tailored to the individual patient and the resources of the care setting.

a. **White blood cell count** with differential and urinalysis and urine culture may assist in diagnosis.

b. A **chest x-ray** may be helpful in patients with pulmonary risk factors (see sec. **III.C.2**) or localizing signs or symptoms.

c. **Blood cultures** are most helpful in patients with high fever or risk factors for endocarditis.

d. An i.v. pylogram may be needed to rule out ureteral damage or obstruction in patients with CVA tenderness, especially in absence of evidence of urinary tract infection (UTI).

e. A **CT scan** may be required to evaluate a patient with persistent fever but without localizing signs or with signs localizing to the abdomen for the presence of an abscess.

f. **Patients with a history of bowel surgery** may require radiologic evaluation [e.g., barium enema, upper gastrointestinal (GI) series, or CT scan] for anastomotic leak or fistula.

C. Sources

1. **Urinary tract infection**

a. The urinary tract is a **common site of infection** in surgical patients, with catheterization as the likely cause of contamination. **Antibiotic prophylaxis** has reduced incidence from as high as 35% to as low as 4%.

b. The majority of UTIs are **lower tract infections. Pyelonephritis** is a rare complication.

c. **Symptoms** of UTI include frequency and urgency in urination and dysuria.

d. **Diagnosis** rests on the appearance of more than 10^5 organisms per mL in a urine culture.

e. **Coliform/organisms** are the cause of the majority of infections. *Escherichia coli* is the most common pathogen; others include *Klebsiella, Proteus,* and *Enterobacter*.

f. **The treatment** is hydration and antibiotics tailored to the pathogen. In uncomplicated UTI, an antibiotic with good *E. coli* coverage should be used until culture results are available. Penicillins, sulfonamides, cephalosporins, and nitrofurantoin have been used with satisfactory results. Patients with a history of recurrent UTI or with conduits or indwelling catheters should be covered for less common pathogens such as *Klebsiella* as well. Sensitivities should be considered in choosing antibiotics.

2. **Pulmonary**

a. **Atelectasis** secondary to alveolar collapse may occur postoperatively. Incentive spirometry, chest physiotherapy, deep-breathing coughing, intermittent positive-pressure breathing, and continuous positive airway pressure have all been used for prevention and treatment of atelectasis.

  b. **Postoperative pneumonia** is associated with hypoventilation and atelectasis.

   (1) **The best preventative measures** are early ambulation, intensive respiratory therapy, and reversal of hypoventilation and atelectasis.

   (2) **Patients at risk for postoperative pneumonia** have an American Society of Anesthesia status of 3 or higher, preoperative hospital stay of 2 days or longer, surgery lasting 3 hours or longer, surgery in the upper abdomen or thorax, nasogastric suction, postoperative intubation, or a history of smoking or obstructive lung disease.

   (3) **Treatment** should be based on risk factors, fever, the presence of purulent sputum, positive sputum or blood cultures, leukocytosis, and physical and radiographic findings consistent with pneumonia.

   (4) The antibiotics chosen to fight the pneumonia should be effective against both **gram-positive** and **gram-negative organisms.** A significant number of hospital-acquired pneumonias are caused by gram-negative organisms that gain access to the respiratory tract through the oropharynx. The risk of gram-negative colonization increases for patients in acute care facilities and has been associated with the presence of nasogastric tubes, preexisting respiratory disease, mechanical ventilation, tracheal intubation, and paralytic ileus.

3. **Phlebitis**

  a. **I.v. catheter-related infections** are common, with a reported incidence of 25% to 35%.

  b. The **i.v. site should be inspected daily** for erythema, pain, and induration. Phlebitis can occur even with close surveillance; studies have shown that many cases of phlebitis manifest initial symptoms more than 12 hours after discontinuation of catheters.

  c. **Prevention methods** including sterile technique during placement and frequent changing of site (every 72 hours) have been shown to significantly decrease the risk of infection.

  d. **Diagnosis** is based on the combination of fever, pain, erythema, induration, and a palpable cord along the vessel.

  e. **Treatment** includes removal of catheter and warm compresses. Phlebitis usually is self-limited and resolves within 3 to 4 days; antibiotic therapy with antistaphylococcal coverage is necessary when catheter-related sepsis has set in.

4. **Wound infection**

  a. **Wound infection rate** for clean cases (infection is not present, there is no break in aseptic technique, no hollow viscous is entered) is 2%; the rate for dirty or infected cases is 40% or more.

  b. **The risk of infection** may increase with several factors.

   (1) **Preoperative shaving** is thought to increase risk of infection.

   (2) **Incidental appendectomy** may increase the rate of infection in clean cases.

   (3) **With increasing lengths of preoperative hospital stay,** wound infection rate increases.

   (4) **Bringing a drain out through the incision** can contribute to infection.

  c. **Wound infections occur** late in the postoperative period, usually after the fourth postoperative day. Fever, erythema, induration, tenderness, and purulent drainage may be present.

  d. **Management** consists of opening, cleaning, and débriding the infected portion of the wound. Dressing changes two to three times daily are necessary to promote healing, development of granulation tissue, and eventual closure by secondary intention. Clean, granulating wounds can often be closed secondarily.

   e. **To decrease the incidence of wound infection,** delayed primary clo-
      sure can be used in already-infected cases.
      (1) **The wound is left open** above the fascia, and sutures are placed
          through the skin and subcutaneous tissues 3 cm apart but not
          tied.
      (2) **Wound care** is begun immediately postprocedure and continued
          until the wound is granulating well.
      (3) **Sutures** can then be tied and staples used to further approximate
          skin edges.
      (4) **Wound infection rate** in high-risk patients may be decreased
          from 23% to 2%.
5. **Pelvic cellulitis**
   a. **Vaginal cuff cellulitis** may be present to some extent in all patients
      who display some erythema, induration, and tenderness at the cuff
      after hysterectomy. Cellulitis is most often self-limited and does not
      require treatment.
   b. **Fever, leukocytosis, and pain** localizing to the pelvis may accompany
      a severe cellulitis in which adjacent pelvic tissues are involved.
      (1) **Broad-spectrum antibiotics** covering gram-positive, gram-negative,
          and anaerobic organisms should be initiated.
      (2) **If fluctuance or a mass is noted at the cuff,** it should be probed
          and opened with a blunt instrument; the cuff can then be left
          open to drain, or a drain can be placed.
   c. **The development of an abscess** in the surgical field or elsewhere in
      the abdominal cavity after gynecologic surgery is uncommon.
      (1) **Contaminated cases** are most likely to lead to the development
          of an abscess, especially when the surgical site is not drained or
          as a secondary complication of a hematoma.
      (2) Most abscesses that do appear are **polymicrobial in nature,**
          caused by pathogens from the vaginal and gastrointestinal tract.
          E. coli, Klebsiella, Streptococcus, Proteus, Enterobacter, and *Bac-
          teroides* have all been isolated.
      (3) **Diagnosis** is sometimes difficult, because abdominal and pelvic
          examinations may not reveal the abscess. Persistent fever and
          increased white blood cell count are seen. Radiologic confirma-
          tion with ultrasound or CT scan is usually needed for diagnosis.
      (4) **Treatment** involves surgical evacuation, drainage, and parenteral
          antibiotics. CT scan–guided drain placement has obviated the need
          for surgical exploration in most circumstances. Broad-spectrum
          antibiotics should be used first and then culturing to refine antibi-
          otic therapy.
IV. **Gastrointestinal complications**
   A. **Preoperative bowel preparation**
      1. **Preoperative bowel preparation is useful on two counts.**
         a. **The reduction of gastrointestinal contents** provides additional room
            in the pelvis and abdomen, facilitating procedures.
         b. **The reduction in the number of pathogenic flora in the colon**
            reduces the risk of infection after surgery and can be carried out when
            colon surgery is anticipated.
      2. **Mechanical bowel preparation** with oral gut lavage using an agent such
         as GoLYTELY and **a clear liquid diet** for 24 hours the day before surgery
         are sufficient precautions when the **colon surgery is not expected.** This
         regimen may be more comfortable and lead to less fluid loss and elec-
         trolyte abnormalities than the combined use of oral magnesium citrate
         and multiple enemas.
      3. **Oral antibiotic regimens,** such as erythromycin base and neomycin or
         metronidazole and neomycin, reduce infection rates from 40% to 5% to
         10% when administered prophylactically before an **anticipated opera-
         tion.** Because the antibiotics are poorly absorbed under these conditions,
         they do not reduce the risk of infection related to vaginal contamination.

Table 24-3. Differential diagnosis between postoperative ileus
and postoperative obstruction

Postoperative ileus	Clinical feature	Postoperative obstruction
Discomfort from distention but not cramping pains	Abdominal pain	Cramping progressively severe
Usually within 48–72 hr of surgery	Relation to previous surgery	Usually delayed, may be 5–7 days for remote onset
Present	Nausea and vomiting	Present
Present	Distention	Present
Absent or hypoactive	Bowel sounds	Borborygmi with peristaltic rushes and high-pitched tinkles
Only if related to associated peritonitis	Fever	Rarely present unless bowel becomes gangrenous
Distended loops of small and large bowels; gas usually present in colon	Abdominal radiographs	Single or multiple loops of distended bowel (usually small bowel) with air-fluid levels
Conservative with nasogastric suction, enemas, cholinergic stimulation	Treatment	Conservative with nasogastric decompression Surgical exploration

From Rock JA, Thompson JD, eds. *Telinde's operative gynecology*, 8th ed. Philadelphia: Lippincott–Raven, 1997. Reprinted with permission.

B. Ileus and small bowel obstruction. Postoperative gastrointestinal dysfunction is a common problem, and differentiating between postoperative ileus and obstruction may be difficult.

   1. **The cause of the arrest and disorganization of gastrointestinal motility** that results in postoperative ileus is unknown. Infection, peritonitis, electrolyte disturbances, extensive manipulation of the GI tract, and prolonged procedures seem to increase the risk of ileus.
   2. **The most common cause of obstruction** of the small bowel following major gynecologic surgery, which occurs in 1% to 2% of cases, is adhesions at the operative site.
   3. **Risk factors** for both ileus and obstruction include infection, malignancy, and a history of radiation therapy.
      a. **Pelvic inflammatory disease** is the most common gynecologic disease process associated with ileus and intestinal obstruction.
      b. **Surgery for pelvic malignancy** can be complicated by postoperative ileus or obstruction.
   4. **The clinical presentation** of ileus may be quite similar to that of obstruction (Table 24-3).
      a. **Nausea, vomiting, and distention** may be present with both.
      b. **Abdominal pain** from obstruction is characterized by progressively more severe abdominal cramps.
      c. **Absent and hypoactive bowel sounds** are more likely to occur with ileus; borborygmi, rushes, and high-pitched tinkles are more characteristic of obstruction.
      d. **Necrosis of the bowel wall,** which will cause progressive leukocytosis and left shift, is a key feature of advancing bowel obstruction.
      e. **Abdominal x-rays** will show distended loops of large and small bowel, with gas present in the colon in the setting of ileus. Single or multi-

ple loops of distended bowel (most often the small bowel) with air-fluid levels are seen in postoperative obstruction.

5. Treatment

a. **Ileus** can be treated with bowel rest, nasogastric suction, and cholinergic stimulation. A longer small-intestinal tube (e.g., Cantor) may also be used. Fluids and electrolytes lost should be adequately replaced. Lack of improvement within 48 to 72 hours requires a search for other causes of ileus, such as ureteral injury, pelvic infection, unrecognized GI tract injury, or persistent fluid and electrolyte abnormalities.

b. **In most cases of obstruction,** the obstruction is partial and will respond to conservative management with bowel rest and nasogastric decompression. Because of the potential for mesenteric vascular occlusion and resulting ischemia or perforation, increasing abdominal pain, progressive distention, fever, leukocytosis, or acidosis should be evaluated with the potential need for surgical exploration and treatment in mind.

C. **Diarrhea** is common following abdominal and pelvic surgery, as the GI tract returns to its normal function and motility. However, prolonged or multiple episodes may represent a pathologic process, such as impending small bowel obstruction, colonic obstruction, or pseudomembranous colitis. *Clostridium difficile*–associated colitis may result from exposure to any antibiotic; stool testing can confirm clinical suspicions. Extended oral metronidazole is needed for adequate therapy. Regardless of the cause of diarrhea, fluid and electrolyte levels should be monitored and replaced as needed.

V. **Thrombosis**

A. **Venous thromboembolism** includes DVT, which usually involves the leg veins, and pulmonary embolism (PE). The incidence of venous thrombosis in the gynecologic patient is 15% (range, 5% to 45%, depending on procedure and associated risk factors). PE is the cause of death in 40% of postoperative deaths in the gynecologic patient.

B. **Risk factors** are circumstances that cause an increase in blood coagulability, venous stasis, and trauma to vessel wall.

C. **Prevention**

1. **Method of prophylaxis** should be chosen on the basis of the patient's risk (Table 24-4).

2. **Factors to consider** include age, weight, procedure (type and length of operation), and comorbid conditions. An age of more than 40 years, obesity greater than 20% of ideal body weight, prolonged surgery, and immobility during pre- and postoperative periods all predispose a patient to DVT and PE. History of thromboembolism, pelvic malignancy, diabetes, heart failure, radiation therapy, and chronic disease also increase the risk of thromboembolic events (Table 24-5).

3. **To significantly reduce the risk of fatal PE,** all large prospective trials have documented the necessity of initiating prophylactic techniques before surgery and continuing them for the duration of the postoperative stay.

4. **A number of methods of prevention/prophylaxis are available.**

a. **Low-dose heparin** has been shown to reduce the risk of thrombi and PE in at-risk patients. In one multicenter study, 5,000 units were administered 2 hours before surgery and every 8 hours afterwards for 7 days, reducing the incidence of thrombi from 25% to 8%. Sixteen deaths from PE were seen in the control group and only two in the treated group. Later studies indicate that a regimen of 5,000 units preoperatively and every 12 hours for 5 days postoperatively may be efficacious as well. These regimens do not significantly alter clotting time and did not increase operative or postoperative bleeding.

b. **Dextran 70 and dextran 40** have shown efficacy similar to low-dose heparin.

c. **Low-molecular-weight heparin** is also an effective preventive therapy, though data on its use for hemorrhagic complications are mixed. Availability, cost, and convenience in each care setting must be considered before choosing the method of prophylaxis.

Table 24-4. Risk categories of thromboembolism in gynecologic surgery

Factor	Risk category		
	Low risk	Medium risk	High risk
Age	<40 yr	≥ 40 yr	≥ 40 yr
Contributing factors			
Surgery	Uncomplicated or minor	Major abdominal or pelvic	Major, extensive malignant disease involved Prior radiation treatment
Weight	Normal	Moderately obese (75–90 kg or >20% above ideal weight)	Morbidly obese (≥115 kg or >30% above ideal weight)
Medical diseases	None	None	Previous venous thrombosis Varicose veins (severe) Diabetes (insulin dependent)
Thromboembolism			
Calf vein thrombosis	2%	10–30%	30–60%
Iliofemoral vein thrombosis	0.4%	2–8%	5–10%
Fatal pulmonary embolism	0.2%	0.1–0.5%	1%
Recommended prophylaxis	Early ambulation and graduated compression stockings	Low-dose heparin or dextran or intermittent pneumatic compression	Dextran or low-dose heparin, intermittent pneumatic compression, or both

From Rock JA, Thompson JD, eds. *Telinde's operative gynecology*, 8th ed. Philadelphia: Lippincott–Raven, 1997. Reprinted with permission.

    d. Compression modalities have also been used for prophylaxis. Studies show an increase in blood velocity as well as a possible decrease in coagulability.
      (1) Graduated compression stockings combined with early ambulation are thought to provide sufficient prophylaxis in the low-risk patient.
      (2) Studies support the use of **external intermittent pneumatic compression devices** as a prophylactic measure in patients at moderate and high risk. Efficacy is similar to low-dose heparin.
      (3) A combination of pharmacologic therapy and external pneumatic compression may be considered in patients at high risk, such as those with morbid obesity or malignancy.
  D. Diagnosis of venous thromboembolism
    1. Deep venous thrombosis
      a. Clinical assessment alone has limited value. Unilateral lower extremity swelling, pain, erythema, and palpable cord may be seen.

Table 24-5. Profile of patient at high risk for venous thrombosis

Factor	Condition
Age	>40 yr
Obesity	
Moderate	75–90 kg or >20% above ideal weight
Morbid	≥ 115 kg or >30% above ideal weight with reduced fibrinolysin and immobility
Immobility	
Preoperative	Prolonged hospitalization; venous stasis
Intraoperative	Prolonged operative time; loss of pump action of calf muscles; compression of vena cava
Postoperative	Prolonged bed confinement; venous stasis
Trauma	Damage of wall of pelvic veins
	Radical pelvic surgery
Malignancy	Release of tissue thromboplastin
	Activation of factor X; reduced fibrinolysin
Radiation	Prior radiation therapy
Medical diseases	Diabetes mellitus
	Cardiac disease; heart failure
	Severe varicose veins
	Previous venous thrombosis with or without embolization
	Chronic pulmonary disease

From Rock JA, Thompson JD, eds. *Telinde's operative gynecology*, 8th ed. Philadelphia: Lippincott–Raven, 1997. Reprinted with permission.

b. **Venography** is the most definitive but also the most invasive method of diagnosis.

c. **^{125}I-labeled fibrinogen scanning** is unreliable in the upper thigh and may take a long time to perform.

d. **Impedance plethysmography** is most specific in the larger veins of the thigh. In the calf, sensitivity is less than 50%.

e. **Doppler ultrasound** (which measures the velocity of blood flow) is also highly sensitive in the larger vessels, such as the lower iliac, femoral, and popliteal. However, sensitivity decreases to less than 60% in the soleal sinuses, the major site of clot formation.

f. **Real-time ultrasound** has shown greater sensitivity than Doppler ultrasound.

g. **Duplex Doppler imaging** combines Doppler examination and real-time ultrasound, enabling the radiologist to visualize the thrombus and measure blood flow through the vessels. Because of the high sensitivity (92%), high specificity (100%), and noninvasive nature of this technique, it has replaced venography as the gold standard for diagnosing DVT.

h. **Serial use** of the diagnostic tests listed above has been shown to significantly improve their sensitivity.

i. **The use of standardized clinical models of pretest probability** in clinical assessment may also improve the sensitivity and specificity of diagnostic tests. In one study by Wells et al. (Table 24-6), pretest probability and normal ultrasonography reliably excluded the presence of venous thrombosis.

j. **Measuring plasma D-dimer,** a fibrin-specific product, is another strategy. In one study, DVT was excluded by the presence of normal plasma D-dimer and a normal result on impedance plethysmography at presentation.

Table 24-6. A clinical model of the pretest probability of deep venous thrombosis*

Major points

Active cancer (ongoing treatment, treatment within previous 6 mo, or palliative therapy)

Paralysis, paresis, or recent plaster immobilization of the leg or foot

Recent bed rest for >3 days, major surgery within 4 wk, or both

Localized tenderness along the distribution of the deep venous system

Swelling of thigh and calf (should be measured)

Swelling of calf to 3 cm more than on symptomless side (measured 10 cm below tibial tuberosity)

Strong family history of deep venous thrombosis (≥ 2 first-degree relatives with a history of deep venous thrombosis)

Minor points

History of recent trauma (within 60 days) to the symptomatic leg

Pitting edema (symptomatic leg only)

Dilated superficial veins (nonvaricose) in symptomatic leg only

Hospitalization within previous 6 mo

Erythema

Clinical probability of deep venous thrombosis

High probability

    ≥ 3 major points and no alternative diagnosis

    ≥ 2 major points, ≥ 2 minor points, and no alternative diagnosis

Low probability

    1 major point, ≥ 2 minor points, and an alternative diagnosis

    1 major point, ≥ 1 minor point, and no alternative diagnosis

    0 major points, ≥ 3 minor points, and an alternative diagnosis

    0 major points, ≥ 2 minor points, and no alternative diagnosis

Intermediate probability

    All other combinations

*Data were adapted from Wells PS, Hirsh J, Anderson DR, et al. Accuracy of clinical assessment of deep-vein thrombosis. *Lancet* 1995;345:1326–30. [Erratum, *Lancet* 1995;346:516.]
From Ginsberg JS. Management of venous thromboembolism. *N Engl J Med* 1996;335:1816–1828. Reprinted with permission.

    2. Pulmonary embolism

        a. The signs and symptoms of PE are varied and may be quite subtle. They include respiratory distress, hypotension, chest pain, fever, hypoxia, and arrhythmias. Laboratory evaluation with arterial blood-gas tests that show an alveolar-arterial gradient may be helpful.

        b. Radionucleotide imaging (a $\dot{V}/\dot{Q}$ scan) is the first step in diagnostic testing. If the results are normal, a diagnosis of PE is excluded; a high probability result is strong evidence of a PE. However, over 50% of patients have nondiagnostic imaging results and need further evaluation. One-fourth of nondiagnostic results occur in patients with PE.

        c. Venous ultrasound or impedance plethysmography should be performed on patients whose $\dot{V}/\dot{Q}$ scan results are nondiagnostic, and PE diagnosed if the results of the second tests are abnormal.

        d. Normal results do not rule out PE. If the test is normal, two options are available: in patients with weak cardiopulmonary reserve, pulmonary

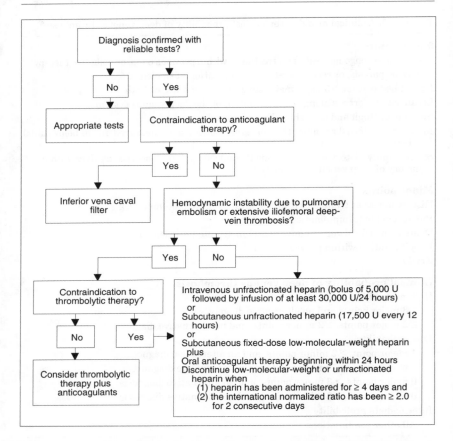

Figure 24-2. Initial management of venous thromboembolism. The initial dose of heparin should be adjusted to achieve an activated partial thromboplastin time in the therapeutic range. In the case of subcutaneous heparin, the activated partial thromboplastin time should be monitored 6 hours after the injection. For patients with extensive deep venous thrombosis or pulmonary embolism, a course of heparin lasting more than 4 days is recommended. (From Ginsberg JS. Management of venous thromboembolism. *N Engl J Med* 1996;335:1816–1828. Reprinted with permission.)

angiography may be performed; in ambulatory patients with good cardiopulmonary reserve, serial venous ultrasonography or impedance plethysmography may be performed.

E. Therapy (Fig. 24-2)

  1. I.v. unfractionated heparin is the generally accepted treatment for DVT. The level of anticoagulation should be closely monitored and may be determined in accordance with local clinical laboratory preferences. **Oral therapy with Coumadin** (preparation of warfarin sodium) may be initiated after symptoms resolve or after 5 to 7 days of i.v. heparin treatment. How long oral anticoagulation should be continued is debated; 4 to 6 weeks is probably adequate when the perioperative period is thought to be the major risk factor for the thromboembolic event.

2. Various algorithms exist for the **administration and monitoring of heparin** (Table 24-7).
3. **Low-molecular-weight heparins** have several advantages over unfractionated heparin, and may replace it in the treatment of venous thromboembolism. The half-lives of low-molecular-weight heparins are longer; the dose response is more predictable, requiring less monitoring; and they may cause less bleeding while producing an equivalent antithrombotic effect.
4. **Thrombolytic therapy** is reasonable in some patients with extensive proximal vein thrombosis or PE, depending on how much time has passed since surgery and the relative risk of bleeding complications.
5. **Placement of a vena caval filter** may be necessary in patients with acute thromboembolism and active bleeding or a high potential for bleeding, patients with a history of multiple venous thrombi who are on medical therapy, and patients with a history of heparin-induced thrombocytopenia.

F. **Potential side effects** of anticoagulant therapy include bleeding, thrombocytopenia, osteoporosis (with long-term heparin-related compounds), and skin necrosis (with coumarins).

1. **Bleeding** that occurs after use of heparin-related compounds can be reversed with protamine; Coumadin-related bleeding can be reversed with vitamin K or with plasma or factor IX concentrates.
2. **Immune, IgG-mediated thrombocytopenia,** which is frequently complicated by the extension of preexisting venous thromboembolism, will appear

Table 24-7. Three published dosing schemes for heparin[a]

Weight-based nomogram[b]

The initial dose is a bolus of 80 U/kg of body weight, followed by an infusion starting at a rate of 18 U/kg/hr. The APTT is measured every 6 hr, and the heparin dose adjusted as follows:

Measured value	Adjustment
PTT <35 sec (<1.2× control value)	80 U/kg as bolus, then increase infusion rate by 4 U/kg/hr
APTT 35–45 sec (1.2–1.5× control value)	40 U/kg as bolus, then increase infusion rate by 2 U/kg/hr
APTT 46–70 sec (>1.5–2.3× control value)	No change
APTT 71–90 sec (>2.3–3× control value)	Decrease infusion rate by 2 U/kg/hr
APTT >90 sec (>3× control value)	Stop infusion for 1 hr, then decrease infusion rate by 3 U/kg/hr

5,000-U bolus dose, followed by 1,280 U/hr[c]

APTT (sec)	Bolus (U)	Stop infusion (min)	Rate of change (mL/hr)	Repeat APTT
<50[d]	5,000	0	+3	In 6 hr
50–59	0	0	+3	In 6 hr
60–85	0	0	0	Next morning
86–95	0	0	−2	Next morning
96–120	0	30	−2	In 6 hr
>120	0	60	−4	In 6 hr

(continued)

Table 24-7. (continued)

Intravenous dose-titration nomogram for APTT[e]

The starting dose is a 5,000-U bolus, followed by 40,000 U/24 hr (if the patient has a low risk of bleeding) or 30,000 U/24 hr (if there is a high risk of bleeding).

	Intravenous infusion[f]		
APTT (sec)	Rate of change (mL/hr)	Change in dose (U/24 hr)	Additional action
≤ 45	+6	+5,760	Repeat APTT in 4–6 hr
46–54	+3	+2,880	Repeat APTT in 4–6 hr
55–85	0	0	None[g]
86–110	–3	–2,880	Stop heparin for 1 hr; repeat APTT 4–6 hr after restarting heparin treatment
>110	–6	–5,760	Stop heparin for 1 hr; repeat APTT 4–6 hr after restarting heparin treatment

APTT, activated partial thromboplastin time.
One mL/hr equals 40 U/hr.
[a]From Ginsberg JS. Management of venous thromboembolism. *New Engl J Med* 1996;335: 1816–1828.
[b]Data are from Raschke RA, Reilly BM, Guidry JR, Fontana JR, Srinivas S. The weight-based heparin dosing nomogram compared with a "standard care" nomogram: a randomized controlled trial. *Ann Intern Med* 1993;119:874–881.
[c]Data are from Cruickshank MK, Levine MN, Hirsh J, Roberts RS, Siguenza M. A standard heparin nomogram for the management of heparin therapy. *Arch Intern Med* 1991;151:333–337.
[d]If the APTT is subtherapeutic despite a heparin dose of at least 1,440 U/hr (36 mL/hr) at any time during the first 48 hr of therapy, the response to an APTT of less than 50 sec is a bolus of 5,000 U and a rate increase of 5 mL/hr.
[e]Data are from Hull RD, Raskob GE, Rosenbloom D, et al. Optimal therapeutic level of heparin therapy in patients with venous thrombosis. *Arch Intern Med* 1992;152:1589–1595.
[f]A heparin sodium concentration of 20,000 U in 500 mL is equal to 40 U/mL.
[g]During the first 24 hr, repeat the APTT every 4 to 6 hr. Thereafter, the APTT is determined once daily, unless the value is in the therapeutic range.

in approximately 3% of patients receiving unfractionated heparin. This complication should be differentiated from the early, benign, transient thrombocytopenia that can occur with therapy. Immune thrombocytopenia should be suspected in a patient who has recently received heparin when the patient's platelet count falls below 100, or less than 50% of baseline, within 5 to 15 days after heparin therapy is begun or sooner.

VI. **Complications of laparoscopic procedures**
   A. **Extraperitoneal insulation of CO$_2$**
      1. **Misplacement of a Veress needle** causes this complication; in most cases, CO$_2$ can be allowed to escape and needle placement attempted again.
      2. **Mediastinal emphysema** is a more uncommon complication that requires observation for respiratory compromise and, in most severe cases, ventilation.
   B. **Vessel injury**
      1. **Etiology and prevention**
         a. **A Veress needle or trocar** may traumatize omental, mesenteric, or major abdominal or pelvic vessels.
         b. **Elevating the anterior abdominal wall** and directing the needle or trocar towards the pelvis during insertion reduces the risk of injury.

   c. Injury of epigastric vessels with accessory trocar placement can generally be avoided.

     (1) Superficial epigastric vessels can usually be identified by transillumination so that injury can be avoided.

     (2) Inferior vessels are deeper, making transillumination difficult; direct laparoscopic visualization and insertion of trocars lateral to the edge of the rectus muscle (6 to 7 cm lateral to midline) will decrease risk of vessel laceration.

  2. Repair and treatment

   a. Irrigation may be necessary to pinpoint source of bleeding.

   b. Injury to small vessels may be treated with coagulation. CO_2 laser treatment is not effective for vessels larger than 2 mm in diameter.

   c. Medium vessel injury is best controlled with bipolar electrocautery; only minimal damage is caused if vessels are grasped before coagulation. A suture or loop ligature can also be placed. If these methods are unsuccessful, laparotomy is necessary.

   d. Injury to a major vessel usually requires laparotomy, transfusion, and vascular repair.

   e. Injury to mesenteric vessels may lead to the compromise of a segment of bowel, requiring resection and repair.

   f. Injury of epigastric vessels during accessory trocar placement can be minimized by several means.

     (1) Pressure can often be used to control superficial vessel bleeding. The trocar sleeve may tamponade bleeding, and turning it may help to compress a vessel. An inflated Foley catheter balloon may be used to impact the puncture site.

     (2) Intracorporeally, **bipolar forceps** can be used to coagulate the bleeding vessel.

     (3) Sutures can be placed through the anterior abdominal wall to stop bleeding. A straight needle or curved urologic needle may facilitate suturing.

     (4) If a hematoma forms, it should be evacuated, the incision explored, and the vessel identified and ligated.

   g. Laceration of the fallopian tube, mesosalpinx, or infundibulopelvic ligament with injury to medium and large vessels may occur. Repairs should be tailored to size of vessel as described above.

C. Bowel injury

  1. Gastric injury is uncommon; risk can be reduced by routine placement of oro- or nasogastric decompression.

  2. Intestinal injury

   a. Etiology and prevention

     (1) Injury may occur during insertion of Veress needle or trocar or during operative procedures.

     (2) Injury is more common in patients with a history of abdominal or pelvic surgery.

     (3) Aspiration with syringe before insulation may permit early recognition of bowel perforation.

     (4) Thermal injury can be caused by inadvertent contact between electrical, thermal, or laser energy and an organ or tissue.

       (a) With electrical injury, the full extent of the damage may not be obvious immediately.

       (b) Laser-induced injury can result from accidentally activating a laser, penetrating too deeply beyond the target, or striking points close to but not on the true target.

   b. Repair and treatment

     (1) Perforation with Veress needle may remain undiagnosed and heal spontaneously.

       (a) If **perforation** is suspected, the needle should be withdrawn and insulation attempted at another site. Once the laparoscope is placed, the site of penetration must be carefully examined.

        (b) **Laparotomy** is not required for most needle injuries, but the injuries should be closely monitored.

    (2) **Hemostatic injury** to the serosa does not need to be repaired.

    (3) **Trocar insertion** often results in injury that must be surgically corrected.

    (4) **If the laparoscope enters the lumen,** it should be left in place to limit soiling and to facilitate identification of the injured site.

    (5) **Small bowel injury** can, in some cases, be repaired laparoscopically with interrupted sutures tied either intracorporeally or externally.

    (6) **Large bowel injury** may be repaired laparoscopically if the patient has had preoperative bowel preparation and there is minimal fecal spill.

    (7) **Laparotomy** is necessary if the surgeon is not experienced in laparoscopic suture technique or if the injury is extensive.

    (8) **Colostomy** is rarely necessary.

D. Bladder injury

  1. Etiology and prevention

    a. Injury **during trocar insertion** is possible.

    b. All patients should have their **bladders drained** after anesthesia has been induced. In procedures anticipated to last longer than 30 minutes, a catheter should be placed for continuous drainage.

  2. Repair and treatment

    a. The **size** of the injury dictates treatment.

    b. **Needle perforations** can be managed expectantly.

    c. **Lacerations less than 5 mm** long will heal spontaneously if the bladder is drained continuously for 4 to 5 days postoperatively.

    d. **Larger injuries** require suturing. This can be attempted laparoscopically by surgeons experienced in laparoscopic suturing technique.

E. Ureteral injury

  1. Etiology and prevention

    a. **Ureteral injuries** are less frequent than bladder injuries.

    b. There is an increased risk with adhesions or endometriosis involving the pelvic sidewalls.

    c. **Preoperative stent placement** can, in some cases, help locate the ureters, thus preventing inadvertent injury.

  2. Diagnosis

    a. **If intraoperative injury** is suspected, i.v. indigo carmine may facilitate identification.

    b. **If ureteral injury** is suspected postoperatively, an i.v. pyelogram should be obtained.

  3. Repair and treatment. The location of the injury will determine which reparative procedure is needed (see sec. **II.A**).

F. Trocar hernia

  1. Trocars greater than 7 mm have increased risk of herniation, and fascial defects should be sutured.

  2. Bowel may be trapped in incisions at time of trocar removal. Direct visualization of the removal of accessory trocars and deflation of pneumoperitoneum, with simultaneous removal of laparoscope and sleeve, will decrease this risk.

Selected Reading

Ginsberg JS. Management of venous thromboembolism. *N Engl J Med* 1996;335:1816–1828.

Sanz LE, ed. *Gynecologic surgery*, 2nd ed. Cambridge: Blackwell Science, 1995.

Gershenson DM, DeCherney AH, Curry SL, eds. *Operative gynecology*. Philadelphia: WB Saunders, 1993.

Rock JA, Thompson JD, eds. *Telinde's operative gynecology*, 8th ed. Philadelphia: Lippincott–Raven, 1997.

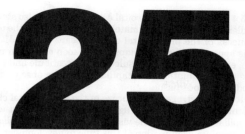

Pediatric Gynecology

Judy M. Lee,
Katherine Miller-Bass,
and Francisco Garcia

I. Gynecologic examination of a child

A. Appropriateness of the examination must be considered in terms of the timing and the type of information needed. The **interview** is the most important aspect in determining the real reason for the visit. The child should be told that the examination is permitted by her caregiver. She also should be advised that if anyone else attempted or attempts to touch her genital area, she should tell her primary caregiver.

B. Patient compliance begins with giving the patient a sense of control over the examination. She can be involved in the examination if given a hand-held mirror. Videocolposcopy has been used as a technique to reduce anxiety in the patient. Use of a drape also facilitates the examination by giving a sense of privacy. A nurse practitioner or physician's assistant should be present at all times and introduced to the patient before the start of the interview. Tools for magnification should be kept on hand.

Those patients traumatized by sexual abuse or previous examinations who refuse to cooperate may have to be examined under anesthesia, depending on whether a pathologic condition is suspected. Otherwise, gaining the confidence of the patient through a series of outpatient visits is advisable.

C. Methods. A detailed and labeled sketch of the external genitalia should be documented in the medical record. A diamond-shaped space can be used to represent the vestibule of a child in the supine position, with the clitoris positioned at 12 o'clock and the posterior fourchette at 6 o'clock. Use of the **supine lateral-spread** method is often sufficient to allow the vestibular structures to be visualized. This involves placing the index finger from each hand or the index and middle finger or thumb and index finger from one hand on both labia majora, lateral to the vestibule and slightly posterior to the vaginal orifice. The tissues are then spread gently until visualization is adequate. The **supine lateral traction** method can be employed by grasping each labium major in the same location by using both hands. Gentle traction is used next, pulling forward, slightly posteriorly and laterally.

D. Prepubertal examination. A general pediatric physical is recommended as is inspection of the external genitalia, visualization of the vagina and cervix, and rectoabdominal palpation. Tanner classification of the external genitalia and breast development should be used. Abdominal examination can be facilitated by placing the child's hand over the examiner's hand. Inguinal examinations may reveal a hernia or gonad. To examine the external genitalia, the child should be placed supine with knees apart and feet touching in the frog-leg position. The child also can sit on her caregiver's lap; the caregiver should sit semireclined with both feet in stirrups. The child's legs are then draped over the caregiver's thighs on either side. If the child is at ease with the use of stirrups, she can be placed in the lithotomy position. A knee-chest position offers the advantage of better visualization of the vaginal canal but can be more anxiety-provoking. Note should be made of perineal hygiene, presence of pubic hair, hymenal configuration, and size of the clitoris. It should not be larger than the average adult clitoris (5.4 mm × 4.4 mm). Introital estrogenization also should be noted. From the toddler years until approximately age 9 or 10 years, the unestrogenized vaginal mucosa of the prepubertal child appears thin, red, and atrophic. Capillary beds appearing like road maps can be seen and often mistaken for inflammation, especially around the sulcus of the vestibule and periurethral area. In areas of inflammation, the capillary beds are obscured by erythema and thickened edematous tissue.

E. **Peripubertal examination.** The estrogenized mucosa of the peripubertal child and of the newborn infant until approximately age 3 years appears moist with a whitish-pink color. Capillary beds cannot be visualized. The tissue is pliable and easily distended. A speculum examination at this time in development can be considered. The examining index finger should be placed through the introitus before use of the speculum. Dropping the knees outward allows the perineal body to relax. Use of the "extinction of stimuli" phenomenon can greatly facilitate a first pelvic examination. This involves using a primary distracting stimulus to detract from a second stimulus, such as pressing the nonexamining finger into the patient's perineum before touching the introitus and having the patient acknowledge the presence of its pressure. In early puberty, a thick, white, cloudy discharge is often present. This is often a physiologic leukorrhea, a result of unopposed estrogen causing vaginal/cervical secretions. This usually occurs before menarche. Proper perineal hygiene should be stressed as *Escherichia coli* colonization is the most common cause of adolescent vulvovaginitis.

II. **Suspected child/sexual abuse**

A. The true **incidence** of child sexual abuse exceeds that reported. The National Incidence Studies conducted most recently in 1993 (NIS-3) have estimated approximately 300,200 children are sexually abused. This is a rate of 45 cases per 10,000 children, which is twice that of the rate of NIS-2 done in 1986 (1). Based on prevalence data, 500,000 new cases of sexual abuse per year are reported in the United States but only 140,000 reports are substantiated (2). Child sexual abuse can be defined as contact or interaction between a child and an adult when the child is being used for the sexual stimulation of that adult or another person. Sexual abuse may also be committed by another minor when that person is either significantly older than the victim or when the abuser is in a position of power or control over that child (3). It includes both sexual contact and noncontact acts such as child pornography and exhibitionism. It has been estimated that one in four girls has been sexually molested by age 16. Girls found to have a vaginal foreign body (VFB) should also undergo an evaluation for sexual abuse.

B. The **medical evaluation** can be extremely anxiety-provoking for the caregiver and child. A lack of control or security can make both feel victimized. Such encounters require utmost sensitivity and respect for family concerns and privacy. In general, children suspected of being victims of abuse should be evaluated by professionals trained in conducting interviews, documenting questions and responses, and collecting necessary evidence.

1. **History.** Questions should be open-ended. Allow sufficient time to establish rapport with the child and avoid a coercive quality to the evaluation. Information must be recorded in the victim's own words. For very young victims with limited verbal skills, techniques such as play-interviews or use of drawings have been used to promote communication. When it is impossible to obtain a history from the victim, the information then must come from relatives, other household members, neighbors, or police officers. Note the child's composure, behavior, and mental state, as well as the interactions with parents and other people. Nonspecific symptoms include night terrors, changes in sleeping habits, and clinging behavior.

2. **Physical examination** reveals findings that vary with the degree of trauma the victim has experienced and the time that has elapsed since the incident. The examination should be complete, extending from head to toe, allowing the child to become accustomed to the touch of the evaluator and the establishment of trust. Use of magnifying devices is essential in enhancing genital findings. The colposcope can be used under regular illumination and with a green filter. A camera attachment allows for collection of photographs that can be added to the medical record and used as evidence.

The anal region must also be inspected as anal abuse is a common form of sexual assault on children. Nonspecific findings associated with poor local hygiene causing superficial lesions must be interpreted with caution and include redness, irritations, abrasions, friability of the posterior fourchette, labial adhesions, hymenal tags or bumps, bruising of the external genitalia, or nonspecific infections. Abnormal physical findings that strongly suggest abuse include hymenal-vaginal or hymenal-perineal tears, enlarged hymenal opening of 1 cm or more, a sexually transmitted disease, or evidence of bite marks on the genitalia or other parts of the body. Definitive findings are that of pregnancy or sperm. Abnormal rectal findings include a diameter greater than 2 cm in the absence of stool in the rectal ampulla, asymmetry of the anus when dilated, an apparently fixed opening, or thickening or smoothing of the skin of the anal verge. Unless vaginal penetration has taken place, the absence of physical findings is common because healing often is complete by the time the child is evaluated.

3. **Collection of evidence.** If the assault occurred within 72 hours of the examination, samples should be collected for the forensic laboratory and handled separately. All collected specimens must be individually packaged, labeled, sealed with special evidence tape, and signed by the appropriate people. A routing slip must be attached. Each label must include patient identification, the specimen, the site from which the specimen was collected, the date and time collected, and the examiner's initials. The specimen package must be given to the police investigator who signs it and a routing slip. Anyone handling the specimen must sign a routing slip as this chain of evidence is crucial for admissibility in court. Items that can be collected for evidence include the clothing that was worn at the time of the assault and combings of the pubic hair for the perpetrator's hair. An examination of semen on the skin and clothing should be done. A UV light can be used to examine the body for secretions. Positive areas can be swabbed with saline-moistened swabs that should be air-dried and put into sterile tubes or clean paper envelopes. Depending on the local forensic laboratory, the swabs may be immediately frozen instead. Several enzymes in semen can be detected to demonstrate its presence. The most commonly used marker is the enzyme acid phosphatase, the activity of which rapidly decreases in the vagina, becoming indistinguishable from normal vaginal enzymes after 72 hours. Motile sperm can be recovered up until 8 hours after an assault. Nonmotile sperm can be found up to 26 hours after an incident. If oral sex was forced, separate swabs should be taken from the perioral skin, gums, tongue, and pharynx. Drops of fluid mixed with a swab can then be air-dried on a slide and either stained or processed as a cytopathology specimen.

C. **Treatment** for the victim consists of addressing the immediate medical needs as well as providing protection against further abuse and psychological support for the victim and her family.

1. **Repair of injuries** depends on the type of injury sustained. Good perineal hygiene with sitz baths should be emphasized. Superficial injuries will resolve within a few days. Any evidence of infection will require use of antibiotics. Small hematomas can be controlled by pressure with an ice pack. Hematomas that continue to expand should be excised, the clots removed, and the bleeding area ligated. Large tears require suturing under anesthesia. Suspected vaginal or rectal lacerations also should be repaired under anesthesia. Bite wounds should be irrigated. Most of these wounds should be left open. A noninfected fresh wound can be primarily closed. Any necrotic tissue should be débrided. After 3 to 5 days, a secondary débridement may be required. If not already immunized, the child should be given a tetanus immunization.

2. Treatment for a **sexually transmitted disease** should be deferred until the results of cultures and serologic tests for syphilis are known. Antibiotic therapy should be instituted only if the child is symptomatic on the initial visit. A repeat VDRL test should be done in 6 weeks to rule out seroconversion.

3. All suspected victims of child abuse should be referred to **child protective services.** Occasionally it is necessary to admit a child to the hospital for safety. Until the question of protection can be answered, it is advisable to provide temporary placement for the child.

4. An essential part of any evaluation for suspected abuse includes providing intensive day-to-day **counseling,** support, and guidance. A trained therapist should be available to help the victim cope with the evaluation process, including the medical treatment and encounters with child protection services and law enforcement agencies. The family also should be offered treatment.

III. Traumatic injuries

A. Trauma by **accident** occurs most frequently to those girls between the ages of 4 and 12 years. Because of the differences in anatomy between a child and an adult, a seemingly innocuous lesion can result in a serious injury. These anatomic differences in the child include the superficial location of the urogenital diaphragm, the intraperitoneal location of the bladder, an underdeveloped perineal body with a thin rectovaginal septum, and the shorter distance between the perineal skin and peritoneal cavity.

1. **Straddle injuries** account for approximately 75% of all genital injuries in young girls. These appear as an area of ecchymosis or hematoma with painful swelling over the labia. Injuries may involve the mons, clitoris, urethra, or anterior portions of the labia minora and labia majora. Injuries to the hymen and injuries extending to the vaginal opening are rarely seen. Hematuria accompanying a perineal lesion warrants a voiding cystourethrogram to rule out bladder or urethral injury. Observation and cold compresses for the first 6 hours, followed by warm sitz baths, often are all that are required for blunt perineal injuries. A urethral catheter, analgesics, and prophylactic antibiotics can be used when a hematoma at the urethral orifice is causing pain and poor urination.

2. **Accidental penetration** occurs most often in 2- to 4-year-olds. It is often the result of falling on a sharp object, usually a pen or pencil. Presentation can include hematuria, vaginal discharge, or bleeding because a puncture wound may not be obvious. Rectal pain or bleeding also can be the presenting complaint. Microscopic hematuria warrants a very careful urethral catheterization. Resistance is an indication for a voiding cystourethrogram instead. In cases of gross hematuria, a catheterization should not be attempted. The child should also undergo a thorough examination with roentgenography, anoscopy, and sigmoidoscopy. Retained foreign bodies in the vagina often present with bloody or purulent discharge. Other symptoms include genital pruritus, abdominal pain, or fever. VFBs may be a previously unrecognized indicator of sexual abuse. VFBs can vary from wads of toilet paper, buttons, and coins to peanuts and crayons. Persistent vaginal discharge in a toddler warrants an examination under anesthesia. Antibiotics should be started before removal. If left undetected, peritonitis can develop from ascending purulent secretions to the fallopian tubes. Because of the general paucity of signs and symptoms, a foreign body often can be found embedded in the vaginal wall by the time the diagnosis is made, requiring a careful examination of the vaginal wall for any defects after the object has been removed. If the thin rectovaginal septum is involved, a temporary colostomy with delayed repair of the vaginal and rectal tissues may be indicated.

3. **Sex-related trauma** to the genital or perineal area is common. In one series, it was responsible for approximately 90% of all pediatric female perineal injuries. Studies of the relationship between childhood sexual abuse and adolescent pregnancy have suggested victims of sexual abuse may be at increased risk for socially deviant behavior, one manifestion of which is pregnancy during their adolescence (4).

4. **Tissue lacerations** may result from gymnastic exercise, waterskiing, or a major motor vehicle accident. Forceful abduction of the legs can result in lacerations of the vaginal orifice that can frequently extend into the fornix.

An examination under general anesthesia must be performed to determine the extent of the injury. Involvement of the rectovaginal septum or extension of the laceration into the peritoneal cavity must be ruled out.

Therapy involves administration of antibiotics, primary surgical repair, and possible use of a temporary colostomy. With massive pelvic fractures such as that found in high-speed, high-impact accidents, severe vaginal or combined urogenital lacerations are common. Management of deep vaginal and rectal perforations involves preoperative antibiotics, proximal diverting colostomy, presacral drainage, washout of the defunctionalized bowel, and closure of the laceration. Postoperative complications can include abscess formation, osteomyelitis, urethral strictures, and fistula formation.

  5. **Clitoral strangulation or ischemia** can be a difficult diagnosis as it is often results from a hair from a caretaker that accidentally wrapped around the base of the organ. Symptoms are that of irritability, engorgement, and possible cellulitis. The outcome depends on the degree of ischemia.

 B. **Management** of pediatric trauma includes a perineal examination for which sedation always should be used if the patient is neurologically and hemodynamically stable. The origin of bleeding must be determined before bimanual examination is performed. In the prepubertal female, a rectal/abdominal examination can be performed instead. In an infant or young girl, a small nasal speculum for visualization of the vagina can be used. A cystoscopic examination for any suspected bladder perforation and an anorectoscopic examination for any suspected anorectal trauma must be performed. Any microscopic hematuria in association with vaginal or vulvar trauma warrants evaluation with computed tomography (CT). Gross hematuria requires an immediate voiding cystourethrogram (VCUG). Penetrating wounds involving intraperitoneal organs require an exploratory laparotomy and, if indicated, any temporary intestinal bypass mechanism. Repair of bladder perforations requires either a suprapubic cystostomy or urethral catheter, depending on the location. Significant urethral injuries should be repaired and a urethral and/or suprapubic catheter placed for decompression. A urethral catheter can be used as both a stent and for decompression in less severe urethral injuries.

IV. **Urinary tract infection (UTI).** Urologic complaints often go hand-in-hand with gynecologic complaints. Obtaining a careful history is very important with regard to voiding patterns, day and night frequency, urgency or stress, quality of the stream, bed-wetting, previous infections, and treatments. Physical examination entails a complete abdominal and external genitalia evaluation; vaginal inspection if indicated; a neurologic assessment including reflexes, perineal sensation, and sphincter tone; and inspection of the lower back for evidence of a spinal abnormality. In adolescents, urologic complaints are essentially abnormalities of childhood that did not resolve or abnormalities relating to the onset of sexual activity. Many genitourinary congenital anomalies are first detected in adolescence secondary to complaints relating to menstrual periods.

 A. The **prevalence** of asymptomatic bacteriuria is influenced by age, sex, and method of diagnosis. One series found 0.9% of infant girls less than 1 year old to have asymptomatic bacteriuria. During the preschool and school years, 0.7% to 1.9% of girls were found to have bacteriuria. Lack of symptoms is due to the low virulence of the bacterial strains, which do not have the ability to adhere to and ascend the uroepithelium. Because asymptomatic bacteriuria in children can be a marker for a renal abnormality, it is recommended that these children be evaluated thoroughly.

 B. **Clinical presentation**
  1. **Cystitis.** Very young children often present with irritability, poor feeding, failure to grow, vomiting, or abdominal distention. Fever may be absent in the neonate. Young children present with failure to be toilet trained at the appropriate age, enuresis, incontinence, frequency, and dysuria. Recurrence of symptoms happen in approximately 10% of these girls. Adolescents present with symptoms similar to that of adults. Hemorrhagic cystitis is more common in adolescents. Most present with an initial onset

of low back pain, urinary frequency, and dysuria that becomes severe. Nausea and a low-grade fever are also common. The differential diagnosis is bacterial vaginitis, especially that associated with bubble baths or soaps.

2. Young children with **pyelonephritis** present with high fevers, abdominal or flank pain, chills, nausea, vomiting, and myalgia. They are often very ill, requiring hospitalization. Young infants, however, usually present with nonspecific findings associated with high fever. Unlike cystitis, a leukocytosis with a left shift can be present. The most common risk factor is **vesicoureteral reflux (VUR)**, estimated at a prevalence of 1% in healthy children. In those with UTIs who have fevers greater than 38.5°C, reflux has been found in 90%. The cause of reflux in the majority of children with VUR is congenital maldevelopment of the ureterovesical junction. The effect of reflux is directly proportional to the presence of an abnormal kidney on the contralateral side, recurrent UTIs, and the grade of the reflux. Reflux is graded from I to V according to severity. In those with severe bladder dysfunction, the normal valve mechanism can be overcome by high pressure. Acute cystitis may produce a transient reflux. In children with a normal bladder and without infection, VUR is a benign condition. VUR has been found to be less common in black children. Other predisposing factors for pyelonephritis are obstruction and severe malformation of the urinary tract. Pyelonephritis can lead to renal scarring in 25% to 30% of children. In this setting, renal scarring usually develops during the first 5 years of life and occurs predominantly at the renal poles with hypertrophy of normal parenchyma. Increased episodes of pyelonephritis increase the incidence of renal scarring. Early and aggressive antibiotic treatment is indicated.

C. **Evaluation** of the child should be undertaken after the first documented UTI. Reinfection occurs within 18 months in up to 40% to 60% of all children. Evidence of an upper UTI warrants a complete radiographic evaluation. Diagnosis of UTI is made by the urine culture. Urinalysis, which can identify inflammatory cells in the urine, can help in initiating treatment. However, it is reliable only 70% of the time. The method of collection depends on the age of the child. The diagnosis of reflux is made by the VCUG. In these children with reflux, the most common urodynamic abnormality is uninhibited bladder contractions. Most low-grade reflux resolves spontaneously with improved bladder function. Renal ultrasound also can be used to assess the upper urinary tract. In children, it has been found to be as sensitive as an intravenous pyelogram (i.v.p.) for the detection of significant renal abnormalities with the exception of uncomplicated duplication anomalies and focal scarring. Older adolescent females with recurrent infection may be best evaluated by an i.v.p. and cystoscopic evaluation with or without a VCUG. Radioisotopic renal scanning can also be used for evaluation of renal scarring, growth, and function. With hydronephrosis in the absence of reflux, mercuroacetylglycylglycine can be used for quantitative assessment of renal function and drainage of the dilated collecting system. Dimercaptosuccinic acid (succimer) is useful for demonstrating renal scarring and establishing the location of acute pyelonephritis.

D. **Bacteriology.** The majority of UTIs are caused by gram-negative organisms, most often by *Escherichia coli*, which is present in 60% to 80% of cases. The most common gram-positive organisms are *Staphylococcus* and *Enterococcus*. The majority of uncomplicated UTIs involve only one organism. Lactobacilli, corynebacteria, and streptococci should be considered contaminants unless the urine was a catheterized specimen or suprapubic aspirate.

E. **Treatment**

1. Treatment of an **acute, uncomplicated lower UTI** involves sulfonamides such as trimethoprim-sulfamethoxazole (TMP-SMX), nitrofurantoin, trimethoprim, and cephalosporins. Fluoroquinolones are best avoided because they have demonstrated toxicity in cartilage. Although controversy exists surrounding the duration of treatment, it is at present recommended that children be treated for 7 to 10 days because of the higher risk of anatomic anomalies. After the first UTI, a child should remain on prophylactic antibi-

otics until a radiographic evaluation is undertaken, usually within 2 to 3 weeks. In older children with pyelonephritis, immediate treatment with oral medications is indicated with close follow-up. TMP-SMX or cephalosporins are often effective. In the younger or very ill child, hospitalization is warranted with immediate initiation of parenteral therapy after the appropriate cultures are obtained. Combination therapy is indicated with broad-spectrum antibiotics such as aminoglycosides or cephalosporins until there is further information regarding the sensitivities of the responsible organism(s). Parenteral therapy is continued until the patient is afebrile for 48 to 72 hours and oral therapy has been instituted for 10 to 14 days. Control cultures should be obtained. Until radiologic evaluation is complete, the child should remain on low-dose prophylaxis.

2. **In managing reflux,** the main goal is to prevent an ascending UTI and renal scarring. Low-grade reflux tends to resolve spontaneously over time. Most resolutions occur within the first few years after diagnosis. The rate of resolution remains constant at approximately 10% to 15% per year. Reflux nephropathy is the most common disorder leading to hypertension in children. Management involves preventing UTIs with daily antibiotic prophylaxis, frequent voiding, and avoidance of constipation. Chemoprophylaxis with TMP-SMX or nitrofurantoin should be prescribed at bedtime as this is the longest time that a child retains urine. A urine culture should be obtained every 3 to 4 months. A radiographic evaluation of the upper urinary tract should be done annually until the reflux disappears.

   Surgical management of reflux involves ureteral reimplantation. Indications are persistent or recurrent infection despite prophylaxis, noncompliance with medical therapy, development of new scarring or failure of renal growth, or persistent significant reflux in adolescent girls. Reimplantation is successful in more than 95% of children.

V. Vulvovaginitis

A. Vulvovaginitis is the most common gynecologic complaint in the prepubertal female. **Vulvovaginal inflammation** accounts for 40% to 50% of visits to a pediatric gynecology clinic. Physiologic changes of the vagina include the initial stimulation of maternal hormones in the newborn period, resulting in a thickened vaginal mucosa and a physiologic leukorrhea. As estrogen levels decrease, the epithelium becomes smooth, thin, and atrophic, with a pH of 6.5 to 7.5. These changes usually take place by 6 weeks postnatally. Because of the neutral pH and lack of estrogenization, these delicate tissues are particularly susceptible to inflammation.

   Risk factors contributing to increased susceptibility are the lack of antibodies that help fight infection, lack of protective hair and labial fat pads, proximity of the rectum to the vagina, relatively small labia minora, and lack of proper hygiene. Other potential risk factors for vulvovaginitis include a small hymenal opening, obesity, preexisting vulvar dermatoses, and systemic illness such as diabetes mellitus. The normal prepubertal vaginal flora include lactobacilli, alpha-hemolytic streptococci, *Staphylococcus epidermidis*, diphtheroid, and gram-negative enteric organisms, especially *E. coli*.

B. **Signs and symptoms** include vaginal discharge staining the underclothing. On occasion, bloodstains are noted. Genital pain, itching, irritation, and dysuria are common. Vulvar burning or stinging may occur when urine comes into contact with irritated, excoriated tissues. On examination, erythema and discharge with an odor may be noted.

C. **Evaluation**

   1. A **history** should be taken before a physical examination. This involves not only getting answers to pertinent questions but gaining the trust of the child and caregiver, especially if the question of sexual abuse arises. The duration, consistency, quantity, and color of the discharge should be noted. Infections with anaerobic bacteria may be accompanied by the presence of a foul odor, and questions should be directed at behavior such as inadequate hygiene including back-to-front wiping,

trauma associated with play, or any genital manipulation with a foreign body or contaminated hands. Close-fitting, poorly absorbent clothing or prolonged exposure to a wet bathing suit may predispose to vulvo-vaginitis. In younger children, the type of diaper and frequency of changes should be noted. Information about recent systemic infections, new medications or lotions, bed-wetting, use of harsh soaps or bubble baths, history of dermatosis, and nocturnal perianal itching should be included in the history.

2. On **physical examination,** a sample of the discharge for microscopic examination and culture should be obtained. In nonrecurrent vulvo-vaginitis with no suspicion of bleeding or a foreign body, a vaginoscopy is not necessary. Presentations for vulvovaginitis are extremely variable, ranging from no discharge to copious secretions. Erythema, edema, and excoriations are commonly noted. Evidence of poor perineal hygiene may be evident, with stool seen in the vulva or between the labia. The config-uration of the hymen should be carefully noted and evaluated for any signs of trauma. The perianal skin should also be examined. The Scotch tape test can be done to test for pinworm infestation. A rectoabdominal examination also may be indicated. Direct collection of vaginal secretions with a regular cotton-tipped swab or saline-moistened urethral swab can be performed. The catheter-in-a-catheter technique involves placing the plastic portion of a no. 14 or 16 i.v. catheter within a shortened no. 12 plastic or rubber urinary catheter. A small syringe filled with 1 to 2 mL saline then is attached and the saline injected into the vagina. The syringe is used to collect the vaginal secretions. Microscopic examination for ova, "clue" cells, trichomonads, and white and red blood cells should be per-formed and the appropriate cultures sent.

D. **Etiology.** The infections that occur in the prepubertal child are often respira-tory, enteric, or sexually transmitted organisms. Respiratory pathogens include *Streptococcus pneumoniae*, a group A beta-hemolytic strep such as *Streptococ-cus pyogenes*, and *Neisseria meningitidis*. *Staphylococcus aureus*, *Branhamella catarrhalis*, and *Haemophilus influenzae* have been responsible for some cases of vaginitis, although they can occur as part of the normal flora. *Shigella* is the most common enteric pathogen, causing a mucopurulent or bloody discharge. In one-fourth or fewer cases, it occurs with an episode of diarrhea. *Candida* is common in the prepubertal stage only in the setting of antibiotic treatment, diabetes mellitus, diapers, or other similar risk factors. Diaper rash is usu-ally a chemical dermatitis. Sexually transmitted organisms include *Neisseria gonorrhoeae*, herpes simplex, human papillomavirus (usually type 6 or 11), *Trichomonas*, and possibly *Gardnerella vaginalis*. *Chlamydia trachomatis*, although associated with sexual abuse, also has been found in some infants who acquired vaginal colonization at birth from a mother with endocervical infec-tion. Persistence of a chlamydial infection after 12 to 24 months of age is unlikely, however, particularly if the child has been treated for upper respira-tory infections or otitis media with erythromycin or TMP-SMX.

E. **Therapy** involves improving perineal hygiene. The majority of vulvovaginal infections result in nonspecific vaginitis, which is often caused by disturbed bacterial homeostasis. This is often a result of suboptimal hygiene. These alter-ations in the flora or host defense mechanisms result in inflammation. A wet preparation shows a mixture of white blood cells, bacteria, and other debris. Sitz or tub baths twice a day for half an hour help eliminate the vaginal dis-charge from vulvar areas. Nonirritating soaps and white cotton underpants should be recommended. Nylon tights, tight blue jeans, and bubble baths should be discouraged. Both the caregiver and child should be instructed about proper front-to-back wiping. The child should be instructed to urinate with her knees apart so that urinary reflux into the vagina is reduced. A hair dryer on cool setting or use of baby powder on the vulva can help with drying. Small amounts of petroleum jelly can be used to protect the vulva. In summer months, prolonged wearing of a wet bathing suit should be discouraged. If symptoms persist after 2 weeks of therapy, the child should be reexamined.

Pinworms should be excluded and can be treated with a single dose of medication, which is repeated 2 weeks later. Mebendazole should not be given to children younger than 2 years. All family members may need to be treated. A 10-day antibiotic course with amoxicillin or a cephalosporin can also be instituted. Vaginoscopy should be considered to exclude a foreign body, neoplasm, or abnormal communication with the gastrointestinal or urinary tract. In unusually persistent cases for which a specific etiology has been ruled out, irrigation of the vagina with a 1% povidone-iodine (Betadine) solution may be helpful. Another approach is prescribing a 2-month course of a small dose of antibiotic at bedtime or three times a week. Estrogen-containing creams can be tried, but only for 3 to 4 weeks at a time. Caution must be exercised as prolonged use with systemic absorption of estrogen can result in iatrogenic precocious puberty. Recurrence often develops when the child has an upper respiratory infection or has failed to use proper hygiene. Obese females are particularly at risk for recurrences. Hymenotomy is curative for those whose vaginitis occurs secondary to a high hymenal opening that impairs vaginal drainage. Other causes include a pelvic abscess and an ectopic ureter.

F. **Pathogens**

1. *N. gonorrhoeae* primarily infects the vagina in the prepubertal child, in contrast to the endocervical infection of an adolescent or woman. The endocervix is closed before the age of 9 or 10 years and, thus, rarely is there an upper tract extension. The most commonly infected sites are the vagina, rectum, pharynx, and conjunctiva. The incubation period is approximately 1 week, with symptoms appearing in 2 to 7 days. Infection with gonococcus results in a copious, purulent discharge that may lead to a severe vulvitis. Neonates present within 3 to 4 days of birth with ophthalmia neonatorum. Infection at more than one anatomic site is common. Positive results for *N. gonorrhoeae* must be confirmed as false-positive cultures have far-reaching consequences. A single i.m. injection of ceftriaxone is the recommended treatment for those with an uncomplicated infection (125 mg for patients weighing less than 45 kg; 250 mg for patients weighing 45 kg or more). An alternative is spectinomycin, 40 mg/kg i.m. If the child is 8 years old or older, doxycycline should be prescribed, 100 mg p.o. b.i.d. for 7 days. Children with complicated gonococcal infections such as arthritis, meningitis, conjunctivitis, or peritonitis should receive a more prolonged course of parenteral ceftriaxone.

2. *Chlamydia* can be acquired by perinatal exposure or by sexual abuse. Perinatal infections have been demonstrated to persist for up to 53 weeks in the vagina and 55 weeks in the rectum. Neonates can present with inclusion conjunctivitis at 5 to 7 days of age, with chlamydial pneumonitis occurring in infancy at about 3 to 11 weeks of age with a history of prolonged cough and congestion. Symptomatic children present with vaginitis, urethritis, and/or pyuria. The diagnosis of *C. trachomatis* can be made by the cell culture technique or by direct immunofluorescence. In light of a positive test result, sexual abuse should be considered but not presumed given the potential for prolonged colonization with perinatally acquired infections. In children older than 24 to 36 months, genital infection is highly associated with sexual abuse. *C. trachomatis* can be treated by erythromycin, 50 mg/kg per day p.o., divided into t.i.d. or q.i.d. for 10 days, for children younger than 8 years of age. Older children can be treated with doxycycline, 100 mg p.o. b.i.d. for 7 days, or with azithromycin, 1 g p.o.

3. **Herpes simplex virus (HSV),** type I or II, also can cause vulvovaginitis. After an incubation period of 2 to 20 days, painful vesicular lesions develop that can ulcerate. Systemic symptoms include fever, nausea, malaise, headache, and inguinal adenopathy. Urinary retention can develop secondary to the intense genital pain. Type I usually presents as an oral infection that can be spread to the genital area with contaminated hands. This may appear as a mild gingivitis or as painful vesicular lesions

of the lips and oral cavity that can ulcerate. Pharyngitis can also develop. HSV-II has been related to genital infections and may be a result of sexual abuse. In either case, an evaluation for sexual abuse must be undertaken. Although uncommon, congenital HSV infection may occur from transplacental passage. Diagnosis is usually made by identifying and culturing suspicious ulcers. These ulcers must be differentiated from that of varicella and recurrent herpes zoster, ammonia dermatosis, trauma, syphilis, Stevens-Johnson syndrome, condyloma, impetigo, or erythema multiforme. Recurrences of herpetic lesions can occur without repeated exposures. Although there are no specific guidelines for treating children, some clinicians use acyclovir to treat those with genital herpes. Others prescribe symptomatic treatment with sitz baths and drying agents. Antibiotics can be prescribed in bacterial superinfection.

4. **Genital warts** are caused by human papillomaviruses, which can be transmitted by perinatal exposure, by sexual abuse, or by close physical contact. Condyloma in children generally presents as flesh-colored verrucous growths that are friable and easily traumatized. These lesions can also be found in the moist mucosal membranes of the urethra, bladder, mouth, and eye. Children can present with vaginal or rectal bleeding, dysuria, vaginal discharge, or painful defecation. Unlike adults who present with labial lesions, prepubertal children tend to present with perianal and periurethral warts. Perianal warts have been strongly associated with additional lesions in the anal canal, which can go undetected and may be a source of recurrence. Vertical transmission often results in laryngeal lesions and is thought to occur by aspiration of infected secretions into the upper airway of a newborn. The majority of perinatally acquired infections are reported in children less than 2 years of age. After the age of 2 years, sexual abuse has been documented in as many as 90% of children being evaluated. Any child, regardless of age, presenting with condyloma acuminatum should undergo an evaluation for sexual abuse. A careful examination of the perianal and periurethral areas is warranted.

   a. The **diagnosis** can be made with application of 3% to 5% acetic acid to suspected lesions. After 10 to 15 minutes, the classic aceto-white appearance of condyloma can be seen. Differential diagnosis includes condylomata lata of secondary syphilis, perineal tumors, urethral prolapse, sarcoma botryoides, and molluscum contagiosum. An examination under anesthesia of the vagina, cervix, periurethral area, and anal canal should also be performed. Biopsies of suspected lesions may be indicated if the diagnosis is uncertain.

   b. **Pathology** of a condyloma is a hyperplastic squamous epithelium with acanthosis, hyperkeratosis, and parakeratosis. Koilocytosis can be present. Given the oncogenic potential of certain subtypes of HPV, children must be followed on a long-term basis, although the exact nature of the follow-up has yet to be defined. Unfortunately, treatment regimens for children are associated with high recurrence rates. Podophyllin resin in dilute solution, 5% to 15%, has been recommended for children. The solution must be removed with soap and water approximately 4 hours after application. Systemic absorption with resultant neurotoxicity has been described in adults and adolescents. Cryotherapy, topical use of 5-fluorouracil cream, and electrosurgical fulguration are other methods of treatment. Use of the carbon dioxide laser has become more frequent because it is less associated with scarring and discomfort. As there is no single best treatment for condyloma, therapy must be individualized for each child.

5. *Trichomonas vaginalis* is a flagellated protozoan dependent on the presence of glycogen, and thus, rarely causes an infection in a nonestrogenic environment. It is rarely seen in patients under 9 years old. During the neonatal period, it can be a relatively common cause of vaginitis. Symptomatic children usually present with copious, yellow-gray frothy discharge and complaints of dysuria and vulvar itching. Given the alkaline

pH and lack of estrogen in the vagina, the urinary tract may often be the primary source of infection. Trichomoniasis is unlikely to be transmitted nonsexually as the organism can only survive for several hours on moist surfaces or in body fluids. Diagnosis is based on seeing motile trichomonads on a wet slide preparation. A child with trichomoniasis should undergo an evaluation for sexual abuse. Treatment involves giving metronidazole, 15 mg/kg per day divided t.i.d. for 7 days.

6. **Bacterial vaginosis** is a mixed infection of *G. vaginalis*, anaerobes such as *Bacteroides* species and *Mobiluncus*, and occasionally genital mycoplasmas. In children it is unclear exactly how often bacterial vaginosis is responsible for vaginitis. It is also unknown whether it can be perinatally transmitted. Symptomatic children often present with a thin white vaginal discharge that has a "fishy" odor. Diagnosis is based on identifying "clue" cells on a wet slide preparation. The whiff test can also be performed by adding a 10% solution of KOH to vaginal secretions in which the fishy odor can be detected. Although bacterial vaginosis can be detected in virginal women, in prepubertal children it is usually sexually transmitted. Thus, children diagnosed with bacterial vaginosis should undergo an evaluation for sexual abuse. Although there are no defined guidelines for treatment in children, some clinicians have used metronidazole in symptomatic children. Ampicillin and amoxicillin may also be of some benefit.

7. Perinatal transmission of **syphilis** often occurs by hematogenous transplacental passage of *Treponema pallidum*. Because there is a latent period between the infection and serologic conversion, an infant may develop congenital syphilis despite negative perinatal serologies. This should be considered when a child presents with possible acquired syphilis at less than 1 year of age. At approximately 21 days after exposure, primary syphilis often presents as a painless genital chancre. These lesions also can present in the oral cavity and perianal area. The differential diagnosis includes condylomata acuminata, trauma, and herpes simplex. Serologic tests are not infrequently negative as the rapid plasma reagin and VDRL test usually take 4 to 8 weeks to convert. The microhemagglutination *T. pallidum* and fluorescent treponemal antibody absorption test can also be negative at the early stages. Darkfield examination should be performed for a definitive diagnosis.

    Secondary syphilis, although uncommon in the pediatric population, usually presents as a skin rash within 1 to several months after the initial exposure. Other possible diagnoses include pityriasis rosea, tinea versicolor, psoriasis, viral illnesses, or a drug reaction. Any child presenting with syphilitic lesions should undergo an evaluation for sexual abuse. Cerebrospinal fluid samples should be obtained in children to rule out congenital syphilis. Any child with congenital syphilis or evidence of neurologic involvement can be treated with penicillin G (200,000 to 300,000 U/kg/day) for 10 to 14 days. Otherwise, treatment can be with 50,000 U/kg of i.m. benzathine penicillin (not to exceed 2.4 million units).

8. **Secondary inoculation** can occur as a result of blood-borne inoculation of the vulva and vagina with organisms causing a primary infection elsewhere in the body. Cultures usually reveal the same organism responsible for the original infection. Treatment depends on the primary source. Good perineal hygiene with sitz or tub baths should be emphasized. Topical corticosteroids can help minimize the inflammatory response. If the vaginal discharge or inflammation persists or recurs after a second course of therapy, then a vaginoscopy is indicated.

    a. *H. influenzae.* The significance of recovering this organism in vaginal secretions is unclear. Symptomatic individuals can be treated with amoxicillin 20 to 40 mg/kg/day p.o. for 7 days.

    b. **Group A beta-hemolytic strep** (*S. pyogenes*) is an important cause of bacterial vulvovaginitis and usually presents 7 to 10 days after a sore throat and upper respiratory tract infection. Children usually present with vaginal bleeding or blood-tinged vaginal discharge. Severe vulvitis is usually associated. Treatment is with penicillin V potassium, 125 to 250 mg p.o. q.i.d. for 10 days.

c. Other **respiratory pathogens** include *S. pneumoniae* and pneumococcus. Treatment is with penicillin V potassium, 125 to 250 mg q.i.d for 10 days.

d. *Shigella* results in a mucopurulent and malodorous vaginal discharge. Diarrhea occurs in less than one-fourth of individuals. Treatment is with trimethoprim, 8 mg/kg/day, and sulfamethoxazole, 40 mg/kg/day, divided b.i.d. p.o. for 7 days.

e. *S. aureus* can be part of the normal vaginal flora. When found in a symptomatic individual, it can be treated with cephalexin, 25 to 50 mg/kg/day p.o. for 7 days; dicloxacillin, 25 mg/kg/day p.o. for 7 days; or amoxicillin/clavulanate potassium (Augmentin), 20 to 40 mg/kg/day p.o. for 7 to 10 days.

9. *Candida* **vulvovaginitis** occurs infrequently in prepubertal girls. History of the infection usually involves a child still in diapers, recent use of an antibiotic, diabetes mellitus, or immunodeficiency. It usually manifests as a white discharge and can be diagnosed by a 10% KOH prep by identifying hyphae and/or spores. If diagnosed in a child without a predisposing condition and especially if recurrent, an evaluation for diabetes or immunodeficiency should be undertaken. Treatment consists initially of a topical antifungal cream such as miconazole. If those are not successful, subsequent treatments consist of intravaginal nystatin liquid or antifungal suppositories that are size appropriate.

10. One-fifth of girls with **pinworms** develop an associated vulvovaginitis. Symptoms include vulvar and perianal itching, particularly at night. The Scotch tape test can be used to diagnose pinworm infestation by recovering the characteristic eggs. Treatment of *Enterobius vermicularis* is with mebendazole, 100 mg p.o. for one dose, for all members of a household except pregnant women and children younger than 2 years.

G. **Congenital anomalies,** such as an ectopic ureter, may result in vulvovaginitis. Anomalous openings onto the perineum or into the vagina or urethra can result in a discharge of clear or infected urine. An i.v.p. can be used to make the diagnosis.

H. **Chemical vaginitis** secondary to the use of new lotions, bubble baths, or harsh soaps can cause irritation of the perineal and vulvar skin. Treatment includes discontinuation of the causative agent, good perineal hygiene, and sitz baths.

I. **Skin disorders** that affect the vulva include psoriasis, eczema, and lichen sclerosus. Dermatologic conditions tend to affect the labia minora and majora rather than the vagina and vestibule. Seborrheic dermatosis also can involve other areas of the body, particularly intertriginous regions. Eczema is characterized by pruritic, dry, and papular-appearing patches of skin. This can be treated by mild, nonfluorinated topical steroid. Lichen sclerosus is a rare disorder of unknown etiology that affects the area around the genitals. Symptoms include itching, soreness, irritation, erythema, dysuria, vaginal bleeding, and discharge. On examination, multiple ivory-colored, polygonal papules can be seen. These papules often coalesce into large plaques that appear atrophic. Purpuric speckling, frank ecchymosis, and secondary infections can be common. Because of the perianal involvement, the rash often gives an hourglass or figure-of-eight pattern. Sexual abuse or vitiligo can be mistakenly diagnosed. Management involves good perineal hygiene. Simple bland ointments with topical antiseptics or antibiotics can be prescribed. If there is no improvement, topical steroids may be instituted.

J. **Adhesive vulvitis** involves fusion of the labia minora, likely caused by the chronic irritation associated with vulvitis. This is common between ages 2 and 6 years. Topical estrogen cream can be applied to the adhesion b.i.d. for 2 to 4 weeks.

K. **Systemic illnesses,** such as varicella, Crohn's disease, Stevens-Johnson syndrome, diabetes, or Kawasaki syndrome, can result in vaginitis.

VI. **Vaginal bleeding** in children is a cause for concern and requires thorough evaluation. It can be caused by vulvar or vaginal irritation or lesions, trauma or sexual abuse, or precocious puberty.

A. **Vulvovaginitis** may cause vaginal bleeding. The causes and management of vulvovaginitis are discussed in detail in sec. **V.**

B. **Urethral prolapse** can sometimes be the cause of bleeding. It is thought to occur after an episode of increased abdominal pressure. The urethral mucosa protrudes through the meatus, forming an annular, hemorrhagic mass that bleeds easily. The average age of onset is 5 years. A short-term course of therapy with estrogen cream is indicated in asymptomatic prolapses. Sitz baths often can be of benefit. In those symptomatic with urinary retention or if the mass is large and necrotic, resection of the prolapsed tissue with insertion of an indwelling catheter for more than 24 hours may be warranted. Antibiotic treatment is necessary if infection occurs. Other urologic disorders with similar presentations include urethral polyps, caruncles, cysts, and prolapsed uterocele.

C. **Dysfunctional uterine bleeding** (DUB) is excessive, prolonged, or erratic bleeding from the endometrium that is not caused by anatomic lesions of the uterus. It is more commonly seen in adolescents than in children. The most common cause of DUB is anovulation, accounting for more than 75% of cases. The average age of menarche is 12.8 years in the United States. However, it can take up to 5 years to establish regular ovulatory cycles. DUB is a diagnosis of exclusion. Blood dyscrasias, organic disorders, and hypothalamic dysfunction should be ruled out. These include thrombocytopenic purpura, platelet disorders, benign intrauterine tumors, threatened abortions, ectopic pregnancy, hydatiform mole, stress, exercise, congenital adrenal hyperplasia, Cushing's syndrome, or thyroid dysfunction. However, the most common cause of anovulation is immaturity of the hypothalamic-pituitary-ovarian axis. The second most common cause is a coagulopathy.

1. **Evaluation** should include a detailed gynecologic, medical, and sexual history. Tanner staging should be performed as should notation of any evidence of an abnormal endocrine effect such as hirsutism, thyromegaly, or galactorrhea. A pelvic examination can help determine an anatomic source of abnormal bleeding or the presence of a foreign body. Laboratory tests should include a complete blood cell count, blood smear, pregnancy test, coagulation profile, thyroid function tests, and prolactin level.

2. **Treatment** depends on the findings. Once other possibilities are ruled out, irregular vaginal bleeding can be controlled with oral contraceptives. In anovulatory bleeding, treatment can consist of only supplying the missing progestin. In oligomenorrhea, withdrawal flow can be induced with medroxyprogesterone acetate, 10 mg p.o. q.i.d., for 10 days/month. If no bleeding commences, further evaluation is necessary. Menometrorrhagia or polymenorrhea can be treated with progestins prescribed for 10 to 14 days for endometrial stabilization after which there is a withdrawal flow. An acute anovulatory episode of bleeding can be controlled with a 50-μg estrogen-progestin oral contraceptive, 1 pill q.i.d. for 1 to 5 days. Once the flow diminishes, the pill can be given once per day for the remaining 21-day cycle, after which a withdrawal bleed should occur. If the bleeding fails to stop after initiation of the q.i.d. dosing, a diagnosis other than anovulation must be considered.

D. **Endometrial shedding** resulting in vaginal bleeding is often associated with precocious puberty, which is defined as the onset of sexual maturation that is younger than 2 standard deviations from the norm. In the United States, sexual precocity is the appearance of secondary sex characteristics before the age of 8 years or the onset of menarche before the age of 10 years.

1. **Causes** of endometrial shedding include a physiologic neonatal withdrawal bleed in the first 2 weeks of life; isolated premature menarche, which is rare without other signs of precocious puberty; iatrogenic/facetious precocious puberty caused by medications containing exogenous estrogens; functional ovarian cysts; ovarian neoplasms; idiopathic preco-

cious puberty; McCune-Albright syndrome; central nervous system (CNS) lesions; or other hormone-producing neoplasms.

2. **Evaluation** should include blood estradiol and gonadotropin levels, a gonadotropin-releasing hormone stimulation test, a pelvic ultrasound and/or CT scan of the abdomen and pelvis to rule out a neoplasm, and if indicated by examination, a CT scan of the head to rule out CNS lesions.

E. **Genital tumors** are relatively uncommon in the prepubertal girl. However, they must be considered part of the differential diagnosis when a patient is found to have a chronic genital ulcer, tissue protruding from the vagina, a malodorous bloody vaginal discharge, or an atraumatic swelling of the external genitalia. Benign tumors of the vulva can cause vulvar bleeding, especially capillary hemangiomas, which usually disappear over time. However, damage to cavernous hemangiomas can result in significant hemorrhage. These are best treated by surgical excision. Sarcoma botryoides (rhabdomyosarcoma) is a fast-growing, aggressive tumor of the genital tract. It is the most common malignant tumor of the genital tract in girls. The peak incidence is before age 2 years, with 90% of patients diagnosed before age 5 years. It arises in the submucosal tissue, spreading beneath an intact vaginal epithelium. The vaginal mucosa then is punctuated by polypoid growths. The hallmark sign is passage of a polypoid mass from the vagina or urethra. Symptoms include vaginal bleeding or discharge and abdominal pain. On examination, an abdominal mass can sometimes be palpated. Diagnosis is made by biopsy. Treatment involves chemotherapy, a combination regimen of vincristine, D-actinomycin, and cyclophosphamide. If the tumor can be resected after chemotherapy, a radical hysterectomy and vaginectomy can be performed. If the tumor is unresectable, radiotherapy can be instituted. Embryonal carcinoma, mesonephric carcinoma, and clear cell adenocarcinoma are often seen in the setting of maternal diethylstilbestrol exposure.

References

1. Sedlak AJ, Broadhurst DB. *Third national incidence studies of child abuse and neglect.* Washington, DC: U.S. Government Printing Office, 1996.
2. Leventhal JM. Epidemiology of sexual abuse of children: old problems, new directions. *Child Abuse Negl* 1998;22:481–491.
3. National Center on Child Abuse and Neglect. *Child sexual abuse. Special report.* Washington, DC: HEW, Children's Bureau, 1978.
4. Stevens-Simon C, Rieichert S. Sexual abuse, adolescent pregnancy, and child abuse. A developmental approach to an intergenerational cycle. *Arch Pediatr Adoles Med* 1994;148:23–27.

Selected Reading

American College of Obstetricians and Gynecologists. *Pediatric gynecologic disorders. ACOG technical bulletin no. 201.* Washington, DC: American College of Obstetricians and Gynecologists, 1995.

Carpenter SEK, Rock JA. *Pediatric and adolescent gynecology.* New York: Raven Press, 1992.

Sanfilipo JS, Muram D, Lee PA, Dewhurst J. *Pediatric and adolescent gynecology.* Philadelphia: WB Saunders, 1994.

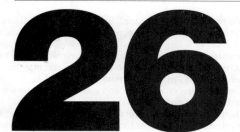

Sexual Function and Dysfunction

Marcela G. del Carmen
and John Murphy

I. **Sexual identity** can be defined by gender identity, sexual orientation, and intention.
   A. **Gender identity** is one's sense of being female or male and usually develops during the second year of life.
   B. **Sexual orientation** is the sex that elicits arousal, either in fantasy or reality.
   C. **Sexual intention** is defined by what the person desires to do with her or his sexual partner.

II. **Normal phases of the sexual response**
   A. **Excitement phase.** In both sexes, muscle tone augments, with a "flush" that initially involves the upper abdomen and then spreads to the breasts. Tachycardia and elevation of blood pressure accompany this phase.
      1. In **women,** excitement may be initiated by visual, psychic, or tactile stimuli. Initially, transudation of the vagina allows for lubrication, which is also promoted by Bartholin's glands. The clitoris increases in diameter at the level of the shaft. The glans clitoridis also swells. The labia majora gape and are displaced toward the clitoris. The inner two-thirds of the vaginal canal expand. Increasing vaginal distention and tenting of the vaginal walls also occur so that the inner vagina swells and changes in color from pink to dark purple. The nipples undergo erection, and the breasts increase in size.
      2. In **men,** this phase may also be initiated by visual, psychic, or tactile stimuli. The penis becomes erect and engorged. The spermatic cords shorten, the testes retract, and the scrotum is thickened and flattened against the body.
      3. The excitement phase is primarily mediated by the **parasympathetic** nerve fibers in both women and men. Consequently, it may be blunted by certain anticholinergic drugs.
   B. **The plateau phase**
      1. In **women,** the outer one-third of the vagina is engorged and swells, thus resulting in a diameter reduction that results in greater friction with intercourse. The inner two-thirds of the vagina are elevated. The uterus increases in size. The clitoris retracts into its hood. The labia continue to engorge.
      2. In **men,** the penis becomes completely engorged and increases in diameter at the coronal ridge. The testes continue to increase in size. Some fluid, from Cowper's glands, enters the urethra. Although this fluid is not semen, it may contain sperm.
      3. In **both women and men,** blood pressure, respiratory rate, pulse, muscle tone, and tension continue to increase.
   C. **The orgasmic phase**
      1. In **women,** the orgasmic response is initiated by rhythmic muscular contractions, followed by uterine contractions that progress from the superior portion of the uterus and move toward the cervix.
      2. In **men,** rhythmic contractions result in contraction of the bulbocavernous muscle. Semen is emptied into the bulbous urethra as the prostate contracts and prostatic fluid mixes with semen. Contractions at the level of the bulb eject the semen.

3. In **both women and men,** neck, abdominal, buttocks, and facial muscles contract. Changes in blood pressure, pulse, and respiration peak and then dissipate.

4. In contrast to the excitement phase, orgasm is primarily mediated by the **sympathetic branch** of the autonomic nervous system and may be influenced by medications such as antihypertensives.

D. **The resolution phase.** Muscle tension and skin and genital engorgement end, with a fading of the sex flush and onset of perspiration.

1. In **women,** the clitoris returns to its previous state, reaching its previous size in 5 to 10 minutes. The nipples appear prominent as an effect of the resolution of the tissue swelling around them. The outer one-third of the vagina decreases in diameter. The uterus returns to its usual size and the cervix descends. Approximately 30 minutes elapse until the unstimulated state is reached. No refractory period has been observed in women.

2. In **men,** loss of erection occurs in two stages. During the first, most of the erectile volume is lost, while in the second, the remaining shrinkage occurs. During this refractory period, men cannot be aroused again. This period lengthens with age and may last from several minutes or hours to days.

III. **History.** Sexual history-taking belongs in the review of systems and should be a part of every gynecologic visit, although the amount of detail may vary with the individual patient. Initially, identifying the patient's vocabulary for her anatomy and experiences should precede more specific questions. Inquiries regarding sexual desire, arousal, orgasm, and satisfaction should be made. An assessment of gender identity and orientation may be helpful.

A. **Problems** with sexual friction should be explored in terms of duration of the concern, best and worst function, and relationship to other factors (e.g., financial problems, losses, medications, illness, surgery, infertility, and contraception). Helpful questions include inquiries about a history of sexual abuse or incest, sexual activity in childhood, and family or religious attitudes toward sex.

B. The **adolescent patient** should be evaluated with regard to menarche, preparation for menses, masturbation, sexual orientation, sexual activity, intercourse, contraception, and protection against sexually transmitted diseases.

IV. **Sexuality and menopause**

A. **Physical and psychological effects of menopause.** Perimenopausal and postmenopausal women may experience a reduction in sexual desire and fantasy, as well as vaginal dryness (often resulting in dyspareunia), which results from slower and decreased lubrication during the arousal phase. Pelvic relaxation, including cystocele, rectocele, uterine prolapse, and decreased vaginal tone may diminish coital pleasure. Muscle and uterine contractions are weaker, often uncomfortable, yielding a markedly less intense orgasmic experience. Sensation may be diminished by skin atrophy and alterations in peripheral nerve endings. If the woman has had a surgical intervention resulting in a tight vagina, difficulties in achieving complete sexual pleasure may arise with a man with a less firm erection.

B. **Management.** It is important to appreciate that menopausal women can still enjoy sexual activity. It is the responsibility of the gynecologist to educate the aging couple about normal changes, to offer hormone replacement therapy, and to discuss noncoital intimacy as a source of pleasure.

C. **Men** may also have decreased sexual activity with aging, with erections requiring more stimulation and taking longer to achieve.

V. **Female sexual dysfunction** may result from orgasmic dysfunction, an inhibited sexual desire, or dyspareunia.

A. **Orgasmic dysfunction** can be divided between women experiencing primary orgasmic problems (patients who have never experienced orgasm) and those with secondary orgasmic problems (women with periods of normal functioning). Women who attain orgasm with stimulation of the clitoris but not with intercourse are not dysfunctional. Approximately 8% to 10% of females in the United States have never experienced orgasm, and 10% achieve it only with fantasy.

1. **Physiology and pathophysiology.** Orgasm can be understood as a genital reflex that is under voluntary control. As with any reflex, inhibition can be learned. Sensory input from the brain and the periphery enter the spinal cord at the level of the sacrum, through the pudendal nerve. The efferent outflow, which involves perivaginal muscle contraction, is mediated at the T-11 to L-2 level.

2. **Functional and psychological factors.** Women with orgasmic dysfunction are unable to progress beyond the plateau phase of sexual response. It is important to note that they may nonetheless experience no difficulties with lubricating adequately and often enjoy lovemaking. Although many women are not sure if they have achieved orgasm, others "fake" it to satisfy their partner. Commonly, women with a primary orgasmic problem experience fears about relationships or sexuality, such as performance anxiety or sexual inhibition. Fear of pregnancy, urinary incontinence, or experiencing pleasure are common.

3. **Treatment.** Successful treatment depends on the ability to allay the patient's anxiety (or anxieties) and to enhance sensory stimulation. Patients with primary orgasmic dysfunction should learn what orgasm feels like. Fantasy can be helpful and self-stimulation may allow the woman to experience sexual arousal. Inquiries should be made about the presence of a trusted partner and guilt-provoking experiences in the patient's past. Masturbating, either alone or with a partner, may be helpful, although prohibitive societal attitudes sometimes are difficult to overcome. Discussion groups may be beneficial for the patient with multiple fears. The final step in treatment protocols involves the transfer of orgasm to a partner experience. Heterosexual women heighten arousal before penetration, often stimulating the clitoris indirectly (during penile thrusting as the hood is pulled back and forth over the clitoris by indirect friction).

B. **Inhibited sexual desire** may be primary (lifelong) or secondary (after a period of normal functioning).

1. Women with a **primary** problem should be assessed by the gynecologist for a history of sexual abuse or trauma in childhood or adolescence. These patients may come from sexually repressive backgrounds and are often involved in an unsatisfactory relationship in which the partner may be unsupportive or even abusive. Treatment involves both psychological and behavioral modifications.

2. Patients with **secondary** problems should be evaluated for the presence of recent life changes (drug/medical problems or losses). These women often report recent problems with a partner, emotional or physical traumas, history of surgical interventions, illnesses, drug or alcohol abuse, or depression. Changes in body image, differences with the attainment of sexual pleasure from their partner, and concerns about pregnancy must also be discussed.

C. **Sexual phobias.** Women with sexual phobias often experience panic or anxiety with the onset of sexual thoughts. These phobias are common in patients developing avoidance patterns; patients are often mistakenly perceived as having a low sexual desire. Treatment is mainly through education, psychotherapy, support, and behavioral desensitization. Pharmacotherapy, in the form of antianxiety medications, is sometimes needed for successful treatment.

D. **Dyspareunia** is defined as pain during sexual intercourse.

1. **History.** Inquiries should be made about a history of trauma or abuse, as well as perceptions of pain with menstruation and childbearing and the patient's association of the latter two to dyspareunia. The interviewer must also inquire about psychological reasons.

2. On **physical examination,** a careful examination of the vaginal opening must be made. Lesions, such as Bartholin's gland abscess, a tender episiotomy scar, or decreased vaginal elasticity that results from aging, can often be elicited with a careful examination. The clitoris should be inspected for the presence of irritations or infections. The vagina should

also be assessed for the presence of infections, sensitivity reactions, atrophic reactions, and decreased lubrication, which may account for dyspareunia. Endometriosis, pelvic inflammatory disease, and ectopic pregnancies have also been associated with painful intercourse.

3. **Treatment** is geared toward managing the specific causative problem.

E. **Vaginismus** occurs in anticipation of penetration of the vagina, and is defined as a painful perivaginal and thigh adductor muscle spasm.

1. **Etiology.** The interviewer should inquire about a history of rape or incest, surgery or trauma to the vaginal area, or medical problems. Vaginismus may be seen in women with little sexual experience, among the young, and those from strict backgrounds. Other etiologies include poor lubrication arising from lack of arousal and sexual phobias.

2. **Treatment.** Gradual vaginal dilation (through the use of dilators or the patient's or partner's finger) is the usual first step in treatment. Some patients require psychotherapy as part of the treatment protocol, especially if the etiology for their vaginismus has a strong psychological component.

VI. **Male sexual dysfunction.** Common problems include reduced or excessive desire, erectile difficulties (problems with arousal), and problems with orgasm (premature ejaculation, inhibited orgasm, or retrograde ejaculation). Psychogenic, organic, or mixed psychogenic and organic factors may be responsible. A careful history should include details about the patient's sexual desires, early life experiences, and the role of his partner. Questions regarding medical illnesses, surgeries, medications, drugs, alcohol, neuropathies, and vasculopathies may help to isolate an organic etiology. Depression, phobias, fear of intimacy or women, and relationship difficulties may also be contributing factors. These forms of dysfunction respond well to behavioral treatments. It is prudent to consult with partners together, so as to help them establish better communication and a more solid relationship. **Organic** causes are treated by addressing the underlying etiology. Several drugs have been associated with sexual dysfunction, including antihypertensives, antipsychotics, central nervous system depressants (such as sedatives, cannabis, alcohol, heroin, and anxiolytics), tricyclic antidepressants, and cimetidine.

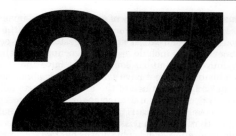

Repeated Pregnancy Loss

Alicia Walsh and
Timothy Hickman

I. Definition. It is generally accepted that 15% to 20% of all clinically documented pregnancies result in spontaneous abortion. Many factors affect the actual risk of miscarriage, including maternal age. For women under 20, miscarriage occurs in 12% of pregnancies. This number increases to 26% for women older than 40. When unrecognized pregnancies are factored into the equation, the spontaneous abortion rate is actually much higher. This often includes losses occurring before the expected onset of menses.

For most women who experience a miscarriage, the recurrence rate is below 30%. In fact, 80% to 90% of women will have a successful pregnancy after a spontaneous abortion. However, some women experience multiple losses. *Repeated pregnancy loss* (RPL) is defined as three consecutive spontaneous abortions before 20 weeks' gestation or a fetal weight less than 500 g. RPL is further divided into *primary*, meaning women without a previous liveborn infant, and *secondary*, for those women with at least one prior liveborn infant. For these women, the recurrence rate for miscarriage has been shown to be as high as 54% after four losses.

Overall, RPL affects 0.5% to 1.0% of pregnant women. There are many purported causes of RPL, but for as many as 50% of women no cause can be identified. Often, multiple factors are determined to play a role.

II. Etiology. Causes of RPL include but are not limited to genetic, anatomic, endocrine, immunologic, infectious, and environmental factors.

A. Genetic

1. **Chromosomal abnormalities** are a common cause of spontaneous abortions. In fact, up to 60% of first trimester miscarriages show a chromosomal abnormality when fetal tissue is tested. These include aneuploidies, trisomies, monosomies, and so forth. Trisomies are detected in almost 50% of miscarriages secondary to chromosomal abnormality. The most common trisomies, in descending order of incidence, are 13, 16, 18, 21, and 22. The single most common abnormality is 45X, which accounts for 25% of all chromosomal abnormalities.

   However, studies of women experiencing RPL show that one miscarriage with documented fetal chromosomal abnormalities does not predict that future losses will also be secondary to chromosomal abnormalities. Abnormal fetal karyotypes are a common cause of single losses but are unlikely to be a major cause of RPL.

2. However, **parental chromosomal abnormalities** may play a role in RPL. Studies have shown that the incidence of chromosomal abnormalities in couples experiencing RPL is 2% to 3%, five to six times higher than the incidence in the general population. The most common abnormality, found in close to 5% of RPL parental karyotypes, is a balanced translocation. Often, the parent is phenotypically normal. The translocation may be passed on in one of three ways: (a) normal karyotype, (b) balanced translocation, or (c) unbalanced translocation, which may be incompatible with life. Other parental chromosomal abnormalities include inversions and mosaicism.

B. Anatomic reasons for RPL can be further divided into congenital and acquired problems.

1. **Congenital problems** encompass a variety of conditions often involving the müllerian genesis. These losses more commonly occur during the second trimester, although losses at earlier stages of gestation can occur. Common uterine abnormalities include septate, bicornuate, didelphic, and, less commonly, unicornuate uteri. Some studies have shown that 27% of women with a history of losses have some anatomic abnormality.

   Unicornuate uterus occurs when one of the müllerian ducts fails to develop. When pregnancy does occur, fetal outcomes are poor. Almost one-half of these pregnancies result in miscarriage and the rest often result in preterm labor, fetal growth retardation possibly secondary to an aberrant blood supply, and malpresentation. A didelphic uterus has two endometrial cavities and two cervices and results from failed fusion of the müllerian ducts. Pregnancy outcome is better in this group. A bicornuate uterus, which consists of two endometrial cavities and one cervix, results from incomplete fusion of the medical walls of the paramesonephric ducts. Almost 60% of these pregnancies result in a liveborn infant. A septate uterus results from failure of resorption of the paramesonephric ducts and is often associated with poor obstetric outcomes. Studies have reported 15% to 28% livebirth rates in women with this type of uterine abnormality.

2. **Acquired anatomic abnormalities** associated with RPL include leiomyomata, intrauterine synechiae, and *in utero* diethylstilbestrol (DES) exposure.

   a. **Fibroids,** particularly submucosal ones, have been purported to cause RPL. These anatomic lesions may result in unfavorable implantation sites and may jeopardize the vascular supply to the placenta. Intramuscular and subserosal fibroids may also be problematic if they are large enough to distort the uterine cavity. One literature review determined that 41% of pregnancies in women with fibroids ended in miscarriage.

   b. **Intrauterine synechiae** most often form after instrumentation of the uterus, although they may occur in cases in which there is an estrogen deficiency. Adhesions are said to account for 5% of RPL cases. Often, these occur after a dilation and curettage in which there is direct trauma to the endometrial cavity. It is purported that these adhesions may interfere with implantation and future vascular supply to the fetus.

   c. **DES-exposed women** have been shown to have poor reproductive outcomes. One study reported a 42% livebirth rate for these women with a majority of losses occurring in the first trimester. *In utero* exposure has been reported to cause multiple anatomic abnormalities, including a T-shaped uterine cavity, a widened lower uterine segment, midfundal constrictions, filling defects, and irregular margins (1). These defects can be seen on hysterosalpingogram in 42% to 69% of DES-exposed women. It has been proposed that these abnormalities may result from DES binding to estrogen receptors during embryologic development of the müllerian system.

   d. **Cervical incompetence** is another anatomic cause of RPL. This is a condition of painless cervical dilation and may be congenital or acquired. Acquired causes include previous cervical surgery (i.e., conization).

C. **Endocrine.** A defect with the corpus luteum known as *luteal phase deficiency* is a proposed cause of RPL. Initial studies showed that perhaps as many as 60% of RPL cases are a result of luteal phase defects, but actual figures are much lower, approximately 40%. In this condition, a deficiency in progesterone causes the endometrial tissue to lag by 2 or more days behind the anticipated histologic age of the tissue. Progesterone production by the corpus luteum is needed to support a pregnancy until the eighth week when the placenta starts to produce the majority of this hormone. Individuals with a luteal phase defect do not produce enough progesterone to support an early pregnancy. Losses tend to occur early, at 4 to 7 weeks' gestation.

Studies show that subclinical diabetes and thyroid disease are unlikely causes of RPL, although women with poorly controlled insulin-dependent diabetes are at an increased risk of spontaneous abortion.

D. **Immunologic** disorders associated with RPL can be further divided into autoimmune and alloimmune factors.

1. In a compilation of studies on women with RPL, 15% were found to have recognizable **autoimmune factors.** The most common antibodies include anticardiolipin antibody, antiphospholipid antibody, and lupus anticoagulant. *In vitro,* these factors cause thrombosis. *In vivo,* they may cause thrombosis and placental infarctions that in turn result in spontaneous abortion. The majority of these losses occur during the second trimester.

2. **Alloimmune factors,** meaning immunity against a foreign entity, are another possible cause of RPL. Some couples experiencing RPL share HLA. This may "preclude the formation of maternal antibodies which normally coat fetal antigens and prevent rejection" (2). This mechanism is a controversial cause of RPL because the sharing of HLA does not always result in poor pregnancy outcomes.

E. **Infectious.** Only a few microbiological agents have been related to RPL. Women experiencing RPL have been shown to be infected with *Ureaplasma urealyticum* and *Mycoplasma hominis* at a higher rate than the general population. Overall, infectious etiologies of RPL are controversial.

F. **Environmental.** It has been shown that tobacco, alcohol, and some drugs are related to RPL. Some chemotherapeutic agents are also a proven cause of pregnancy loss. Ionizing radiation, anesthetic gases, and some heavy metals are other possible causes of spontaneous abortion in women exposed to these agents. Many dermatologic preparations, especially those containing vitamin A derivatives, cause spontaneous abortions.

G. **Unknown.** In as many as 50% to 60% of women experiencing RPL there is no identified cause.

III. **Diagnosis.** Although RPL is defined as three consecutive pregnancy losses, a physician need not wait for three losses to start a diagnostic workup. In particular, for older couples without children, it may be wise to start a workup after two losses. Also, it is important to do a complete workup, as some couples will have multiple reasons for RPL.

A complete history is the first step. A detailed family history should be taken, including reproductive outcomes and medical illnesses. An occupational history should also be elicited to determine exposure to various chemicals. This should be followed by a thorough examination, including cultures for *Chlamydia,* gonorrhea, *Mycoplasma,* and *Ureaplasma.* Blood tests, including thyroid function tests, a random or fasting glucose, antiphospholipid antibody, lupus anticoagulant, and anticardiolipin antibody, should be ordered. A karyotype of each partner is helpful in locating translocations, inversions, and mosaicisms. Karyotypes of fetal tissue may also be obtained but may be of limited value.

To diagnose a luteal phase defect, a timed endometrial biopsy should be obtained in two consecutive cycles. A histologic lag of 2 or more days is considered significant. Some practitioners obtain a midluteal serum progesterone, although the sensitivity is considered low by many. A serum progesterone above 10 ng/dL points to a low probability of an out-of-phase endometrial biopsy. These results should be read carefully as different pathologists may record varying results for biopsy dating and several studies have reported a histologic lag in endometrial tissue in women with no history of pregnancy loss.

To exclude anatomic abnormalities several studies may be performed. Begin with a good physical examination and imaging studies, including a hysterosalpingogram, pelvic ultrasound, computed tomography scan, or magnetic resonance imaging. In the operating room, an examination under anesthesia, hysteroscopy, and a diagnostic laparoscopy may be performed.

IV. **Treatment.** As mentioned earlier, as many as 50% of women will have no cause found for their RPL. For these patients, supportive measures are the best treatment. Cases in which a cause for RPL is diagnosed can often be treated.

A. When **genetic causes** for RPL are diagnosed, it becomes important to involve genetic counseling as part of any treatment plan. The rate of recurrence of miscarriage often will depend on the actual genetic abnormality discovered. Some couples with a known translocation or inversion can have a good pregnancy outcome. Others may need to turn to sperm or oocyte donation to avoid lethal abnormalities in their offspring. Details of donation can be found in Chap. 28.

B. Treatment for **anatomic abnormalities** often involves surgery. Hysteroscopic removal of uterine septa and synechiae has resulted in good pregnancy outcomes for many couples. Some physicians will also place an intrauterine device after resection of synechiae and place the patient on oral estrogen to help prevent reformation of adhesions. If surgery is decided on for uterine abnormalities, such as fibroids and unicornuate uterus, it should clearly be discussed with the couple that some studies have shown no difference in pregnancy outcome for patients treated surgically versus those treated with expectant management. Also, some women with anatomic abnormalities, even without treatment, have a fair to good rate of pregnancy success.

C. **Endocrine abnormalities** can often be treated with replacement therapy. Researchers are currently undecided whether phase deficiency will affect pregnancy outcome. Many studies have shown no benefit in treating luteal phase defects. However, some physicians use progesterone as either intravaginal suppositories (25 mg b.i.d. starting the third day after ovulation and continuing for 8 to 10 weeks), as i.m. injections, or orally administered micronized progesterone. It should be mentioned that as many as 60% to 70% of women diagnosed with a luteal phase deficiency will carry a viable infant with the next pregnancy. Other endocrine abnormalities, such as thyroid disorders and diabetes, should be corrected.

D. When an **infection** is diagnosed, the appropriate antibiotic therapy should be instituted. *Chlamydia* and gonorrhea can be treated with 1 g of azithromycin orally and 125 mg of ceftriaxone i.m., respectively. Infections with *Mycoplasma* and *Ureaplasma* are treated with doxycycline, 100 mg b.i.d. orally for 10 days. Clindamycin, 300 mg t.i.d. orally for 7 to 10 days, can be used for patients who are pregnant or allergic to doxycycline. Both partners should be treated to prevent reinfection.

E. **Environmental** factors should be addressed. Women who smoke or drink alcoholic beverages should be encouraged to abstain from these activities. If exposed to environmental toxins, individuals should try to eliminate or reduce exposure.

References

1. Patton PE. Anatomic uterine defects. *Clin Obstet Gynecol* 1994;37:705–721.
2. The American Fertility Society. *Guidelines for practice: recurrent pregnancy loss.* Birmingham, AL: The American Fertility Society, 1993.

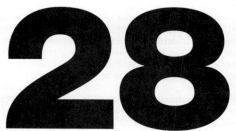

Infertility and Assisted Reproductive Technologies

Supriya Varma and
Endrika Hinton

I. Infertility

A. Incidence. In 1988, of all reproductive-age (15 to 44 years old), married couples in the United States, 8.4% (over 5 million couples) were infertile; 2.2 million had primary infertility, and 2.9 million had secondary infertility. Female age adversely impacts fertility; the rate of infertility is 7% in women ages 20 to 24 years and 29% in women ages 40 to 44 years.

B. Causes
  1. **Anovulation:** 10% to 15%
  2. **Pelvic factors:** 30% to 40%
  3. **Cervical factors:** 10% to 15%
  4. **Male factors:** 30% to 40%
  5. **Unexplained:** 10%

C. Evaluation. The initial assessment begins with an extended fertility history and examination, ideally with both partners present. Age, previous pregnancy, and menstrual, sexual, sexually transmitted disease, and infertility histories should be elicited. A sexual history includes the frequency and timing of intercourse, impotence, dyspareunia, and the use of lubricants. Ten percent of patients will have no identifiable cause of infertility. In normal sexually active couples, the fecundity rate (achieving pregnancy within one menstrual cycle) is 20% per month, so the importance of both timing and frequency should be stressed. The elements of a basic infertility evaluation include the following:

  1. **Semen analysis.** The sample should be collected after a 48-hour abstinence period and evaluated within 1 hour of ejaculation. If abnormalities are present, the patient should be referred to a urologist specializing in infertility to be evaluated for reversible causes of male-factor infertility. Normal parameters are as follows:
     a. **Volume** ≥ 1 mL
     b. **Concentration** ≥ 20 million spermatozoa/mL
     c. **Initial motility** $> 50\%$
     d. **Normal morphology** $> 60\%$

  2. The **basal body temperature (BBT) chart** is a simple means of determining whether ovulation has occurred. The woman's temperature is taken with a regular thermometer upon awakening, before any activity, and recorded daily on the standard graph. Progesterone rises after ovulation through a central thermogenic effect increases the basal temperature by approximately 0.6°F, creating a biphasic temperature curve.

  3. The **postcoital test (PCT/Huhner test)** allows direct analysis of sperm and cervical mucus interaction, and provides a rough estimate of sperm quality. When the male partner is unable to produce a specimen for routine semen analysis, this test may serve as rudimentary evaluation of the male factor. The test is scheduled in the periovulatory period (day 12 to 14) of a 28-day menstrual cycle. The couple is asked to have intercourse after 48 hours of sexual abstinence, and the mucus is examined within 2 to 8 hours. Although interpretation of the PCT is subjective, a finding

of 5 to 10 progressively motile spermatozoa per high-power field and clear acellular mucus with a spinnbarkeit of 8 cm generally excludes a cervical factor. The **causes of an abnormal PCT** include cervical stenosis, varicosities, hypoplastic endocervical canal, poor timing, and male factors.

4. The **hysterosalpingogram (HSG)** allows assessment of uterine and fallopian tube contour and tubal patency. It is performed in the early follicular phase, within 1 week of cessation of menstrual flow, to minimize the chances of interrupting a pregnancy. The procedure is performed by injecting a radio-opaque dye through the cervix and monitoring its progress through the reproductive tract to the peritoneal cavity. First, a small amount of dye (1 to 2 cc) is injected, to visualize the uterine cavity. Then more is injected, forcing a radio-opaque dye through the fallopian tubes and out into the peritoneal cavity. Fluoroscopic images are taken of the uterine cavity to demonstrate dye spill. Permanent radiographic films are made. Prophylactic antibiotics (e.g., doxycycline, 100 mg p.o. b.i.d.) are advisable when the patient has a history of pelvic inflammatory disease or when hydrosalpinges are identified during the study.

5. An **endometrial biopsy** evaluates the response of the endometrium to progesterone. A luteal phase defect (LPD), may result from inadequate estrogen priming or from progesterone secretion. The biopsy also documents ovulation; the endometrium can be dated within 2 to 3 days. To determine whether the biopsy is in phase, count back from the first day of the menses (considered day 28). The test is usually performed on day 22 to 24 of the menstrual cycle. The date of the biopsy and the subsequent period are used to determine whether an LPD is present. The **risks** of the procedure are minimal, but include infection, bleeding, interruption of pregnancy, and uterine perforation.

6. A **diagnostic laparoscopy** assesses peritoneal and tubal factors such as endometriosis and pelvic adhesions, as well as allowing corrective surgery. Laparoscopy should be scheduled in the follicular phase, as with HSG, and is the final step in the patient's evaluation, unless the HSG was suspicious for abnormalities. Instillation of dye through the fallopian tubes (chromotubation) should be performed to document tubal patency. The basic workup should be reviewed with the couple to discuss provisional diagnosis and treatment options. Hysteroscopy may also be included to ensure no subtle abnormalities were missed on the HSG.

D. **Treatment of anovulation.** Agents currently available for the management of anovulation include the following:

1. **Clomiphene citrate (CC)** is useful in women with oligomenorrhea and amenorrhea with intact hypothalamic-pituitary-ovarian axes. If the patient is anovulatory, CC is often used before diagnostic procedures continue. This synthetic, nonsteroidal estrogen agonist-antagonist increases the release of gonadotropin-releasing hormone (GnRH) and subsequent luteinizing hormone (LH) and follicle-stimulating hormone (FSH) release. It is usually given in a dose of 50 mg/day, beginning 5 days after the onset of spontaneous menses for a duration of 5 days. A sustained rise in BBT or an elevation in serum progesterone greater than 1.5 ng/mL, assayed 2 weeks after the last dose of CC, provides presumptive evidence of ovulation.

   a. **Most treatment regimens** start with 50 mg/day for 5 days. If ovulation fails to occur, the dose is increased to 100 mg/day. Human chorionic gonadotropin (hCG), 5,000 IU to 10,000 IU, may be used additionally to stimulate an LH surge. Eighty percent of couples will conceive in the first three cycles after treatment.

   b. **Potential side effects** are vasomotor flushes, blurring of vision, urticaria, pain, bloating, and multiple gestation (5%; usually twins).

2. **GnRH, human menopausal gonadotropin (hMG), FSH, and bromocriptine** are used primarily in women who fail to respond to CC or who have hypogonadotrophic amenorrhea, unexplained infertility or prolactin disorders. These agents are more expensive, and the regimens are more complicated for both the patient and the physician. Prescription of these drugs should be left to gynecologists trained in their use.

a. **GnRH** is used most successfully in patients with hypothalamic amen-orrhea. It is administered either i.v. or s.q., in a pulsatile fashion (60- to 90-minute pulses), by an infusion pump. This method of delivery mimics normal GnRH pulses. Successful ovulation rates are 75% to 85%, and cumulative pregnancy rates are 78% to 85%. The main advantage over hMG is decreased incidence of hyperstimulation syn-drome and multiple gestation.

b. **hMG** and **purified follicle-stimulating hormone** are useful in patients who do not achieve pregnancy with CC and patients with endometrio-sis or unexplained infertility. Ideally, the agents are administered after the entire infertility evaluation has been completed. Doses are given via i.m. injections over a 7- to 11-day period and result in ovarian hyperstimulation. A preparation for s.q. injection is also available (Fertinex). Follicle maturation is monitored using sonography and ser-ial estradiol levels. Once adequate follicle size (16 to 18 mm) is achieved, hCG is administered to induce ovulation. The major **risks** include ovarian hyperstimulation, multiple gestation (30%), and, arguably, potential ovarian malignancy.

c. **Bromocriptine** is used primarily to induce ovulation in patients with hyperprolactinemia; its use in euprolactinemic patients remains con-troversial. Bromocriptine is a dopamine agonist that directly inhibits pituitary secretion of prolactin, thereby restoring normal gonadotropin release. The usual starting dose is 2.5 mg q.h.s. This dosage is increased to 2.5 mg b.i.d. gradually, to prevent dopaminergic side effects, which include nausea, diarrhea, dizziness, and headache. If oral administra-tion cannot be tolerated, vaginal administration is recommended. A response is usually seen in 2 to 3 months, and in 80% of hyperpro-lactinemic patients, ovulation and pregnancy result. CC is added to the regimen if ovulation does not occur within 2 to 3 months after begin-ning treatment.

E. **Male factor infertility.** Although the gynecologist does not treat male patients directly, therapies to treat male factor infertility often involve hormonal manipulation in the female partner. Fortunately, the initiation of intracyto-plasmic sperm injection has revolutionized therapies for male infertility. As long as viable sperm can be retrieved by ejaculation, epididymal aspiration, or testicular biopsy, successful pregnancy can usually be achieved. Men with abnormal semen parameters should be evaluated by a urologist to ensure no correctable causes or medical conditions requiring attention are present.

F. **Endometriosis** occurs in 40% of infertile women; it is diagnosed and its stage determined by laparoscopy. The American Society of Reproductive Medicine has formulated a uniform system of classification that divides the disease into minimal, mild, moderate, and severe endometriosis. Endometriosis has a neg-ative impact on fertilization, and once diagnosed it should be treated med-ically or surgically before instituting infertility therapy. Treatment may include surgical fulguration or medical therapies such as GnRH agonists, danazol, and continuous oral contraceptive pills, all of which prevent preg-nancy. If fertility is desired, observation, hMG, or FSH may be employed in mild cases and *in vitro* fertilization (IVF) or gamete intrafallopian transfer in severe cases.

G. **Infections** of the female and male genital tracts have been implicated as causes of infertility. Chlamydia and gonorrhea are the major pathogens. How-ever, *Ureaplasma urealyticum* and *Mycoplasma hominis* have also been impli-cated. If *U. urealyticum* and *M. hominis* are identified by culture, the patient should be treated with doxycycline, 100 mg p.o. b.i.d. for 7 days. This has been shown to increase the pregnancy rate in patients with primary infertility.

H. **Tubal factor** infertility has increased with increased incidence of salpingitis. Tubal disease can be divided into proximal and distal disease.

1. **Proximal tubal obstruction** is identified on HSG. However, tubal spasm may mimic proximal obstruction, and obstruction should be confirmed by laparoscopy. Treatment consists of tubal cannulation, microsurgical tubocornual reanastomosis, or IVF.

2. **Distal tubal disease** or distortion can be seen on HSG and laparoscopy. The success of corrective surgery depends on the extent of disease. Contraindications to surgical reconstruction include absent rugal folds and thick, fixed tubal wall.

3. **Extent of tubal disease**
   a. **Mild.** Hydrosalpinx is narrower than 15 mm, with positive rugal pattern and no peritubal or periovarian adhesions. The pregnancy rate postneosalpingostomy is 80%.
   b. **Moderate.** Hydrosalpinx is 15 to 30 mm, with lack of rugal pattern and periovarian and peritubular adhesions without fixation. The pregnancy rate postneosalpingostomy is 31%.
   c. **Severe.** Hydrosalpinx is wider than 30 mm, with frozen pelvis, obliteration of the cul-de-sac, and no fimbria. The pregnancy rate postneosalpingostomy is 16%. Laparoscopic and open reconstructive surgery have similar success rates of approximately 25%.

II. **Assisted reproductive technologies.** The first child successfully conceived by IVF was born in the 1970s. Since then, the number of assisted-reproduction programs in the United States has increased to more than 200.
   A. **Definitions**
      1. **IVF** refers to extraction of oocytes followed by fertilization in the laboratory and transcervical transfer of embryos into the uterus.
      2. In **gamete intrafallopian transfer,** extraction of oocytes is followed by the transfer of gametes into the fallopian tube by laparoscopy.
      3. **Zygote intrafallopian transfer** refers to the placement of embryos into the fallopian tube after oocyte retrieval and fertilization.
      4. In **intracytoplasmic sperm injection of a single spermatozoon,** spermatozoa are injected into the oocytes, and the resulting embryos are transferred transcervically into the uterus.
   B. **Indications for IVF**
      1. **Tubal conditions** that indicate IVF are, primarily, large hydrosalpinges, absence of fimbria, severe adhesive disease, repeated ectopic pregnancies, or failed reconstructive surgical therapy.
      2. Stages I through IV of **endometriosis** are increasingly considered major indications for IVF. Stage III and stage IV disease are associated with significantly lower pregnancy rate, which is attributable to poor oocyte quality.
      3. **Unexplained infertility** applies to couples who have failed to conceive after 2 to 5 years of regular intercourse and in whom no definite abnormality can be detected.
      4. **Male factor infertility** is one of the major indications for IVF. IVF is necessary in men with sperm counts lower than 2 million/mL. Additional parameters, such as lowered sperm motility or abnormal morphology, are associated with further reduction in fertilizing ability.
   C. **Ovulation stimulation agents and protocols for IVF.** The agents most commonly used to stimulate multiple ovarian follicles are hMG and purified FSH.
   D. **Monitoring ovarian response**
      1. **Follicle number and size** are monitored with transvaginal sonography and estradiol levels.
      2. Once **optimal follicle size** is achieved, a single injection of hCG is given to induce final follicular maturation, after which ovulation will occur within 36 hours.
   E. **Oocyte retrieval, culture fertilization, and transfer**
      1. The two major **techniques of oocyte retrieval** are ultrasound-guided follicular puncture and laparoscopic oocyte retrieval. The former is the most widely used technique. Ultrasonically guided vaginal oocyte retrieval is performed 34 to 36 hours after hCG injection.
      2. **Oocyte fertilization.** Approximately 50,000 to 100,000 motile spermatozoa are added to each dish containing an oocyte. Fertilization is documented by the presence of two pronuclei. At that stage, most embryos are cryopreserved for an unlimited period, with a survival rate of 75%.

3. **Embryo transfer** is most commonly carried out 48 to 80 hours after retrieval at the four- to ten-cell stage. In general, no more than four to five embryos are transferred to limit the risk of multiple gestation and to optimize pregnancy rates. The actual number of embryos transferred depends on the individual's age and other risk factors for multiple pregnancy. It is common practice to supplement the luteal phase with progesterone by vaginal suppository, beginning the day of oocyte release and continuing into the twelfth week of pregnancy.

F. **Retrieval and pregnancy results**
1. Most programs have **delivery rates** of approximately 20% for women under the age of 40 years who are not affected by male factor infertility. The risk of ectopic pregnancies is 4% to 5%, and the risk of heterotopic pregnancies is 1%. Multiple gestation rate is approximately 30% (25% twins and 5% triplets).
2. The cumulative **pregnancy rates** are as follows:
   a. **One cycle:** 13%
   b. **Two cycles:** 25%
   c. **Three cycles:** 38%
   d. **Four cycles:** 47%
   e. **Five cycles:** 49%
   f. **Six cycles:** 58%

Selected Reading

Mosher WD, Pratt WF. Fecundity and infertility in the United States: incidence and trends. *Fertil Steril* 1991;56:192.

World Health Organization. *Laboratory manual for the examination of human semen and sperm—cervical interaction.* Cambridge, MA: Cambridge Univ. Press, 1992.

Adashi EY. Clomiphene citrate initiated ovulation: a clinical update. *Semin Reprod Endocrinol* 1986;4:255.

Padilla SI, Person GK, McDonough PG, Reindollar RH. The efficacy of bromocriptine in patients with ovulatory dysfunction and normoprolactinemic galactorrhea. *Fertil Steril* 1985;44:695.

Ho Yuen, Pride S. Induction of ovulation with exogenous gonadotropins in anovulatory infertile women. *Semin Reprod Endocrinol* 1990;8:1861.

Batzofin JG, Marrs RP, Serafini PC, et al. Assisted reproductive treatments for male factor infertility. *Probl Urol* 1987;1:430.

Kaupila A. Changing concepts of medical treatment of endometriosis. *Acta Obstet Gynecol Scand* 1993;72:324.

Olive DL, Schwartz LB. Endometriosis. *N Engl J Med* 1993;328:1759.

Mahadevan MM, Trouson AO, Leeton JF. The relationship of tubal blockage, infertility of unknown cause, suspected male infertility, and endometriosis to success of in vitro fertilization and embryo transfer. *Fertil Steril* 1983;40:755.

Jones HW Jr, et al. Three years of in vitro fertilization at Norfolk. *Fertil Steril* 1984;42:826.

Hurst BS, Schlaff WD. Andrologic parameters for in vitro fertilization and embryo transfer. In: Damewood MD, ed. *The Johns Hopkins handbook of IVF and ART.* Boston: Johns Hopkins University Press, 1990.

Trounson AO, Mohr LR, Wood C, Leeton JF. Effect of delayed insemination on in-vitro fertilization, culture and transfer of human embryos. *J Reprod Fertil* 1982;64:285–294.

Tarlatzis BC. Oocyte collection and quality. *Assist Reprod Rev* 1992;2:16.

Tan SL, et al. Cumulative conception and live birth after in-vitro fertilization. *Lancet* 1992;339:1390.

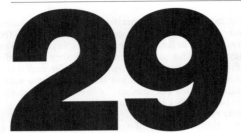

Amenorrhea

Greg Kaufman,
Laura Castleman, and
Howard A. Zacur

I. **Definition and epidemiology.** Amenorrhea is an absence of spontaneous menses during the reproductive years. Amenorrhea is physiologic during lactation and pregnancy.
   A. **Primary amenorrhea** refers to absence of menses in girls aged 16.5 years with secondary sex characteristics, or in girls aged 14 years without secondary sexual characteristics. Primary amenorrhea occurs in fewer than 0.1% to 2.5% of reproductive-age women.
   B. **Secondary amenorrhea** refers to absence of menses for 3 to 6 months or more in women who have previously menstruated. Prevalence rates of secondary amenorrhea in the general population have been reported to range between 1% and 5%.

II. **Clinical presentation**
   A. The **history** should include questions about the following:
      1. Pubertal milestones and menstrual history
      2. Abnormalities of growth and development
      3. Diet, exercise, or weight change
      4. Drug use (antipsychotics, hormonal contraceptives, antihypertensives, narcotics)
      5. Systemic disease, including hypothyroidism, adrenal insufficiency, growth hormone (GH) excess
      6. Previous surgery
      7. Galactorrhea, hirsutism
      8. Past gynecologic or obstetric problems (hemorrhage, dilatation and curettage, infection)
      9. Family history of genetic abnormalities
   B. The **physical examination** should include assessment of the following:
      1. Height and weight proportions (height of less than 60 inches suggests gonadal dysgenesis)
      2. Signs of **thyroid disease** [protuberant eyes, enlarged thyroid (most often hypothyroid), puffy face, thick tongue or lips, heat or cold intolerance]
      3. **Secondary sexual characteristics**
         a. **Thelarche** is breast development. Thelarche occurs, on average, at 10.8 years of age and indicates estrogen exposure.
         b. **Adrenarche** is reflected by pubic and axillary hair development. Adrenarche occurs, on average, at 11 years of age and indicates ovarian and adrenal androgen production and end-organ androgen response.
      4. **Decrease in breast size or vaginal dryness,** indicating decreasing estrogen exposure (or increasing androgen exposure; see Chap. 33)
      5. **Presence of a cervix,** which confirms the presence of a uterus

III. **Differential diagnosis and treatment.** Although gonadal failure is the most frequent cause of primary amenorrhea, anorexia nervosa is the most common cause of amenorrhea overall in teenagers. Uterovaginal agenesis is the second most common cause of primary amenorrhea. Of women with secondary amenorrhea who are not pregnant, 49% to 62% have hypothalamic disorders, including polycystic ovary (PCO), 7% to 16% have pituitary disorders, 10% have ovarian disorders, and 7% have Asherman's syndrome.

Table 29-1. Signs and symptoms of Turner's syndrome[a]

Sexual infantilism
Short stature
Webbed neck
Cubitus valgus (deviation of the elbow away from body midline on extension)
Shield chest with wide-set nipples
Pigmented nevi
Low-set ears
High-arched palate
Streak gonads

[a]Increased risk of skeletal, renal, and cardiac anomalies in one-third of cases

A. **Primary amenorrhea.** An easy way to approach the clinical diagnosis of primary amenorrhea is to separate patients into four categories (described in decreasing order of frequency).

1. **Secondary sexual characteristics absent, cervix present.** This category accounts for one-half of patients with primary amenorrhea. Affected patients are deficient in estrogen, either from failure of gonadal development or from a central defect.

a. **Primary ovarian disorders.** Defective or absent ovarian function with sex chromosome abnormalities causes gonadal dysgenesis. A primary ovarian disorder is the most common etiology of primary amenorrhea, accounting for 30% to 40% of patients. Affected patients present with elevated gonadotropin levels [follicle-stimulating hormone (FSH) levels greater than 40 mIU/mL], and usually have streak gonads. The genetic distribution is roughly as follows: 50%, 45,XO; 25%, mosaics; 25%, 46,XX. In individuals with a Y chromosome, a 20% incidence of dysgerminoma and gonadoblastoma exists; gonadectomy is recommended for affected patients. Development of secondary sex characteristics can be a symptom of steroid-producing tumors.

(1) **Turner's syndrome.** Gonadal dysgenesis associated with 45,XO is the most common chromosomal abnormality found in spontaneous abortions. Fewer than 0.3% of affected fetuses survive to term, for an incidence of 1 in 2,000 to 3,000 live births. The defect usually is not inherited. Affected individuals commonly may present with primary amenorrhea and short stature (Table 29-1). Workup includes a karyotype to confirm 46,X as a single cell line; mosaics that include the Y chromosome can appear clinically like Turner's syndrome but are treated as outlined in sec. III.A.1.a.(2). These patients have streak gonads.

(2) **Pure gonadal dysgenesis** comprises the karyotypes 46,XY (Swyer syndrome) and 46,XX. The disorder may be inherited. Patients present with primary amenorrhea, eunuchoid habitus, normal stature, and infantile internal and external female genitalia; one-third have major cardiovascular or renal abnormalities. Some patients with 46,XX may have a few ovarian follicles, develop breasts, or menstruate for several years; neurosensory deafness is common.

(3) **Chromosomal mosaics.** Individuals with the karyotypes X/XX, X/XXX, or X/XX/XXX have a low incidence of physical stigmata. Affected patients tend to be short and may undergo premature menopause; 20% have enough estrogen to menstruate. The clinical presentation of individuals with the karyotypes XO/XY, XO/XYY, or XO/XY/XYY ranges from a syndrome similar to that of typical gonadal dysgenesis to ambiguous genitalia to phenotypic maleness.

(4) **Structural abnormalities of the sex chromosome.** Patients with 46,XX can have a deletion of short-arm 46,XXp-. Their clinical presentation is similar to that of patients with Turner's syndrome. Other patients may have a deletion of long-arm 46,XXq-. Such individuals have primary amenorrhea, sexual infantilism, streak gonads, usually normal stature, and no somatic abnormalities.

b. **Central nervous system, hypothalamic, or pituitary failure.** Low gonadotropin and estradiol production may cause primary or secondary amenorrhea. Affected patients fail to bleed after progesterone challenge.

(1) **Anatomic lesions** of the hypothalamus or pituitary include tumors (adenoma, microadenoma, craniopharyngioma, germinoma, glioma, teratoma, endodermal sinus tumor); infectious lesions (tuberculosis, sarcoidosis, encephalitis, Hand-Schüller-Christian disease causing eosinophilic granulomas, hemosiderosis); lesions resulting from surgery, irradiation, or trauma; stenosis of the aqueduct of Sylvius; empty sella syndrome; and internal carotid artery aneurysms.

(2) **Kallmann's syndrome** is an inherited disorder characterized by the absence of gonadotropin-releasing hormone (GnRH) because of a lack of neurons originating from the olfactory bulb. The absence of GnRH results in an absence of FSH and luteinizing hormone (LH) secretion. Patients present with anosmia, cleft lip, and sometimes congenital deafness. Treatment consists of hormone replacement. Exogenous gonadotropins can induce ovulation.

(3) **Anorexia nervosa or bulimia.** Weight loss from extreme dieting or binging and purging represents a common cause of secondary amenorrhea among young women. Patients are often white, middle- to upper-class girls or women younger than 25 years, who present with hypothermia, hypotension, bradycardia, hyperkeratinemia, and constipation. Treatment primarily consists of psychiatric and medical support. Patients have normal to low gonadotropin secretion, which is thought to result from diminished GnRH secretion.

(4) **Exercise-induced amenorrhea** may be caused by suppression of GnRH release by elevated β-endorphin and catechol estrogens.

(5) **Constitutional delay of puberty,** a persistence of prepubertal hypothalamic suppression, is a diagnosis of exclusion. Initial treatment is reassurance, followed by hormone replacement therapy for bone growth and psychological development.

(6) **Hyperprolactinemia** interrupts gonadotropin secretion, probably by causing hypothalamic dysfunction.

c. **Endocrinopathies.** 17α-hydroxylase deficiency (46,XX) is a very rare cause of primary amenorrhea. In this condition, progesterone cannot be converted to cortisol, which results in decreased cortisol levels with elevated adrenocorticotropic hormone (ACTH), progesterone, and aldosterone. Affected patients also have decreased sex steroid levels. Patients present with sexual infantilism, hypertension, and hypokalemic alkalosis. Treatment involves estrogen and glucocorticoid replacement.

d. **General workup and treatment** for patients with absent secondary sexual characteristics and cervix present is as follows:

(1) **Measure FSH.** If the FSH level is greater than 40 mIU/mL and the patient is younger than 30 years, perform a peripheral white blood cell karyotype. If a Y chromosome is present, excise the gonads. If a 46,XX karyotype is present, measure electrolyte and serum progesterone levels to rule out 17α-hydroxylase deficiency (hyponatremia, hypokalemia, progesterone greater than 3 ng/mL, 17α-hydroxyprogesterone less than 0.2 ng/mL, and deoxycorti-

costerone greater than 17 ng/100 mL). Replace estrogen-progesterone to develop secondary sexual characteristics and prevent
osteoporosis and cardiac disease. If a 17α-hydroxylase deficiency
is detected, corticoids also must be replaced.

(2) If FSH is low, the patient has a central nervous system (CNS), hypothalamic, or pituitary deficit; **measure serum prolactin.** Regardless of the prolactin level, consider cranial computed tomography
or magnetic resonance imaging to rule out a tumor. Because all
affected individuals are 46,XX, performing a karyotype is unnecessary. Initially, administer estrogen-progesterone to foster secondary
sexual characteristics. GH can help patients with gonadal dysgenesis. Usually, GH treatment is administered in consultation with a
pediatric endocrinologist. To promote fertility, ovulation is induced
with human menopausal gonadotropins or pulsatile GnRH. For
patients with gonadal dysgenesis, donor eggs are required.

2. **Secondary sexual characteristics and cervix present.** Patients in this
category may present with primary or secondary amenorrhea. One-third
of affected patients with primary amenorrhea have breasts and a uterus;
one-fourth of these have hyperprolactinemia.

a. **CNS or hypothalamic causes**

(1) **Anatomic lesions,** listed in sec. **III.A.1.b.(1)** may appear with or
without secondary sexual characteristics.

(2) **Drugs affecting prolactin levels.** Prolactin stimulators include
anesthetics; psychotropics (phenothiazines, tricyclic antidepressants, opiates); hormones such as estrogen, oral contraceptive
preparations (effects should not last more than 6 months), and
thyrotropin-releasing hormone; antihypertensives (α-methyldopa,
reserpine); and antiemetics (sulpiride, metoclopramide). Prolactin
inhibitors include levodopa and dopamine. Many of these medications can also cause amenorrhea without significantly changing prolactin levels.

(3) **Stress, exercise, and eating disorders** are described in sec.
III.A.1.b.

(4) **Polycystic ovarian syndrome** is described in Chap. 33, sec. **IV.A.**

(5) **Functional hypothalamic amenorrhea.** Patients with functional
hypothalamic amenorrhea have dysfunctional LH pulsatility,
probably from an abnormality in GnRH pulsatility.

b. **Pituitary causes** are described in sec. **III.A.1.b.** The differential diagnosis for secondary amenorrhea also includes Sheehan's syndrome,
which results from obstetrical hemorrhage.

c. **Ovarian causes** should be considered if patients have elevated
gonadotropin and low estradiol levels.

(1) **Radiation and chemotherapy,** especially alkylating agents, can
injure ovaries, decreasing the number of oocytes. Unaffected
gonads have no increased risk of congenital anomalies.

(2) **Premature ovarian failure** is follicular depletion before age 40.
In 30% to 50% of cases, premature ovarian failure is associated
with autoimmune disorders such as Hashimoto's thyroiditis.

(3) **Ovarian resistance syndrome.** In patients with this syndrome,
primordial follicles fail to progress despite elevated gonadotropins.

(4) **Polycystic ovarian syndrome** is described in Chap. 33, sec. **IV.A.**

(5) **Infection, vascular injury, or cystectomy** also can deplete follicles and lead to amenorrhea.

d. **Uterine causes.** Patients with uterine disorders are the only group
with amenorrhea and present breasts and cervix who show normal
endocrinologic findings. Intrauterine adhesions can obliterate the
endometrial cavity, causing Asherman's syndrome. Usually, intrauterine adhesions result from previous endometrial curettage after pregnancy, although they can be caused by other surgical procedures as

well as by infection. Examination reveals difficulty in passing a sound into the uterine cavity. Hysteroscopy can best confirm the diagnosis.
  e. **Workup** of patients with primary amenorrhea in whom secondary sexual characteristics and cervix are present is the same as that for patients with secondary amenorrhea (see sec. **III.B.2**).
3. **Secondary sexual characteristics present, cervix absent**
  a. **Androgen insensitivity** (testicular feminization syndrome) is the third most common cause of primary amenorrhea. Affected patients are 46,XY and have an X-linked dominant or recessive trait that causes a testosterone receptor defect. Patients produce müllerian duct inhibitory factor and have normal-functioning testes with a complete absence of internal female genitalia. Affected patients have a blind vaginal pouch, abundant breast tissue, scant axillary and pubic hair, and normal external female genitalia. Androgen insensitivity results in an increased concentration of LH, probably because of a lack of feedback inhibition of the hypothalamic-pituitary axis. The increased LH and androgen levels causes affected patients' estradiol levels to be higher than those of normal men.
  b. **Müllerian anomalies or agenesis** (Mayer-Rokitansky-Küster-Hauser syndrome) affects a group of 46,XX patients and occurs in 1 in 4,000 to 5,000 female infants. The disorder is the second most frequent cause of primary amenorrhea, accounting for 15% of cases, and appears to be sporadic, not inherited. Affected patients have normal, functioning ovaries but only rudimentary uterine anlagen and no vaginas. Increased incidences of renal, skeletal, cardiac, and other congenital abnormalities are associated with müllerian anomalies.
  c. **Diagnosis and treatment**
    (1) Obtain karyotype and testosterone level.
    (2) Patients who have normal body hair and a normal female testosterone level have uterine agenesis. A karyotype should be obtained if uterine agenesis is suspected because this disorder's clinical appearance may resemble that of male pseudohermaphroditism. Individuals with uterine agenesis are sterile and have no need for hormonal supplementation. An i.v. pyelogram should be performed to rule out renal anomalies. Treatment may also include vaginal mechanical dilation or reconstruction.
    (3) Patients with androgen insensitivity usually have been raised as girls. After breast development and epiphyseal closure, the gonads should be removed and estrogen should be replaced. Testicular malignancy is extremely rare in affected patients younger than 20 years.
4. **Secondary sexual characteristics and cervix absent.** Patients in this category account for less than 1% of cases of primary amenorrhea. Affected patients are 46,XY but have an abnormality in testosterone synthesis. The production of müllerian inhibitory factor causes internal female organs to regress. The differential diagnosis includes 17α-hydroxylase deficiency (46,XY), 17,20-desmolase deficiency, and agonadism. Affected patients have elevated gonadotropin levels and low-normal female testosterone levels and require testicular removal and estrogen administration. Because these patients do not have a uterus, they do not require progesterone when given estrogen replacement therapy.
B. **Secondary amenorrhea** usually stems from problems in the CNS, but ovarian and uterine disorders may also occur.
  1. **Differential diagnosis.** The etiology of secondary amenorrhea is very similar to that of primary amenorrhea with present cervix and secondary sexual characteristics described in sec. **III.A.2**.
  2. **Workup**
    a. Rule out pregnancy and hyperprolactinemia.
    b. If the **prolactin level is elevated,** evaluate thyroid function with thyroid-stimulating hormone and free thyroxine. Primary hypothyroidism

may cause elevated thyroid-stimulating hormone and prolactin levels resulting in amenorrhea and galactorrhea.

  c. Measure FSH and LH levels.

    (1) If both LH and FSH are within the normal range as measured in mIU, the diagnostic categories of either hypothalamic dysfunction or functional ovarian hyperandrogenism (polycystic ovarian syndrome) are likely.

    (2) If the LH concentration is twice or more than twice that of the FSH concentration, PCO is the diagnosis.

    (3) If both the LH and the FSH concentrations are low normal, hypothalamic dysfunction is the diagnosis.

    (4) If both the LH and the FSH concentrations are elevated, ovarian failure is the diagnosis.

  d. Measure 17-hydroxylase (OH) progesterone and progesterone concentrations to rule out late-onset adrenal hyperplasia (LOAH).

    (1) If the 17-OH progesterone level exceeds 200 ng/dL and the patient has not ovulated (progesterone concentration is lower than 3 ng/mL), perform ACTH stimulation testing to diagnose LOAH.

    (2) A 17-OH progesterone concentration exceeding 1200 ng/dL occurring 30 minutes after i.v. administration of 0.25 mg synthetic ACTH (Cortrosyn) is diagnostic for LOAH.

  e. A **progesterone challenge test** (100 to 200 mg i.m. of progesterone in oil or medroxyprogesterone acetate, 10 mg p.o. qd for 10 days) is administered to induce uterine withdrawal bleeding. This will occur if the endometrial lining has been sufficiently exposed to estradiol (greater than 30 pg/nL). Failure to induce uterine bleeding by this test implies a low estrogen level, most likely due to a hypothalamic or pituitary problem or that the uterine lining has been scarred (Asherman's syndrome).

3. Treatment

  a. Dopamine agonist therapy (bromocriptine or cabergoline) may be given to hyperprolactinemic patients to normalize prolactin and restore cyclical ovulation and menses. This therapy is particularly useful if pregnancy is desired. Alternatively, depending on individual circumstances, these patients may be observed or given medroxyprogesterone acetate on a cyclical basis to induce withdrawal bleeding or given oral contraceptive pills if properly informed of the risks and benefits and monitored clinically.

  b. Women with PCO may be treated with combination oral contraceptive pills or cyclical medroxyprogesterone acetate to cause cyclical uterine withdrawal bleeding if pregnancy is not desired. Ovulation-inducing drugs (e.g., clomiphene citrate) may be provided if pregnancy is desired.

  c. For women with premature menopause or who have low estrogen levels (i.e., who fail to respond to a progesterone challenge test) due to a hypothalamic pituitary problem, estrogen replacement therapy may be provided.

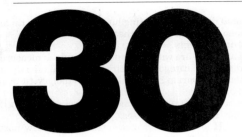

Pubertal Disorders

Marcela G. del Carmen
and John Murphy

I. **Precocious puberty.** Physically, the first sign of puberty may be either thelarche (breast development) or pubarche (pubic hair development). Average age at menarche is 12.7 years. Regardless of the time of onset of thelarche, the interval between breast development and menarche is 2.3±1.0 years. Bone age is a better marker for the onset of puberty than chronologic age. Puberty begins at a bone age of 11 years, whereas menses usually begin by bone age of 13 years. In North America, sexual precocity is defined as the appearance of any sign of secondary sexual characteristics at less than 8 years of age (more than 3.0 standard deviations below the mean).

A. **Complete isosexual precocity,** also known as *true* or *central precocious puberty,* is the result of premature activation of the pulsatile hypothalamic gonadotropin-releasing hormone (GnRH) mechanism. *Isosexual* refers to secondary sexual characteristics appropriate for the child's sex. Because the pituitary secretes luteinizing hormone (LH) and follicle-stimulating hormone (FSH), both breast and pubic hair development occur as a result of ovarian androgen stimulation.

1. **Idiopathic precocious puberty** may manifest in infancy and is more common in girls (age of onset is 6 to 7 years) than in boys. Inquiries about a family history of early maturation should be made because true precocious puberty may be transmitted in an autosomal recessive fashion, particularly in boys.

    a. **Physical findings** in girls include breast development and pubic hair, enlargement of the labia minora, and maturation of the vaginal mucosa. Usually, the progression of secondary sexual characteristics occurs more rapidly than in normal puberty. The child may experience a course of development that fluctuates between progression and regression. Some girls may experience spontaneous regression, while others may have persistence of secondary sexual characteristics.

    b. **Hormones.** The stimulation of gonadal steroids leads to an increased secretion of growth hormone (GH) and serum insulin-like growth factor–I, which in turn results in rapid growth. In milder cases, girls have a slower progression of bone age and maintain their target heights. Although ovulation may occur early in childhood, true precocious puberty does not result in premature menopause. Plasma concentrations of gonadotropin and gonadal steroids, the LH response to GnRH, and the LH pulse's frequency and amplitude are in the pubertal range.

2. **Central nervous system (CNS) tumors** that result in true precocious puberty are equally prevalent among boys and girls. Astrocytomas; ependymomas; optic or hypothalamic gliomas, which are often associated with neurofibromatosis; tuberous sclerosis; suprasellar cyst; sarcoid granuloma; postcranial radiation for leukemia or other tumors; and craniopharyngiomas may result in true precocious puberty.

    a. **Pathophysiology.** The mechanism that causes precocious puberty is hypothesized to be either a mass effect of the growth, which impinges on the pathway that inhibits the GnRH pump in childhood; or a result of the cranial radiation used for the treatment of the growth. Hamartomas of the tuber cinereum (not true neoplasms, but congenital midline spherical masses emerging from the third ventricle) have ectopic GnRH-secreting cells that mediate a pulsatile release of GnRH. These hamartomas may cause seizures, mental retardation, behavioral disturbances, headaches, visual changes, and dysmorphic syndromes.

  b. **Treatment.** The location of tumors leading to precocious puberty makes their surgical removal difficult. Management usually involves radiation, chemotherapy, or both. Hamartomas are slow-growing tumors and can be followed for change in size with computed tomographic (CT) scans or magnetic resonance imaging (MRI). Manifestations of precocious puberty can be treated with GnRH agonists.

3. **Other CNS disorders** such as hydrocephalus, encephalitis, brain abscess, static cerebral encephalopathy, sarcoid granulomas, hypothalamic tuberculous granulomas, and head trauma (associated with cerebral atrophy or focal encephalomalacia) can result in true precocious puberty. Arachnoid cysts, which emerge *de novo* as a consequence of infection, can cause precocious puberty (possibly with an associated GH deficiency). The propensity for patients with von Recklinghausen's disease (neurofibromatosis type 1) to develop CNS tumors may lead to precocious puberty.

4. **Congenital adrenal hyperplasia (CAH).** Patients with CAH who either have been undertreated or have started treatment late may undergo early puberty. Patients in whom CAH or virilizing tumors have been treated may develop precocious puberty after the lowering of androgen levels [if their skeletal age has reached 11 to 13 years (see sec. **III. A.1**)].

5. **Primary hypothyroidism** may result in premature breast development, which regresses after the initiation of thyroid hormone replacement. The absence of a growth spurt may help to establish hypothyroidism as the cause of premature development.

B. **Incomplete isosexual precocity,** also known as *pseudoprecocious puberty* or *GnRH-independent sexual precocity*, is characterized by extrapituitary secretion of gonadotropins or gonadal steroid secretion that is independent of GnRH pulsatile stimulation.

1. **Autonomous ovarian follicular cysts** are the most common form of estrogen-secreting masses in children. Large follicular cysts often manifest as abdominal pain or a mass, commonly after torsion or as an incidental finding on pelvic sonography. Plasma levels of estradiol may be elevated. Urine estrogen levels may also be in the early pubertal range. Exploratory laparotomy or laparoscopy is sometimes necessary to differentiate between these benign cysts and a possible malignant ovarian neoplasm. Removal or rupture of a hormonally active (estradiol-secreting) cyst may result in correction of the precocity, while intervention for a non–hormonally active cyst may have no effect. Autonomously secreting cysts are not associated with increased LH pulsatile secretion or with a pubertal response of LH to GnRH.

2. **Ovarian tumors** (2% to 5%) may cause precocious puberty. Approximately 60% of ovarian tumors causing precocious puberty are granuloma cell tumors; the remainder are arrhenoblastomas, thecomas, lipid cell tumors, and cysts. Only approximately 3% of patients with granuloma cell tumors die of their disease. Approximately 80% of these tumors can be palpated on bimanual exam and fewer than 5% are bilateral. While LH and FSH levels usually are suppressed in patients with ovarian tumors, their plasma concentration of estradiol is usually elevated. Sonography of the ovary facilitates the diagnosis. Subsequent to surgical removal of the tumor, measurements of plasma levels of estradiol may be used to screen for metastasis (in patients younger than 9 years, an elevated estradiol suggests recurrence or metastasis).

3. **Peutz-Jeghers syndrome** consists of mucocutaneous pigmentation and gastrointestinal polyposis and is also associated with a rare sex cord tumor. The tumor's estrogen secretion may result in feminization and incomplete sexual precocity. Although rare, epithelial tumors of the ovary, dysgerminomas, or Sertoli-Leydig cell tumors have been found in patients with Peutz-Jeghers syndrome. Girls with Peutz-Jeghers syndrome should be evaluated with serial pelvic sonography for the presence of gonadal tumors.

4. **McCune-Albright syndrome** is characterized by irregular hyperpigmented macules (café au lait spots), polyostotic fibrous dysplasia (progressive bone disorder), and GnRH-independent sexual precocity. At least two of these three features must be present to make the diagnosis of McCune-Albright syndrome. The bone disorder can involve any bone and may cause facial asymmetry or hyperostosis. Although the autonomous hyperfunction most commonly involves the ovary, the adrenals, the thyroid, the parathyroids, and the pituitary may also be involved. Because of factors secreted by the bone lesions, hypophosphatemic vitamin D–resistant rickets or osteomalacia may also be seen. With involvement of the skull, optic or auditory nerve compression resulting in blindness or deafness, facial asymmetry, or ptosis may be seen.

   a. **Pathophysiology.** Sexual precocity results from an autonomous luteinized follicular cyst. The ovaries are composed of multiple follicular cysts, among which one is often large or dominant. The response of LH to GnRH is prepubertal (nonpulsatile). The pubertal pattern of LH pulses is initially absent, but when the bone age approaches 12 years, the GnRH pulse mechanism is activated and ovulation is established, which results in a progression from GnRH-independent to GnRH-dependent puberty.

   b. **Treatment.** GnRH agonists are not effective therapy for this disorder. Aromatase inhibitors, such as medroxyprogesterone, have been shown to help.

5. **Adrenal disorders** such as adenomas can secrete estrogen alone and give rise to sexual precocity. Patients in whom CAH has been untreated may exhibit virilization as well as some breast development. Estrogen-secreting adrenal carcinomas may also produce other hormones that result in heterosexual precocity. See sec. III.A.1 for further details.

C. **Contrasexual precocity** results from increased androgen levels and leads to inappropriate virilization. In girls, virilization is an indicator of organic disease (with the exception of premature adrenarche).

1. **Congenital adrenal hyperplasia** is discussed in sec. III.A.1.

2. **Cushing's disease** that results from an adrenal carcinoma may manifest as growth failure with or without virilization, obesity, striae, and moon facies.

3. **Arrhenoblastoma** is the most common virilizing ovarian tumor. Even less frequently seen in children are lipoid cell tumors of the ovary and gonadoblastoma.

D. **Patient assessment** must include a careful history and physical examination.

1. **History.** Inquiries should be made about birth trauma, encephalitis, changes in personality, headaches, visual changes, seizures, abdominal pain, urinary or bowel changes, increased appetite, and use of medications or creams. In most cases, information about the age of onset of precocious puberty is not helpful in establishing a diagnosis. Also, the age of pubertal onset in the patient's mother, sisters, and grandmothers should be ascertained. Vaginal bleeding is often the first symptom of McCune-Albright syndrome. Patients with true precocity and incomplete isosexual precocity may present with a history of irregular bleeding. Any family history of neurofibromatosis and tuberous sclerosis should be noted. The child's growth pattern should be recorded in a chart because accelerated growth and bone age may help to distinguish between premature thelarche and true precocious puberty (a growth spurt correlates with the onset of precocious puberty).

2. **Physical examination.** On examination, evidence of papilledema, visual field defects, or café au lait spots should be sought. The child's head circumference should be measured and recorded. Note the size and texture of the thyroid gland, and inquire about any hair or skin changes. Closely inspect the breasts and external genitalia, and note the degree of breast, pubic, and axillary hair growth and the appearance of the vaginal mucosa. Ovarian masses are often easily palpated, and ultrasonography may be helpful because patients with true precocity often have slightly enlarged ovaries with multiple follicle cysts. In girls with McCune-Albright syndrome, a simple ovarian cyst may be seen with ultrasound.

3. **Laboratory testing** depends on the initial evaluation. An extensive workup is indicated in the presence of vaginal estrogenization and acceleration of linear growth. If premature thelarche is found, however, an x-ray film of the wrist to document bone age and a vaginal smear for estrogen effect are indicated. A skeletal survey is indicated for patients in whom the McCune-Albright syndrome is suspected. Bone lesions may be detected by bone scan before they are apparent radiographically. As chronologic age approaches 6 years, however, the GnRH pulse generator is established and ovulatory cycles ensue. A CT scan or MRI is often helpful in diagnosing CNS abnormalities such as hamartomas of the hypothalamus.

   a. **Baseline values.** Between 1 and 2 years of age, LH levels range from 0.6 to 1.3 ng/mL and FSH ranges from 1.9 to 3.2 ng/mL, and dehydroepiandrosterone sulfate (DHEA-S) levels are usually less than 50 ng/mL. Plasma estradiol levels are between 11 and 18 pg/mL (40 to 60 pmol/L). From 3 to 4 years of age, LH ranges from 1.1 to 2.0 mIU/mL, and FSH from 1.0 to 1.7 mIU/mL, with estradiol ranging from 14 to 26 pg/ml (51 to 95 pmol/L). At age 6, usual ranges of LH are observed to be between 1.1 and 4.3 mIU/mL, FSH between 1.0 and 2.0 mIU/mL, and estradiol levels are usually 20 pg/mL (73 pmol/L).

   b. **GnRH stimulation.** True precocity, gonadotropin-independent precocity, and premature thelarche may be differentiated with a GnRH stimulation test. After 150 μg GnRH is administered i.v., blood is drawn at 15-minute intervals. The pubertal response, seen in patients with normal pituitary function, is a rise in plasma LH to a peak of about 50 mIU/mL at 15 to 30 minutes. Patients with pituitary insufficiency show a diminished (prepubertal) response to GnRH. In patients with gonadotropin-independent precocity, ovarian tumors, or premature thelarche, a prepubertal response to the GnRH test can be expected.

   c. **Findings.** In patients with precocious puberty, bone age is greater than height age. Both gonadotropin and gonadal steroid concentrations in the plasma, as well as the LH response to GnRH and the frequency and amplitude of LH pulses, are in the normal pubertal range. In fact, although affected children may initially be tall, they have a short final height as a result of early epiphyseal closure. LH and FSH levels, associated with the sleep cycle in early puberty, may not be of significant diagnostic value if obtained during the daytime. In the early stages of true precocity, low daytime levels of gonadotropins may be found. High estradiol (100 to 200 pg/mL) and low gonadotropin levels indicate an estrogen-secreting cyst or tumor. High LH levels may signal a gonadotropin-producing tumor or choriocarcinoma [which secretes human chorionic gonadotropin (hCG) and cross-reacts with LH on the standard assay]. A urine or serum pregnancy test would detect such a rise in hCG. Elevated LH alone does not lead to isosexual precocity in the absence of increased estrogen secretion. In true precocity, nocturnal pulses of LH and FSH are evident. Affected patients show a pubertal response to the GnRH test. Most patients with precocious puberty have an age-appropriate response to DHEA-S. An estrogen excess (higher than 40% superficial cells) on vaginal smear suggests an estrogen-secreting granuloma cell tumor. It is crucial to determine the date of the last menstrual period in studying a vaginal smear. Elevated estradiol levels are seen in 50% of patients with theca-granulosa cell tumors. In the luteal phase of isosexual precocity and in ovarian thecomas, increased levels of serum progesterone and urinary pregnanediol are evident.

E. **Treatment** varies according to the diagnosis. Ovarian tumors require surgical removal. Ovarian cysts may spontaneously regress or may require aspiration. In cases of recurrent cysts, cystectomy may be indicated. In patients with McCune-Albright syndrome, treatment of an ovarian cyst will fail to produce a regression of puberty. In central precocity, ovarian cysts should be observed because gonadotropin suppression is likely to result in their regression. GnRH agonists have been shown to suppress precocious puberty by selectively and reversibly suppressing LH and FSH, restoring estradiol to its prepubertal level, and mediating the regression (or preventing progression) of breast development and the cessation of menses. GnRH-agonist therapy is also effective for treating patients with precocity secondary to hypothalamic hamartomas and optic nerve gliomas (associated with neurofibromatosis). Patients with sexual precocity may manifest mood swings, impulsivity, and aggressiveness, all of which are ameliorated by GnRH therapy. It is important to inform patients that their development is *early*, not *abnormal*. GnRH agonists will not lead to a decrease in estradiol levels or regression of puberty in girls with the following disorders: McCune-Albright syndrome, gonadotropin-independent puberty, and cyclic gonadal steroid production.

F. **Follow-up** depends on the diagnosis. Patients undergoing treatment with GnRH agonists require close monitoring of bone age, vaginal cytology (for maturation index), physical examination findings, and growth records. Incomplete estrogen suppression by GnRH may lead to a further decrease in final height. If growth rate and bone age correlate and the vaginal smear is unestrogenized, the patient can be followed by her primary care physician at 3-month intervals to assess progression of sexual development. A pediatric endocrinologist should be consulted in cases of accelerated growth rate, advanced bone age, and vaginal estrogenization. Patients whose onset of puberty occurs after age 6 and whose prognosis for adult stature is favorable without intervention may require only careful follow-up, reassurance, and counseling. Medroxyprogesterone (Depo-Provera) may be used to induce cessation of menses.

II. **Thelarche** is unilateral or bilateral breast development. Without other signs of sexual maturation, early breast development is referred to as *premature thelarche*. It commonly occurs by age 2 and is rare after age 4. Usually a regression of the breast enlargement occurs after a few months. It may persist, however, for several years or until the onset of puberty. In about 50% of patients, breast development lasts 3 to 5 years. Nipple development is usually absent. In general, affected patients have bilateral breast bud enlargement to about 2 to 4 cm without nipple or areolar changes. Statural growth is normal. Premature thelarche may often be unilateral, and sonography of the ovaries may be required to rule out malignant conditions. Plasma estrogen levels may be elevated, and a urocystogram may demonstrate an estrogen effect on squamous epithelial cells in the urine. In affected patients, FSH serum concentrations may be in the pubertal range, with an FSH to LH ratio that is higher than in normal individuals or in girls with central precocious puberty. The LH response to GnRH is prepubertal. Ovarian sonography often reveals one or several cysts that appear and disappear with changes in the size of the breasts. The uterus, however, remains prepubertal in size.

A. **Patient assessment** includes a review of medications or creams used recently. Application of topical conjugated estrogens (Premarin) for longer than 2 to 3 weeks may result in breast changes. On examination, the appearance of the vaginal mucosa, breast size, and presence of a pelvic mass on rectal examination should be noted. The uterus should not be enlarged, and growth charts should document a rate within the previously established percentile for height and weight. A vaginal smear or urocystogram to assess estrogenization and a pelvic ultrasound study should be obtained.

B. **Treatment** is directed toward reassurance and follow-up to confirm that the-larche is not the first manifestation of precocious puberty. A careful and complete physical examination, as well as linear growth and bone age measurements, should be obtained at each visit. Breast biopsy is usually contraindicated because breast bud removal may impair future normal development. It is important to reassure the patient and her parents that, in most cases, pubertal development ensues at a normal, adolescent age.

III. **Ambiguous genitalia** must be evaluated with a careful history, physical examination, and laboratory tests. Based on the karyotype, two groups of patients with ambiguous genitalia can be distinguished: XX neonates and XY neonates. Patient assessment must include measurement of the stretched phallus from the pubis to the tip, with attention to the location of the urethra (perineal versus penile), the degree of labial-scrotal fold fusion, and the presence or absence of gonads in the scrotum or inguinal rings. A digital rectal examination may reveal the presence of a cervix (usually easily palpable at birth secondary to stimulation by placental estrogen *in utero*). In female infants, an anogenital ratio (anus to fourchette or anus to base of clitoris) greater than 0.5 may indicate labioscrotal fusion.

A. **The XX neonate**

1. **Congenital adrenal hyperplasia** results from the excessive production of adrenal androgens caused by increased levels of adrenocorticotropin hormone (ACTH). Sustained levels of ACTH cause overstimulation of the adrenals and overproduction of adrenal androgens, resulting in virilization. These disorders are autosomal recessive and manifest as varying degrees of virilization, depending on the degree of enzymatic block.

   a. **Etiology.** The most common cause of CAH (95%) is 21-hydroxylase deficiency, in which decreased aldosterone secretion may result in only virilization or salt-losing hyponatremia, or may produce hyperkalemia and shock if severe. Virilization is the result of 17-hydroxyprogesterone (an androgen precursor) production, which leads to excess secretion of adrenal androgens.

   b. **Diagnosis.** Patient assessment may reveal clitoromegaly, postvaginal fusion with wrinkling or pigmentation of the scrotal sac, and absence of a proper vesicovaginal septum (which results in a urogenital sinus). A genetic female may show a penile urethra as well as fully male external genital phenotype, with the exception of testes. The salt-losing form of CAH usually is associated with more severe virilization. A male neonate may be discharged before the diagnosis is made, before the onset of the life-threatening hyponatremia that can result in shock and death. Virilized female neonates who do not manifest salt loss may go undiagnosed for years, until hyponatremia and shock occur when they are stressed, or until pubic hair, lower voice, abnormal muscular hyperplasia, or excessive growth develops within the first year of life. Unlike children with central precocious puberty, male patients with CAH have prepubertal testes (smaller than 2.5 cm) and female patients exhibit a rather severe degree of virilization. The diagnosis of 21-hydroxylase deficiency should be considered in any child with ambiguous genitalia in the absence of palpable testes; a phenotypic male without palpable testes; a male child with ambiguous genitalia and a history of severe vomiting, hypoglycemia, and shock; and a boy with premature virilization (or a girl, at any age, with any degree of virilization).

2. **Female pseudohermaphroditism** is defined as the presence of normally developed ovaries and müllerian structures with ambiguous external genitalia. *In utero*, the external genitalia feminize in the absence of testes. Therefore, a female fetus exhibits masculinization if exposed to androgens. Exposure to androgens after 12 weeks' gestation, after separation of the vagina and the urogenital sinus, results in clitoral hypertrophy. Earlier exposure leads to retention of the urogenital sinus and labioscrotal fusion; a penile urethra from labial fusion forms if exposure occurs early enough in differentiation. The uterus and the fallopian tubes are normal, even with severe masculinization, because regression of the mül-

lerian duct requires anti-müllerian hormone, formally referred to as *müllerian inhibiting factor*, secretion by the fetal testes, an event that is not mimicked by androgens. Occasionally, ambiguous external genitalia may be a consequence of non-androgen–induced disturbances in differentiation such as an anterior abdominal wall defect.

B. **True hermaphroditism** must include evidence of both ovarian and testicular tissue in either the same or the opposite gonad. The presence of gonadal stroma in the absence of oocytes is insufficient to designate the rudimentary gonad as an ovary. Evidence of a few oocytes in a streak gonad accompanying testicular tissue on the contralateral side is also insufficient to make this diagnosis.

   a. **Physical findings** may reveal evidence of either female or male external genitalia, often ambiguous. As a result of the size of the phallus, 75% of affected children are raised as males. Hypospadias is common, with a penile urethra seen in some cases. The patient may present with cryptorchidism and an inguinal hernia that may contain a uterus (seen in most cases) or gonad. Regardless of the external genitalia, the ipsilateral genital duct will develop in a fashion that is consistent with the gonad. In patients with an ovotestis, the genital duct usually develops in a female fashion. Breast development is seen in puberty, with menses developing in approximately 50% of patients. Although spermatogenesis is rare, ovulation often occurs; pregnancy and childbirth have been reported in patients with a 46,XX karyotype. In an ovotestis, ovarian function is often normal, with a normal cyclic pattern of FSH and LH production. Testicular function is usually abnormal.

   b. **Diagnosis.** True hermaphroditism must be considered in any patient with ambiguous genitalia. Approximately 70% of patients are X chromatin–positive. Approximately 60% are 46,XX, 12% are 46,XY, and 13% have a 46,XX/46,XY karyotype. A 46,XX/XY karyotype in conjuction with ambiguous genitalia is a strong indicator of true hermaphroditism, although the presence of a 46,XX or 46,XY karyotype does not rule it out. After all forms of pseudohermaphroditism have been excluded, the diagnosis of true hermaphroditism can be established with histologic evidence of both ovarian and testicular tissue.

   c. **Treatment** is based on the patient's age at diagnosis and on evaluation of the internal and external genitalia. In infants without an established gender identity, either a female or a male assignment can be made. From a 46,XX patient assigned a male gender, all müllerian and ovarian structures should be removed. The testis or testicular tissue in an ovotestis has an increased risk of malignant transformation. 46,XX true hermaphrodites raised as boys should undergo gonadectomy, prosthetic testes implants, and hormonal replacement at puberty. In the case of a 46,XX/46,XY chimera or a 46,XY true hermaphrodite with a testis on one side and a contralateral ovary and adequate phallus size, an attempt should be made to retain a histologically unremarkable testis in the scrotum and raise the patient as a boy. In such cases, the risk of malignancy may be higher than in normal patients. True hermaphrodites raised as girls must undergo removal of all testicular tissue. The risk of neoplastic transformation in retained ovarian tissue in such patients remains unclear. In older patients, gender identity assignment should be consistent with the sex of rearing. All dysgenetic and discordant tissue must be removed, with plastic repair of the external genitalia. Gonadal hormone treatment is recommended at puberty.

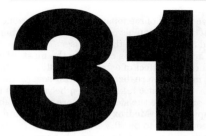

Menopause and Hormone-Replacement Therapy

Samuel Del Rio and
Edward E. Wallach

I. **Menopause** occurs after a woman's last spontaneous menstrual period. The **climacteric** is the entire transition from the reproductive to the postreproductive era of a woman's life. Menopause is only one of several events that occur during the climacteric.

A. **Age at menopause.** The median age of women at menopause is 51.3 years, although age at menopause ranges from 48 to 55 years. No correlation exists between age of menarche and age of menopause.

1. Only current smoking can be identified as a cause of **early menopause,** resulting in an advance in occurrence of approximately 1.5 years.

2. In contrast, **premature ovarian failure** is defined as the cessation of ovarian function in women younger than 40 years. Premature ovarian failure is characterized by secondary amenorrhea with elevated levels of follicle-stimulating hormone (FSH), luteinizing hormone (LH), or both. Ovarian failure may be induced by exposure to external irradiation or cytotoxic chemotherapy. Ovarian function may be terminated by viral infection or surgery. In a large percentage of cases, the cause of the failure is unknown; these cases are referred to as *idiopathic ovarian failure.*

B. **Etiology and diagnosis**

1. **Endocrinology.** Reduction in ovarian function during the climacteric is associated with the cessation of ovulation and a decline in ovarian estrogen and androgen production. Because of the decreased estrogen production, levels of FSH rise. The ovary contains its greatest number of oocytes at around the fifth month of gestation when about 7 million oocytes are present. At birth, the number of oocytes is estimated at about 1 to 2 million, and by menarche this number falls to 400,000. By the time of menopause, only a few hundred or thousand oocytes remain in the ovary.

2. **Testing.** When any doubt exists about the diagnosis of menopause, other causes of secondary amenorrhea must be ruled out. Laboratory studies should include a serum pregnancy test, serum prolactin level to rule out a prolactin-producing pituitary tumor, and serum FSH level. The best time to measure serum FSH is during days 2 to 4 of a normal menstrual period. Ideally, FSH is measured twice, 2 weeks apart, to avoid a mid-cycle FSH peak. An elevation in FSH level to 15 to 20 mIU/mL is associated with early ovarian failure. For perimenopausal women on oral contraceptives, FSH is measured late in the pill-free week. When the serum FSH exceeds 40 mIU/mL, the patient can be switched to hormone-replacement therapy (HRT).

3. **Workup** should include evaluation of liver function, breast examination, mammography if the patient is older than 50 years or if otherwise indicated, and pelvic examination, Pap smear, endometrial sampling if indicated by abnormal bleeding, and blood pressure and weight measurement.

C. **Signs and symptoms**

1. **Vasomotor instability** causes the hot flash, characterized by a sudden reddening of the skin over the head, neck, and chest, accompanied by a feeling of intense body heat and concluding with profuse perspiration.

a. Incidence. Seventy-five percent of menopausal women experience hot flashes. Eighty percent of those who have hot flashes endure them for longer than 1 year and 50% for longer than 5 years.

b. Treatment. Estrogen administration is currently the most effective treatment for hot flashes. The effect of estrogen usually is not immediate. The full benefit may not be realized until after several months of therapy. For women who cannot take estrogen because it is medically contraindicated or because the side effects are unacceptable, a few alternative therapies exist. Medroxyprogesterone acetate, 150 mg/month i.m., has been shown to be 90% effective in the treatment of hot flashes. Clonidine (0.05 to 0.15 mg/day), propranolol (60 mg/day), and belladonna alkaloids (Bellergal) also have been shown to be somewhat effective in the treatment of hot flashes.

2. Urogenital atrophy. The vagina, vulva, urethra, and trigone of the bladder all contain large numbers of estrogen receptors, and all of these structures undergo atrophy when estrogen levels are reduced during menopause.

a. Vulvar and vaginal effects. The atrophic vulva loses most of its collagen, adipose tissue, and water-retaining ability and becomes flattened and thin. Sebaceous glands remain intact, but secretions decrease. Vaginal shortening and narrowing occur, and the vaginal walls become thin, lose elasticity, and become pale in color. The atrophic vagina secretes less, causing vaginal dryness. Dyspareunia is the most common complaint related to vaginal atrophy. As for hot flashes, the mainstay of therapy is systemic or local estrogen.

b. The effect of estrogen deficiency on the urethra and bladder is associated with **urethral syndrome,** which is characterized by recurrent episodes of urinary frequency and urgency with dysuria. Estrogen relieves urgency, urge incontinence, and dysuria and may protect against recurrent lower urinary tract infections. Estrogen does not, however, improve stress incontinence.

3. Irregular uterine bleeding. Because of the changing hormonal milieu, complaints of irregular bleeding are very common during the climacteric. If an episode of bleeding occurs more often than 21 days, lasts longer than 8 days, is very heavy, or occurs after a 6-month interval of amenorrhea, particularly if such bleeding occurs in an irregular pattern, then an evaluation must be undertaken to rule out neoplasm (see Chap. 32, sec. **III**).

4. Osteoporosis describes a condition of diminishing bone mass and subsequent skeletal fractures. *Osteoporosis* is defined as a fall in bone mass of more than 2.5 standard deviations (SDs) below the mean for young adults. The spine (vertebral crush fractures), hip (femoral neck and intertrochanteric fractures), and wrist (Colles' fractures) are very common sites of fractures associated with osteoporosis. For each reduction in bone mass of 1 SD, the risk of fracture doubles. The four most widely used methods for assessing bone density are single-photon absorptiometry, dual-photon absorptiometry, dual-energy x-ray absorptiometry, and quantitative computed tomography.

a. Pathophysiology. Menopausal osteoporosis is primarily a result of a dominance of osteoclastic activity. Estrogen deficiency causes an increased rate of skeletal remodeling, with an increase in resorption that is greater than the increase in bone formation.

b. Risk factors associated with osteoporosis include female gender, white or Asian race, family history of osteoporosis, early menopause (natural or surgical), sedentary lifestyle, low weight for height, tobacco and alcohol use, and low calcium intake.

c. Treatment

(1) Estrogen is the best studied agent for prevention of postmenopausal osteoporosis and has U.S. Food and Drug Administration (FDA) approval. Case-control studies have demonstrated that HRT for at least 6 years reduces the risk of hip fractures and Colles' fractures by 50%. Cohort studies have also shown that long-term HRT reduces the incidence of vertebral deformities in postmenopausal women by about 90%. If HRT is stopped, the risk for fracture of the hip may return to near baseline 6 or more years after cessation of treatment.

(2) **Bisphosphonates** are a new class of drugs analogous to the physiologically occurring inorganic pyrophosphates. Bisphosphonates are resorption inhibitors. **Alendronate** (Fosamax), 10 mg/day, may be used in postmenopausal women for the treatment of osteoporosis. Daily treatment with oral alendronate progressively increases the bone mass of the spine, hip, and total body and reduces the risk of vertebral fractures, the progression of vertebral deformities, and height loss in postmenopausal women with osteoporosis.

(3) **Calcitonin,** a polypeptide hormone, inhibits bone resorption by a direct inhibitory action on the activity of osteoclasts and is approved by the FDA for the treatment of osteoporosis. Because calcitonin is degraded when taken orally, a parenteral route must be used. A nasal form, nasal salmon calcitonin (Miacalcin) has been used effectively in the treatment of postmenopausal osteoporosis. Calcitonin, in both injectable and nasal spray preparations, is also effective in preventing early postmenopausal bone loss. Dietary supplementation with vitamin D (400 to 800 IU/day) and calcium (800 to 1,000 mg/day) is recommended.

II. **Benefits and risks of hormone-replacement therapy**
   A. **Atherosclerosis and cardiovascular disease (CVD).** CVD is the leading cause of death in women. One in three women dies from CVD. In contrast, one in nine women develops breast cancer. Many studies indicate that for women on estrogen replacement therapy, the risk of heart disease is reduced by about 50%. In one report, the use of estrogen was associated with a 12% to 19% decrease in serum levels of unfavorable low-density lipoprotein cholesterol and a 9% to 13% increase in favorable high-density lipoprotein cholesterol (1). These effects occur with both oral and nonoral ethinyl estradiol, and with oral, but not vaginal, conjugated estrogens. The transdermal patch has not been shown to have the same beneficial effect on lipids as other routes of delivery. One study demonstrated that long-term use of postmenopausal estrogen (mean length of estrogen use was 17.1 years) was associated with reduced overall mortality risk (2). This risk reduction occurred primarily through a reduction in cardiovascular-related deaths.

   B. **Malignancy.** For a woman who is 50 years old, the lifetime risk of developing endometrial cancer is approximately 2.5%, and the risk of dying from endometrial cancer is less than 1%. It is well established that estrogen therapy without concomitant progestogen is associated with endometrial hyperplasia and an increased risk of endometrial cancer. Adding a progestogen to estrogen replacement therapy significantly reduces the risk of endometrial disease associated with unopposed estrogen. The duration of progestogen administration per cycle is very important; at least 12 days each month of progestogen administration are required to forestall the development of endometrial abnormalities.

   C. **Contraindications** to HRT include pregnancy, estrogen-dependent neoplasms, distant or recent history of breast cancer, recent endometrial cancer, undiagnosed vaginal bleeding, acute vascular thrombosis or emboli, and severe liver disease.

      1. After undiagnosed vaginal bleeding, acute vascular thrombosis or emboli, or acute liver disease has resolved, HRT may be prescribed. After liver or thromboembolic disease, a nonoral route of HRT administration may be preferable to an oral route because transdermally administered estrogen has no effect on hepatic protein synthesis, particularly of clotting factors.

      2. As do postmenopausal women with breast cancer, many women suffer the effects of estrogen deficiency after treatment for endometrial cancer. Because of the theoretical risk that dormant cancer cells may be activated

by HRT, however, women traditionally have not been offered HRT after treatment for endometrial cancer. Many experts believe that for women with a history of endometrial cancer, the proven risks of long-term estrogen deficiency far outweigh the presumed risks of taking estrogen, and reports suggest that HRT can be prescribed safely after treatment for endometrial cancer (3).

3. A history of ovarian or cervical cancer is not a contraindication to HRT. Similarly, the presence of known cardiovascular disease, diabetes, or hypertension is not a contraindication to HRT. On the contrary, the presence of risk factors for vascular disease is becoming an indication for HRT.

References

1. Miller VT, Muesing RA, LaRosa JC, Stoy DB, Phillips EA, Stillman RJ. Effects of conjugated equine estrogen with and without three different progestogens on lipoproteins, high-density lipoprotein subfractions, and apdipoprote in A-I. *Obstet Gynecol* 1991;77:235–240.
2. Ettinger B, Friedman GD, Bush T, Quesenberry CP Jr. Reduced mortality associated with long-term postmenopausal estrogen therapy. *Obstet Gynecol* 1996;87:6–12.
3. Creasman WT, Henderson D, Hinshaw W, Clarke-Pearson DL. Estrogen replacement therapy in the patient treated for endometrial cancer. *Obstet Gynecol* 1986;67:326–330.

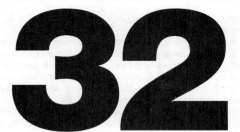

Abnormal Uterine Bleeding

Ralph Zipper and
Edward E. Wallach

I. **Physiology of the normal menstrual cycle.** In the early follicular phase, follicle-stimulating hormone (FSH) increases, leading to estradiol secretion. With increased estradiol levels, FSH levels fall. The dominant follicle, however, continues to secrete estradiol. Luteinizing hormone's (LH) responsiveness to gonadotropin-releasing hormone (GnRH) is selectively amplified by estradiol levels until, finally, plasma estradiol levels of 200 to 300 pg/mL initiate the mid-cycle gonadotropin surge. The surge is also facilitated by progesterone that is produced by ovarian granulosa cells. After ovulation occurs, estradiol levels decrease, and plasma progesterone levels rise with the formation of the corpus luteum. In the absence of increased human chorionic gonadotropin (hCG) from a conceptus, the corpus luteum involutes, and progesterone and estradiol levels fall off again before the next cycle begins.

II. **Etiology and pathophysiology of dysfunctional uterine bleeding.** Abnormal uterine bleeding is the second most common complaint evaluated by gynecologists, after vaginal infection. Although normal menstrual bleeding is defined as cyclic menstruation every 22 to 34 days that lasts fewer than seven days, for practical purposes, any patient who complains of passage of clots or a change in menstrual pattern may be considered to have abnormal uterine bleeding. Because patients have different thresholds for changing pads and tampons, and because they have differing absorbencies, pad and tampon counts are an unreliable method of quantifying blood loss. Furthermore, although abnormal uterine bleeding is the most common cause of anemia in women younger than 40 years, the majority of affected patients are not anemic, and thus hemoglobin levels are no more reliable than pad and tampon counts in diagnosing abnormal uterine bleeding. The diagnosis must be based on the subjective complaints of the patient. The evaluation of abnormal uterine bleeding should be guided by patients' individual risks for specific underlying abnormalities, and identical abnormalities may require different treatments in different patient populations.

A. **Definitions**
   1. **Polymenorrhea** is uterine bleeding at intervals of fewer than 22 days.
   2. **Oligomenorrhea** is uterine bleeding at intervals of more than 34 days.
   3. **Hypermenorrhea (menorrhagia)** is menses lasting longer than 6 days.
   4. **Metrorrhagia** is bleeding at irregular intervals.
   5. **Menometrorrhagia** (polymenorrhea-hypermenorrhea) is heavy, irregular bleeding.
   6. **Intermenstrual bleeding** is bleeding between regular menses.

B. **Classification.** The causes of abnormal uterine bleeding may be categorized as either organic or nonorganic. Organic causes include reproductive tract disease, systemic disease, and pharmacologic alterations. Nonorganic causes cannot be measured readily or definitively linked to the abnormal bleeding pattern (physical or emotional stress, weight change, diet, etc.).
   1. **Reproductive tract disease**
      a. **Leiomyomata.** Leiomyomata (fibroids) are the most common uterine neoplasm. These benign smooth muscle tumors are found in 20% to 30% of patients older than 30 years and are uncommon in younger

patients. The most common bleeding pattern associated with leiomyomata is hypermenorrhea.
  b. **Polyps.** Endometrial polyps are generally benign lesions that are found in less than 2% of premenopausal patients who undergo dilatation and curettage (D&C). Benign cervical polyps are found in up to 4% of patients undergoing routine speculum examination. Although cervical polyps are commonly asymptomatic, associated symptoms most commonly include intermenstrual bleeding and postcoital spotting.
  c. **Carcinomas.** Endometrial carcinoma is rare in patients younger than 40 years and uncommon in the perimenopausal years. Fewer than 1% of patients aged 40 to 55 years who undergo D&C for abnormal uterine bleeding have endometrial carcinoma (see Chap. 37). Cervical carcinoma, however, is a disease of both women of reproductive age and postmenopausal women. Although it is rarely the cause of abnormal bleeding, it must be considered in the differential diagnosis. Almost all cervical lesions that cause abnormal bleeding are visible on examination. The most common bleeding patterns associated with cervical carcinoma are intermenstrual and postcoital bleeding.
  d. **Infection.** Abnormal bleeding is not a common presenting symptom of either endometritis or cervicitis. If present, bleeding associated with endometritis is most commonly intermenstrual, and bleeding with cervicitis is postcoital.
2. **Systemic disease or disorder**
  a. **Disorders of coagulation.** Coagulopathies may lead to abnormal uterine bleeding, often by exacerbating another underlying mild abnormality such as fibroids. Coagulopathies, however, are a relatively rare cause of abnormal uterine bleeding. Von Willebrand's disease is the most common inherited bleeding disorder in women (occurring in up to 1 in 1,000 patients). Other entities such as idiopathic thrombocytopenic purpura, hypersplenism, and hematologic malignancy (e.g., leukemia) may also be associated with abnormal uterine bleeding.
  b. **Endocrinopathies that cause anovulation.** Anovulation can create an environment of unopposed estrogen. In the absence of progestin, the endometrium eventually breaks down, which may or may not lead to the formation of hyperplasia. Hypothyroidism and hyperprolactinemia are common disorders that can lead to anovulation (see Chap. 29, sec. **III.A.1.c**).
  c. **Liver failure.** Decreased metabolism of estrogen and decreased clotting factor synthesis may lead to endometrial glandular and stromal breakdown, which may or may not produce endometrial hyperplasia. Anovulation may also ensue. Menometrorrhagia is common.
  d. **Morbid obesity.** Peripheral conversion of androstenedione to estrone occurs in adipose tissue. Increased estrogen levels may lead to endometrial glandular and stromal breakdown, which may or may not lead to hyperplasia. Elevated estrogen levels also may lead to anovulation, which can compound the problem by decreasing progesterone secretion.
  e. **Pregnancy.** Uterine bleeding occurs in as many as 30% of first-trimester pregnancies. Therefore, etiologies such as threatened abortion, incomplete abortion, and ectopic pregnancy must always be considered in a patient with abnormal uterine bleeding, and a pregnancy test must be performed.
3. **Pharmacologic alterations.** Various medications may cause abnormal uterine bleeding. Any medication that acts upon the hypothalamic-pituitary axis can lead to anovulation and abnormal bleeding.
  a. **Psychotropic medications.** Certain medications used in the treatment of psychiatric patients can affect the hypothalamic-pituitary axis. Antidepressants are among the commonly used medications associated with anovulation. The antipsychotics can also interfere with normal menstrual cycle.

b. Hormonal contraception

(1) Levonorgestrel implants. Sixty percent to 80% of patients experience irregular bleeding during the first year of levonorgestrel implant (Norplant) use.

(2) Medroxyprogesterone. Approximately 30% of patients taking medroxyprogesterone (Depo-Provera) experience irregular bleeding during the first year. After the first year, 75% of patients on medroxyprogesterone are amenorrheic.

(3) Combination oral contraceptive preparations (OCPs). Intermenstrual ("breakthrough") bleeding is experienced by 10% to 30% of patients during the first month of OCP use, and by 1% to 10% during the subsequent 2 months. With chronic use, abnormal bleeding may result from atrophy.

(4) Progestational agents. High doses of progesterone often are used in the treatment of abnormal uterine bleeding and endometrial hyperplasia. Prolonged use of these agents may result in endometrial atrophy, which itself often can cause abnormal uterine bleeding.

4. **Dysfunctional uterine bleeding.** Abnormal uterine bleeding without a demonstrable organic cause (see sec. II.B.1–3) is categorized as dysfunctional uterine bleeding (DUB). This diagnosis is made only if an organic etiology is neither identified nor suggested by history and physical examination.

   a. **Anovulation.** The predominant cause of DUB is anovulation. By definition, this anovulation is not secondary to a demonstrable organic cause (see sec. II.B.1–3). Anovulation is multifactorial and related to alterations of the hypothalamic-pituitary ovarian axis. Anovulation associated with polycystic ovarian disease (PCOD) and other forms of hyperandrogenism lack a discrete organic etiology, and associated bleeding abnormalities may be considered to be DUB (see Chap. 33, sec. IV.A). Anovulation results in continued estrogen production in the absence of corpus luteum formation. The endometrium is exposed to unopposed estrogen, leading to overgrowth that may exceed blood supply. Glandular and stromal breakdown ensues, resulting in bleeding.

   b. **Ovulation.** Occasionally, DUB may be associated with ovulatory cycles. A persistent corpus luteum, which does not regress in 12 to 14 days, may result in DUB. Menorrhagia without a demonstrable cause may be classified as DUB.

III. **Diagnosis.** With the exception of DUB, the nomenclature of diagnosis should reflect the pathologic etiology of the abnormal bleeding (e.g., menometrorrhagia secondary to leiomyomata, or hypermenorrhea-polymenorrhea secondary to hypothyroidism).

A. **Patients younger than 40 years.** Many younger patients present with a complaint of 1 or 2 months of abnormal bleeding. At this point, it is appropriate to limit management to a pregnancy test and reassurance (pregnancy and anovulation are very common, and malignancy is rare). Patients with persistent or severe bleeding must undergo further evaluation.

   1. **History.** A thorough history may reveal the underlying pathology.

      a. **Menstrual history and pattern of bleeding.** Specific questions should address frequency and duration of menses, the presence of clots, and postcoital spotting. Different patterns may suggest specific pathologies (see sec. II.B).

      b. **Medications.** All medications used by the patient, including birth control, must be recorded (see sec. II.B.3).

      c. **Factors associated with anovulation.** Has the patient had a change in weight, diet, or exercise patterns? Is she encountering any new psychosocial stressors?

      d. **Signs or symptoms of endocrinopathy.** Are any signs or symptoms of thyroid disease present? Are signs or symptoms of pituitary micro- or macroadenoma (i.e., galactorrhea or mass effect) present?

    e. **Bleeding diathesis.** Does the patient experience frequent nosebleeds or excessive dental bleeding or bruise easily? Is there a family history of a bleeding disorder (see sec. **II.B.2**)?

    f. **Known reproductive tract disease.** Many patients are already aware of diagnoses such as leiomyomata uteri, and time can be saved by asking about these disorders at the outset of the investigation.

2. **Physical examination**

    a. **General appearance.** Assess for obesity, asthenic habitus, manifestations of hypothyroidism, PCOD habitus, virilization, cushingoid habitus, and signs of liver disease.

    b. **Skin and mucous membranes.** The conjunctiva and dependent areas of the body should be examined for petechiae and ecchymoses. The skin also should be inspected for signs of androgen excess (i.e., acne or hirsutism).

    c. **Thyroid.** The thyroid should be examined for nodules or enlargement.

    d. **Speculum examination** should include a survey for gross lesions of the lower reproductive tract, including polyps, myomas, condylomata, and cervical neoplasia. Biopsy of suspected intraepithelial lesions or carcinoma should be ordered (colposcopy should be scheduled). Gonorrhea and chlamydia cultures should be performed if signs of cervicitis exist (friability or mucopus). A Pap smear should be obtained if one has not been obtained within an acceptable time frame. When examining patients for acute vaginal hemorrhage, fornices should be examined for traumatic lacerations.

    e. **Bimanual examination.** An enlarged uterus may signify leiomyomata or pregnancy. An adnexal mass may represent a functional cyst or neoplasm. Because rectal bleeding can be mistaken for vaginal bleeding, a rectal exam should be performed with occult blood testing (unless bimanual exam confirms a gynecologic etiology) as well as an inspection for hemorrhoids.

3. **Laboratory tests, studies, and procedures.** A pregnancy test is mandatory for all pre- and perimenopausal patients and should be performed before the history and physical examination. A hematocrit or hemoglobin test should also be obtained. If a complete blood cell count (CBC) can be obtained at no additional cost, it should be ordered (rare cases of significant thrombocytopenia may be discovered). Other laboratory studies are not routinely indicated. Specific findings on history and physical exam, however, may indicate additional testing.

    a. **Signs or symptoms of androgen excess.** Because the therapy for PCOD or hyperandrogenism is geared toward alleviation of symptoms, multiple tests aimed at confirming these diagnoses are frequently unnecessary. Androgen-secreting adrenal and ovarian neoplasms and prolactinomas, however, may masquerade as PCOD. Therefore, serum testosterone, dehydroepiandrosterone sulfate, and prolactin levels should be determined. It is important to remember, however, that prolactin can be mildly elevated in patients with PCOD; in primary hyperprolactinemia, the prolactin elevation is significant and unaccompanied by the increase in serum testosterone often seen with PCOD or hyperandrogenism. Testosterone levels higher than 150 ng/dL are consistent with stromal hyperthecosis or neoplasm, whereas lower values are more consistent with PCOD. If virilization is accompanied by signs or symptoms of Cushing's disease, a 24-hour free urinary cortisol study should be performed.

    b. **Signs or symptoms of hyperprolactinemia.** A serum prolactin concentration should be ordered. A historical review of the patient's medications is indicated before beginning a workup. Many medications can cause hyperprolactinemia (psychotropic medications, oral contraceptives, H_2 blockers, opiates). Prolactin may also be elevated secondary to pregnancy, hypothyroidism, PCOD, and renal failure. These entities should be ruled out before considering a radiologic study of the sella or pituitary.

c. **Signs or symptoms of hypothyroidism.** A thyroid-stimulating hormone (TSH) level should be ordered. This is the most sensitive test for the detection of hypothyroidism. Both a TSH level and a thyroxine value are necessary, however, to diagnose uncommon central hyperthyroidism.

d. **Signs, symptoms, or family history of bleeding diathesis or abnormal uterine bleeding refractory to therapy.** A CBC with differential count screens for idiopathic thrombocytopenia purpura, hypersplenism, and hematologic malignancy should be obtained. A partial thromboplastin time (PTT) and ristocetin cofactor identify von Willebrand's disease. Findings from these two tests are not consistently abnormal; therefore, the tests should be repeated if the index of suspicion is high. Patients with abnormal uterine bleeding refractory to therapy have an increased incidence of reproductive tract disease, which should be further investigated (see sec. **III.A.3.h**).

e. **Signs or symptoms of liver failure.** Transaminases (aspartate and alanine aminotransferase), alkaline phosphatase, bilirubin, and prothrombin time are obtained by ordering the standard Chem 12 [Sequential Multiple Analyzer (SMA) 12] system. Although some of these parameters may normalize with severe disease, prothrombin time will remain prolonged, and clinical manifestations will persist.

f. **Increased risk of endometrial cancer.** Patients diagnosed with dysfunctional uterine bleeding who are morbidly obese, have hypertensive diabetes, or have a family history of cancer should undergo endometrial sampling. Patients younger than 30 years may undergo a trial of symptomatic therapy (i.e., hormonal) before undergoing endometrial sampling. Endometrial sampling should also be considered for any patient older than 30 years with DUB refractory to standard therapies (see sec. **III.A.3.h**). Office sampling of the endometrium is expensive, and a tissue sample is not required in the diagnosis and treatment of abnormal uterine bleeding in the majority of patients younger than 40 years. Endometrial biopsy should be reserved for specific cases in which patients are at risk.

g. **Immunocompromised status suggestive of tuberculous endometritis.** Immunocompromised patients are at increased risk of contracting tuberculosis. If endometritis is suspected, tuberculous endometritis must be considered. These patients should undergo a purified protein derivative skin test with anergy panel. An endometrial sample should be examined for tuberculosis if a patient's test results are positive or the patient is anergic or from an area of the world in which tuberculosis is endemic.

h. **Dysfunctional uterine bleeding refractory to therapy.** Patients of any age with DUB that is refractory to therapy have high incidences of unrecognized leiomyomata and endometrial polyps; therefore, such patients should be evaluated using ultrasound, sonohysterography, or hysteroscopy. If a lesion is not demonstrated by such a study, an endometrial biopsy should be performed.

B. **Premenopausal patients older than 39 years**
1. **History and physical examination.** The history and physical examination are identical to those described in sec. **III.A.1,2**, but particular attention is paid to menopausal signs and symptoms as well as to risk factors for endometrial carcinoma.
2. **Laboratory tests, studies, and procedures.** A pregnancy test and a CBC are mandatory; other laboratory tests are ordered only when indicated (see sec. **III.A.3**). Because the incidence of endometrial cancer may be as high as 3% in this patient population, unless bleeding is secondary to nonendometrial reproductive tract disease (i.e., leiomyomata), an endometrial biopsy should be considered. Clinical judgment, however, must be applied. A perimenopausal patient without risk factors for endometrial cancer need not undergo biopsy for bleeding suggestive of a single anovulatory cycle. Although obtaining a biopsy sample from a patient younger

than 40 years may be justified, failing to obtain such a sample from a patient older than 39 years must be justified. Endometrial biopsy should be performed in an office setting. D&C offers no significant diagnostic advantage (see sec. **III.D**). Although ultrasound may obviate the need for endometrial biopsy in postmenopausal patients (see sec. **III.D.4**), only rarely does it do so in premenopausal patients, who rarely have an atrophic endometrium. Therefore, ultrasound assessment unnecessarily increases the cost of the workup and usually should be avoided (see sec. **III.A.3.h**).

C. **Postmenopausal patients.** Because the incidence of endometrial carcinoma may be as high as 10% among women with postmenopausal bleeding, thorough evaluation is required. Any uterine bleeding in a postmenopausal patient who is not receiving hormone-replacement therapy (HRT) must be considered abnormal. Any change in the bleeding pattern of a patient receiving HRT, except for the evolution of amenorrhea, should be considered abnormal. Bleeding occurring before day 11 of the progestogen phase of cyclic therapy usually is considered abnormal. Any bleeding after the first year of continuous hormone replacement regimens also should be evaluated.

   1. **History.** A focused history is performed.
      a. **Establish postmenopausal status.** How long has the patient been amenorrheic? Does she have menopausal signs or symptoms?
      b. **Hormone replacement.** Is the patient receiving hormone replacement therapy? Is she on a continuous or cyclic regimen? Has the patient been taking the progestogen?
      c. **Bleeding pattern.** Bleeding before day 11 of cyclic HRT is abnormal. Although spotting during the first year of continuous HRT may be considered normal, if such spotting represents a new symptom, it must be evaluated. Any change in bleeding pattern should also be evaluated. Bleeding patterns of patients who are not receiving HRT can also be helpful. Blood found only on toilet paper suggests anal or rectal bleeding. Postcoital bleeding suggests cervical disease or vaginal atrophy, and spontaneous vaginal bleeding suggests endometrial pathology.
   2. **Physical examination**
      a. **General appearance.** Patients are observed for signs of estrogen excess (obesity) or deficiency (atrophy).
      b. **Speculum examination.** Atrophic vaginitis and vaginal lacerations are possible sources of bleeding. Gross lesions of the cervix or vagina should prompt biopsy. Unless recently obtained, a Pap smear should be performed. After the speculum is removed, the anus should be surveyed for hemorrhoids.
      c. **Bimanual examination.** A rectovaginal examination should be performed. Anal and rectal lesions such as hemorrhoids or fissures may be identified. A test for occult rectal bleeding should also be obtained.
   3. **Laboratory tests, studies, and procedures.** A CBC and either an ultrasound or an endometrial sample examination is mandatory unless a vaginal, rectal, or cervical source of the bleeding has been identified. An abdominal or transvaginal ultrasound may be used to assess the thickness of the endometrial stripe. Endometrial stripes larger than 5 mm warrant biopsy (see sec. **III.D.4**). Stripes as large as 8 mm may be acceptable for patients on HRT (see sec. **III.D.4**).

D. **Methods of endometrial assessment.** Assessment of the endometrium is almost never needed for patients younger than 30 years (see sec. **III.A.3**). Although endometrial assessment may be indicated in patients aged 30 to 40 years, the physician must justify the decision (i.e., bleeding refractory to therapy or risk factors for carcinoma). In premenopausal patients older than 40 years, the endometrium should be assessed if abnormal bleeding occurs. The physician must justify failure to assess the endometrium in this patient population (e.g., first episode of oligohypermenorrhea in a thin patient). Postmenopausal bleeding and abnormal bleeding during HRT always merit an assessment of the endometrium.

1. **D&C.** Although a simple procedure, D&C has several disadvantages, perhaps the most significant of which is that it is performed in an operating room with the use of anesthesia. Therefore, the procedure is expensive and associated with the inherent risks of anesthesia. Uterine perforation may occur, especially when D&C is performed in a postmenopausal patient. Although safer, simpler, and less expensive methods of endometrial sampling are now available, many clinicians continue to perform D&C. Numerous investigators have demonstrated that office sampling techniques may be as effective as D&C (see sec. **III.D.2,3**). Moreover, the suggestion that D&C is therapeutic for DUB has never been conclusively demonstrated.
2. **Office biopsy.** Office sampling with the Novak curette or Pipelle or Vabra aspirator is both simple and safe. Complications are extremely rare. These procedures are much less costly than D&C. Numerous studies have shown these techniques to be of comparable sensitivity to D&C. Some investigators have also noted a lower incidence of tissue insufficient for diagnosis (TID) with these techniques, compared with D&C. Although some clinicians perform a D&C after office sampling returns TID, this practice is not well founded. If the uterine cavity is clearly entered during office sampling, it is rare that a subsequent D&C significantly alters the diagnosis (i.e., confirms a diagnosis of atypia or carcinoma after office sampling has yielded TID).
3. **Hysteroscopy and biopsy.** With appropriate equipment and patient selection, hysteroscopy can be performed in an office setting. Complications are rare (less than 1%). Although less expensive than D&C, office hysteroscopy with biopsy is more time consuming and expensive than blind sampling techniques (see sec. **III.D.2**). It has been suggested that hysteroscopy with biopsy is the most sensitive technique for the evaluation of the endometrium. This relatively high degree of sensitivity, however, is limited to the diagnosis of polyps, myomata, and other neoplasms and is associated with a decrease in specificity. Furthermore, hysteroscopic impression is imprecise. The incidence of discrepancy between hysteroscopic impression and directed biopsy may approach 20%. As many as 19% of biopsy-proven hyperplasias and   of biopsy-proven carcinomas are unsuspected at the time of hystero   Based on the inaccuracy of hysteroscopic impression, it is pruden   form a random sampling of the endometrium concurrently.
4. **Ultrasound.** Ultrasound is useful   assessment of postmenopausal bleeding because more than 50%   ted patients' bleeding is secondary to endometrial atrophy.   ing such patients ultrasonographically can prevent the discon   expense of a tissue diagnosis. Although ultrasound is sensitive   iagnosis of leiomyomata, this diagnosis is usually made by hist   hysical examination. Numerous authors have examined his   rrelations with ultrasound endometrial stripe measurements   lane endometrial stripe measurements of less than 6 mm (lane) represent an atrophic endometrium, and pathologic le   ly are found. A transvaginal sonogram measurement of less t   has a sensitivity, specificity, positive predictive value, and ne   dictive value of 100%, 75%, 90%, and 100%, respectively. Th   trasound assessment of the patient with postmenopausal blee   bviate the need for endometrial sampling in as many as 5(es. Patients on cyclic HRT should be scanned immediately   progestogen phase of their cycle (days 1 to 3).
5. **Sonohysterography (SHG).** SHG   es the installation of a sterile solution (usually crystalloid) into   erine canal during ultrasonography. SHG is the most sensitive   vasive method of diagnosis for endometrial polyps and submucous   mata; its sensitivity approaches that of hysteroscopy. Unlike hyster   py, however, directed biopsy is difficult. Therefore, the indications   sonohysterography are limited. If office hysteroscopy is impossible,   IG is a safe and simple alterna-

tive for the evaluation of the patient with DUB refractory to therapy, which has a high incidence of polyps and myomata. Sonohysterography is also useful if a previous study has not enabled differentiation of a polyp or submucous myoma from a thickened endometrial stripe and is especially helpful when endometrial sampling is impossible or contraindicated. SHG is also a reasonable alternative to office hysteroscopy if hysteroscopic biopsy or polypectomy is impossible in this setting. SHG may be used to avoid hysteroscopy in an operating room for patients with DUB refractory to therapy (see sec. **III.A.3.h**). Patients with negative SHG findings should undergo endometrial sampling to rule out neoplasia.

IV. Treatment
A. Patients younger than 40 years
1. **Reproductive tract disease**
   a. **Leiomyomata.** Hormonal manipulation in the form of OCPs, progestational agents, or GnRH agonists can be considered.
      (1) **OCPs** are easy to use. In addition to decreasing mean blood loss, OCPs have contraceptive and noncontraceptive benefits (see Chap. 19, sec. **I.D**).
      (2) For patients desiring fertility or patients in whom OCPs are contraindicated, a **progestogen** may be used by itself. Most commonly, medroxyprogesterone acetate (5 to 10 mg) is prescribed for the last 10 days of the cycle.
      (3) Patients for whom OCP or progestogen therapy has failed may be considered for treatment with a **GnRH agonist.** GnRH agonists create a pseudomenopausal state, and patients experience associated menopausal signs and symptoms. The negative effect of GnRH agonists on the lipid profile and bone density limit the duration of their use to 6 months or less generally.
      (4) **Nonsteroidal antiinflammatory drugs** (NSAIDs) have been shown to decrease the mean blood loss in ovulatory patients with menorrhagia. Commonly, naproxen sodium (Naprosyn) is administered for 3 to 8 days, beginning with menses. NSAIDs usually are combined with hormonal agents. The antifibrinolytic agents epsilon-aminocaproic acid and tranexamic acid have demonstrated similar success to NSAIDs; side effects, however, limit their use.
      (5) **Surgery** remains the definitive treatment of leiomyomata and may be selected for patients unresponsive to pharmacologic interventions. Surgical options include myomectomy, endometrial ablation, and hysterectomy. As many as 25% of patients who undergo myomectomy eventually undergo a hysterectomy. Endometrial ablation produces a satisfactory decrease in bleeding in more than 80% of patients. Only myomectomy preserves fertility, however, and only hysterectomy offers definite cure.
   b. **Polyps.** Polyps are readily treated by simple polypectomy. Hypermenorrhea associated with endometrial polyps may respond to hormonal or NSAID therapy.
   c. **Endometritis.** Endometritis should be treated with a 10- to 14-day course of antibiotics. Doxycycline is the antibiotic of choice. If the infection is refractory to therapy or associated with signs of adnexal inflammation, therapy for pelvic inflammatory disease such as cefoxitin is warranted.
   d. **Endometrial hyperplasia**
      (1) **Typical hyperplasia.** Treatment should be continued for 4 to 6 months, at which time an endometrial biopsy should be obtained to confirm regression of the hyperplasia. In the absence of attempts at conception, these patients should probably be maintained on cyclic monthly progestin withdrawal or OCPs to prevent recurrence. An endometrial biopsy should also be repeated if abnormal bleeding persists during treatment or recurs. An

endometrial biopsy should be repeated if abnormal bleeding persists or recurs.

(2) **Atypical hyperplasia** requires treatment because in approximately 23% of cases, atypical hyperplasia progresses to carcinoma. Hysterectomy is an acceptable first-line treatment. As many as 25% of uteri removed in the treatment of atypical hyperplasia harbor a focus of well-differentiated carcinoma. For patients who wish to retain their fertility, progestational therapy is an acceptable approach. Continuous megestrol acetate regimens may achieve up to 100% response rates. Acceptable dosing regimens range from 20 to 40 mg b.i.d. Preliminary data suggest that even lower doses may be effective. Treatment is continued for 6 months, with endometrial biopsies performed at 3 and 6 months. Dosing is increased if regression is not observed. Progesterone withdrawal regimens are not consistently effective and should not be used in the treatment of atypical hyperplasia; they may, however, be useful in preventing recurrence.

e. **Carcinoma.** Total abdominal hysterectomy with bilateral salpingo-oophorectomy and staging is the standard therapy for endometrial or cervical cancer. Postoperative radiation is offered to certain patients at high risk for recurrence or metastasis. Radiation is an acceptable first-line treatment of patients who are poor surgical candidates.

2. **Systemic disease.** Although the first line of treatment is aimed at the underlying disease (i.e., thyroxine for hypothyroidism or bromocriptine for prolactinoma), additional therapy may be required to treat the abnormal bleeding until the underlying disease is well controlled (see sec. **IV.A.1**). When medical management fails, endometrial ablation or more definitive surgical treatment may be considered.

a. **Endocrinopathies.** Abnormal uterine bleeding is usually secondary to anovulation in patients with endocrinopathies. Treatment of bleeding is therefore identical to that of DUB (see sec. **IV.A.4**).

b. **Morbid obesity or liver disease.** Morbidly obese patients or patients with liver disease suffer from estrogen excess and should be treated with a progestational agent or OCPs (see sec. **IV.A.1.a**).

c. **Disorders that affect coagulation.** Initially, OCPs or progestin is administered (see sec. **IV.A.1.a**). If this initial treatment is ineffective, a continuous regimen of OCPs or Depo-Provera is used in an attempt to produce atrophy and amenorrhea.

3. **Pharmacologic alterations.** Whenever possible, the inciting agent should be discontinued. If discontinuation is impossible, therapy is tailored to the underlying pathophysiology. Most psychotropic medications cause abnormal uterine bleeding by inducing anovulation. Therefore, therapy is identical to that for DUB (see sec. **IV.A.4**). Bleeding during the first year of Norplant use is often a result of anovulation and can be treated in a similar fashion. Bleeding after chronic progestin exposure (including OCPs) is secondary to endometrial atrophy and can be treated with estrogen supplementation.

4. **Dysfunctional uterine bleeding.** Affected patients suffer from anovulation and abnormal bleeding resulting from estrogen excess at the level of the endometrium. Patients may be effectively treated with OCPs or progestogens as described in sec. **IV.A.1.a**. Patients desiring fertility may be treated effectively with ovulation induction. The abnormal bleeding in PCOD is usually anovulatory and can be treated accordingly. However, endometrial hyperplasia can occur in PCOD because of unopposed estrogen exposure.

B. **Premenopausal patients older than 39 years.** Endometrial sampling usually is performed before therapy is initiated (see sec. **III.B.2, III.D**). Therapies are similar to those for patients younger than 40 years (see sec. **IV.A**), except that OCPs should not be used for patients who smoke more than 15 cigarettes per day.

C. **Postmenopausal patients** should never be treated before the endometrium is assessed. The endometrium may be sampled or an ultrasound may be obtained (see sec. **III.D.4**).

1. **Atrophic endometrium.** Treatment is not required for atrophic endometrium. If treatment is desired, estrogen therapy should be initiated. Patients on HRT may increase their estrogen dose by 50% to 100% for several months. Patients who are not on HRT may be started on cyclic HRT (the progestin may be withheld for the first 2 months). Patients with atrophic endometrium that is refractory to therapy may have a polyp and should be evaluated with hysteroscopy or SHG (see sec. **III.D.3,5**).

2. **Proliferative endometrium.** Treatment is not required for proliferative endometrium. If treatment is desired, patients should receive cyclic hormonal therapy. Patients already on cyclic HRT may increase their progestational dose by 50% to 100%.

3. **Hyperplastic endometrium.** Contrary to cases of hyperplastic endometrium in pre- and perimenopausal patients, the inciting milieu in older patients is usually permanent. Therefore, these patients always should be treated with a continuous progestational therapy. Serial biopsies also should be performed, as described in sec. **IV.A.1.d.** Because of the high incidence of endometrial carcinoma associated with atypical hyperplasia in postmenopausal patients and the need for chronic progestational therapy to ensure a durable cure, hysterectomy should be considered strongly in postmenopausal patients with atypical hyperplasia. When megestrol is used to treat atypical hyperplasia, therapy should be continued for at least 6 months (see sec. **IV.A.1.d**).

4. **Carcinoma.** Treatment of endometrial and cervical cancers is the same as described in sec. **IV.A.1.e.**

V. **Acute vaginal hemorrhage.** Occasionally, patients experience severe vaginal bleeding. These patients usually present to the emergency department. Under such circumstances, endometrial sampling is inappropriate.

A. **History and physical examination.** An abbreviated history and physical exam is performed (see sec. **III.A–C**). Particular attention is paid to menstrual history and reproductive tract disease, as pregnancy and leiomyomata are by far the most common offenders. It is also necessary to look for vaginal tears from coitus or trauma and rectal bleeding, which are other common causes of acute vaginal hemorrhage.

B. **Laboratory studies.** A pregnancy test, CBC, prothrombin time, and activated partial thromboplastin time should be obtained.

C. **Therapy.** Intravenous fluid resuscitation should be initiated immediately. If anemia is severe and bleeding persists, blood transfusion should be initiated. Two units of packed red cells are usually sufficient.

1. **History and physical examination findings consistent with endometrial atrophy.** Patients on chronic megestrol acetate therapy occasionally present with vaginal hemorrhage. Patients bleeding from endometrial atrophy may be treated with conjugated estrogens (Premarin), 25 mg i.v. every 2 to 4 hours (up to four doses). Antiemetics also should be administered. Patients may continue to take oral Premarin or OCPs. After 2 weeks of Premarin therapy, progestin should be added (patients who remain on unopposed estrogen therapy require yearly assessment of the endometrium). An OCP taper also may be used as the primary therapy (see sec. **V.C.3**).

2. **History and physical examination findings consistent with endometrial hyperplasia.** Often, morbidly obese patients present with signs and symptoms of endometrial hyperplasia. Initiate an OCP taper or high-dose continuous progestin therapy. Megestrol, 20 mg, can be given twice each day and should be continued for at least 1 month. An endometrial sample should be obtained after the bleeding is controlled.

3. **History and physical examination findings inconsistent with pathologic etiology or consistent with myomata.** An OCP taper usually controls the bleeding. No data suggest a superiority of any available formulation or taper regimen. A common approach is to administer four tablets/day for 4 days, three tablets/day for 4 days, two tablets/day for 4 days, then one tablet each day for a total of 2 months (omitting placebo

pills). Patients are then continued on OCP therapy, with normal monthly withdrawal. Patients are encouraged to continue taking OCPs for at least 4 months. Because OCP tapers are associated with significant nausea and vomiting, the dose should be divided throughout the day and antiemetics should be provided. Premarin i.v. is an acceptable alternative for patients who cannot tolerate oral medication (see sec. **V.C.1**). Bleeding usually is controlled within 48 hours.

4. **Pregnancy.** Acute vaginal hemorrhage associated with pre-viable pregnancy usually is caused by incomplete abortion. Such hemorrhages in first trimester pregnancies are best treated with suction curettage. Ring forceps may be used to remove products of conception lodged in the cervix, which often significantly attenuates bleeding. Second trimester incomplete abortions are best treated with dilatation and evacuation (D&E). Patients who experience incomplete abortion who undergo suction curettage or D&E should receive antimicrobial prophylaxis (e.g., doxycycline, 100 mg before the procedure). If any signs of infection are present, broad spectrum coverage with i.v. cefotetan and doxycycline or triple antibiotics should be initiated. I.v. antibiotics are continued until the patient has remained afebrile for at least 24 hours. The management of viable pregnancies is well described in the obstetric literature.

5. **Bleeding requiring surgical intervention.** Surgical intervention is indicated if blood loss cannot be replaced with transfusion or if bleeding shows no signs of abating after 48 hours. D&C should be performed, though it may provide only temporary attenuation and should be followed by hormonal therapy. The patient should provide informed consent for hypogastric artery ligation and hysterectomy, which are the next lines of therapy should D&C fail. If available, hypogastric artery embolization may be considered as an alternative to ligation.

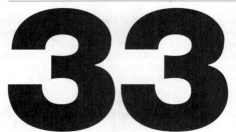

Hyperandrogenism

Supriya Varma,
Endrika Hinton, and
Howard A. Zacur

I. Definition and description

A. Hyperandrogenism describes the finding of an elevated plasma or serum concentration of androgen or any manifestation of the biological activity of excess androgen hormone.

B. Hirsutism is a clinical example of a manifestation of the biological activity associated with elevated levels of androgen hormones. *Hirsutism* refers to the growth of dark terminal hair on the face, chest, back, lower abdomen, and upper thighs.

   1. Types of hair growth. At birth, all hair follicles on skin surfaces of the body produce fine, unpigmented hair known as lanugo hair. With age, some of these hair follicles on particular areas of the body produce thick, darkly pigmented hair in response to androgen exposure. This thick, dark hair is called terminal hair. The remaining hair follicles produce villus hair, which is finer than terminal hair and not as darkly pigmented. For example, hair follicles on the lower arms and legs do not respond to androgen stimulation and continue to produce villus hair.

   2. Hypertrichosis. Excessive growth of villus hair may caused by genetic factors or exposure to drugs such as phenytoin (Dilantin). This type of excessive villus hair growth is called hypertrichosis and should not be mistaken for hirsutism.

C. Acne. Infections of the pilosebaceous glands adjacent to hair follicles result in the formation of dermal abscesses, called *acne*. These skin lesions may exist on the surface of the skin or within the dermis. The lesions within the dermis are known as pustular acne. Because of the ability of androgen hormones to stimulate secretions from pilosebaceous glands, it has long been believed that development of severe cases of acne is a manifestation of excessive androgenic hormone activity. Pustular acne involving the face and back is thought to result from excessive androgen stimulation.

D. Oily skin. Release of secretions from pilosebaceous glands in response to androgen stimulation may result in excessive skin oiliness.

E. Voice changes. Human vocal cords thicken in response to androgen exposure. This thickening is irreversible. Thickened vocal cords result in lowering of the tone of the voice.

F. Male body habitus. Hypertrophy of major muscle groups, such as arm and leg muscles, occurs in response to androgen exposure. Not only do muscle cells become larger in response to androgen exposure, but their number increases as well. Hypertrophy of major muscle groups results in the development of what is commonly described as male body habitus.

G. Male pattern baldness. Recession of frontal hair, as well as loss of hair in the temporal regions of the scalp and the crown of the head, is commonly seen in men as they age and occurs in response to androgen hormones. The fact that excessive androgen activity stimulates hair growth on some parts of the body while causing hair loss from others remains unexplained.

H. Enlargement of the clitoris. Enlargement of the clitoris may occur in response to excessive androgen exposure. Enlargement of the clitoris is a dose-dependent event and is irreversible.

I. **Virilization.** *Virilization* refers to androgenic hormone activity that, in addition to hirsutism, may result in deepening of the voice, male body habitus development, male pattern baldness, clitoromegaly, and reduction of breast size.

II. **Androgenic hormones.** Androgenic hormones include those that stimulate terminal hair growth and cause voice and muscle changes, hair loss, clitoral enlargement, and reduction in breast size. Well-known androgens include testosterone and androstenedione. A well-known androgen hormone precursor is dehydroepiandrosterone sulfate.

  A. **Testosterone.** In women, testosterone is produced in equal amounts by the adrenal gland and the ovary. Secretion of testosterone by the adrenal glands and ovaries accounts for 50% of testosterone found in the circulation. The remainder of the circulating testosterone is produced by peripheral conversion of androstenedione, secreted by the adrenal gland and ovaries, to testosterone. Normal circulating concentrations of testosterone in women range from 20 to 75 ng/dL. This range is far lower than the testosterone concentrations found in men, which range from 300 to 800 ng/dL. Testosterone is the most potent androgenic hormone.

  B. **Androstenedione.** Androstenedione is produced in equal amounts by the adrenal glands and the ovaries. It is a less potent androgen than testosterone, but can produce androgenic biologic effects when present in excess amounts.

  C. **Dehydroepiandrosterone (DHEA).** DHEA and its sulfate (DHEAS) are produced almost exclusively by the adrenal gland. DHEA is metabolized quickly, so measurement of its concentration does not accurately reflect adrenal gland activity. DHEAS, in contrast, has a long half-life, so measurement of its activity reflects adrenal gland activity. Normal levels of DHEAS in women are 38 to 338 μg/dL. DHEA and DHEAS are accurately referred to as precursors of androgens.

III. **Diagnosis of hyperandrogenism**

  A. **Physical and pelvic examination.** Hyperandrogenism may be diagnosed if biologic signs of androgen excess are present. These signs include excessive sexual hair growth, male pattern baldness, deepening of the voice, enlargement of the clitoris, reduction in breast size, and male muscular development.

  B. **Laboratory evaluation.** Measurements of serum or plasma androgens may be obtained to diagnose hyperandrogenism. Serum or plasma testosterone and androstenedione levels are commonly measured. DHEAS is an androgen precursor, but DHEAS levels often are ordered to detect excessive adrenal gland activity. Levels of metabolites of testosterone may also be ordered. Production of 3α-androstenedione, which is a metabolite of dihydrotestosterone, has been postulated to correlate with the conversion of testosterone to dihydrotestosterone by the enzyme 5α-reductase. Increased activity of this enzyme, which is present in hair follicles, has been suggested as the cause of hirsutism when the circulating concentration of testosterone is normal.

IV. **Causes of hyperandrogenism.** Five causes of hyperandrogenism have been identified: hyperandrogenemic chronic anovulation syndrome, late-onset adrenal hyperplasia, tumors of the ovary or adrenal glands, Cushing's syndrome, and idiopathic or drug-induced processes.

  A. **Hyperandrogenemic chronic anovulation syndrome.** Stein and Leventhal in 1935 described seven women who were amenorrheic, obese, and hirsute and who had cystic ovaries. From this initial description, the term *Stein-Leventhal syndrome* was used to identify other similarly affected women. Because of the cystic changes found within the ovaries of affected patients the terms *polycystic ovarian syndrome*, or *polycystic ovarian disease* (PCOD), are also used to describe these patients. Orderly follicular development, which ultimately leads to the emergence at monthly intervals of a dominant follicle that releases an oocyte, does not occur routinely in patients with PCOD. Although follicle development occasionally proceeds to ovulation in affected patients, development of the follicle to only its initial growth stage is common. As a consequence, the ovarian cortex becomes populated with numerous small follicles, or "cysts," in these patients. This effect may be induced in the ovaries of unaffected women who are exposed to persistently elevated androgen levels. The hyperandrogenemic state is believed to be a cause of incomplete follicular development. As a result of these observations, the term *hyperandrogenemic chronic ovulation syndrome* is preferred to other terms to describe these patients.

1. **Symptoms.** Patients with hyperandrogenemic chronic ovulation syndrome present with hirsutism, oligomenorrhea, menorrhea, obesity, infertility, and pelvic pain. All or only some of these symptoms may be present. Virilization is not a common finding in affected patients.

2. **Pathogenesis.** The cause of hyperandrogenemic chronic ovulation syndrome remains unknown. Abnormalities of the hypothalamic pituitary axis and the ovarian or adrenal steroidogenic pathway have been suggested as possible explanations for this condition.

   a. At the level of the hypothalamic pituitary axis, an increase in the frequency and amplitude of luteinizing hormone (LH) pulses has been recorded in affected patients. An increase in the ratio of the plasma or serum concentrations of LH to follicle-stimulating hormone from 1 to greater than 2 is observed in patients with hyperandrogenemic chronic ovulation syndrome. Disordered regulation of hypothalamic pituitary secretion of gonadotropin-releasing hormone is believed to be the cause of this increase in ratio.

   b. Increased secretion of androgens from the ovary and adrenal gland in patients with hyperandrogenemic chronic ovulation syndrome also has been observed. This increased secretion may result from stimulation of thecal cells by LH to produce androgens. Increased resistance to insulin often is observed in affected patients. It has been suggested that the extra insulin may bind to insulin-like growth factor receptors within the ovary, which may amplify the androgen-stimulating effect of LH on thecal cells.

   c. Increased secretion of androgen from the adrenal gland has also been suggested as a cause of hyperandrogenemic chronic ovulation syndrome. The mild elevation of DHEAS levels frequently seen in these patients has been cited as supporting evidence for this theory. Unfortunately, studies designed to detect adrenal gland enzyme deficiencies or excesses that could cause excessive secretion of androgens in patients with hyperandrogenemic chronic anovulation have identified such disorders in only a small number of patients.

B. **Late-onset adrenal hyperplasia.** The adrenal enzyme 21-hydroxylase (21-OH) converts progesterone to deoxycorticosterone, or 17-hydroxylase (17-OH) progesterone to deoxycortisol. A deficiency in the activity of this enzyme causes a decrease in cortisol production, resulting in increased pituitary secretion of adrenocorticotropic hormone (ACTH). Increased stimulation of the adrenal gland by ACTH may result in the production of increased amounts of the deoxycortisol precursor 17-OH progesterone. Androstenedione is produced from 17-OH progesterone by the enzyme 17α-hydroxylase-17,20-desmolase. Androstenedione is in turn converted to testosterone by 17-ketosteroid reductase. Increased levels of 17-OH progesterone result in increased secretion of androstenediol and testosterone from the adrenal gland. Elevated basal levels of 17-OH progesterone and increased release of 17-OH progesterone by the adrenal gland in response to ACTH stimulation are seen in patients with late-onset adrenal hyperplasia. Only 3% to 5% of hyperandrogenemic patients can be shown to have a partial deficiency in 21-hydroxylase. This percentage is approximately the same as the expected prevalence of partial 21-OH deficiency in the general white population. Therefore, late-onset adrenal hyperplasia is not a common cause of hyperandrogenemic chronic anovulation syndrome.

C. **Androgen-producing ovarian or adrenal tumors.** Tumors of the ovary or adrenal gland that secrete androgens are quite rare. The presence of an androgen-producing tumor is suspected on the basis of clinical findings. Virilization, particularly virilization of rapid onset, often is observed in the presence of an androgen-producing tumor. A serum or plasma concentration of testosterone that exceeds 200 ng/dL warrants concern about the presence of an ovarian or adrenal androgen-producing tumor. A concentration of DHEAS exceeding 1,000 μg/dL causes concern about an adrenal androgen-producing tumor. Palpation of an adnexal mass in a virilized individual with only a mildly elevated testosterone level also suggests the presence of an ovarian androgen-producing tumor.

D. Cushing's syndrome. Excessive adrenal gland steroidogenesis may occur either as a result of glandular hyperfunction or in response to excessive stimulation by ACTH. If glandular hyperfunction is causative, the disorder is defined as *adrenal hyperplasia resulting in Cushing's syndrome*, whereas if excessive stimulation by ACTH is responsible, the disorder is referred to specifically as *Cushing's disease*, which is caused by a pituitary adenoma that secretes ACTH. Patients with Cushing's syndrome usually are identified easily clinically because of moon facies, increased nuchal fat (buffalo hump), abdominal striae, facial erythema, and truncal obesity. Increased 24-hour urinary excretion of free cortisol and inability to suppress fasting serum or plasma cortisol levels to less than 5 μg/dL 12 hours after oral administration of 1 mg of dexamethasone are laboratory tests used to confirm the diagnosis of Cushing's syndrome. Patients with Cushing's disease are identified by magnetic resonance imaging of the pituitary gland and by high-dose dexamethasone-suppression tests.

E. Idiopathic and drug-induced hirsutism. Idiopathic hirsutism is diagnosed in individuals who are hirsute but who do not demonstrate abnormal findings on the standard laboratory tests ordered to identify known causes of hirsutism. Although estimates vary depending on the study cited, it is estimated that perhaps 5% to 15% of all hirsute patients may be said to have idiopathic hirsutism.

   1. Because the presence of hirsutism is a biological manifestation of hyperandrogenism, the inability to identify a specific androgen that is elevated in patients with idiopathic hirsutism may reflect simply a lack of knowledge about the androgen responsible.

   2. An alternative explanation is based on the hypothesis that patients with idiopathic hirsutism demonstrate increased skin sensitivity to androgens. In particular, it has been suggested that patients with idiopathic hirsutism convert testosterone to greater quantities of dihydrotestosterone than normal because of increased activity of the converting enzyme 5α-reductase. Despite an initial report in support of this hypothesis, follow-up studies have failed to corroborate this result.

   3. Occasionally drug ingestion may be responsible for hirsutism. Use of danazol, a 17α-ethinyl derivative of testosterone, for treatment of endometriosis and methyltestosterone for hormone replacement are two examples of drugs that may cause hirsutism.

V. Consequences of hyperandrogenism

A. Hirsutism and acne. Hirsutism is a common consequence of hyperandrogenism. Acne is another direct consequence of hyperandrogenism. The adverse psychological reaction by a patient to severe acne may be profound.

B. Lipid changes. Subjects with hyperandrogenism exhibit lowered high-density lipoprotein cholesterol and increased low-density lipoprotein cholesterol compared with controls. The cause of this altered lipid profile may be the insulin resistance commonly observed in hirsute patients with hyperandrogenemic chronic anovulation syndrome, rather than the hyperandrogenism itself.

VI. Treatment of hirsutism or hyperandrogenism. Treatment of the patient with hirsutism or hyperandrogenism depends on the cause of the hirsutism and whether the patient desires to become pregnant.

A. Hyperandrogenemic chronic ovulation syndrome. Treatment of patients with hyperandrogenemic chronic ovulation syndrome depends on their desire to conceive.

   1. If pregnancy is not desired, therapy is directed toward stopping the development of new hair growth, removing existing excessive hair growth, and regulating the menstrual cycle.

   a. Combination oral contraceptive agents. Oral contraceptive preparations (OCPs) diminish circulating gonadotropin levels and increase sex hormone–binding globulin (SHBG) levels. Lowering of gonadotropin levels results in decreased ovarian androgen secretion, producing lower circulating levels of androgens. Increasing SHBG results in less free testosterone available for conversion to dihydrotestosterone in the hair follicle. Lowered total and free androgen levels in women treated with OCPs cause a reduction in the formation of new androgen-dependent hair growth and androgen-stimulated acne.

  b. **Spironolactone.** Spironolactone, a steroid compound that is an aldosterone antagonist, was originally dispensed as an antihypertensive agent. Its activity as an antiandrogen was detected after men receiving the compound developed gynecomastia. It is now known that spironolactone inhibits the binding of dihydrotestosterone to its receptor. Spironolactone also inhibits androgen synthesis by inhibiting 17-hydroxylase and 17,20-lyase. After 6 months of therapy at 100 to 200 mg/day, reduction in the diameter of terminal hair and cessation of new terminal hair growth is observed. Because of potential adverse effects on the development of the external genitalia of male fetuses, spironolactone should be used together with contraception in sexually active women.

  c. **Flutamide** is a nonsteroidal antiandrogen that blocks the binding of androgen to its receptor. Flutamide was developed initially for the treatment of prostate disease. When administered in a dosage of 250 mg/day, decreased terminal hair diameter and cessation of new hair growth is observed. Some individuals receiving this drug have developed serious hepatotoxicity.

  d. **Finasteride** is an inhibitor of type II 5α-reductase. Finasteride was developed initially as a treatment for prostate hypertrophy and cancer. By inhibiting 5α-reductase, the drug decreases dihydrotestosterone activity at the hair follicle. Two types of 5α-reductase enzyme activity exist, type I and type II. Although finasteride treatment prevents new hair growth and decreases the terminal hair shaft diameter, it does not appear to completely inhibit type I 5α-reductase, which is the type present in the skin.

2. **If pregnancy is desired** by individuals with hyperandrogenemic chronic ovulation syndrome, assistance with ovulation induction frequently is required. This assistance may be provided by using the oral medication clomiphene citrate or by systemic administration of gonadotropins.

  a. **Clomiphene citrate.** Clomiphene citrate seems to act by blocking the binding of estrogen to its receptor in the hypothalamus. Clomiphene citrate usually is administered orally in doses of 50 to 100 mg/day for 5 days. Monitoring the patient using a basal body temperature chart, pelvic ultrasound, or measurement of serum progesterone 14 days after the last clomiphene tablet is taken can document ovulation.

  b. **Gonadotropins.** Direct stimulation of the ovary to induce ovulation is achieved by injecting gonadotropins i.m. or s.q.

B. **Late-onset adrenal hyperplasia**

  1. Individuals diagnosed with late-onset adrenal hyperplasia may be treated by administering **glucocorticoid agents** to restore ovulation. This treatment also reduces circulating androgen levels. Glucocorticoid administration is therefore appropriate therapy for infertility or hirsutism in individuals with late-onset adrenal hyperplasia.

  2. Alternatively, the same **hormone therapy** indicated for individuals with hyperandrogenemic chronic anovulation may be used in individuals with late-onset adrenal hyperplasia. OCPs or antiandrogens may be used successfully to treat hirsutism. Ovulation-inducing drugs may also be used to treat infertility.

C. **Androgen-producing ovarian or adrenal tumors** usually are treated surgically. Depending on the type of tumor, additional treatment with chemotherapy or radiation therapy may be required.

D. Cushing's syndrome. Surgery of the pituitary or adrenal gland may be required to treat Cushing's disease or adrenal hyperplasia causing Cushing's syndrome.

E. Idiopathic hirsutism. The same medications used to treat hirsute patients with hyperandrogenemic chronic anovulation may be used to treat patients with idiopathic hirsutism.

Selected Reading

Azziz R, Zacur HA. Polycystic ovary syndrome. In: Zacur HA, Wallach EE, eds. *Reproductive medicine and surgery*. St. Louis: Mosby, 1995:230.

Stein IF, Leventhal ML. Amenorrhea associated with bilateral polycystic ovaries. *Am J Obstet Gynecol* 1935;29:181.

Zacur HA. Prolactin abnormalities in polycystic ovarian syndrome. In: Azziz R, Nestler JE, DeWailly D, eds. *Androgen excess disorders in women*. Philadelphia: Lippincott–Raven, 1997:287.

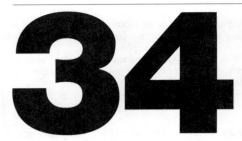

Cervical Intraepithelial Neoplasia

Joelle Osias and
Edward Trimble

I. Epidemiology

   A. Incidence. Approximately 15,000 new cases of cervical cancer are reported each year in the United States. Before mass cervical cancer screening was initiated in the 1950s, diagnosis of cervical cancer usually was delayed until the onset of clinical symptoms. More than 60% of all cases were inoperable at the time of presentation. Today, unfortunately, one-half of women who develop cervical cancer have never been screened or have been screened at intervals of more than 3 years. The risk of cervical cancer is shown in Table 34-1 (1–4).

   B. Etiology. Although epidemiologic risk factors are well known, little is known of the pathobiology of cervical carcinogenesis. The two major independent risk factors for the development of cervical cancer are lifetime number of sexual partners and smoking. The risk of invasive cervical cancer is higher by twofold in smokers than in nonsmokers. The number of cigarettes smoked also seems to correlate with disease severity, with an increased risk of high-grade disease in women who smoke more than half a pack of cigarettes per day (5). Other risk factors include sexual activity before the age of 16 years, sexually transmitted diseases [including human papillomavirus (HPV) and herpes], low socioeconomic status, oral contraceptive use, human immunodeficiency virus infection, and immunosuppression.

II. Terminology and definitions. The terminology used to define preinvasive lesions of the cervix has changed as physicians' understanding of the pathobiology of precursor lesions has evolved. Preinvasive cervical lesions of the cervix originally were divided into two separate categories: dysplasia and carcinoma *in situ*. Traditionally, the classification of Pap smear results was based on numerical class designations: class I, normal; class II, atypical and reactive changes; class III, cells with atypical features suggestive but not diagnostic of malignancy; class IV, atypical cells strongly suggestive of malignancy; and class V, malignant cells.

   A. Cervical intraepithelial neoplasia (CIN). The hypothesis that all types of cervical dysplasia represent a continuum of a single disease process led to the development of CIN terminology. The microscopic features of CIN are thought to represent infection that results in a loss of normal differentiation and maturation of squamous epithelium and proliferation abnormalities of the basal and parabasal layers. The histologic grading is based on the proportion of the epithelium occupied by undifferentiated basal type cells. The three grades of precursor lesions recognized are CIN I (mild dysplasia), CIN II (moderate dysplasia), and CIN III (severe dysplasia and carcinoma *in situ*). The microscopic features of dysplasia include disordered maturation, nuclear hyperchromatism, increased nuclear to cytoplasmic ratio, pleomorphism, mitoses, and dyskeratosis.

   B. The Bethesda system. More recently, studies have shown that CIN does not represent a continuum of a single biological process but two separate disease entities with different biological behaviors. One entity is a viral lesion with a low likelihood of progression to malignancy; the other is a preneoplastic process limited to the epithelium but with definite malignant potential. On the basis of clinical behavior and molecular biological findings, the decision

Table 34-1. Lifetime risk of cervical cancer

Uninvestigated	1 in 100
HSIL, untreated for 20 yr	1 in 3
LSIL and surveillance	1 in 500
After treatment for CIN (all grades)	1 in 250

CIN, cervical intraepithelial neoplasm; HSIL, high-grade squamous intraepithelial lesion; LSIL, low-grade squamous intraepithelial lesion.
From McIndoe WA, McLean MR, Jones RW, Mullins PR. The invasive potential of carcinoma in situ of the cervix. *Obstet Gynecol* 1984;64:451–458. Reprinted with permission.

was made to adopt a new terminology that more accurately reflects current knowledge of precancerous lesions of the cervix. In December 1988, the Bethesda system for reporting cervicovaginal cytologic diagnoses was developed. The Bethesda system divides cervical lesions into two basic categories: low-grade squamous intraepithelial lesions (LSILs) and high-grade squamous intraepithelial lesions (HSILs). LSIL consolidates HPV cellular changes with those of CIN I. It represents a heterogeneous group of epithelial lesions that are thought to have little likelihood of progressing to cervical cancer. HSIL includes moderate dysplasia (CIN II) and severe dysplasia or carcinoma *in situ* (CIN III), suggesting a definite malignant potential.

   C. **Specimen adequacy.** If a cytology specimen is reported to be "unsatisfactory for evaluation," the Pap smear should be repeated. If a specimen is reported to be "satisfactory but limited by ...," the test may or may not be repeated, depending on the clinical situation. Specifically, the absence of a transformation zone component (endocervical cells or metaplastic squamous cells) should not be the only criterion for repeating the test. Data in the literature conflict with regard to using the presence of endocervical cells as a means of predicting the presence of a significant lesion. Cross-sectional studies demonstrate that smears with endocervical cells have a higher percentage of abnormalities than those without endocervical cells. Longitudinal studies that have followed women whose initial smears lacked endocervical cells, however, have not shown an increased detection of abnormalities on subsequent smears that contained endocervical cells, as would be expected had the first smear been associated with a higher false-negative rate (6). The 1992 National Cancer Institute (NCI) workshop on this topic concluded that if no clinical suspicion of a premalignant lesion exists in a patient with a satisfactory Pap smear result but with an inadequate transformation zone component, and if the patient's clinical history and examination findings are otherwise negative, routine follow-up is satisfactory.

 III. Molecular and epidemiologic evidence suggests that **infection with HPV** of certain types is a major risk factor for invasive cancer.

   A. **HPV screening.** HPV DNA has been detected in 80% to 90% of preinvasive and invasive carcinomas. HPV DNA also is found, however, in a high percentage of women with a normal cervix. Infection of the cervix or vagina with one or more of over 20 genital types of HPV is common, particularly among young, sexually active women. Sensitive polymerase chain reaction screening has shown that between 17% and 40% of women are positive for the HPV. A cohort study showed that the risk of developing CIN has a direct relationship to HPV infection. They showed that the cumulative incidence of CIN at 2 years after HPV DNA is confirmed was 28% among women with positive test results for HPV and 3% among those without detectable HPV DNA. The risk was highest among women with HPV types 16 and 18. Because of the high prevalence of HPV in cytologically normal women, however, general HPV screening has limited value. The long latency period between initial exposure to HPV and the development of cervical cancer and the small fraction of women with HPV who develop cervical dysplasia suggest that other factors must play an important part in carcinogenesis.

B. **HPV typing.** Clinically, HPV infection can manifest as cervical condylomas, and a dramatic increase in the incidence of both condylomas and CIN has occurred in recent years. HPV DNA typing reveals that most condylomas contain HPV types 6 and 11. The typical cytologic change seen in HPV infection is koilocytosis, which is characterized by an enlarged cell with a clear zone around the nucleus, producing a perinuclear halo. The cytologic changes induced by HPV overlap with those of CIN I and are now categorized as LSIL. HPV typing has shown that subtypes 6, 11, 31, and 35 predominate in CIN I. Subtypes 16, 18, and 33 (higher risk) predominate in CIN II and III and in low-grade CIN lesions that progress to malignancy. Type 16 is found in 50% of invasive cancers. The finding of HPV DNA, particularly of a high-risk type (16, 18, 31, 33, 35, 39, 45, 51, 52, 56, or 58), in the cervical specimen of a woman with a positive Pap smear test finding makes it more likely that the underlying lesion is a squamous intraepithelial lesion rather than a benign reactive process (4). The finding of a low-risk HPV type (6, 11, 42, 43, 44), which rarely is found in cancers in nonimmunosuppressed women, suggests that the lesion is not likely to progress (7). Although it is not possible to predict the future contribution of HPV testing to clinical practice, preliminary studies suggest that HPV typing could be clinically relevant.

IV. **The risk of progression of CIN to invasive cancer** increases with the grade of the lesion, but the behavior of CIN in any individual case remains unpredictable.
A. **HPV.** Low-grade lesions appear to have a high likelihood of regression. Evidence suggests, however, that high-risk HPV types are likely to be found in low-grade lesions that progress to invasive cancer. Most investigators have shown that low-grade lesions that contain a type of HPV that is not associated with cancer or return a negative result for HPV have little potential for progression. Greenberg and colleagues have shown that HPV types associated with cancer induced low-grade dysplasias to progress to high-grade dysplasias in approximately 9% of cases. None of the low-grade lesions without HPV or with only HPV types not associated with cancer progressed to CIN III.
B. **Pathophysiology.** Pathologically, nearly all CIN lesions arise in the transformation zone of the cervix. The transformation zone represents the area of glandular epithelium that undergoes a process of squamous metaplasia. Maximal metaplasia occurs during fetal development, adolescence, and first pregnancy. Metaplasia during adolescence is stimulated by a decrease in the vaginal pH. Cells actively undergoing metaplasia are vulnerable to carcinogens, which may explain the epidemiologic association between age of intercourse and cervical cancer. The anterior lip is affected more often than the posterior lip. CIN lesions may extend up the endocervical canal and involve endocervical glands.
V. **The Pap smear test and other diagnostic tools.** Management of cervical intraepithelial lesions is based on a combination of cytology, colposcopy, and directed biopsy.
A. **Cytology.** The goal of cervical cytology screening is to reduce the incidence of cervical cancer by detecting and treating preinvasive lesions. The Pap smear has evolved into an effective cancer screening test that allows millions of women to have potentially precancerous cervical lesions discovered and treated in a timely fashion.
1. **Screening** for cervical cancer is based on two principles: squamous cancers of the female genital tract have a well-defined preinvasive stage, and identifying precancerous lesions that have a high risk of progression can lead to early intervention and prevention of invasive cancer. The American Cancer Society and the American College of Obstetricians and Gynecologists recommend that women who are sexually active or have reached the age of 18 undergo an annual Pap smear and pelvic examination. After three or more consecutive satisfactory smear findings, the test may be performed less frequently at the discretion of the physician. It is important, however, that patients be informed that the Pap smear is not infallible. Rates of false-negative findings for CIN of 20% have been reported.

False-negative findings most commonly result from inadequate sampling, poor processing, and laboratory error.

2. **Technique.** A Pap smear is performed by placing a wooden spatula against the external os and rotating the spatula through 360 degrees. A cytobrush is inserted into the external os and rotated 180 degrees. The method of using the spatula combined with the cytobrush yields a greater number of endocervical cells and improves detection of CIN lesions. The material obtained by the cervical spatula and cytobrush is spread on a glass slide and immediately placed in fixative, usually 95% ethanol.

3. **Atypical findings.** Infection, inflammatory or reparative changes, and the effects of irradiation can result in atypical smears suggestive but not diagnostic of CIN. These smears must be repeated after a suitable interval of 3 to 6 months and after antibiotic therapy, if appropriate.

4. **Positive findings.** Every patient with a Pap smear finding that suggests HSIL (CIN II or CIN III) should be referred for colposcopy.

B. **Cervicography.** After staining the cervix twice with 3.0% to 5.0% acetic acid, two photographs (cervicograms) are taken. Cervicography is a useful adjunct to cytology because it may detect lesions that are not identified by cytology. Cervicography is limited in its ability to detect endocervical lesions, is less useful in older women than younger, and is of limited value in women whose transformation zones are not fully visible. Cervicograms are placed into one of four categories: negative, atypical, positive, and technically unsatisfactory. An atypical cervicogram suggests the presence of a minor lesion. A positive cervicogram mandates colposcopy. Some evidence suggests that the combination of cervicography and cytology improves the chances of detecting lesions and helps in triaging patients for colposcopy (8).

C. **Colposcopy.** The most important tasks in managing patients with cervical dysplasia are to rule out invasion and to determine the extent and distribution of the lesion. The colposcope is a stereoscopic, binocular magnifying instrument that allows examination of the cervix at magnifications ranging from six- to fortyfold. Some colposcopes have a green filter that allows better definition of vascular architecture by absorbing red light, thus making blood vessels appear black and more prominent. Colposcopy is inadequate to evaluate disease in the endocervical canal.

1. **Technique.** Acetic acid, 3.0% or 5.0%, is applied to the cervix. Acetic acid removes mucus and dehydrates cells. The more protein in the cell, the whiter it becomes. Normal squamous epithelium remains pink because it is glycogen rich and is not modified by acetic acid. Areas with the most pronounced colposcopic abnormalities are sampled using a small punch biopsy instrument.

2. **Abnormal or unsatisfactory results.** Abnormal features that may represent CIN include epithelium that whitens with application of acetic acid ("acetowhite"), mosaicism, and punctations. In a satisfactory colposcopic examination, the entire transformation zone as well as the full extent of the lesion is visualized. An examination designated unsatisfactory indicates that the transformation zone was not completely visualized or that the full extent of the lesion was not visualized. Under such circumstances, a cone biopsy is required, especially if a repeat Pap smear shows persistent dysplasia. Abnormal areas should prompt biopsy. Bleeding can be controlled with silver nitrate sticks or Monsel's solution (ferric sulfate).

3. Many physicians perform an **endocervical curettage** (ECC) as part of the colposcopic assessment of patients with abnormal Pap smear findings. ECC helps to evaluate the endocervical canal and to exclude the diagnoses of invasive carcinoma, unsuspected adenocarcinoma *in situ* (AIS), and invasive adenocarcinoma. Alternatively, an endocervical brush can be used to sample the endocervical canal.

VI. **Management of patients with LSILs** remains a dilemma. Approximately 2.5 million women in the United States have low-grade cytologic abnormalities of the cervix (4). It has been estimated that, in the United States, $35 billion was spent on the workup and treatment of women with mild cytologic abnormalities in 1994.

A. **Principles for evaluation.** The biological behavior of low-grade cervical lesions remains uncertain. Most Pap smear findings suggestive of LSIL, however, represent lesions that regress spontaneously. Some women with LSIL have or develop a precancerous lesion; most patients with LSIL on cytology results, however, suffer from a subclinical HPV infection and have only a small risk of developing cancer of the cervix. Between 20% and 30% of women with smear results indicating mild dysplasia have a high-grade lesion. Studies have shown a lack of correlation between cytology and histology, according to which approximately one-third of women with mildly abnormal smears have underlying CIN III (9). Such women usually are identified by continued cytologic surveillance. The clinical challenge is to distinguish the small minority of patients with LSIL that will progress to cancer from the large majority of patients with LSIL that will persist unchanged or regress spontaneously.

  1. A review of nine prospective studies from the literature reported between 1969 and 1988 showed that progression of LSIL to invasive disease occurs over 11 to 24 months. In 1987, the American College of Obstetricians and Gynecologists suggested that until tests are developed that enable physicians to distinguish lesions with progressive potential from lesions without progressive potential, HPV-associated lesions should be treated as if they were destined to progress. As a consequence, many clinicians have come to adopt the standard of care that requires patients with atypical squamous cells of undetermined significance (ASCUS) or LSIL to undergo colposcopy and directed biopsy.

  2. Nasiell and colleagues studied the behavior of mild cervical dysplasia during long-term follow-up. In this retrospective study of 550 women whose first smear suggested CIN I, a colposcopic examination was performed after a mean cytologic surveillance of 3 years. At colposcopy and biopsy, 66% of lesions were found to have regressed to normal, 22% had persisted as CIN I, and 16% had progressed to CIN II. In two patients who were lost to follow-up, invasive disease had developed by the time colposcopy was performed. The authors concluded that if regression rates are significant and surveillance identifies high-risk patients, early referral for colposcopy is not mandatory (6).

B. **Strategies for evaluation.** Two opposing policies exist for workup of LSIL. The first policy is routine referral for colposcopy, followed by frequent cytologic surveillance and either referral for repeat colposcopy if the dysplasia persists or reversion to a routine cervical screening program if cytology reverts to normal. The second policy is selective referral for colposcopy of women who are likely to fail to appear for follow-up cytologic surveillance. The advantage of routine colposcopy referral for women with a mild cytologic abnormality is that colposcopy identifies patients with a relatively high-grade lesion who may be missed by a policy of follow-up with cytology.

  1. **Surveillance with Pap test every 4 to 6 months for 2 years.** A strategy of cytologic surveillance is reasonable only if the prevalence of HSIL among the patient population being treated is low. Retrospective studies suggest that women who are successfully followed by cytology do not have an increased risk of cervical cancer if a biopsy is performed when cytologic abnormalities persist (10). It is absolutely paramount that patients managed in this fashion be considered reliable for follow-up. If follow-up smears show persistent dysplasia, colposcopy and directed biopsy are indicated. After three consecutive negative Pap smear results that are satisfactory for evaluation, the patient can be returned to a routine screening protocol.

  2. **HPV testing and cervicography** are newer techniques that may help to identify high- and low-risk patients.

  3. **Immediate colposcopic assessment after a cervical smear showing any kind of squamous intraepithelial lesion.** Advantages of routine colposcopy are that it enables prompt histologic diagnosis and decreases the problem of noncompliance. Potential adverse effects of routine colposcopy

include overtreatment and increased anxiety in some women while they are undergoing repeated smears.

C. **Follow-up.** After histologic confirmation of LSIL, if the entire transformation zone and lesion are seen, the lesion can be excised or ablated or the patient can be monitored carefully with no treatment.

    1. **Excision or ablation** should be considered for patients who are not likely to return for follow-up. Carbon dioxide laser or cryotherapy is used for ablation. Currently, the favored method for excision is the loop electro-surgical excision procedure (LEEP), which is preferred because it is both diagnostic and therapeutic. Before an ablative procedure is performed, biopsy samples must be obtained to evaluate the extent of the lesion and rule out invasion.

    2. **Monitoring with no treatment.** Because 60% of LSILs regress spontaneously, follow-up is an appropriate management strategy for compliant patients (11–13).

VII. **ASCUS.** Fifty percent of women with invasive cancer who present after cervical screening have had atypical findings on their Pap smears. Invasive cancer occurs in 0.1% of patients with atypical findings on Pap smear. Ten percent to 20% of women with atypical findings on Pap smear have high-grade CIN or invasive cancer at the time the smear is obtained. An ASCUS Pap smear finding has a higher probability of representing invasive cancer than an LSIL Pap smear finding.

A. **Incidence.** Variation exists among criteria used by different laboratories to designate ASCUS. The clinician is encouraged to communicate directly with the cytopathologist when necessary to fully explain the diagnosis of ASCUS. ASCUS corresponds to the previously used terms "atypia," "inflammatory atypia," or "class II." According to the 1992 NCI workshop, a diagnosis of ASCUS may be expected in no more than 5% of routine Pap smears. In high-risk populations with a higher prevalence of squamous intraepithelial lesions a correspondingly higher prevalence of ASCUS is to be expected.

B. **Follow-up**

    1. **Unqualified results.** Ordering follow-up Pap tests without colposcopy is an acceptable strategy if the diagnosis of ASCUS is not qualified further or if the cytopathologist favors a reactive process. In patients who are monitored using repeat Pap tests, compliance is a key component of successful management. The Pap test should be repeated every 4 to 6 months for 2 years until three consecutive negative (and adequate) Pap smear results have been returned, at which point the patient can revert to routine screening protocols. If a second ASCUS result is obtained during the 2-year follow-up period, the patient should be considered for colposcopic evaluation. Women with a diagnosis of unqualified ASCUS associated with severe inflammation should be reevaluated, preferably after 2 to 3 months.

    2. **Infections.** If specific infections such as chlamydia or gonorrhea or vaginitis caused by *Candida* or *Trichomonas* is identified, treatment with antibiotics is appropriate. The use of antibiotic creams in the absence of a specific diagnosis is not indicated.

    3. **Postmenopausal patients.** A diagnosis of ASCUS in a postmenopausal woman who is not receiving hormone-replacement therapy (HRT) has different implications than the same diagnosis in a woman of reproductive age. In postmenopausal women, atrophic cells have the appearance of parabasal cells with a high nuclear to cytoplasmic ratio and may suggest a neoplastic process; topical estrogen cream often assists in the differential diagnosis. If the Pap test result is still equivocal after an appropriate trial of estrogen therapy, the patient should be referred for colposcopy.

    4. **Results favoring neoplasm.** If the diagnosis of ASCUS favors a neoplastic process the patient should be managed as if she had a diagnosis of LSIL. If the patient with ASCUS is at high risk because of previous positive Pap test findings or poor compliance, colposcopy is indicated.

VIII. **Atypical glandular cells of undetermined significance (AGUS).** The biology of glandular precursor lesions is not clear. Until recently, AIS was thought to be rare, but preinvasive glandular disease and invasive adenocarcinoma are being recognized more frequently. AIS and endocervical glandular atypia frequently are detected in women aged 35 to 39 years and may involve one quadrant of the cervix or may be multifocal with skip lesions along the endocervical canal.

A. **Assessment.** An association between the squamous neoplasia and AIS exists, and it is postulated that HPV may be a common etiologic agent. The association may result from benign changes in endocervical or endometrial cells in reaction to AIS. Ninety percent of glandular disease occurs within 25 mm of the squamocolumnar junction. Unlike squamous lesions, glandular lesions of the cervix may be multifocal, and skip lesions are common. Although helpful, ECC can miss up to half of all endocervical lesions (14). If the cytopathology report indicates a suspicion of AIS, the endocervical canal should be evaluated; the evaluation is probably best accomplished by a cone biopsy.

B. **Follow-up** of AGUS is not established. One option is to repeat the Pap smear using a cytobrush. Endocervical and endometrial curettage and hysteroscopy may be useful in evaluating patients with AGUS. A persistent finding of AGUS that is not adequately interpreted after these procedures warrants a cone biopsy.

IX. Identifying **HSILs** should be the primary aim of cytology screening programs to maximize health gain. Overinvestigating and overtreating many young women with minor epithelial abnormalities is not cost effective and can lead to increased morbidity. All patients with cytologic evidence of HSIL on Pap smear should be referred for colposcopy and directed biopsy. Most affected women have CIN grades II and III and require treatment. After biopsy to confirm the presence of a high-grade lesion and delineation of the distribution of the lesion, excisional or ablative therapy aimed at removal or destruction of the entire lesion and the transformation zone usually is performed.

X. **Management of intraepithelial lesions during pregnancy.** Nearly 86% of all cervical abnormalities that occur during pregnancy are classified as LSILs, most of which are attributable to the HPV. The remaining 14% are HSILs. The incidence of invasive carcinoma in pregnant women ranges from 1 in 250 to 1 in 5,000. The pregnant state, with its hormonal and vascular changes, does not affect the natural history of an invasive cervical cancer even if it is stratified for stage, and no evidence that CIN progresses more rapidly to invasive cancer in pregnant patients than in nonpregnant patients exists (15) (Fig. 34-1).

XI. **Cone biopsy** can be performed using a scalpel, a small spot laser beam, or loop diathermy. The morbidity of conization is proportional to the size and length of the cone; adverse effects include cervical stenosis, incompetence, and decreased fertility caused by excision of the gland-bearing part of the endocervix that produces mucus at ovulation. A significant rate (approximately 10%) of hemorrhage requiring hospital readmission and occasional blood transfusion also is associated with cone biopsy. Indications for the procedure include the following conditions:

A. CIN II or III with a lesion that extends beyond view into the endocervical canal

B. Cytologic or colposcopic suggestion of microinvasive or invasive disease

C. A Pap smear showing HSIL with normal findings on colposcopic examination and an abnormal ECC result

D. Suspicion of adenocarcinoma that is raised by Pap smear findings

E. An unreliable patient, for whom follow-up cannot be guaranteed

XII. **Treatment of patients with a mildly abnormal Pap smear result.** There is disagreement about whether histologically confirmed, persistent LSIL should be treated. Some believe that little justification for local therapy exists. Viral changes are often extensive and difficult to treat without extensive tissue ablation. Because recurrence is likely, careful surveillance is often recommended. A small proportion (10% or less) of patients with persistent LSIL subsequently are shown to have HSIL.

XIII. **Local therapy.** For patients with a preinvasive lesion that is confirmed cytologically and completely visualized colposcopically and in which invasion has been ruled out, local therapy is appropriate. Persistent disease usually is diagnosed within 12 months. The main advantage of local therapy is that most patients can

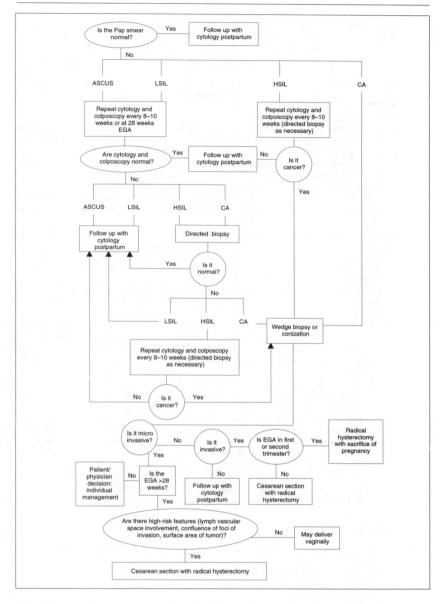

Figure 34-1. Triage algorithm used for managing pregnant women with abnormal cervical cytologic findings. Colposcopy of a pregnant cervix can be challenging even for an experienced colposcopist. Second opinions from gynecologic oncologists are often requested in these cases. ASCUS, atypical squamous cells of undetermined significance; CA, cytologic abnormalities; EGA, estimated gestational age; HSIL, high-grade squamous intraepithelial lesions; LSIL, low-grade squamous intraepithelial lesions. This algorithm is based, in part, on textual information in Campion MJ, Sedlacek TV. Colposcopy in pregnancy. *Obstet Gynecol Clin North Am* 1993;20:153–163. (From Harper DM, Roach MSI. Cervical intraepithelial neoplasia in pregnancy. *J Fam Pract* 1996;42:79–82. Reproduced with permission.)

be treated on an outpatient basis, without general anesthesia. Tissue destruction must extend to a depth of 6 to 7 mm. Most commonly quoted series indicate a 90% success rate after first treatment. Most gynecologists recommend sexual abstinence for 4 weeks after local therapy to allow healing of the transformation zone. The patient is asked to present for reassessment in 6 to 8 weeks and is followed with Pap smears every 3 to 4 months until three consecutive negative Pap smear results have been obtained, at which point the patient may be monitored with annual Pap smears. Methods of local therapy include cryotherapy, carbon dioxide laser, and LEEP.

A. Cryotherapy. A nitrous oxide cryoprobe is used. Application of the probe to the cervix produces an iceball that must extend 5 mm beyond the edge of the lesion. Contact may be improved by using a lubricant. Results are best when a double-freeze technique is used: 3 minutes of freezing, 5 minutes of thawing, 3 minutes of refreezing. Complications include uterine spasm producing a low pelvic ache and, occasionally, a feeling of faintness. A success rate of over 90% has been reported with cryotherapy. Patients should be warned that they will have a profuse watery discharge, which is sometimes bloodstained and unpleasant, for up to 3 weeks.

B. Carbon dioxide laser. Tissue is vaporized by conversion of cellular water to steam. The treatment usually can be undertaken satisfactorily in an outpatient setting using local anesthesia. Burning is the sensation most commonly experienced by patients during the procedure. Secondary hemorrhage is an unusual but recognized complication.

C. LEEP, also known as *large loop excision of the transformation zone*, has become a popular tool for evaluating patients because it is both diagnostic and therapeutic.

  1. Common **indications** include cytologic or colposcopic evidence of HSIL (CIN II or III); unsatisfactory colposcopy results in the presence of a Pap smear showing HSIL, persistent LSIL (CIN I), or LSIL in a patient with high risk of noncompliance; and the necessity of ruling out the invasive cancer of AIS.

  2. Technique. LEEP can be performed on an outpatient basis under local anesthesia using local infiltration of 1% lidocaine, with or without epinephrine; the use of a vasoconstrictor can be helpful in decreasing bleeding. Removing the specimen in one piece is preferable. Patients with CIN extending to the margin of resection should be followed with close cytologic surveillance and colposcopy rather than retreated immediately. If the limits of the lesion and the transformation zone are not entirely visible, cervical conization should be performed. The morbidity rates associated with LEEP are relatively low; bleeding and discomfort are common short-term sequelae of LEEP. Long-term effects on fertility and obstetric morbidity have not been clearly defined. The success rate is greater than 90%.

References

1. Campion MJ, Reid R. Screening for gynecologic cancer. *Obstet Gynecol Clin North Am* 1990;17:695–727.
2. Christopherson WM, Lundin FE Jr, Mendez WM, Parker JE. Cervical cancer control: study of morbidity and mortality trends over a twenty-one-year period. *Cancer* 1976;38:1357–1366.
3. Brinton LA, Hamman RF, Juggins GH, et al. Sexual and reproductive risk factors for invasive squamous cell cervical cancer. *J Natl Cancer Inst* 1987;79:23–30.
4. Kurman RJ, Henson DE, Herbst AL, Noller KL, Schiffman MH. Interim guidelines for management of abnormal cervical cytology. *JAMA* 1994;271:1866–1869.
5. Trevathan E, Layde P, Webster LA, et al. Cigarette smoking and dysplasia and carcinoma *in situ* of the uterine cervix. *JAMA* 1983;250:499–502.
6. Mitchell H, Medley G. Longitudinal study of women with negative cervical smears according to endocervical status: Victorian Cytology Service, Melbourne, Australia. *Lancet* 1991;337:265–267.

7. Lorincz AT, Reid R, Jenson AB, Greenberg MD, Lancaster W, Kurman RJ. Human papilloma virus infection of the cervix: relative risk association of 15 common anogenital types. *Obstet Gynecol* 1992;79:328–337.

8. Reid R, Greenberg MD, Lorincz A, et al. Should cervical cytologic testing be augmented by cervicography or human papilloma virus deoxyribonucleic acid detection? *Am J Obstet Gynecol* 1991;164:1461–1471.

9. Giles JA, Hudson EA, Crow J, Williams D, Walker P. Colposcopic assessment of the accuracy of cervical cytology screening. *Br Med J* 1998;316:1099–1102.

10. Flannelly G, Kitchener H. Every woman with an abnormal cervical smear should be referred for treatment: debate. *Clin Obstet Gynecol* 1995;38(3):585–591.

11. Montz FJ, Bradley JM, Fowler JM, Nguyen L. Natural history of the minimally abnormal Papanicolaou smear. *Obstet Gynecol* 1992;80:385–388.

12. Nasiell K, Roger V, Nasiell M. Behavior of mild cervical dysplasia during long term follow up. *Obstet Gynecol* 1986;67:665–669.

13. Brown MS, Phillips GL. Management of the mildly abnormal Pap smears: a conservative approach. *Gynecol Oncol* 1985;22:149–153.

14. Andersen W, Frierson H, Barber S, Tabbarah S, Taylor P, Underwood P. Sensitivity and specificity of endocervical curettage and the endocervical brush for the evaluation of the endocervical canal. *Am J Obstet Gynecol* 1988;159:702–707.

15. Harper D, Roach M. Cervical intraepithelial neoplasia in pregnancy. *J Fam Pract* 1996;42:79–83.

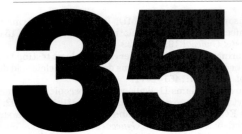

Vulvar and Vaginal Cancers

Cornelia Liu Trimble
and Edward Trimble

I. **Vulvar neoplasms.** It is estimated that 3% to 4% of all primary malignancies of the female genital tract develop on the vulva.

   A. **Squamous carcinoma** is the most common type of histopathology found in vulvar carcinoma, comprising over 85% of cases. Squamous carcinomas of the vulva have one of two distinct etiologies: either associated with or not associated with human papillomavirus (HPV).

      1. **Vulvar carcinoma associated with HPV** tends to occur in younger women than carcinoma not associated with HPV, and risk factors are similar to those for cervical carcinoma, including early age at first intercourse, multiple lifetime sexual partners, and cigarette smoking. Like squamous cancers of the cervix, this type of vulvar carcinoma is associated with an intraepithelial precursor lesion, vulvar intraepithelial neoplasia (VIN). HPV types most commonly found in these lesions are 16 and 18. Because VINs tend to be multifocal, colposcopy of the entire lower genital tract, including the cervix, vagina, and vulva, is warranted.

        a. **Pathological features.** Like cervical dysplasia, vulvar dysplasia may involve only the deeper layers of the epidermis and rete pegs (VIN 1). As cellular atypia progresses, lack of maturation of the nucleus and cytoplasm is seen in cell layers closer to the surface (VIN 2). Full-thickness atypia is called VIN 3. Grossly, VIN 3 lesions are slightly elevated, rough, and delineated and are white, red, or brown in color.

        b. **Assessment.** Initial evaluation should include vulvar colposcopy and full-thickness biopsy. After the diagnosis of VIN has been confirmed, the lesion should be removed with a wide local excision. Occasionally, laser ablation is used for a lesion close to the urethra or clitoris. The rate of progression from VIN to invasive vulvar cancer is low; progression also appears to be slow, over years to decades.

      2. **Vulvar carcinoma not associated with HPV** tends to occur in older women. Affected patients often give a history of pruritus. No known precursor lesion develops, although either lichen sclerosus or squamous hyperplasia often are found near these cancers, which are usually unifocal.

      3. **Treatment** of small vulvar carcinomas may be initially surgical; larger lesions, particularly those close to the urethra, vagina, or rectum, are treated best initially with primary chemoradiation, which generally enables more conservative surgery that preserves function and body image. For smaller lesions, the primary surgery generally is tailored to the lesion. The procedure, which is more conservative than a traditional radical vulvectomy, has been termed a radical local excision, or partial vulvectomy. The lateral margins should be 1 to 2 cm, and the deep margin should extend to the urogenital diaphragm. Inguinal lymph node dissection is reserved for lesions with invasions of 3 mm or deeper, or lesions with lymphovascular invasion. Inguinal node dissection is unilateral for lateralized lesions and bilateral for central lesions. Adjuvant pelvic radiation therapy is indicated for patients with more than two affected inguinal lymph nodes.

B. Basal cell carcinomas constitute 2% to 3% of all vulvar carcinomas and occur most commonly in postmenopausal white women. Most patients experience pruritus. Grossly, these lesions appear as a whitish nodule or plaque. The prognosis is good, despite a roughly 20% risk of local recurrence. Metastases to the inguinal lymph nodes are rare; wide local excision is usually sufficient treatment.

C. Verrucous carcinoma is a variant of squamous carcinoma that occurs in post-menopausal women. The tumors of verrucous carcinoma are large, fungating masses that may present as mistakenly diagnosed condyloma acuminata resistant to treatment. Because the histologic appearance of verrucous carcinoma so closely resembles normal squamous epithelium, a sufficiently deep biopsy must be obtained for diagnosis. It is prudent to include a good clinical history with the specimen. Although lymph node metastasis is exceedingly rare, tumor recurrence is common. Treatment consists of radical local excision. Radiation is contraindicated because it may induce increased aggression in malignant activity.

D. Melanomas constitute the second most common primary malignancy of the vulva, with a peak frequency in the sixth to seventh decades of life. The lesions of melanomas are typically raised, with irregular pigmentation and irregular borders. The lesions are found with roughly equal frequency on the labia majora and on mucosal surfaces. Prognosis largely depends on tumor thickness and on the presence or absence of lymph node involvement. Radical local excision is recommended for the primary lesion. The role of regional lymphadenectomy is not well defined.

E. Paget's disease of the vulva is rare. Most affected patients are in their seventh or eighth decade of life and experience local irritation and pruritus. The lesion has slightly raised edges and is red, with islands of white epithelium. The lesions are sharply demarcated and often have foci of excoriation and induration. Unlike Paget's disease of the breast, in the majority of cases no underlying adenocarcinoma is found. An adenocarcinoma of the underlying sweat glands is found in 15% to 20% of patients who have intraepithelial Paget's disease.

    1. If the disease is limited to the epithelium, its clinical course may be both prolonged and indolent. Wide local excision is the mainstay of treatment. While grossly wide surgical margins are indicated, the use of frozen section evaluation of margins at the time of operation is a subject of controversy. Although recurrence is common when the surgical margins show positive findings, the histology on permanent section is more accurate than that possible on frozen section.

    2. If an underlying adenocarcinoma is identified, the patient should undergo radical excision and inguinal lymphadenectomy. The prognosis in patients with lymph node involvement is poor.

F. Sarcomas of the vulva are rare.

    1. Leiomyosarcomas are the most common of the vulvar sarcomas. These lesions develop most frequently in the labium majus or in the region of Bartholin's glands. Standard treatment includes radical local excision. An effective chemotherapeutic agent has not yet been developed for this disease.

    2. Rhabdomyosarcoma is the most common soft tissue tumor of childhood. In 20% of cases, the pelvis or genitourinary system is involved. In such cases, the vagina is more frequently affected than the vulva. Combination chemotherapy generally is used as primary treatment, followed by conservative surgery.

    3. Alveolar soft part sarcoma most frequently involves the soft tissue of extremities in young adults. Very rarely, alveolar soft part sarcoma can involve the vulva. Standard therapy consists of radical local excision.

    4. Dermatofibrosarcoma protuberans is a low-grade sarcoma that rarely occurs in the vulva. This lesion may appear initially as an indurated plaque on which multiple firm, reddish or bluish nodules may appear.

Although the lesion may recur locally, systemic metastases are uncommon. Standard therapy consists of radical local excision.

   5. **Malignant fibrous histiocytoma,** although uncommon, is the second most common vulvar sarcoma in adults. The tumor involves deep soft tissue and skeletal muscle. The patient presents with a solitary mass that grows relatively rapidly. Although first-line therapy consists of radical local excision, radiation therapy has been reported to decrease the rate of local recurrence.

II. **Vaginal neoplasms.** The majority of vaginal neoplasms are squamous cell lesions. It is thought that most vaginal squamous cell lesions are associated with HPV infection. Patients with malignant squamous lesions of the cervix and vulva are at increased risk of having vaginal lesions as well. Careful examination and colposcopy of the vagina should be performed on patients in whom a vulvar or cervical cancer is diagnosed. The spectrum of squamous lesions parallels that of squamous lesions in the cervix or vulva and ranges from vaginal intraepithelial lesions (VAINs, classified as VAIN 1, 2, or 3, depending on the thickness of the atypia) to invasive vaginal carcinoma. VAINs may be treated with local excision, laser ablation, or topical 5-fluorouracil cream. Early-stage vaginal cancer may be treated with local excision, brachytherapy, or both, whereas advanced-stage vaginal cancer is treated best with radiation therapy.

   A. **Clear cell carcinomas** of the vagina are uncommon. In women exposed to diethylstilbestrol (DES) *in utero*, particularly before 18 weeks' gestation, however, careful surveillance of the vagina and cervix is prudent. DES was used until 1972 to treat pregnant women thought to be at risk for miscarriage. Although most patients with DES-related clear cell carcinoma of the vagina are diagnosed between the ages of 18 and 24 years, the oldest reported patient with a clear cell primary cancer of the vagina was 42 years old at the time of diagnosis.

      1. **Diagnosis.** The most frequent location of clear cell adenocarcinoma is the upper one-third of the vagina. Many clear cell adenocarcinomas occur on the anterior surface and may present as a submucosal nodule. Therefore, it is necessary to rotate the speculum 90 degrees to visualize the anterior vaginal wall in addition to performing a careful bimanual examination. Many patients present with abnormal bleeding or vaginal discharge. The most important prognostic factor is stage at diagnosis.

      2. **Treatment.** Small tumors limited to the vagina may be treated with partial vaginal excision and brachytherapy. Larger tumors or tumors close to the cervix may require partial vaginectomy, radical hysterectomy, and pelvic lymph node dissection. Patients with high-stage disease are treated with radiation.

   B. **Sarcoma botryoides** occurs most often in children younger than 5 years. In this group, sarcoma botryoides is the most common vaginal neoplasm. As the age of the patient increases, the most common site of occurrence moves distally. The most common presenting symptom is vaginal bleeding. The lesion manifests as one or more polypoid excrescences that are pinkish-red and translucent. Conservative surgery after neoadjuvant chemoradiation is the current standard of treatment.

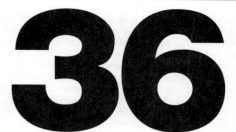

Cervical Cancer

Robert Bristow
and Albert Steren

I. Epidemiology

A. Incidence. Cervical cancer is the second most common cancer among women worldwide, following breast cancer. Carcinoma of the uterine cervix is the third most common malignant gynecologic neoplasm in the United States. Mortality and incidence rates for cervical cancer have declined in most developed countries, with declines being attributed to the introduction of screening with the Pap smear (see Chap. 34). The American Cancer Society estimated that in 1995 there were 15,800 new cases of invasive cervical carcinoma diagnosed in the United States, with 4,800 deaths due to this disease. The mean age for diagnosis of cervical cancer is 52.2 years, and the distribution of cases is bimodal, with peaks at 35 to 39 years and 60 to 64 years.

B. Risk factors

1. Race. The rate of cervical cancer among African-Americans remains about twice as high at all ages as among whites. The incidence is also approximately two times higher for Hispanic Americans and even higher for Native Americans, while Asian groups experience rates similar to or lower than whites. These differences are at least partially accounted for by the strong inverse association between cervical cancer incidence and socioeconomic factors. When socioeconomic differences are controlled for, the excess risk of cervical cancer among African-Americans is substantially reduced from over 70% to less than 30%. Racial differences are also apparent in survival; 57% of all African-Americans with cervical cancer survive 5 years, compared with 69% of all whites with the disease.

2. Sexual and reproductive history. First intercourse before the age of 16 is associated with a twofold increased risk of cervical cancer compared with women with first intercourse after the age of 20. Cervical cancer risk is also directly proportional to the number of lifetime sexual partners. These characteristics of sexual behavior are considered measures of a sexually transmitted infectious pathogen involved in cervical neoplasia. However, there may be evidence indicating that both early age at first coitus and number of sexual partners have independent effects. Similarly, increasing parity appears to be a separate risk factor even after controlling for socioeconomic and reproductive characteristics. In contrast, there is little evidence to support an association between age at menarche, age at menopause, or character of menses and carcinoma of the cervix.

3. Cigarette smoking has emerged as an important etiologic factor in cervical carcinoma. The increased risk for smokers is approximately twofold, with a dose-response relationship to duration and intensity of smoking.

4. The data on oral **contraceptive use** and cervical cancer is complicated by the correlation between oral contraceptive use and sexual behavior, patterns of screening, potential surveillance bias, selection bias, and the inability to control for human papillomavirus (HPV) in earlier studies. Thus, interpretation of studies showing increased and decreased risks remains difficult, and data should be interpreted with caution. Use of barrier methods of contraception, especially those that combine both mechanical and chemical protection, have been shown to lower the risk of cervical cancer, presumably because of reduced exposure to infectious agents.

5. **Male partner contribution.** The sexual histories of the male partners of women with cervical cancer may be etiologically important. In several studies, the husbands of cervical cancer patients have reported significantly more sexual partners when compared with control husbands. In addition, husbands of affected women have also been more likely to report a history of venereal infections, early sexual experiences, affairs during marriage, and visits to prostitutes. Although it is possible that males may carry and transmit the etiologic agent, evidence for this hypothesis has been difficult to demonstrate.

6. **Immunosuppression.** Cell-mediated immunity appears to be a factor in the development of cervical cancer. Immunocompromised women [e.g., renal transplant, human immunodeficiency virus (HIV) infected] may not only be at higher risk of developing the disease but also demonstrate more rapid progression from preinvasive to invasive lesions. HIV-positive patients also appear to have more advanced disease at diagnosis than HIV-negative patients.

C. **Etiology.** Evidence supports the significant role of **HPV** infection in the etiology of cervical neoplasia. These DNA tumor viruses colonize mucosal or cutaneous epithelium and induce hyperproliferation, which results in the formation of warts at the site of infection. Based on differences in DNA sequencing, more than 70 different types of HPV have been identified, more than 20 of which are known to infect the anogenital tract. HPV types 16, 18, 31, 45, 51–53, and 56 are associated with invasive carcinoma. HPV DNA (predominantly types 16, 18, and 31) has been isolated from 80% to 100% of cervical carcinomas.

II. **Detection and prevention**

A. **Screening.** Cervical neoplasia is presumed to be a continuum, from dysplasia to carcinoma *in situ* to invasive carcinoma. For this reason, screening for cervical cancer with the use of exfoliative cytology (Pap smear) can have significant effects on the incidence, morbidity, and mortality from invasive disease by facilitating the eradication of precursor lesions. A single negative Pap smear may decrease the risk of developing cervical cancer by 45%, and nine negative smears during a lifetime decreases the risk by as much as 99%. Eddy, using a mathematical model, indicated that in women 35 to 64 years of age, screening intervals of 10, 5, and 3 years reduced the incidence of invasive cervical cancer by 64%, 84%, and 91%, respectively (1).

B. **Prevention**

1. **Current methods.** Protection from sexually transmitted disease and cessation of smoking both decrease risks of cervical cancer and should be encouraged.

2. **Potential methods**

a. **Chemoprophylaxis.** Given the prolonged preinvasive phase of the accessibility of the cervix, chemo prevention of precursor lesions is promising.

b. **HPV vaccine.** The significant role of HPV infection has stimulated investigators to pursue the development of vaccines that could be used in prevention as well as treatment efforts. An efficacious vaccine could conceivably eradicate cervical cancer as a public health issue.

III. **Clinical presentation**

A. **Presenting symptoms.** The most common symptom of cervical cancer is abnormal vaginal bleeding or discharge. Abnormal bleeding may take the form of postcoital spotting, intermenstrual bleeding, or heavy menstrual bleeding (menorrhagia). Serosanguinous or yellowish vaginal discharge, at times foul-smelling, may occur with particularly advanced and necrotic carcinomas. Pelvic pain may result from locally advanced disease or tumor necrosis. Extension to the pelvic sidewall may cause sciatic pain or back pain associated with hydronephrosis. Metastatic involvement of the iliac and paraaortic lymph nodes can extend into the lumbosacral nerve roots and also present as lum-

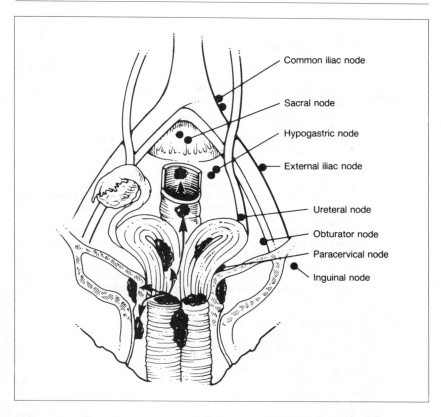

Figure 36-1. Possible sites of direct extension of cervical cancer to adjoining organs or metastases to regional lymph nodes. The uterus, cervix, and vagina are depicted bisected and opened to reveal the possible sites of tumor implantation. (From Scott JR, DiSaia PJ, Hammond CB, Spellacy WN. *Danforth's obstetrics & gynecology*, 7th ed. Philadelphia: Lippincott–Raven, 1997:909. Reprinted with permission.)

bosacral back pain. Bladder or rectal invasion by advanced stage disease may produce urinary or rectal symptoms (e.g., hematuria, hematochezia).
- **B. Physical findings.** Cervical carcinoma most commonly appears as an exophytic cervical mass that characteristically bleeds on contact. With endophytic tumors the neoplasm develops entirely within the endocervical canal and the external cervix may appear normal. In these cases, bimanual examination may reveal a firm, indurated, often barrel-shaped cervix. Cervical cancer may also take the form of a small, shallow, ulcerative crater.
- **C. Spread of disease** (Fig. 36-1)
  - **1. Direct extension**
    - **a. Paracervical and parametrial extension.** The lateral spread of cervical cancer occurs through the cardinal ligament, and significant involvement of the medial portion of this ligament may result in ureteral obstruction. Tumor cells commonly spread through parametrial lymphatic vessels to expand and replace parametrial lymph nodes. These individual tumor masses enlarge and become confluent, eventually replacing the normal parametrial tissue. Less commonly, the

central tumor mass reaches the pelvic sidewall by direct contiguous extension of the tumor from the cervix through the cardinal ligament.

   b. Vaginal extension. The upper vagina is frequently involved (50% of cases) when the primary tumor has extended beyond the confines of the cervix. Anterior extension through the vesicovaginal septum is most common, often obliterating the dissection plane between the bladder and underlying cervical tumor and making surgical therapy difficult or impossible. A deep posterior cul-de-sac can represent an anatomic barrier to direct tumor spread from the cervix and vagina to the rectum posteriorly.

   c. Bladder and rectal involvement. Anterior and posterior spread of cervical cancer to the bladder and rectum is uncommon in the absence of lateral parametrial disease. Twenty percent of patients with clinical stage IIIB disease have biopsy-proven bladder invasion.

  2. Lymphatic spread of cervical carcinoma follows an orderly and reasonably predictable pattern. The most commonly involved, in descending order of incidence, are the obturator, external iliac, and hypogastric lymph node groups (see Fig. 36-1). The parametrial, inferior gluteal, and presacral lymph nodes are less frequently involved. Secondary nodal involvement (common iliac, paraaortic) rarely occurs in the absence of primary nodal disease. The percentage of involved lymph nodes increases directly with primary tumor volume. Rarely, retrograde lymphatic embolization may occur to the inguinal lymph nodes. In patients with clinically advanced or recurrent disease, metastatic disease may be detected in the scalene nodes.

IV. Staging

  A. Clinical staging. In 1995, the International Federation of Gynecology and Obstetrics (FIGO) revised the clinical staging of cervical carcinoma (Table 36-1 and Fig. 36-2). The most notable changes were for stage IA1 (microinvasive carcinoma), which is now defined as stromal invasion no greater than 3.0 mm in depth and no wider than 7.0 mm. This new definition reflects data indicating that patients with less than 3.0 mm of invasion are at very low risk of metastatic disease and may be treated more conservatively (Table 36-2). The second significant change in the clinical staging system was the inclusion of stages IB1 and IB2, reflecting the prognostic importance of tumor volume for macroscopic lesions limited to the cervix. The distribution of patients by clinical stage is 38% stage 1, 32% stage II, 26% stage III, and 4% stage IV.

    FIGO's clinical staging system for cervical carcinoma is based on clinical evaluation (inspection, palpation, colposcopy), radiographic examination of the chest, kidneys, and skeleton, and endocervical curettage and biopsies as needed. Lymphangiograms, arteriograms, computed tomographic (CT) scan findings, magnetic resonance imaging, and laparoscopy and laparotomy findings should not be used for clinical staging (Table 36-3). Routine laboratory studies should include a complete blood cell count, electrolyte and chemistry panel, and urinalysis.

    Evaluation of disease extent. The clinical stage is determined by inspection and palpation of the cervix, vagina, and pelvis and by examination of extrapelvic areas, specifically the abdomen and supraclavicular lymph nodes. It is important to palpate the entire vagina to determine whether disease is limited to the cervix (IB), extends to the upper two-thirds of the vagina (IIA), or also involves the lower one-third of the vagina (IIIA). Tumor extension into the parametrial tissue (IIB) or to the pelvic sidewall (IIIB) is best appreciated on rectovaginal examination. Examination under anesthesia is preferred. When there is doubt concerning which stage a tumor should be assigned, the earlier stage is chosen. Once a clinical stage has been determined and treatment has begun, subsequent findings on either extended clinical staging or surgical exploration should not alter the assigned stage. Assignment of a more advanced stage during treatment will result in an

Table 36-1. Staging for carcinoma of the cervix uteri (FIGO, 1995)

Stage	Description	Comments[a]
Stage 0	Carcinoma *in situ*, intra-epithelial carcinoma.	
Stage I	The carcinoma is strictly confined to the cervix.	The diagnosis of both stage IA1 and IA2 cases should be based on microscopic examination of removed tissue, preferably a cone, which must include the entire lesion. The lower limit of stage IA2 should be measurable macroscopically (even if dots need to be placed on the slide prior to measurement), and the upper limit of stage IA2 is given by measurement of the two largest dimensions in any given section. The depth of invasion should not be more than 5 mm taken from the base of the epithelium, either surface or glandular, from which it originates. The second dimension, the horizontal spread, must not exceed 7 mm. Vascular space involvement, either venous or lymphatic, should not alter the staging but should be specifically recorded, as it may affect treatment decisions in the future.
Stage IA	Invasive cancer identified only microscopically. All gross lesions, even with superficial invasion, are stage IB cancers. Invasion is limited to measured stromal invasion with maximum depth of 5 mm and width of 7 mm.[a]	
Stage IA1	Measured invasion of stroma no greater than 3 mm in depth and no wider than 7 mm.	
Stage IA2	Measured invasion of stroma greater than 3 mm and no greater than 5 mm in depth, and no wider than 7 mm.	
Stage IB	Clinical lesions confined to the cervix or preclinical lesions greater than stage IA.	Lesions of greater size should be classified as stage IB. As a rule, it is impossible to estimate clinically whether a cancer of the cervix has extended to the corpus or not. Extension to the corpus should therefore be disregarded. A patient with a growth fixed to the pelvic wall by a short and indurated but not nodular parametrium should be assigned to stage IIB. It is impossible, at clinical examination, to decide whether a smooth and indurated parametrium is truly cancerous or only inflammatory. Therefore, the case should be placed in stage III only if their parametrium is nodular on the pelvic wall or if the growth itself extends to the pelvic wall.
Stage IB1	Clinical lesions no greater than 4 cm.	
Stage IB2	Clinical lesions greater than 4 cm.	
Stage II	The carcinoma extends beyond the cervix but has not extended to the pelvic wall. The carcinoma involves the vagina but not as far as the lower one-third.	
Stage IIA	No obvious parametrial involvement.	
Stage IIB	Obvious parametrial involvement.	
Stage III	The carcinoma has extended to the pelvic wall. On rectal examination, there is no cancer-free space between the tumor and the pelvic wall. The tumor involves the lower one-third of the vagina. All cases with a hydronephrosis or nonfunctioning kidney are	The presence of hydronephrosis or nonfunctioning kidney due to stenosis of the ureter by cancer permits a case to be allotted to stage III even if, according to the other findings, the case should be assigned to stage I or stage II.

(continued)

Table 36-1. (continued)

Stage	Description	Comments
	included unless they are known to be due to other causes.	
Stage IIIA	No extension to the pelvic wall.	
Stage IIIB	Extension to the pelvic wall and/or hydrone-phrosis or nonfunc-tioning kidney.	
Stage IV	The carcinoma has extended beyond the true pelvis or has clinically involved the mucosa of the bladder or rectum. A bullous edema as such does not permit a case to be allotted to stage IV.	The presence of bullous edema, as such, should not permit a case to be assigned to stage IV. Ridges and furrows in the bladder wall should be interpreted as signs of sub-mucous involvement of the bladder if they remain fixed to the growth during palpation (i.e., examination from the vagina or the rectum during cystoscopy). A finding of malignant cells in cytologic washings from the urinary bladder requires further examination and biopsy from the wall of the bladder.
Stage IVA	Spread of the growth to adjacent organs.	
Stage IVB	Spread to distant organs.	

FIGO, International Federation of Gynecology and Obstetrics.
[a]The depth of invasion should not be more than 5 mm taken from the base of the epithelium, either surface or glandular, from which it originates. Vascular space involvement, either venous or lymphatic, should not alter the staging.
From Shingleton HM, Orr JW. *Cervical cancer*. Philadelphia: JB Lippincott Co, 1995. Reprinted with permission.

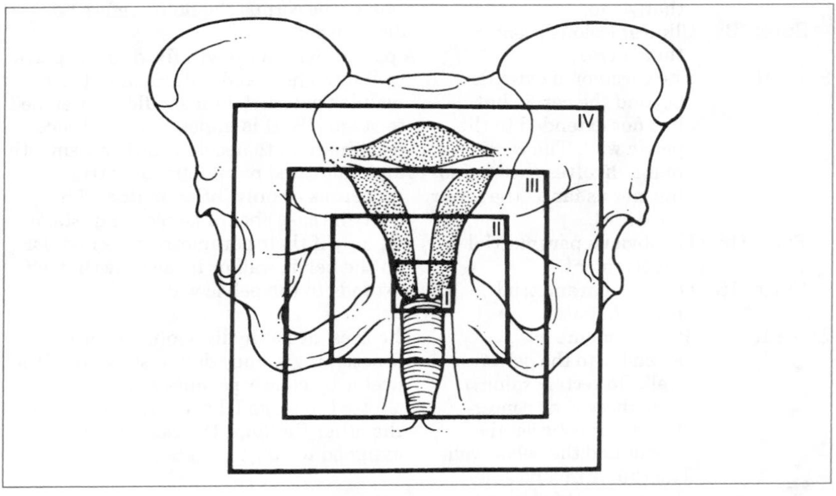

Figure 36-2. Clinical stages of carcinoma of the cervix. In stage I, only the cervix is involved. In stage II, the parametrium or upper two-thirds of the vagina is involved. In stage III, the malignancy extends to the pelvic sidewalls or involves the lower one-third of the vagina. In stage IV, areas beyond the true pelvis are involved. (From Scott JR, DiSaia PJ, Hammond CB, Spellacy WN. *Danforth's obstetrics & gynecology*, 7th ed. Philadelphia: Lippincott–Raven, 1997:910. Reprinted with permission.)

Table 36-2. Incidence of pelvic and paraaortic nodal metastasis by stage

Stage	Positive pelvic nodes (%)	Positive paraaortic nodes (%)
Ia1	0	0
Ia2		
(1–3 mm)	0.6	0
(3–5 mm)	4.8	<1
Ib	15.9	2.2
IIa	24.5	11
IIb	31.4	19
III	44.8	30
IVa	55	40

From Berek JS, Hacker NF, eds. *Practical gynecologic oncology,* 2nd ed. Baltimore: Williams & Wilkins, 1994. Adapted with permission.

Table 36-3. Staging procedures

Physical examination[a]	Palpate lymph nodes
	Examine vagina
	Bimanual rectovaginal examination (under anesthesia recommended)
Radiologic studies[a]	I.v. pyelogram
	Barium enema
	Chest x-ray film
	Skeletal x-ray film
Procedures[a]	Biopsy
	Conization
	Hysteroscopy
	Colposcopy
	Endocervical curettage
	Cystoscopy
	Proctoscopy
Optional studies[b]	Computed tomographic scan
	Lymphangiography
	Ultrasonography
	Magnetic resonance imaging
	Radionucleotide scanning
	Laparoscopy

[a]Allowed by International Federation of Gynecology and Obstetrics (FIGO).
[b]Information that is not allowed by FIGO to change the clinical stage.
From Berek JS, Hacker NF, eds. *Practical gynecologic oncology,* 2nd ed. Baltimore: Williams & Wilkins, 1994. Adapted with permission.

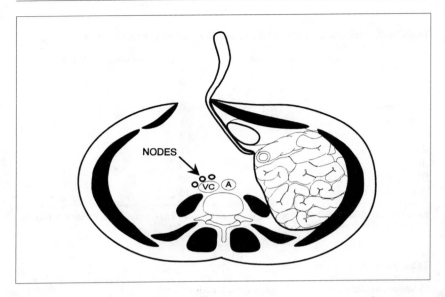

Figure 36-3. Representation of the abdominal contents in the peritoneal envelope displaced to the patient's left, allowing dissection of nodes between the renal vessels and the bifurcation of the iliac vessels. A, aorta; VC, vena cava. (From Shingleton HM, Orr JW Jr. *Cancer of the cervix: diagnosis and treatment.* New York: Churchill Livingstone, 1995:110. Reprinted with permission.)

apparent, but deceptive, improvement in the results of treatment for early-stage disease.

B. **Surgical staging.** The 1995 FIGO staging classification for cervical cancer is based on pretherapy clinical findings. Only the subclassifications of stage I (IA1, IA2) require pathologic assessment. Discrepancies between clinical staging and surgicopathologic findings range from 17.3% to 38.5% in patients with clinical stage I disease to 42.9% to 89.5% in patients with stage III disease. This has led some to emphasize surgical staging of cervical carcinoma to identify occult tumor spread, determine the presence of extrapelvic disease, and offer adjunctive or extended field radiation therapy. Transperitoneal surgical staging procedures followed by abdominopelvic irradiation is associated with appreciable complications, particularly enteric morbidity. The extraperitoneal surgical approach can be performed through a paraumbilical or paramedian incision and allows accurate assessment of disease status (Fig. 36-3). It is associated with few complications, and does not significantly delay institution of radiation therapy. The role of laparoscopic surgical staging for cervical cancer is yet to be determined.

V. **Prognostic variables**

A. **Tumor characteristics.** Prognostic variables directly related to surgicopathologic tumor characteristics and their effect upon survival were compiled by the National Cancer Institute's Surveillance, Epidemiology, and End Results program for the period 1973 to 1987 (2). This study, which includes 17,119 cases of invasive cervical cancer, indicates that FIGO stage, tumor histology, histologic grade, and lymph node status are all independent prognostic variables relating to survival. In addition, tumor volume and depth of invasion have also been shown to have a significant impact on survival (Table 36-4).

Table 36-4. Prognostic variables: tumor characteristic

Characteristic	5-year survival
Stage[a]	
IA	97.0%
IB	78.9%
IIA	54.9%
IIB	51.6%
IIIA	40.5%
IIIB	27.0%
IV	12.4%
Histology[a]	
Squamous	67.2%
Adenocarcinoma	67.7%
Adenosquamous	54.9%
Grade[a]	
Well-differentiated	74.5%
Moderately differentiated	63.7%
Poorly differentiated	51.4%
Lymph node status[a]	
Negative	75.2%
Positive pelvic	45.6%
Positive paraaortic	15.4%
Tumor volume[b]	
<2 cm	90%
>2 cm	60%
>4 cm	40%
Depth of invasion[c,d]	
<10 mm	86–94%
11–20 mm	71–75%
>20 mm	60%

[a]From ref. 2, with permission.
[b]From Hatch KD. Cervical cancer. In: Berek JS, Hacker NF, eds. *Practical gynecologic oncology*, 2nd ed. Baltimore: Williams & Wilkins, 1994.
[c]From ref. 3, with permission.
[d]3-year survival.

1. **Stage.** Clinical stage of disease at the time of presentation is the most important determinant of subsequent survival regardless of treatment modality. Five-year survival declines as FIGO stage at diagnosis increases from stage IA (97%) to stage IV (12.4%). Significant declines in survival are seen for every stage compared with stage IA.
2. **Histology.** There are conflicting data on the influence of histologic subtype on tumor behavior, prognosis, and survival. Adenosquamous carcinoma is associated with lower survival rates compared with similar stage squamous tumors and adenocarcinomas.
3. **Histologic grade.** Significant decreases in 5-year survival rates are associated with histologic grades of moderately differentiated (63.7%) and poorly differentiated (51.4%) compared with well-differentiated tumors (74.5%).
4. **Lymph node involvement.** Among surgically treated patients, survival is directly related to the number and location of lymph node metastases.

For all stages of disease, when both pelvic and paraaortic lymph nodes are negative, 5-year survival is 75.2%. Survival decreases to 45.6% with positive pelvic nodes, while involvement of paraaortic nodes lowers 5-year survival to 15.4%. Patients with bilateral pelvic lymph node involvement have a worse prognosis than those with unilateral disease. The recurrence rate is 35% for patients with one positive node, 59% with two or three, and 69% with more than three positive nodes.

5. **Tumor volume.** Lesion size is an important predictor of survival independent of other factors. Larger tumor volume is associated with higher rates of parametrial involvement and decreased survival. For stages IB through IIB, 5-year survival decreases from 84.9% to 69.6% when the parametria are involved with tumor.

6. **Depth of invasion.** Survival is also strongly correlated with depth of tumor invasion into the stroma, with 3-year survival rates of 86% to 94% for depths less than 10 mm, 71% to 75% for 11 to 20 mm, and 60% for 21 mm of invasion (3).

B. **Host factors**

1. **Age.** Whether younger women have a lower survival rate than older women with the same stage of cervical cancer remains controversial. Some investigators have reported lower 5-year survival rates in women younger than 35 to 40 years (4,5). However, most studies have no matched controls and do not control for tumor volume within stage. Other investigators have found no survival difference for women above or below the age of 35 for squamous carcinomas and adenocarcinomas, but decreased survival for younger women with adenosquamous tumors (6).

2. **Anemia.** The incidence of pretreatment anemia (Hgb 12 g/dL) increases with advancing stage of disease, occurring in 25%, 33%, and 45% of patients with stages I, II, and III disease, respectively. Anemia is associated with more frequent pelvic recurrences and decreased survival, primarily due to the higher incidence of failed radiation therapy in these patients. Tumor hypoxia is the proposed mechanism of radioresistance in the presence of anemia. Transfusion to a Hgb 10 g/dL, as well as appropriate vitamin and mineral supplementation, should be considered before beginning radiation therapy. Another prognostic hematologic parameter is thrombocytosis ($>400,000/mm^3$), which has been associated with decreased survival after controlling for cell type, stage, and age.

3. **Coexisting medical conditions.** Coexistent medical problems such as diabetes or hypertension are frequently associated with significant vascular disease and potentially contribute to both tumor hypoxia and decreased blood supply to normal pelvic tissues. Patients with such conditions are subject to a higher incidence of treatment complications, pelvic recurrence, as well as decreased survival. Pelvic inflammatory disease produces a reactive vasculitis, which when combined with radiation therapy can lead to higher incidence of intestinal complications.

VI. **Pathology** (Table 36-5)

A. **Microinvasive carcinoma (MICA).** MICA is a lesion not apparent clinically that is diagnosed by histologic examination of a cone biopsy or hysterectomy specimen that includes the entire lesion. Involvement of the cone margins by invasive carcinoma or even a high-grade intraepithelial lesion precludes a diagnosis of MICA, because deeper invasion may exist higher in the endocervix. Histologically, MICA is characterized by the presence of irregularly shaped tongues of epithelium projecting from the base of an intraepithelial lesion into the stroma. The FIGO staging system of cervical carcinoma separates microscopic lesions into stage IA1 (measured invasion of stroma ≤3.0 mm in depth and no wider than 7.0 mm) and stage IA2 (stromal invasion of 3.1 to 5.0 mm and <7.0 mm). Lymph vascular involvement does not alter classification. The Society of Gynecologic Oncologists (SGO) has defined MICAs as neoplastic epithelium invading the stroma in one or more places to a depth of 3.0 mm or less below the basement membrane of epithelium and in which lymph or blood vascular involvement is not demonstrated. Lesions fulfilling

Table 36-5. Modified World Health Organization histologic classification of epithelial tumors of the uterine cervix

Squamous cell carcinoma
  Microinvasive squamous cell carcinoma
  Invasive squamous cell carcinoma
  Verrucous carcinoma
  Warty (condylomatous) carcinoma
  Papillary squamous cell (transitional) carcinoma
  Lymphoepithelioma-like carcinoma
Adenocarcinoma
  Mucinous adenocarcinoma
    Endocervical type
    Intestinal type
    Signet ring type
  Endometrioid adenocarcinoma
    Endometrioid adenocarcinoma with squamous metaplasia
  Clear cell adenocarcinoma
  Minimal deviation adenocarcinoma
    Endocervical type (adenoma malignum)
    Endometrioid type
  Serous adenocarcinoma
  Mesonephric carcinoma
  Well-differentiated villoglandular adenocarcinoma
Other epithelial tumors
  Adenosquamous carcinoma
  Glassy cell carcinoma
  Mucoepidermoid carcinoma
  Adenoid cystic carcinoma
  Adenoid basal carcinoma
  Carcinoid-like tumor
  Small cell carcinoma
  Undifferentiated carcinoma

From Kurman RJ. *Blaustein's pathology of the female genital tract,* 4th ed. New York: Springer–Verlag, 1995. Adapted with permission.

the SGO criteria of MICA have virtually no potential for either metastases or recurrence because lymph vascular involvement is associated with a higher incidence of pelvic node metastases. Therefore, this definition appears to be the most useful for guiding clinical management.

  B. **Invasive squamous cell carcinoma.** Squamous cell carcinoma is the most common histologic type of cervical cancer, comprising 75% to 90% of cases in most series. Because of their frequency, most information regarding etiology and epidemiology is pertinent only to the more common squamous lesions.

    1. **Grade.** Histologic differentiation of cervical carcinomas is divided into three grades. Grade 1 tumors are *well-differentiated* with mature squamous cells, often forming keratinized pearls of epithelial cells. Mitotic activity is low. *Moderately well-differentiated* carcinomas (grade 2) have higher mitotic activity and less cellular maturation accompanied by more

nuclear pleomorphism. Grade 3 tumors are composed of *poorly differentiated* smaller cells with less cytoplasm and often bizarre nuclei. Mitotic activity is high.

2. **Subclassification.** Squamous cell carcinomas are also subclassified according to cell type (or degree of differentiation). The most commonly used descriptive evaluation divides squamous cell carcinomas into *large cell keratinizing, large cell nonkeratinizing,* and *small cell* types. Small cell squamous carcinomas should not be confused with small cell anaplastic carcinomas, which resemble oat cell carcinoma of the lung and are generally associated with reduced survival rates. Categorizing squamous carcinomas of the cervix by keratin status is of questionable utility as there is no universal agreement on the prognostic significance of this distinction.

3. **Variants of squamous cell carcinomas.** *Verrucous carcinoma* is a distinct type of extremely well-differentiated squamous cell carcinoma that microscopically appears exophytic, with an undulating hyperkeratotic surface composed of rounded papillary projections that lack central fibrovascular cores. The lack of fibrovascular cores is particularly useful in discriminating these tumors from giant condylomata acuminata, which display prominent fibrovascular cores. *Papillary squamous cell carcinoma* is a rare variant of squamous carcinoma. The cells have the appearance of a high-grade squamous intraepithelial lesion with hyperchromatic nuclei and scant cytoplasm, resembling transitional cell carcinoma of the urinary bladder.

C. **Adenocarcinoma.** Grossly, cervical adenocarcinoma may appear as a polypoid or papillary exophytic mass. Conversely, diffuse cervical enlargement may be the only indication that an endophytic lesion is present. In approximately 15% of adenocarcinomas, the lesion is located entirely within the endocervical canal and escapes visual inspection. Histopathologically, cervical adenocarcinomas may exhibit a variety of glandular patterns composed of diverse cell types.

1. **Mucinous adenocarcinoma.** Mucinous adenocarcinoma is the most common type of cervical adenocarcinoma. There are three histologic variants of mucinous adenocarcinomas that may occur alone or in combination. Endocervical-type adenocarcinomas are composed of cells with basal nuclei and abundant pale, granular cytoplasm that resemble cells of the normal endocervical mucosa. These tumors tend to be well- or moderately differentiated and mucin production may be plentiful. Intestinal-type lesions are composed of cells that are histologically similar to those of adenocarcinomas of the colon. Mucin production is less prominent and the cell tends to be pseudostratified. The signet ring type is the third histological variant of mucinous adenocarcinoma; however, it rarely occurs in a pure form and is usually admixed with cells of the endocervical or intestinal types.

2. **Endometrioid carcinoma.** Endometrioid carcinomas, accounting for up to 30% of cervical adenocarcinomas, are composed of cells resembling those of typical adenocarcinomas of the uterine corpus. The cells usually have oval nuclei that are arranged perpendicular to the basement membrane of the gland and contain little or no mucin. Endometrioid carcinomas should be distinguished from endometrial adenocarcinoma extending to the endocervix, if possible.

3. **Clear cell carcinoma.** Clear cell carcinoma accounts for approximately 4% of adenocarcinomas of the cervix. The gross appearance of these tumors varies from nodular, reddish lesions to small, punctate ulcers. Histologically, tumor cells are characterized by abundant, clear cytoplasm. Clear cell carcinomas that develop in the absence of diethylstilbestrol (DES) exposure occur most commonly in postmenopausal women and may arise in either the endocervix or ectocervix. Women developing clear cell carcinomas after previous DES exposure tend to be young and have primarily ectocervical lesions.

4. **Minimal deviation adenocarcinoma (MDA).** MDA, or adenoma malignum, is reported to represent 1% of cervical adenocarcinomas. It is a well-differentiated tumor, characterized by cytologically bland, but architecturally atypical glands that vary in size, shape, and depth of stromal penetration. MDA lesions are more likely than other types of cervical adenocarcinoma to precede or develop coincidentally with an ovarian carcinoma.

D. **Other malignant epithelial tumors**

1. **Adenosquamous carcinoma.** Primary cervical carcinoma with both malignant-appearing glandular and squamous elements is referred to as adenosquamous carcinoma. This entity should not be confused with adenocarcinoma and its histologically benign squamous differentiation. The clinical behavior of these tumors is controversial. Julian et al. observed that patients with adenosquamous carcinoma of the cervix have lower 5-year survival rates than patients with squamous carcinoma of comparable stage (7). However, other investigators have reported improved survival for adenosquamous carcinoma compared with squamous carcinoma and pure adenocarcinoma (8).

2. **Glassy cell carcinoma** represents approximately 1% of cervical cancers and is characterized by large cells with a distinctive "ground glass" or granular cytoplasm. The prognosis and clinical course of these tumors are similar to other poorly differentiated carcinomas.

VII. **Treatment**

A. **General management by stage.** Surgery and radiation therapy are the two therapeutic modalities most commonly used to treat invasive cervical carcinoma. In general, primary surgical management is limited to stages I and IIA. There are several advantages to surgical therapy that make it an attractive option, particularly for younger women. Surgery allows for a thorough pelvic and abdominal exploration, which can identify patients with a disparity between the clinical and surgicopathologic stages. These patients can be offered an individualized treatment plan based on their disease status. Surgery also permits conservation of the ovaries with their transposition out of subsequent radiation treatment fields. Radical hysterectomy results in vaginal shortening; however, with sexual activity, gradual lengthening will occur. Fistula (urinary, bowel) formation and incisional complications related to surgical treatment tend to occur early in the postoperative period and are usually amenable to surgical repair. Other reasons for the selection of radical surgery over radiation include concomitant inflammatory bowel disease, previous radiation for other disease, and the presence of a simultaneous adnexal neoplasm.

Radiation therapy, on the other hand, can be used for all stages of disease and most patients regardless of age, body habitus, or coexistent medical conditions. Preservation of sexual function is significantly related to the mode of primary therapy. Pelvic irradiation produces persistent vaginal fibrosis and atrophy, with loss of both vaginal length and caliber. In addition, ovarian function is lost in virtually all patients undergoing tolerance-dose radiation therapy to the pelvis. Fistulous complications associated with radiation therapy tend to occur late and are more difficult to repair secondary to radiation fibrosis, vasculitis, and poorly vascularized tissues.

1. **Stage IA1.** The five-year survival rate of these patients approaches 100% with primary surgical therapy. In the absence of lymph vascular space invasion, the incidence of pelvic lymph node metastases is 0.3%. Extrafascial hysterectomy is adequate treatment of this group of patients. Conization may be used selectively if preservation of fertility is desired, provided that the surgical margins are free of disease. Lymph vascular involvement increases the risk of pelvic node metastases to 2.6%. Pelvic lymphadenectomy and extrafascial hysterectomy should be performed in these cases. If enlarged pelvic nodes are encountered, the procedure can be converted to a modified radical (class II) hysterectomy. In medically inoperable patients, stage IA carcinoma can be effectively treated with radiation.

Table 36-6. Squamous cell carcinoma of the cervix, dose–tumor volume relation: average dose radiation (cGy) required to obtain 90% control in treated area

Tumor volume	Dose (cGy)
<2 cm	5,000
2 cm	6,000
2–4 cm	7,000
4–6 cm	7,500–8,900
6 cm	8,000–10,000

From Shingleton HM, Orr JW. *Cancer of the cervix: diagnosis and treatment.* New York: Churchill Livingstone, 1995:160. Reprinted with permission.

2. **Stage IA2.** Microinvasive carcinoma with stromal invasion of 3.1 to 5.0 mm is associated with positive pelvic lymph nodes in 3.9% to 8.2% of cases. The preferred treatment of these lesions is modified radical (class II) hysterectomy with pelvic lymphadenectomy.
3. **Stages IB1, IB2, IIA.** Radical surgery (class III hysterectomy) or adequate irradiation is equally effective in treating stages IB and IIA carcinoma of the cervix. Numerous uncontrolled studies support the merits of either modality, with no significant difference in survival or pelvic tumor control. Five-year survival rates of 85% for stage IB and 70% for IIA have been reported for both primary surgical and radiation treatment.

   Management of patients with bulky stage I disease (IB2) should be individualized. Most of the available survival data for cervical cancer was published before the FIGO subclassification of stage IB (IB1 and IB2). Expansion of the upper endocervix and lower uterine segment can distort cervical anatomy and lead to suboptimal placement of intracavitary radiation sources. Consequently, the central failure rate is 17.5% in patients with cervical lesions greater than 6 cm treated with irradiation alone. One approach is to combine external irradiation (4,000 cGy) with a single intracavitary implant followed in 6 weeks by extrafascial hysterectomy. While many clinicians confine the use of radical hysterectomy to patients with small IB (<3–4 cm) or IIA lesions, there is evidence that acceptable survival rates can be obtained for patients with bulkier disease confined to the cervix with primary surgical treatment. Five-year survival ranges from 73.6% to 82.0% after radical hysterectomy and bilateral pelvic lymphadenectomy for cervical lesions greater than 4 cm. Survival decreases to 66% at 5 years for lesions greater than 6 cm.
4. **Stages IIB, III, IVA, IVB.** Radiation therapy is the treatment of choice for patients with stage IIB and more advanced disease. Radiation therapy for invasive cervical cancer is given as a combination of external and intracavitary therapy. The average total dose required to control disease within the treated area in 90% of cases ranges from 5,000 cGy for lesions less than 2 cm to more than 8,000 cGy for tumor volumes exceeding 6 cm (Table 36-6). Long-term survival rates with irradiation therapy alone are approximately 70% for stage I, 60% for stage II, 45% for stage III, and 18% for stage IV. Patients with stage IVB disease are usually treated with chemotherapy alone or chemotherapy in combination with local irradiation. These patients have a uniformly poor prognosis regardless of treatment modality.
B. **Surgical management**
   1. **Types of hysterectomy.** There are five distinct variations or classes of hysterectomy used in the treatment of cervical cancer (Table 36-7).
      a. **Class I** hysterectomy refers to the standard *extrafascial total abdominal hysterectomy*. This procedure ensures complete removal of the

Table 36-7. Types of abdominal hysterectomy

Type of surgery	Intrafascial	Extrafascial type I	Modified radical type II	Radical type III
Cervical fascia	Partially removed	Completely removed	Completely removed	Completely removed
Vaginal cuff removal	None	Small rim removed	Proximal 1–2 cm removed	Upper one-third to one-half removed
Bladder	Partially mobilized	Partially mobilized	Mobilized	Mobilized
Rectum	Not mobilized	Rectovaginal septum partially mobilized	Mobilized	Mobilized
Ureters	Not mobilized	Not mobilized	Unroofed in ureteral tunnel	Completely dissected to bladder entry
Cardinal ligaments	Resected medial to ureters	Resected medial to ureters	Resected at level of ureter	Resected at pelvic sidewall
Uterosacral ligaments	Resected at level of cervix	Resected at level of cervix	Partially resected	Resected at postpelvic insertion
Uterus	Removed	Removed	Removed	Removed
Cervix	Partially removed	Completely removed	Completely removed	Completely removed

From Perez CA. Uterine cervix. In: Perez CA, Brady LW, eds. *Principles and practice of radiation oncology,* 2nd ed. Philadelphia: JB Lippincott Co, 1992. Reprinted with permission.

cervix with minimal disruption to surrounding structures (bladder, ureters).

  b. **Class II** hysterectomy is also referred to as a *modified radical hysterectomy.* This procedure involves dissection of the ureters from the parametrial and paracervical tissues down to the ureterovesical junction. This permits removal of all parametrial tissue medial to the ureters as well as the medial half of the uterosacral ligament and proximal 1 to 2 cm of vagina. This operation may be performed with pelvic lymphadenectomy.

  c. In **class III** hysterectomy or *radical abdominal hysterectomy* the ureters are completely dissected from within the paracervical tunnel, and the bladder and rectum are extensively mobilized. Establishment of the paravesical and pararectal spaces facilitates the removal of all the parametrial tissue out to the pelvic sidewall, complete resection of the uterosacral ligaments, and excision of the upper one-third to one-half of the vagina (Fig. 36-4). Bilateral pelvic lymphadenectomy may be performed either before or after radical hysterectomy, at the discretion of the surgeon.

  d. **Class IV/class V.** A class IV or *extended radical hysterectomy* includes removal of the superior vesical artery, periureteral tissue, and up to three-fourths of the vagina. In a class V or *partial exenteration operation* the distal ureters and portion of the bladder are resected. Class IV and class V procedures are rarely performed today because patients with disease extensive enough to require these operations can be more adequately treated using primary radiation therapy.

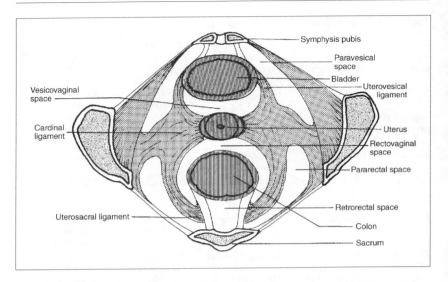

Figure 36-4. The pelvic ligaments and spaces. (From Dunnihoo DR. *Fundamentals of gynecology and obstetrics*, 2nd ed. Philadelphia: JB Lippincott Co, 1992:28. Reprinted with permission.)

    2. Complications of radical abdominal hysterectomy
        a. Acute complications. Radical abdominal hysterectomy with bilateral pelvic lymphadenectomy can lead to all of the acute complications associated with a major surgical procedure. Modern surgical techniques and anesthesia have reduced the operative mortality rate to 0.6%. Febrile morbidity is common and is reported to occur in 25% to 33% of patients after radical hysterectomy. The major causes include pulmonary atelectasis, urinary tract infections, wound infections or hematomas, and pelvic cellulitis. Potentially lethal pulmonary embolism occurs in 1% to 2% of patients. Ureterovaginal and vesicovaginal fistulas occur in 2% and 0.9% of patients, respectively.
        b. Bladder dysfunction. The most commonly observed subacute and chronic complication after radical hysterectomy is urinary dysfunction resulting from partial denervation of the detrusor muscle during excision of the paracervical and paravaginal tissue. In the early postoperative period, patients experience a loss of bladder sensation and inability to initiate voiding. Various degrees of long-term urinary dysfunction are seen, ranging from a hypertonic low-compliance bladder to a hypotonic bladder subject to overdistension. Extensive paravaginal dissection may also result in a denervated, atonic urethra with resultant stress urinary incontinence.
        c. Pelvic lymphocyst. Pelvic lymphocyst formation occurs in 2.0% to 6.7% of patients following radical hysterectomy and pelvic lymphadenectomy. Most lymphocysts are asymptomatic and do not require intervention. However, occasionally lymphocysts may produce pelvic pain, ureteral obstruction, or partial venous obstruction with thrombosis. In these cases, prolonged percutaneous drainage or surgical excision may be indicated. Closed suction drainage of the retroperitoneum has long been employed after pelvic lymphadenectomy in an effort to decrease the incidence of lymphocyst formation. However,

several studies of patients suggest that the use of closed suction drainage offers no advantage compared with leaving the retroperitoneal space open (9,10), and it may in fact increase the incidence of postoperative complications and lengthen hospital stay without decreasing the incidence of pelvic lymphocyst formation.

3. Surgical adjuvant therapy

a. Radiation following radical hysterectomy and pelvic lymphadenectomy. Data are limited concerning the efficacy of postoperative whole pelvic irradiation in patients at high risk of recurrence after radical hysterectomy and pelvic lymphadenotomy. Postoperative adjuvant radiation therapy has been advocated for patients with microscopic parametrial invasion, pelvic lymph node metastases, deep cervical invasion, and positive or close surgical margins. Morbidity is acceptable, provided the total dose is limited to 4,500 to 5,000 cGy in divided fractions. However, lymphedema has been reported in up to 23.4% of patients receiving combined surgery and radiation therapy. Postoperative radiation therapy has been shown to reduce the rate of pelvic recurrence after radical hysterectomy in high-risk patients. Although there are no controlled studies, retrospective data suggest that postoperative irradiation after radical hysterectomy may provide a modest gain in survival in patients with three or more positive pelvic lymph nodes. No survival benefit has been demonstrated for patients with one or two positive lymph nodes receiving postoperative radiation therapy compared with receiving surgery alone.

b. Neoadjuvant chemotherapy. The administration of chemotherapeutic agents before or after radical hysterectomy has been termed neoadjuvant chemotherapy. Cisplatin, bleomycin, and vinblastine has been the most extensively studied combination. Preoperative chemotherapy offers the advantage of increasing the operability of initially large, unresectable tumors. Complete clinical response rates range from 17% to 44%, with overall response rates of 80% to 90%. In addition to increasing in surgical resectability, preoperative chemotherapy also decreases the number of positive pelvic lymph nodes and improves 2- and 3-year survival rates compared with historical controls. Chemotherapy following radical hysterectomy has also been advocated when histopathologic analysis reveals nodal metastases, lymph vascular space invasion, positive surgical margins, parametrial extension, or poorly differentiated histology; however, the long-term survival benefits of this approach are yet to be established.

C. Radiation therapy. External-beam irradiation is usually delivered from a linear accelerator. The purpose of external therapy is to decrease the tumor volume and reduce the anatomic distortion produced by larger tumors, allowing optimization of subsequent intracavitary therapy. Thin patients can be treated with two opposing anteroposterior ports. Larger patients require the addition of two lateral ports to achieve optimal dose distribution within the pelvis. Once external therapy has been completed, brachytherapy can be delivered using a variety of intracavitary techniques including intrauterine tandem and vaginal colpostats, vaginal cylinders, or interstitial needle implants. Complications of radiation therapy can be divided into acute (those occurring during or immediately after therapy) and chronic (those that occur months to years after completing therapy).

1. Acute complications of radiation therapy

a. Uterine perforation may occur at the time of intracavitary therapy and if unrecognized may cause significant blood loss, radiation damage, and peritonitis. Ultrasound or CT scanning can be used to locate the uterine tandem if perforation is suspected. Laparoscopy can also be used if perforation cannot be excluded by noninvasive studies. Appropriate management consists of removal of the implant and broad-spectrum antibiotics if signs of infection are evident.

b. **Proctosigmoiditis** occurs in up to 8% of patients undergoing radiation therapy for cervical cancer, usually in those receiving more than 5,000 cGy of external-beam radiation. Symptoms of proctosigmoiditis include abdominal pain, diarrhea, and nausea. Management consists of antispasmodics, a low-gluten and low-lactose diet, and steroid enemas. Severe cases may require hyperalimentation and diverting colostomy.

c. **Acute hemorrhagic cystitis** occurs in approximately 3% of patients receiving radiation therapy for cervical cancer. Symptoms can usually be controlled with bladder irrigation, antispasmodics, and antibiotics as necessary.

2. **Chronic complications of radiation therapy**

a. **Vaginal stenosis** has been reported in up to 70% of patients receiving radiation therapy for cervical cancer. The severity of stenosis can be minimized by continued sexual activity, use of vaginal dilators, and conjugated estrogen vaginal cream.

b. **Rectovaginal and vesicovaginal fistulas** each complicate approximately 1% of cases of cervical cancer treated with irradiation. Proctosigmoidoscopy or cytoscopy should be used to visualize the fistula site, and biopsy specimens should be taken from the edge of the fistula to rule out recurrent tumor. Diversion of the fecal (colostomy) or urinary (percutaneous nephrostomy) stream is usually required to allow adequate healing (3 to 6 months) before surgical repair. Bulbocavernosus or omental flaps can be used to provide a new vascular supply to the irradiated operative site.

c. **Small bowel obstruction** occurs in approximately 2% of patients undergoing definitive radiation therapy for cervical cancer and is more common in those patients with vascular disease or who have undergone previous abdominal surgery. The most common site of small bowel obstruction is the terminal ileum, which is relatively fixed within the radiation field by the cecum. Mild or partial small bowel obstruction can be treated conservatively with nasogastric suction, blood and electrolyte replacement, and total parenteral nutrition. Complete small bowel obstruction or cases recalcitrant to conservative therapy require surgical treatment.

D. **Chemotherapy**

1. **Single-agent chemotherapy** is used to treat patients with extrapelvic metastases as well as those with recurrent tumor who have been previously treated with surgery or irradiation and are not exenteration candidates. Cisplatin has been the most extensively studied agent and has demonstrated the most consistent clinical response rates. Although there is some variation among different studies, single-agent cisplatin results in a complete response in 24% of cases, with an additional 16% of patients demonstrating a partial response. However, in most series, responses to cisplatin are short-lived (3 to 6 months). Ifosfamide, an alkylating agent similar to cyclophosphamide, has produced overall response rates as high as 29% in cervical cancer patients; however, such efficacy has not been confirmed by all investigators. Other agents demonstrating at least partial activity against cervical cancer include carboplatin, doxorubicin, vinblastine, vincristine, 5-fluorouracil (5-FU), methotrexate, and hexamethyl melamine.

2. The most active **combination chemotherapy** regimens used to treat cervical cancer all contain cisplatin. The agents most commonly used in combination with cisplatin are bleomycin, 5-FU, mitomycin C, methotrexate, cyclophosphamide, and adriamycin. Overall objective response rates vary between 0% and 65%, while clinical complete response rates range from 0% to 36%. Despite these significant response rates, median duration of survival is only 4 to 10.5 months. Consequently, there is little objective evidence to suggest that combination chemotherapy is superior to single-agent treatment with cisplatin in the overall survival of patients with advanced or recurrent cervical cancer.

3. **Chemoradiation.** The use of combination chemoradiation therapy is based on the theory of synergistic cell kill—the therapeutic effect of two treatment modalities in combination will be greater than if the effects of the two modalities individually are simply added together. Specific chemotherapeutic agents that have been combined with radiation to treat cervical cancer are 5-FU, hydroxyurea, and cisplatin. A study by the Gynecologic Oncology Group (GOG) indicates that cisplatin alone is more effective than hydroxyurea and more tolerable than the combination of cisplatin/5-FU/hydroxyurea as a concomitant chemoradiation regimen for locally advanced cervical cancer. When combined with radiation, weekly cisplatin reduces the 2-year risk of progression by 43% (2-year survival = 70%) for stage IIB through state IVA cervical cancer.

E. **Posttreatment surveillance.** Among patients with recurrent cervical cancer, recurrence is detected within 1 year in 50% of cases and within 2 years in more than 80%. Pelvic examination and lymph node evaluation, including supraclavicular nodes, should be performed every 3 months for 2 years and then every 6 months for an additional 3 years. Because over 70% of women with pelvic recurrence will have abnormal cervical/vaginal cytology, appropriate cytologic smears should be obtained at the time of each routine examination. An annual chest x-ray is indicated to detect pulmonary metastases. If a palpable pelvic mass is detected or symptoms suggest urinary obstruction, a CT scan of the abdomen and pelvis with intravenous contrast should be obtained to rule out recurrent tumor and delineate ureteral involvement. CT-guided fine-needle aspiration (FNA) cytology can then be performed to confirm recurrent disease.

F. **Treatment of recurrent cervical cancer.** Cervical cancer detected within the first 6 months after therapy is often termed *persistent cancer*, whereas that diagnosed later is usually referred to as *recurrent disease*. Appropriate treatment for recurrent cervical cancer is dictated by the site of recurrence and the modality of primary therapy. Generally, patients in whom recurrent cervical cancer develops after primary surgery should be considered for radiation therapy. Conversely, surgical treatment should be considered for those patients with recurrent disease after initially receiving irradiation. Patients who have had suboptimal or incomplete primary irradiation may be candidates for additional radiation therapy; however, the risk of urinary or enteric fistula formation is usually prohibitive. Interstitial implant radiation techniques may minimize the dose to the bladder and rectum and produce acceptable disease control if the recurrence is small and confined to the central pelvis. Distantly metastatic recurrent tumor is not amenable to therapy modality alone and is an indication for palliative chemotherapy, radiation therapy, or both.

Only patients with recurrent tumor confined to the central pelvis are candidates for surgical intervention. Total hysterectomy is inadequate treatment for patients who have centrally recurrent cervical cancer. Approximately 15% of patients with recurrent cervical cancer will have a small-volume central pelvic recurrence. These patients can be treated with radical hysterectomy with 5-year survival rates approaching 30% to 50%; however, the inability to accurately assess tumor volume may be associated with failure in situations in which a more radical procedure may have resulted in cure. Additionally, radical hysterectomy after tolerance doses of radiation therapy is associated with a 20% to 50% rate of ureteral strictures, urinary fistulas, and other serious complications. Therefore, pelvic exenteration is usually the procedure of choice for centrally recurrent cervical cancer.

1. **Preoperative considerations.** A thorough investigation should be undertaken to rule out extrapelvic metastases. Abdominopelvic CT scan can identify enlarged paraaortic lymph nodes and liver metastases. Physical examination includes palpation of inguinal and supraclavicular lymph nodes. Suspicious areas should be biopsied by FNA with CT guidance if necessary. Other contraindications are shown in Table 36-8. Pelvic sidewall involvement may be difficult to differenti-

Table 36-8. Preoperative contraindications to exenteration in patients with recurrent cervical cancer

---

Absolute

    Extrapelvic disease

    Triad of unilateral leg edema, sciatica, and ureteral obstruction

    Tumor-related pelvic sidewall fixation

    Bilateral ureteral obstruction (if secondary to recurrence)

    Severe, life-limiting medical illness

    Psychosis or the inability of the patient to care for herself

    Religious or other beliefs that prohibit the patient from accepting transfusion

    Inability of physician or consultants to manage any or all intraoperative and postoperative complications

    Inadequate hospital facilities

Relative

    Age older than 75 years

    Large tumor volume (>4 cm)

    Unilateral ureteral obstruction

    Metastasis to the distal vagina

From Shingleton HM, Orr JW. *Cancer of the cervix: diagnosis and treatment.* New York: Churchill Livingstone, 1995:265. Adapted with permission.

ate from radiation fibrosis on physical examination. Although many lesions may seem to be clinically nonresectable during examination, the philosophy of most gynecologic oncologists is that the operating room is the court of last resort; in the absence of documented extracervical disease, most women should be considered surgical candidates. In most series, approximately 25% of patients with recurrent cervical cancer are deemed satisfactory candidates for exenterative surgery. Thorough preoperative psychological and nutritional preparation are essential to optimize outcome.

  2. **Operative approaches**

    a. **Anterior exenteration** is indicated for the treatment of recurrent cervical cancer limited to the cervix, anterior vagina, and bladder, or a combination. The procedure combines radical cystectomy with radical hysterectomy and vaginectomy. A negative proctoscopic examination does not exclude tumor involvement of the rectal serosa or muscularis; consequently, the decision to limit the procedure to anterior resection must be based on intraoperative findings.

    b. **Posterior exenteration** combines abdominal perineal resection of the rectum with radical hysterectomy and vaginectomy and is indicated for lesions confined to the posterior fornix and rectovaginal septum. Using surgical stapling devices, low-rectal reanastomosis can be accomplished in approximately 70% of cases.

    c. **Total pelvic exenteration** is most often required for recurrent cervical cancer. The procedure involves the *en bloc* excision of the bladder, uterus, rectum, and vagina. A continent urinary diversion can be created using a segment of ascending colon and terminal ileum with a buttressed ileocecal valve providing the continence mechanism (Indiana pouch, Miami pouch). Reconstruction of the pelvic floor can be accomplished with the use of an omental pedicle flap. A neovagina can be created by a variety of techniques including gracilis or bulbocavernosus myocutaneous flaps. Vaginal reconstruction using a transverse rectus abdominus musculocutaneous flap also gives excellent functional results.

3. **Survival.** With modern surgical techniques and intensive care unit support, perioperative mortality does not exceed 7% in recent series. With proper patient selection and surgical judgment, 5-year survival rates after pelvic exenteration range from 45% to 61% in recent large series.

VIII. Special problems

A. Cervical cancer in pregnancy. Depending on the patient's socioeconomic status and the hospital's referral base, cervical cancer occurs in 0.02% to 0.90% of all pregnancies (1 in 110 to 1 in 5,000). Conversely, 0.1% to 7.6% of all cervical cancer patients are pregnant at the time of diagnosis. Cervical cancer coincident with pregnancy poses complex diagnostic and therapeutic decisions that may jeopardize both mother and fetus.

1. **Diagnosis.** Cervical cytologic screening should be part of routine antenatal care. Endocervical canal sampling with the cytobrush has been shown to significantly increase cytologic specimen adequacy without an associated increase in adverse pregnancy events. Colposcopy is indicated for abnormal cervical cytology. Directed biopsy should be performed when high-grade intraepithelial lesions or microinvasion is suspected. Cervical conization is generally performed in pregnancy only for diagnostic, rather than therapeutic, purposes. Conization is indicated in any patient whose cytologic smear or biopsy suggests invasive carcinoma when a diagnosis of invasive disease may result in a treatment or delivery modification. An unsatisfactory colposcopy is not an indication for conization unless the cervical cytology is highly suspicious for microinvasive carcinoma. Conization should only be performed in the second trimester because of the increased risk of perioperative hemorrhage and spontaneous pregnancy loss (as high as 33%) associated with first trimester procedures.

2. **Pretreatment evaluation.** Pregnant women with cervical cancer should undergo the same pretreatment metastatic evaluation as nonpregnant women. It should be noted that urinary tract dilatation normally associated with pregnancy may mimic obstructive uropathy. Because the bimanual examination may be difficult in pregnancy, magnetic resonance imaging may be useful to delineate extracervical disease while minimizing fetal radiation exposure.

3. **Treatment.** Traditionally, vaginal delivery of pregnant cervical cancer patients has been avoided because of the theoretical potential for dissemination of tumor cells during cervical dilatation. However, overall survival after vaginal delivery (52.9%) is not significantly different from that after abdominal delivery (46.1%). Although these data are not adjusted for gestational age and tumor volume, the risk of tumor dissemination is probably only theoretical. Hemorrhage remains a significant risk of vaginal delivery in patients with large cervical carcinomas, and in these cases abdominal delivery is advisable.

   a. **MICA.** In patients with stages IA1 and IA2 disease there appears to be no harm in delaying definitive therapy until after fetal maturity has been attained. Patients with less than 3 mm of invasion and no lymph vascular space involvement may be followed to term and delivered vaginally. Extrafascial hysterectomy can then be performed 4 to 6 weeks later if further childbearing is not desired. Patients with 3 to 5 mm of invasion or lymph vascular invasion can also be safely followed until fetal maturity has been reached. However, surgical treatment should include a modified radical hysterectomy with pelvic lymph node dissection performed either at the time of cesarean delivery or 4 to 6 weeks postpartum. Radiation therapy is associated with survival rates comparable to surgical treatment.

   b. **Stages IB1, IB2, and IIA.** In patients having large volume cervical cancer, a delay in therapy in excess of 6 weeks may be detrimental to the mother's chance of survival. If the diagnosis is made after 20 weeks' gestation, consideration may be given to postponing therapy until fetal viability, as neonatal intensive care allows salvage rates of about 80% for infants born at 28 weeks. Standard treatment consists of classic cesarean delivery followed by radical hysterectomy and pelvic and paraaortic lymph node dissection; however, this procedure is associated with increases in both operative time and blood loss compared with nonpregnant patients. Radiation therapy results in equivalent survival rates and may be preferable for patients who are poor surgical candidates.

   c. **Advanced-stage disease.** Radiation therapy is indicated for patients with stages IIB to IV or poor surgical candidates with smaller volume disease. When advanced carcinoma is diagnosed in the second trimester, consideration may be given to delaying therapy until fetal viability. If the fetus is viable, it should be delivered by classic cesarean section and radiation treatment begun postoperatively. When radiation therapy is employed during the first trimester, the fetus should be left *in situ*, as spontaneous abortion will occur in 70% of cases before the administration of 4,000 cGy. Pyometra can occur infrequently.

   4. **Prognosis.** Five-year survival is not significantly different for patients with stages I and II disease whether they are diagnosed during the first, second, or third trimester. Pregnancy has no known adverse survival effects on the ultimate prognosis of patients with cervical cancer. However, diagnosis at a late gestational age or postpartum is associated with more advanced clinical stage and correspondingly poor long-term survival rates.

B. **Incidental cervical carcinoma found at simple hysterectomy.** Occasionally, invasive cervical carcinoma will be incidentally discovered in the surgical specimen after simple extrafascial hysterectomy has been performed. Unless disease is limited to stage IA1, microinvasive carcinoma (<3 mm) without lymph vascular involvement, simple hysterectomy is inadequate treatment, as the parametrial soft tissue, vaginal cuff, and pelvic lymph nodes may still harbor residual tumor. Additional treatment is dictated by the patient's age, the volume of disease, and the status of the surgical margins of resection.

   1. **Surgery.** Although it may be technically difficult to perform an adequate radical resection after previous simple hysterectomy, reoperation should be considered in selected clinical situations, particularly for young patients in whom ovarian preservation is desired. Radical postsimple hysterectomy surgery for invasive cervical cancer generally includes radical parametrectomy, resection of the cardinal ligaments, excision of the vaginal stump, and pelvic lymphadenectomy. Use of postoperative adjuvant radiation therapy is dictated by surgical and pathologic findings. Survival after successful reoperation for patients with stage I disease is comparable to that of patients treated primarily with radical hysterectomy.

   2. **Radiation therapy.** Cervical carcinoma at the margins of resection after simple hysterectomy or the presence of gross residual tumor are absolute indications for radiation therapy. These patients have a much less favorable prognosis than patients without residual tumor and patients with comparable disease who have been appropriately staged and treated with radiation alone. Radiation therapy is also well-suited for older patients and for those who are poor surgical candidates. Survival after radiation therapy correlates with the volume of disease, the status of the surgical margins, and the delay between simple hysterectomy and institution of radiation treatments. Five-year survival is 95% to 100% for patients with microscopic disease, while 82% to 84% of those with macroscopic disease and negative margins survive 5 years. If the surgical margins of resection are microscopically involved with carcinoma, 5-year survival ranges from 38% to 87%; survival drops to 20% to 47% for patients with gross residual tumor.

C. **Carcinoma of the cervical stump.** With few indications for subtotal hysterectomy today, invasive carcinoma of the cervical stump is not commonly seen. Patients with a true carcinoma of the cervical stump have a significantly better prognosis than patients with a coincidental cervical lesion undiscovered at the time of hysterectomy. A period of 2 years is commonly used to differentiate true from coincidental lesions. The natural history and patterns of spread of carcinoma of the cervical stump are similar to those of carcinoma of the intact uterus. The diagnostic evaluation, clinical staging, and principles of treatment are also unchanged. In appropriate surgical candidates, early-stage disease can be treated with simple or radical trachelectomy with or without pelvic lymphadenectomy, depending on the volume of disease. Advanced-stage disease is treated with radiation therapy. However, the lack of a uterine cavity, into which a tandem containing two or three radiation sources is usually inserted, can make intracavitary treatment more difficult. If the length of the cervical canal is less than 2 cm, use of a uterine tandem may be impossible. In this case, vaginal ovoids can be used alone or in combination with external beam therapy to complete the recommended dosimetry.

D. **Adenocarcinoma.** Adenocarcinoma of the cervix accounts for approximately 10% to 15% of all invasive cervical neoplasms. Similar to squamous carcinomas, tumor size, depth of invasion, and histological tumor grade have been identified as predictors of pelvic lymph node metastases and overall survival. Although cervical adenocarcinomas have been reported to have a worse prognosis than similar-stage squamous carcinomas, this difference may be due, at least in part, to the tendency of adenocarcinomas to grow endophytically and establish a large tumor volume before clinical detection. Local tumor extension as well as lymph node metastases are reported to occur comparatively earlier in adenocarcinomas than in squamous carcinomas (11). When cervical adenocarcinomas and squamous carcinomas are comparatively matched by patient age, clinical stage, tumor volume, and treatment method, survival outcomes are not significantly different between histologic subtypes (12).

   Treatment for patients with stage IB1 or smaller adenocarcinoma of the cervix may be determined by the same indications as for squamous carcinoma. The management of stage IB2–IIA lesions is controversial. There does not appear to be significant survival advantage when radiation therapy is followed by adjunctive extrafascial hysterectomy. However, Moberg et al. reported on 138 patients with stages IB and IIA cervical adenocarcinoma and found that combined treatment consisting of intracavitary radiation and followed by radical hysterectomy and pelvic lymphadenectomy resulted in superior survival compared with patients treated with radiation therapy alone (13). The incidence of residual adenocarcinoma after combined therapy with intracavitary radiation and radical hysterectomy has been reported to be as high as 30%, compared with only 11% for squamous carcinomas treated in similar fashion (14). Such high rates of persistent disease after radiation may be an argument in favor of combined therapy for bulky stage I and stage II adenocarcinomas.

E. **Small cell carcinomas** of the uterine cervix are similar to small cell "neuroendocrine" tumors of the lung and other anatomic locations. These tumors are clinically aggressive, demonstrating a marked propensity to metastasize locally and to distant sites. At the time of diagnosis, disease is often widely disseminated, with bone, brain, and liver being the most common sites. The workup should include bone marrow aspiration biopsy of the iliac crest and bone, liver, and brain imaging studies to rule out metastatic spread. Because of the high metastatic potential of small cell carcinomas, local therapy alone (surgery, radiation, or both) rarely results in long-term survival. Multiagent chemotherapy, in combination with external beam and intracavitary radiation therapy, is the standard therapeutic approach. The two most commonly used chemotherapeutic regimes are vincristine, adriamycin, cyclophosphamide (Cytoxan), and etoposide and cisplatin.

F. **Bilateral ureteral obstruction** and uremia can occur secondary to lateral extension of cervical cancer within the pelvis. Women with ureteral obstruction resulting from untreated cervical cancer or recurrent disease after primary surgical therapy are candidates for radiation therapy. When there is no evidence of distant metastatic disease, urinary stents may be placed percutaneously and radiation therapy instituted with curative intent. If the ureteral obstruction precludes stent placement, urinary diversion may be accomplished by way of percutaneous nephrostomy tubes. In patients with metastatic disease beyond the radiation treatment field, ureteral stent placement and palliative radiation therapy coupled with systemic chemotherapy may result in median survival rates of up to 17 months. In patients previously treated with maximum-dose radiation therapy, bilateral ureteral obstruction is due to radiation fibrosis in only 5% of cases; recurrent carcinoma is the cause of obstruction in the vast majority of cases. The management of patients with recurrent disease is more complex. Additional radiation therapy will lead to troublesome fistula formation and bowel complications. Distant metastatic disease precludes exenterative surgery and limits the therapeutic options for these patients. Some have suggested that these patients should not undergo urinary diversion as uremia may be a more preferable method of expiration than hemorrhage or progressive cachexia with severe pelvic pain. Nevertheless, ureteral stent placement or urinary diversion with percutaneous nephrostomy tubes are effective in alleviating bilateral obstruction.

G. **Cervical hemorrhage.** Profuse vaginal bleeding from large cervical malignancies is a challenging therapeutic situation. Generally, conservative measures to control cervical hemorrhage are preferable to emergency laparotomy and vascular (hypogastric artery) ligation. Attention must first be directed toward the stabilization of the patient with appropriate intravenous fluid and blood product replacement. Immediate control of cervical hemorrhage can usually be accomplished with a vaginal pack soaked in Monsel's solution (ferric subsulfate). Topical acetone (dimethyl ketone) applied with a vaginal pack placed firmly against the bleeding tumor bed has also been used successfully to control vaginal hemorrhage from cervical malignancy (15). Definitive control of cervical hemorrhage can be accomplished with external radiation therapy of 180 to 200 cGy/day if the patient has not previously received tolerance doses of pelvic irradiation. Alternatively, arteriography can be used to identify the bleeding vessel(s) followed by Gelfoam or steel coil embolization. Vascular embolization has the disadvantage of producing a hypoxic local tumor environment and potentially compromising the efficacy of subsequent radiation therapy.

References

1. Eddy GL. Screening for cervical cancer. *Ann Int Med* 1990;113:214–216.
2. Kosary CL. FIGO stage, histologic, histologic grade, age and race as prognostic factors in determining survival for cancers of the female gynecological system: an analysis of 1973–87 SEER cases of cancers of the endometrium, cervix, ovary, vulva, and vagina. *Semin Surg Oncol* 1994;10:31–46.
3. Delgado G, Bundy BN, Fowler WC Jr, et al. A Prospective surgical pathological study of stage I squamous carcinoma of the cervix: a Gynecologic Oncology Group study. *Gynecol Oncol* 1989;35:314–320.
4. Stehman FB, Bundy BN, DiSaia PJ, Keys HM, Larson JE, Fowler WC. Carcinoma of the cervix treated with radiation therapy. I. A multi-variate analysis of prognostic variables in the Gynecologic Oncology Group. *Cancer* 1991;67:2776–2785.
5. Stanhope CR, Smith JP, Wharton JT, Rutledge FN, Fletcher GH, Gallager HS. Carcinoma of the cervix: the effect of age on survival. *Gynecol Oncol* 1980;10:188–193.
6. Baltzer J, Lohe KJ, Kopcke W, Zander J. Histological criteria for the prognosis in patients with operated squamous cell carcinoma of the cervix. *Gynecol Oncol* 1982;13:184–194.
7. Julian CG, Daikoko NH, Gillespie A. Adenoepidermoid and adenosquamous carcinoma of the uterus. *Am J Obstet Gynecol* 1977;128:106–116.
8. Kilgore LC, Soong SJ, Gore H, Shingleton HM, Hatch KD, Partridge EE. Analysis of prognostic features in adenocarcinoma of the cervix. *Gynecol Oncol* 1988;31:137–153.

9. Jensen JK, Lucci JA III, DiSaia PJ, Manetta A, Berman ML. To drain or not to drain: a retrospective study of closed-suction drainage following radical hysterectomy with pelvic lymphadenectomy. *Gynecol Oncol* 1993;51:46–49.
10. Patsner B. Closed-suction drainage versus no drainage following radical abdominal hysterectomy with pelvic lymphadenectomy for stage IB cervical cancer. *Gynecol Oncol* 1995;37:232–234.
11. Hopkins MP, Schmidt RW, Roberts JA, Morely GW. Gland cell carcinoma (adenocarcinoma) of the cervix. *Obstet Gynecol* 1988;72:789–795.
12. Shingleton HM, Gore H, Bradley DH, Soong SJ. Adenocarcinoma of the cervix. I. Clinical evaluation and pathologic features. *Am J Obstet Gynecol* 1981;139:799–814.
13. Moberg PJ, Einhorn N, Silfversward C, Soderberg G. Adenocarcinoma of the uterine cervix. *Cancer* 1986;57:407–410.
14. Kjorstad KE, Bond B. Stage IB adenocarcinoma of the cervix: metastatic potential and patterns of dissemination. *Am J Obstet Gynecol* 1984;150:297–299.
15. Patsner B. Topical acetone for control of life-threatening vaginal hemorrhage from recurrent gynecologic cancer. *Eur J Gynecol Oncol* 1993;14:33–35.

Selected Reading

Berek JS, Hacker NF, eds. *Practical gynecologic oncology*, 2nd ed. Baltimore: Williams & Wilkins, 1994.
DiSaia PJ, Creasman WT. *Clinical gynecologic oncology*, 4th ed. St. Louis: Mosby–Yearbook, 1993.
Hoskins WJ, Perez CA, Young RC. *Principles and practice of gynecologic oncology*. Philadelphia: JB Lippincott Co, 1992.
Knapp RC, Berkowitz RS, eds. *Gynecologic oncology*, 2nd ed. New York: McGraw-Hill, 1993.
Kurman RJ. *Blaustein's pathology of the female genital tract*, 4th ed. New York: Springer–Verlag, 1995.
Morrow CP, Curtin JP. *Synopsis of gynecologic oncology*, 5th ed. New York: Churchill Livingstone, 1998.
Shingleton HM, Orr JW. *Cervical cancer*. Philadelphia: JB Lippincott Co, 1995.

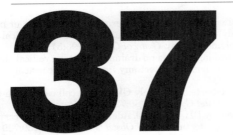

Cancer of the Uterine Corpus

Thomas Randall and
Edward Trimble

Endometrial Cancer

I. **Epidemiology**
   A. Endometrial cancer is the most common gynecologic malignancy and the fourth most common cancer in women in the United States. In 1995, 31,000 cases of endometrial cancer were reported in the United States. Endometrial cancer is the eighth most common malignant neoplasm worldwide. Cancer of the uterine corpus appears to be a disease of affluent societies and countries with Westernized lifestyles, with wide intercountry variations in incidence and mortality. Incidence ranges from 5.9 per 100,000 in Shanghai, China, to 44 per 100,000 among white women in the San Francisco Bay area. Three-fourths of women with endometrial cancer are postmenopausal, whereas only 5% are aged 40 years or younger. Three-fourths of affected women present with a tumor confined to the uterus, and the majority of these patients do well, with an overall 5-year survival rate of 83%. A significant minority, however, have advanced or recurrent disease at presentation, and approximately 6,000 women die of endometrial cancer yearly in the United States. Age-adjusted mortality rates are 5.7 per 100,000 women in Denmark, 2.6 per 100,000 in the United States, and lowest in Hong Kong, at 1.4 per 100,000.
   B. **Risk factors and etiology.** The etiology of endometrial cancer is hypothesized to be a hormone-mediated process; this hypothesis is supported by laboratory, clinical, and epidemiologic data. Unopposed estrogenic stimulation of the endometrium is found with unopposed estrogen therapy, chronic anovulation, obesity, diabetes mellitus, nulliparity, and late menopause (after age 52); all of these conditions are commonly recognized risk factors for endometrial cancer. The risk increases with increased obesity and with a truncal distribution of body fat. Patients receiving tamoxifen appear to be at the same risk as those who are treated with unopposed estrogen. Hypertension frequently is found in patients with endometrial cancer but does not appear to be an independent risk factor. Increased exposure to progesterone and decreased estrogens are found to decrease the risk of endometrial cancer. Accordingly, multiparity, use of oral contraceptives, and cigarette smoking have been reported to decrease the risk of endometrial cancer.

II. **Detection and prevention**
   A. **Screening**
      1. **Population.** The low incidence of endometrial cancer and the frequent presentation of precursor and early-stage lesions because of vaginal bleeding render general screening for endometrial cancer a low-yield activity. A high-risk population that may benefit from screening can be identified on the basis of known risk factors. Women receiving unopposed estrogen; obese women; nulliparas; women with polycystic ovarian disease, chronic anovulation, granulosa cell tumors, or a history of breast or colon cancer; women with a family history of breast, ovarian, endometrial or colon cancer; women receiving tamoxifen; or women with a com-

bination of these risk factors may be at high enough risk to warrant routine asymptomatic screening, although definitive data to support such screening are not currently available.

2. **Tools.** Cost and patient discomfort limit the utility of all three of the methods used for screening, except in symptomatic or high-risk patients.

   a. **Endometrial biopsy** has demonstrated high sensitivity and specificity in detecting endometrial cancer.

   b. **Endovaginal ultrasound** has been proposed as a screening tool. The incidence of endometrial neoplasia was found to be quite low in postmenopausal women with endometrial stripes measuring 3 to 5 mm; conversely, patients with stripes larger than 10 mm had a 10% to 20% incidence of endometrial hyperplasia or neoplasia.

   c. **Office hysteroscopy** also enables evaluation of the uterine lining and cavity.

B. **Prevention**

1. **Oral contraceptives** may decrease the risk of endometrial cancer.
2. **Maintenance of proper weight** decreases the risk of endometrial cancer.
3. **Avoidance of unopposed estrogen** decreases the risk of endometrial cancer.
4. **Timely detection of precursor lesions.** Endometrial hyperplasias, especially those with atypia, are highly associated with the presence of a cancer or progression to a cancer (see sec. **III**).
5. **Management of endometrial hyperplasia.** The risk of endometrial hyperplasia progressing to endometrial cancer is based on the architectural complexity of the lesion (simple or complex) and, to a greater extent, the presence of cytologic atypia.

   a. **Simple hyperplasia and complex hyperplasia** can be treated with progestational agents and careful pathologic follow-up.

   b. **Hyperplasia with atypia** should be considered a premalignant lesion, especially in postmenopausal patients. Simple extrafascial hysterectomy is the treatment of choice for most women. Progestational agents can reverse most hyperplastic lesions, but progestational therapy must be continued as long as risk factors persist and requires serial endometrial biopsies to confirm its success. Therefore, hormonal therapy generally is offered to poor surgical candidates or to patients who decline surgical therapy.

III. **Presentation and diagnosis**

A. **Signs and symptoms.** At least 90% of patients with endometrial cancer present with symptoms of abnormal uterine bleeding, abnormal vaginal discharge, or leukorrhea. The presence of endometrial or glandular cells on a Pap smear warrants further evaluation for endometrial cancer, particularly if cytologic atypia is present or if the patient is postmenopausal.

B. **Indications for endometrial biopsy (EMB), dilatation and curettage.** Patients with postmenopausal bleeding or abnormal pre- or perimenopausal bleeding, and postmenopausal patients with upper genital tract infection and abnormal vaginal discharge or endometrial cells on Pap smear, should be evaluated with a careful pelvic examination, Pap smear, endocervical curettage, and an EMB in the office. Because the accuracy of EMB results is approximately 90%, patients at high risk for endometrial cancer who show a negative EMB result should undergo a fractional dilatation and curettage, performed on an inpatient basis. Alternatives to fractional dilatation and curettage include transvaginal ultrasound and office hysteroscopy.

IV. **Staging and prognosis**

A. **Clinical.** Patients who are unable to undergo primary surgery are staged according to the 1971 International Federation of Gynecology and Obstetrics (FIGO) criteria. Because many patients, when staged surgically, are found to have more extensive disease than that of their clinical stage, all patients who are able to undergo surgery are now staged by primary surgical staging according to the 1988 FIGO criteria. If a diagnosis of endometrial cancer has been made, it is not necessary to perform an examination under anesthesia or fractional curettage in an inpatient setting, or to sound the uterus before definitive surgery.

B. Surgical. All patients who are able to undergo laparotomy are staged according to the 1988 FIGO criteria. The extent of surgery and the selection of any adjuvant treatments are based on intraoperative findings, including thorough evaluation of the hysterectomy specimen. Surgical staging is indicated for patients at risk of occult extrauterine disease: that is, patients with more than a superficially invasive grade 1 lesion (see sec. **V.B** for staging procedure).

C. Histology. The major histologic types of endometrial cancer are endometrioid, mucinous, serous, clear cell, and undifferentiated.

    1. Type I and type II cancers. More than 80% of endometrial cancers are endometrioid in type. Endometrioid endometrial adenocarcinomas are subdivided on the basis of degree of differentiation, percentage of solid component, and nuclear atypia into grades 1, 2, and 3. The patient's survival is greatly affected by the grade of the lesion, with an overall 5-year survival rate of 62%. The other histologic types—clear cell, papillary serous, mucinous, squamous, and undifferentiated—make up the remaining 10% to 15% of endometrial cancer and are associated with a poor prognosis regardless of grade, with 5-year survival rates in the range of 30% or less in most studies. Several authors, noting this distinction between endometrioid and other types of lesion, have divided endometrial cancer into type I and type II lesions. Type I, representing well- and moderately differentiated endometrioid carcinoma, is thought to result from an estrogen-dependent process that progresses from hyperplasia through cellular atypia to cancer. Type II appears to arise *de novo* and is thought to be caused by an unknown carcinogen or carcinogens.

    2. Endometrial clear cell carcinomas are histologically identical to those arising in the vagina, cervix, and ovary and in early stages appear to have a prognosis similar to that of grade 3 endometrioid adenocarcinomas.

    3. Uterine papillary serous carcinoma is histologically similar to serous ovarian carcinoma. The tumor tends to occur in older women, has a high propensity for intraabdominal spread, and is refractory to most standard therapies.

D. Prognostic factors

    1. Surgical stage. Five-year survival rates according to surgical staging are as follows: stage I, 75%; stage II, 60%; stage III, 30%; and stage IV, 10%.

    2. Risk of recurrence for patients with stage I disease is strongly affected by grade and depth of invasion.

    3. Malignant peritoneal washings are associated with a higher stage and, therefore, a higher risk of recurrence.

    4. Nonendometrioid histologic findings are associated with worse prognoses than endometrioid adenocarcinoma.

    5. Patient age. Young patients tend to fare better than older patients because of an increased prevalence of better-differentiated, lower-stage lesions.

    6. Estrogen and progesterone receptors, when present, are independently favorable prognostic factors.

    7. Lymphatic space invasion, tumor size of greater than 2 cm, and DNA aneuploidy all confer an increased risk of recurrence.

V. Clinical management

A. Preoperative evaluation. Endometrial cancer is typically a disease of women in their 60s and 70s who have coexisting medical problems including obesity, hypertension, and diabetes mellitus. The evaluation of a woman with endometrial cancer should include a thorough history, physical examination, EMB (or review of material from prior biopsy), indicated laboratory studies, and radiologic evaluation. The remainder of the evaluation should focus on assessing operative risk. More sophisticated studies such as proctoscopy, barium enema, computed tomographic (CT) scan, or magnetic resonance imaging should be reserved for clinical situations in which advanced disease is suspected or a precise diagnosis is unclear.

B. Disease clinically confined to the uterus. All patients with endometrial cancer who are medically able should undergo laparotomy through an adequate incision, including extrafascial hysterectomy, bilateral salpingo-oophorectomy (BSO), and thorough exploration of the pelvis and abdomen. A vertical incision facilitates proper surgical staging. Washings should be sent for cytologic examination. Prophylactic measures to prevent the spill of malignant cells into the vagina or peritoneal cavity do not appear to be beneficial. The size, location, grade, and depth of myometrial invasion of the lesion should be determined intraoperatively.

    1. **Selective pelvic and paraaortic lymphadenectomy** should be performed (in patients able to undergo more extensive surgery) if any of the following is present: grade 3 differentiation, grade 2 differentiation with a bulky lesion, type II histology such as serous or clear cell carcinoma, invasion of more than 50% of the myometrium, cervical extension, or evidence of extrauterine metastases, including palpable lymphadenopathy. The absence of lymphadenopathy on radiological studies or on exploration does not obviate the necessity of performing lymph node sampling. Many surgeons perform omental biopsy when they perform lymph node sampling.

    2. **Vaginal hysterectomy and operative laparoscopy.** Patients with well-differentiated lesions who are at increased medical risk for complications of abdominal surgery may be treated with vaginal hysterectomy. Operative laparoscopy may be performed to facilitate adnexectomy and lymph node sampling in some of these patients. Controlled studies have not yet been undertaken to determine the comparability of laparotomy and laparoscopy in this setting.

C. Clinically advanced disease. Patients with palpable cervical extension of endometrial cancer may be treated with radical hysterectomy and surgical staging. Alternatively, preoperative radiation may be given and followed in 6 weeks by extrafascial hysterectomy. In either case, the patient should be carefully surgically staged, and all detectable tumor should be resected.

    1. **Patients with metastases to the vagina or parametrium** should be treated with radiation, usually a combination of external-beam and brachytherapy, followed in 6 weeks by extrafascial hysterectomy. A patient with a newly diagnosed endometrial carcinoma and a pelvic mass should undergo primary surgery, which allows the mass to be diagnosed and directs further therapy. Patients who are found to have stage III endometrial cancer should undergo as complete a cytoreduction as possible.

    2. **If extrapelvic metastases are found,** the treatment should be tailored to the individual patient. Most patients undergo hysterectomy, which may increase control of pelvic disease and limit vaginal bleeding. Additional surgery may be performed to control symptoms such as bowel obstruction. Most patients are treated with systemic therapy; those with hormone receptor–positive tumors commonly are treated with progestins, while those with hormone receptor–negative tumors are given doxorubicin (Adriamycin) or platinum-based chemotherapy.

D. Adjuvant therapy. Patients with stage I to II disease are evaluated postoperatively to determine whether they are likely to benefit from adjuvant radiotherapy. Adjuvant radiation therapy has been shown to decrease pelvic recurrence but has not been shown to improve overall survival. Patients with myometrial invasion of greater than 50%, cervical or lower uterine segment involvement, lymph space invasion, grade 3 differentiation, or type II histology usually are offered whole pelvic irradiation (typically 5,000 cGy external beam in fractionated doses). If positive paraaortic nodes and no distant metastases are present, extended-field irradiation (whole pelvic radiation with an aortic "chimney") is offered. Some centers offer vaginal cuff radiation to patients with low- or intermediate-risk disease. Patients who have positive peritoneal cytologic findings and no other evidence of metastases may be offered whole abdominal radiation or systemic chemotherapy.

E. Follow-up. Most patients are evaluated at 3- to 6-month intervals for 2 years. The patient is assessed for the development of recurrent disease or for the development of a second primary tumor, especially breast cancer. After 2 years, the patient may be seen every 6 months to 1 year. A study has shown that routine CT scans and chest x-ray studies do not effectively detect preclinical recurrences.

F. Recurrent disease. The overall survival rate of recurrent endometrial cancer is less than 30%. Patients who have small, localized lesions, have not received radiation, or whose disease recurs more than 3 years after initial presentation have a more favorable prognosis than other patients. Treatment is based on the location of the disease and on previous therapy. Surgery, including exenteration, may be appropriate for patients with isolated pelvic tumors. Radiotherapy may be offered to patients who have not previously received it or to control symptoms at distant sites, such as bone or brain. Other patients must be treated with systemic chemotherapy or progestins.

Uterine Sarcomas

I. Epidemiology. Sarcomas of the uterus are uncommon, comprising 3% of uterine cancer cases. Of these cases, 50% are carcinosarcomas (CS), 40% are leiomyosarcomas (LMS), and 8% are endometrial stromal sarcomas (ESS), and the majority are adenosarcomas. A number of other sarcomas of the uterus have been described but are not discussed here.

  A. Carcinosarcoma. Patients with CS have a median age at diagnosis of 62 years. The risk factors for CS are similar to those for adenocarcinoma of the endometrium: nulliparity, obesity, and diabetes. One in ten patients with CS has a history of exposure to radiation, although this ratio varies among different studies and different regions.

  B. Leiomyosarcoma. Patients with LMS have an average age at diagnosis of 53 years. No clear risk factors have been identified, although 20% of patients with LMS are nulliparous.

  C. Endometrial stromal sarcoma usually is found in postmenopausal women. No risk factors are described for ESS.

II. Histology. Uterine sarcomas traditionally are divided into pure sarcomas, which contain only malignant stromal elements, and mixed sarcomas, which contain both sarcomatous and malignant glandular elements. Each of these two groups can also be described as homologous, containing only elements native to the uterus, or heterologous, containing extrauterine tissue such as striated muscle. The endometrial stromal sarcomas are pure homologous sarcomas. CS is a mixed sarcoma that has both homologous and heterologous variants; leiomyosarcomas are pure sarcomas that also have both homologous and heterologous variants. The presence of heterologous elements does not affect prognosis.

III. Staging. No official staging system exists for uterine sarcomas. Most clinicians use the 1988 FIGO surgical staging system for adenocarcinoma of the endometrium. Clinical staging of the tumors is unreliable.

IV. Diagnosis

  A. Carcinosarcoma. Patients with CS most frequently present with postmenopausal bleeding. Many patients also have pelvic or abdominal pain or an abnormal vaginal discharge. Half of affected women are found to have a polypoid mass protruding through the cervical os; occasionally, patients present with uterine contractions as they deliver a polypoid mass from the endometrial cavity into the vagina. Endometrial biopsy usually confirms the diagnosis. Unlike in endometrial carcinoma, patients with CS frequently present with advanced disease; 10% to 20% of patients with CS present with extrapelvic metastases.

  B. Endometrial stromal sarcoma. Patients with ESS usually present with abnormal uterine bleeding or with pelvic pain. The diagnosis usually can be confirmed by endometrial biopsy.

  C. Leiomyosarcoma. Patients with LMS tend to present with menometrorrhagia or postmenopausal bleeding. The symptoms of LMS are indistinguishable from those of benign leiomyomata, and the diagnosis usually is made after hysterectomy. In a study at Los Angeles County–University of Southern California Medical Center, 0.7% of patients undergoing surgery for leiomyomata were found to have LMS. The risk of LMS increased slightly with age, but other factors thought to assist in the diagnosis, such as the rapid growth of a solitary myoma, were not specific for LMS in this study. Evidence suggests that color-flow Doppler studies may aid in the preoperative diagnosis of LMS, but the validity of this technique and its applicability to the general population remain to be demonstrated.

V. Management

A. Initial management. Uterine sarcomas should be managed initially by exploratory laparotomy through a vertical incision with total abdominal hysterectomy, BSO, and peritoneal washings. All traces of resectable tumor should be removed. Surgical staging using omentectomy and lymph node sampling is controversial because the information gained is often more useful prognostically than therapeutically. Staging facilitates the management of patients who appear intraoperatively to have stage I or II disease because the presence of metastases affects whether and how the patient is treated postoperatively.

B. Management of low-grade lesions. LMS and ESS have low-grade counterparts that often carry a benign prognosis; clinical management of these counterparts therefore may be more conservative than that of frank sarcomas.

1. **Endometrial stromal tumors** are divided into endometrial stromal nodules, low-grade ESS, and high-grade ESS. Endometrial stromal nodules have fewer than five mitoses per high-powered field, pushing boundaries, minimal cytologic atypia, and no evidence of lymph vascular space invasion. The tumors are benign and can be treated with hysterectomy or even myomectomy. Low-grade ESS have similar histologic characteristics to endometrial stromal nodules, except that growths into lymphatic and vascular spaces are found. The clinical behavior of low-grade ESS is difficult to anticipate from the histologic appearance of the specimen, and adjuvant treatment with either progestins or pelvic irradiation is warranted.

2. **Smooth muscle tumors** include intravenous leiomyomatosis, benign metastasizing leiomyomas, and disseminated peritoneal leiomyomatosis. All of these tumors tend to be estrogen-responsive, and treatment with progestins or with oophorectomy in addition to hysterectomy is appropriate. LMS also must be distinguished from leiomyomas of uncertain malignant potential, which are cellular myomas with four to nine mitoses per high-powered field and no cytologic atypia. Leiomyomas of uncertain malignant potential may be treated by hysterectomy, or even by myomectomy alone.

C. Adjuvant treatment

1. **Carcinosarcoma.** The most effective adjuvant therapy for patients with stage I or II CS has not yet been determined. A current trial randomizes patients with optimally debulked CS to whole abdominal and pelvic radiation therapy or treatment with ifosfamide and cisplatin. Patients with distant metastases can be treated with chemotherapy. Hormonal therapy has little effect in CS.

2. **Leiomyosarcoma.** More than one-half of patients with LMS experience recurrence. The tumor tends to resist both radiation and hormonal therapy. Chemotherapy with doxorubicin hydrochloride (Adriamycin) and ifosfamide has a moderated (25%) response.

3. **Endometrial stromal sarcoma.** Pelvic radiation is recommended for patients with stage I ESS. Patients with more advanced disease should receive progestins or tamoxifen if their tumors are hormone receptor–positive and Adriamycin-based chemotherapy if their tumors are hormone receptor–negative.

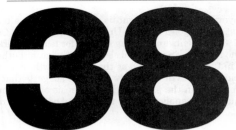

Ovarian Cancer

Linda Duska and
Annette Bicher

I. Epithelial ovarian cancer accounts for 90% of all cases of ovarian cancer. The tumors are derived from the coelomic epithelium, or mesothelium.

   A. Epidemiology. Ovarian cancer is the fifth most common malignancy in American women. In the United States it is the leading cause of death from gynecologic cancer. Ovarian cancer is the seventh most common malignancy worldwide.

      1. Incidence and mortality. Ovarian cancer currently has the highest fatality-to-case ratio of all the gynecologic malignancies. In 1998, approximately 25,400 new cases of ovarian cancer will be diagnosed and 14,500 women will die from their disease (1). For women in the United States, lifetime risk of developing the disease is approximately 1 in 70, or 1.4%. Epithelial ovarian cancer is common in women younger than 40 years, increases to a peak in women aged 60 to 64 years, then decreases, as shown in Fig. 38-1. The incidence of ovarian cancer shows wide geographic variation, with the highest incidence rates (11.5 to 15.3 per 100,000 women) in Scandinavian countries, Israel, and North America; and the lowest rates (3.3 to 7.8 per 100,000 women) in developing countries and Japan. The incidence of ovarian cancer has remained stable over the last three decades in high-risk (developed) countries, whereas increasing incidence has been reported in low-risk (developing) countries (Fig. 38-2).

      2. Risk factors. The causes of ovarian cancer are poorly understood, but several factors have been associated with an increased or decreased risk of the disease.

         a. Individual risk and protective factors. Age over 40 years, white race, nulliparity, infertility, history of endometrial or breast cancer, and family history of ovarian cancer consistently have been found to increase the risk for invasive epithelial cancer. Parity, oral contraceptive (OC) use, history of breast-feeding, tubal ligation, and hysterectomy have been associated with decreased risk of ovarian cancer. The relationship of a number of additional factors to the risk of ovarian cancer has not been well elucidated; these factors include age of menarche, age of menopause, use of fertility drugs, estrogen replacement therapy, talc use, dietary factors, lactose intolerance, and history of mumps and other infectious diseases.

         b. Family history. An association between ovarian cancer and a family history of ovarian cancer and other malignancies including breast, endometrial, colon, and prostate cancer has been reported in the literature. Although the lifetime risk for American women is estimated to be 1.4%, women who have one first-degree relative with ovarian cancer have a 5% risk, and women with two first-degree relatives with ovarian cancer have a 7% risk of developing ovarian cancer (2). A very small subset of women with two first-degree relatives with ovarian cancer have one of the three distinct autosomal dominant syndromes that have been termed *familial ovarian cancer*: site-specific ovary, breast-ovary, and Lynch II syndromes. (Lynch syndromes are heredi-

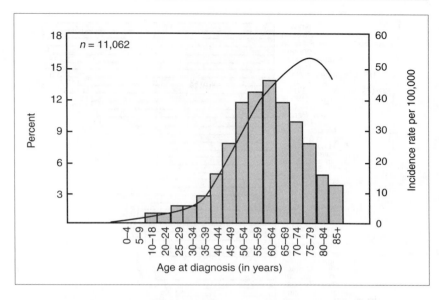

Figure 38-1. Ovarian cancer incidence rates by age, 1973 to 1982. (From Yancik R, Ries LG, Yates JW. Ovarian cancer in the elderly: an analysis of surveillance, epidemiology, and end results program data. *Am J Obstet Gynecol* 1986;154:639–647. Reprinted with permission.)

tary nonpolyposis colorectal cancers. Lynch I is colorectal cancer. Lynch II families have associated endometrial, ovarian, and other cancers.) These syndromes can involve the breast, ovary, colon, and endometrium. The risk of developing ovarian cancer for a woman with two or more affected first-degree relatives and whose family carries familial ovarian cancer has been estimated to be 40% to 50%. The hereditary ovarian cancer syndromes are rare, accounting for less than 1% of all reported ovarian cancer cases. The recent identification of the breast and ovarian cancer susceptibility gene (*BRCA1*) is an important advance in the field of genetic epidemiology. This gene has been linked to familial breast cancer and may be linked to the breast-ovary and site-specific ovarian cancer syndromes. Several genes for Lynch II syndrome have also been identified. Screening tests for these genes are available.

c. **Environmental factors** may play a role in ovarian cancer. An association between diet and ovarian cancer was suggested on the basis of the geographic variation of ovarian cancer incidence and mortality. Some have suggested that diets high in animal fat increase the risk of ovarian cancer. Decreased risk has been associated with higher intake of total vegetables, vitamin A, and vitamin C. An association between talc use and ovarian cancer has been proposed; the epidemiologic data, however, remain inconclusive.

d. **Reproductive factors** play an important role in ovarian cancer risk. Increasing parity decreases the relative risk of developing ovarian cancer. Nulliparity has been associated with an increased risk of ovarian cancer. The use of OCs also has been associated with a decreased relative risk. Increasing duration of OC use has been associated with decreasing risk, and evidence suggests that the protective effect of OC

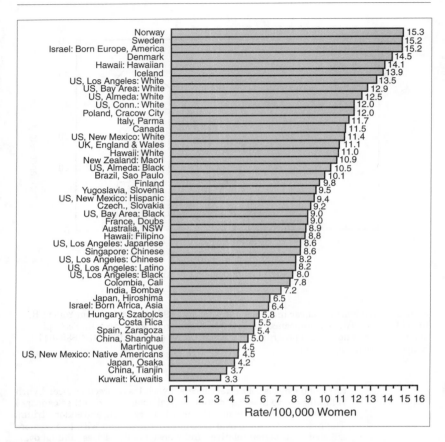

Figure 38-2. Age-adjusted incidence rates of ovarian cancer in selected populations, 1978 to 1982. Rates adjusted to the world standard population. (From Tortolero-Luna G, Mitchell MF, Rhodes-Morris HE. Epidemiology and screening of ovarian cancer. *Obstet Gynecol Clin North Am* 1994;21:3, with data from Muir C, Waterhouse J, Mack T, et al. *Cancer incidence in five continents*. Lyon: IARC, 1987:892–893. Reproduced with permission.)

use persists for 10 or more years after discontinuation of use. Women with a history of breast-feeding have been reported to have a lower risk for ovarian cancer than nulliparous women and parous women who have not breast-fed. Women with a history of difficulty conceiving have been found to have an elevated risk of ovarian cancer; the association remains inconclusive, however, because the multitude of causes of infertility have not been separated clearly in studies. In addition, the risk of nulliparity has been difficult to separate from the risk of difficulty conceiving. The use of fertility drugs has not yet been associated clearly with an elevated risk of ovarian cancer. Tubal ligation or hysterectomy with ovarian preservation both lower the risk of ovarian cancer.

3. **Etiology.** The etiology of ovarian cancer is multifactorial. Three main hypotheses have been proposed to explain the pathogenesis: the inces-

sant ovulation, gonadotropin, and pelvic contamination theories. The first two theories have received the most support from epidemiologic data. The possibility that a combination of these hypothetical etiologies occurs during the complex process of carcinogenesis has also been suggested, and future results from studies should help to clarify the issue.

   a. **The incessant ovulation hypothesis** postulates that repeated minor trauma to the epithelial surface of the ovary caused by continuous ovulation increases the likelihood of ovarian cancer. The protective effects of ovulation suppression by parity, OC use, lactation, and pelvic surgery support this hypothesis. The differences in protective effect provided by pregnancy and OC use, however, undermine this hypothesis.

   b. **The gonadotropin hypothesis,** which postulates that exposure of the ovary to continuously high circulating levels of pituitary gonadotropin increases the risk of malignancy, is supported by the protective effects of parity and OC use and the increased risk observed with fertility drugs. The protective effect of lactation, which increases follicle-stimulating hormone, however, is inconsistent with the gonadotropin hypothesis. The lack of association of ovarian cancer with late age of menopause also is inconsistent with both the incessant ovulation and the gonadotropin hypotheses.

   c. **The pelvic contamination theory** suggests that carcinogens may come into contact with the ovary after passing through the genital tract. Although the protection afforded by tubal ligation and hysterectomy supports this hypothesis, the significant role of other reproductive factors is not explained by the pelvic contamination theory.

B. **Detection and prevention**

   1. **Criteria for effective screening tools.** Early ovarian cancer is a silent and often asymptomatic disease. An effective screening test must have sufficient specificity, sensitivity, and positive predictive value for the disease it is employed to detect. To screen large populations of women, the screening test must also be cost-effective. A sufficiently high positive predictive value is difficult to achieve for a disease with such a low incidence as ovarian cancer (compared with breast cancer, which occurs in 1 of 9 women, ovarian cancer occurs in 1 of 70). Currently, no available screening test has sufficient positive predictive value for early-stage ovarian cancer.

   2. **Routine yearly pelvic examination** is currently in use for the general population as a screening tool. The rectovaginal pelvic examination, however, does not have sufficient sensitivity to diagnose early disease.

   3. **CA-125,** first described in the 1980s, is an antigen expressed by 80% of nonmucinous epithelial ovarian cancers. A level greater than 35 U/mL is considered abnormal. In premenopausal women, however, CA-125 levels may also be elevated in a number of benign conditions, including pelvic inflammatory disease, endometriosis, pregnancy, and hemorrhagic ovarian cysts. In addition, approximately 50% of women with early ovarian cancer have a normal CA-125 level (3). Other markers for ovarian cancer include CA-19-9, CA-15-3, OVX1, *Her-2/neu* and human chorionic gonadotropin (hCG) fragments, and the use of combinations of these markers in screening tests has been investigated; an appropriately sensitive and specific combination, however, has not been identified.

   4. **Transvaginal ultrasound** also has been considered as a screening tool, in combination with color Doppler imaging. Unfortunately, transvaginal ultrasound has a poor positive predictive value when used to screen the general population. In one metaanalysis, ultrasound findings led to 32 surgeries for each case of ovarian cancer identified (4). If the use of ultrasound as a screening tool is limited to high-risk populations (postmenopausal patients or women with a significant family history), then 17 surgeries are required to find one case of stage I cancer. Multimodal screening using CA-125 with sonogram has been evaluated and found not to be an efficacious general screening tool.

5. **Current recommendations for screening** include a comprehensive family history and annual rectovaginal pelvic examination for women with no significant family history of ovarian cancer (3). Women with two or more first-degree relatives with ovarian cancer have a 3% chance of having a familial ovarian cancer syndrome, which carries a 40% lifetime risk of ovarian cancer; these women should be examined and counseled by a gynecologic oncologist. Women with a familial ovarian cancer syndrome should undergo annual rectovaginal pelvic examination, CA-125 determination, and transvaginal ultrasound. Most authors agree that after women at high risk for ovarian cancer complete their childbearing, they should undergo prophylactic oophorectomy. Participation in a clinical trial for screening should be encouraged. *BRCA1* testing, if available, helps to identify patients at highest risk of hereditary ovarian cancer.

6. **Prevention**

   a. If a woman is undergoing pelvic surgery for other reasons, **prophylactic removal of the ovaries** may be considered to eliminate her risk of future ovarian cancer almost entirely (although the risk of peritoneal cancer still exists after removal of both ovaries). The associated risk of premature menopause, with its potential for bone loss and heart disease, must be weighed against the risk of developing ovarian cancer.

   b. Because their use has been shown to be protective, a number of authors suggest encouraging the use of **OCs.** High-risk groups may be the most appropriate candidates for OC prophylaxis.

   c. **Potential methods.** No chemoprophylactic agents are currently available for ovarian cancer. Because of the difficulty in detecting early stages of ovarian cancer, designing a chemo prevention trial is difficult. High-risk groups such as nulliparous women taking infertility drugs may be sufficiently well defined to allow chemo preventive interventions. Retenoids may be a reasonable choice, given the antiproliferative effects they have shown (5).

C. **Pathology of epithelial ovarian cancer.** Epithelial tumors are thought to arise from the surface epithelium of the ovary, which is closely related to the coelomic epithelium lining the peritoneal cavity. The tumors are classified by cell type and behavior as benign, borderline [low malignant potential (LMP)], or malignant. Borderline tumors are associated with a small risk of recurrence, may have invasive implants, and may decrease survival. Malignant tumors recur, metastasize, and decrease survival.

   1. **Serous tumors.** The serous histologic subtype is the most common, accounting for 46% of all epithelial ovarian tumors. The mean age of patients at diagnosis is 56 years. The epithelium resembles the normal lining of the fallopian tube. Seventeen percent of serous tumors are borderline, and 33% are malignant. Thirty-three percent of borderline tumors are bilateral, and carcinomas are bilateral in 33% to 67% of cases.

   2. **Mucinous tumors** are lined by cells that resemble the cells of the endocervical glands. Eighty percent of all ovarian mucinous tumors are benign; malignant mucinous ovarian tumors are quite rare. Less than 5% of mucinous tumors are malignant, and 16% are borderline. The mean age of patients diagnosed with malignant tumors is 52 years. Mucinous tumors can become quite large, filling the abdominal cavity. Malignant tumors are commonly bilateral (although borderline mucinous tumors are bilateral in only 8% of cases).

   3. **Endometrioid tumors** account for 6% to 8% of epithelial tumors. Most endometrioid tumors are malignant. Twenty percent may be borderline. The mean age of patients diagnosed with malignant tumors is 57 years. A significant proportion of cases have been associated with endometrial adenocarcinoma, and 10% of cases are associated with endometriosis.

   4. **Clear cell carcinomas** account for 3% of ovarian cancers. These tumors are the ovarian neoplasms most commonly associated with hypercalcemia and hyperpyrexia. Histologically, hobnail-shaped cells are characteristic

of the clear cell carcinomas. The mean age of patients diagnosed with clear cell carcinoma is 53 years. Clear cell adenocarcinoma is bilateral in 13% of cases. Clear cell carcinomas also have been associated with endometrial cancer and endometriosis.

5. **Malignant Brenner tumors** are very rare and are defined as a benign Brenner tumor associated with an invasive component of another type of carcinoma.

D. **Natural history**

1. **Precursor lesions.** The pathogenesis of epithelial ovarian cancer, which may develop *de novo* from benign lesions, or from changes in borderline, LMP tumors, is unknown. The concept of ovarian intraepithelial neoplasia is neither well understood nor universally accepted.

2. **Pattern of metastasis.** Ovarian cancer can spread by direct extension, by exfoliation of cells into the peritoneal cavity (transcoelomic spread), via the bloodstream, or via the lymphatic system. The most common pathway of spread is believed to be transcoelomic. Cells from the tumor are shed into the peritoneal cavity and circulate, following the path of the peritoneal fluid up the paracolic gutters, along the intestinal mesenteries, and up to the diaphragm. Commonly, the omentum also is involved. Essentially all peritoneal surfaces are at risk. Lymphatic spread to the pelvic and paraaortic lymph nodes can occur. Hematogenous spread to the liver or lungs can occur in advanced disease.

E. **Clinical evaluation**

1. **Presentation.** Approximately 80% of patients diagnosed with epithelial ovarian cancer have advanced (stage III or greater) disease. Although some women with early disease experience symptoms, including pelvic pain or pressure, most women are asymptomatic. Often, the symptoms that develop are vague, and include abdominal bloating, early satiety, weight loss, constipation, anorexia, and irregular menstrual bleeding. On physical examination, a pelvic mass is an important sign of disease (Fig. 38-3). Some authors have suggested that a palpable ovary in a postmenopausal patient should be evaluated further, although this suggestion is controversial. Later, abdominal distention may develop, and chest examination may reveal evidence of pleural effusion.

2. **Evaluation of pelvic mass** varies depending on age and index of suspicion. After the decision to proceed to surgical evaluation is made, the preoperative evaluation should include a full history and physical examination. Additional tests, including serum CA-125, pelvic ultrasound, barium enema to rule out primary bowel disease in postmenopausal women, mammogram, Pap smear, complete blood cell count, electrolytes and liver function tests, electrocardiogram and chest radiograph, pulmonary function tests, arterial blood gas, and echocardiogram, should be performed on the basis of a patient's risk factors, the suspicion of malignant disease, and the patient's underlying medical status. Surgery should be preceded by a thorough preparation of the bowel.

F. **Staging.** The assigned stage of disease is based on surgical and pathologic findings (Table 38-1). The importance of complete surgical staging in developing a proper treatment plan and prognosis cannot be overemphasized. In a cooperative national study in which 100 patients with apparent stages I and II disease underwent additional surgical staging, 28% of stage I patients were staged up, and 43% of stage II patients were staged up. The surgical staging procedure involves exploring the abdomen and pelvis through a vertical incision; taking washings from the pelvis, gutters, and diaphragm; taking multiple biopsies of peritoneal sites including pelvic sidewalls, surfaces of the rectum and bladder, cul-de-sac, lateral abdominal gutters, and diaphragm; removing the infracolic omentum, and sampling the pelvic and paraaortic lymph nodes. In addition, a total abdominal hysterectomy and bilateral salpingo-oophorectomy are performed. Debulking, also called *cytoreduction*, is defined as removal of as much tumor as possible during the initial operation. Optimal debulking implies that tumor nodules of no greater diameter than 1 to 2 cm are left

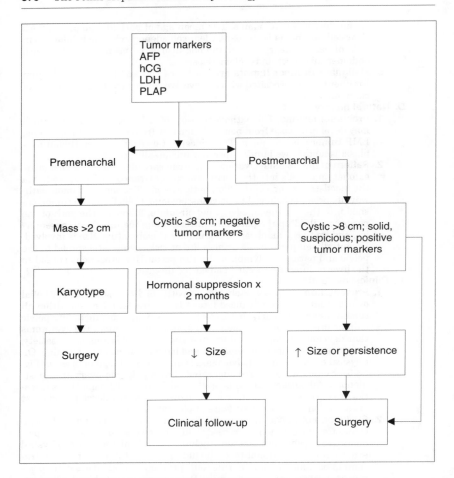

Figure 38-3. Evaluation of a pelvic mass in young female patients. AFP, alpha-fetoprotein; hCG, human chorionic gonadotropin; LDH, lactate dehydrogenase; PLAP, placental alkaline phosphatase. (From Berek JS, Hacker NF, eds. *Practical gynecologic oncology*, 2nd ed. Baltimore: Williams & Wilkins, 1994:381. Reprinted with permission.)

behind. Aggressive attempts at cytoreduction have been shown to improve long-term survival (6).

G. **Prognostic factors.** The overall 5-year survival rate of ovarian cancer is 25% but individual prognoses vary depending on stage, grade, histology of the tumor, and amount of residual disease remaining after initial debulking surgery.

  1. **Stage.** The 5-year survival rate of patients with epithelial ovarian cancer correlates directly with tumor stage. Patients with stage I disease have a 90% 5-year survival rate. This rate assumes that the patient has been surgically staged thoroughly and that microscopic disease in the abdomen has not been missed. Stage II patients have a 5-year survival rate of 80%. Patients with stages III and IV disease have 5-year survival rates of 15% to 20% and less than 5%, respectively.

  2. **Grade and histologic type.** Histologic type historically has not been thought to be important in terms of prognosis. Some studies, however,

Table 38-1. FIGO staging of primary carcinoma of the ovary (1985)

FIGO stage	Tumor characteristics
Stage I	Growth limited to the ovaries.
Stage IA	Growth limited to one ovary; no ascites; no tumor on the external surface; capsule intact.
Stage IB	Growth limited to both ovaries; no ascites; no tumor on the external surfaces; capsule intact.
Stage IC	Tumor either stage IA or IB but with tumor on surface of one or both ovaries; or with capsule ruptured; or with ascites present containing malignant cells; or with positive peritoneal washings.
Stage II	Growth involves one or both ovaries with pelvic extension.
Stage IIA	Extension or metastases to the uterus or tubes.
Stage IIB	Extension to other pelvic tissues.
Stage IIC	Tumor either stage IIA or IIB, but with tumor on surface of one or both ovaries; or with capsule ruptured; or with ascites present containing malignant cells; or with positive peritoneal washings.
Stage III	Tumor involves one or both ovaries with peritoneal implants outside the pelvis and/or positive retroperitoneal or inguinal nodes. Superficial liver metastasis equals stage III. Tumor is limited to the true pelvis but with histologically proven malignant extension to small bowel or omentum.
Stage IIIA	Tumor grossly limited to the true pelvis with negative nodes but with histologically confirmed microscopic seeding of abdominal peritoneal surfaces.
Stage IIIB	Tumor of one or both ovaries with histologically confirmed implants of abdominal peritoneal surfaces, none exceeding 2 cm in diameter; nodes are negative.
Stage IIIC	Abdominal implants >2 cm in diameter or positive retroperitoneal or inguinal nodes.
Stage IV	Growth involves one or both ovaries, with distant metastases. If pleural effusion is present, there must be positive cytology to allot a case to stage IV. Parenchymal liver metastasis equals stage IV.

FIGO, International Federation of Gynecology and Obstetrics.
From ref. 6, adapted with permission.

have indicated that clear cell carcinomas are associated with a worse prognosis than other histologic cell types. Histologic grade is clearly a prognostic factor. The overall 5-year survival for patients with grade 1 epithelial malignancies is 40%, compared with 20% for grade 2 cancers and 5% to 10% for grade 3 cancers.

3. **The volume of residual disease after debulking** surgery correlates with survival. Patients in whom optimal cytoreduction is achieved (no tumor mass >2 cm in diameter) have improved survival rates.

4. **Biological factors.** Tumor ploidy has been shown to be an independent prognostic variable, with one study showing a median survival period of 5 years for diploid tumors, versus a median survival period of 1 year for aneuploid tumors. Some studies have shown a correlation of proliferation fraction by flow cytometry with prognosis. In addition, some investigators have shown a correlation of the expression of the *Her-2/neu* oncogene with poorer prognosis; others have not clearly substantiated this finding, however, and further study is required.

H. **Treatment** of epithelial ovarian cancer depends on whether the disease is considered to be early or late, as well as whether the histology is borderline or malignant.

  1. **LMP,** or borderline, tumors show a different behavior pattern from their malignant counterparts. Overall, borderline tumors comprise 4% to 14% of all ovarian malignancies. Approximately 15% of all epithelial ovarian malignancies are borderline tumors. Borderline tumors most commonly are of the serous or mucinous histologic subtypes. Unlike their malignant counterparts, borderline tumors often are found in younger patients, with mean patient age at diagnosis ranging from 40 to 53 years (compared with 61 years for malignant tumors). The majority of affected patients present with early-stage disease, although 20% show intraabdominal spread (7), and should be treated with surgical staging and debulking as for epithelial malignant tumors. Mucinous borderline tumors may be associated with a concurrent appendiceal primary tumor, and affected patients also should undergo appendectomy. Because of the indolent growth of borderline tumors, controversy exists about the need for subsequent chemotherapy or radiation therapy. If disease recurs, it recurs an average of 10 years after initial diagnosis, and resection can be performed again at the time of recurrence. Most patients die with the disease rather than of the disease. In addition, early-stage disease in women who want to maintain fertility may be treated with unilateral salpingo-oophorectomy, or even with unilateral cystectomy, with good results. Patients who present with stage I disease have a 99% 5-year survival rate.

  2. **Early-stage malignant disease** (stages I and II) may be divided into favorable and unfavorable categories. Patients with stage IA or IB disease and with grade 1 tumors are considered to have a favorable prognosis. Patients with moderately or poorly differentiated tumors of any stage, stage IC, or stage II disease are considered to have an unfavorable prognosis. Patients with an unfavorable disease designation have a relapse rate of at least 20%. In contrast, patients with favorable disease have a 5-year survival of 94% to 96%.

     a. **Surgical therapy.** Initial surgical therapy is necessary for establishing a histologic diagnosis and appropriate staging. A full staging procedure is particularly important for patients with disease that appears to be confined to the pelvis (8). About one-third of such patients are staged up by the results of a complete surgical evaluation. After a full staging procedure, only 10% to 15% of patients with epithelial ovarian cancer are found to have stage I or II disease. Patients with apparent stage I disease may wish to preserve the uterus and one ovary for future childbearing. If the tumor is localized and has favorable histologic characteristics (i.e., grade 1 tumor), such an option may be considered after appropriate counseling of the patient by a gynecologic oncologist. The remainder of the surgical staging should be performed, however, to ensure that the disease is indeed confined to the pelvis. After the procedure, the woman should be followed closely with pelvic examinations and CA-125 measurements. Total abdominal hysterectomy and bilateral salpingo-oophorectomy should be performed after childbearing is completed.

     b. **Chemotherapy.** For patients with early-stage disease and favorable prognostic factors, no chemotherapy is indicated. Patients with unfavorable prognostic factors should receive postoperative chemotherapy. Chemotherapy may be single agent, such as single agent melphalan, platinum, or paclitaxel, or a platinum-based combination regimen. The appropriate chemotherapy regimen for patients with early-stage disease still is being evaluated in clinical trials.

     c. **Radiation.** Patients with early-stage disease have been treated with whole abdominal radiation or intraperitoneal radiocolloids (^{32}P), resulting in decreased disease-free periods but with identical overall 5-year survival rates, compared with surgical therapy. Radiologic methods, however, currently are used only in the setting of clinical trials.

3. **Advanced disease** always requires an effort at optimal surgical debulking and a course of chemotherapy after initial surgery to improve patients' chances for survival.

   a. **Primary cytoreductive surgery,** or debulking, is the most important treatment of advanced disease. No universal agreement on the precise definition of optimal debulking has been reached. Different authors use different measures of residual disease in their definition of optimal; these values range from 1 to 2 cm. The measurement of residual disease does not represent the total volume of tumor cells left behind, but merely the diameter of the largest residual nodule. For example, a patient with one unresected nodule measuring 2.5 cm is not optimally debulked, whereas a patient with miliary studding of the entire peritoneal cavity with residual tumor implants is considered to be optimally debulked.

   b. **Combination chemotherapy** most often is used as postoperative treatment for advanced epithelial ovarian cancer. Combination chemotherapy with six courses of cisplatin or carboplatin plus paclitaxel is the treatment of choice for patients with advanced disease. Courses are given every 3 to 4 weeks, with monitoring of tumor status by physical examination, CA-125 levels, and imaging studies if appropriate.

      (1) **Cisplatin** acts by binding to DNA and producing cross-links and DNA adducts. Important side effects include severe nausea and vomiting, dose-related nephrotoxicity, ototoxicity, peripheral neuropathy, and myelosuppression.

      (2) The mechanism of action of **carboplatin** is the same as that of cisplatin; the side effects, however, differ greatly. The most important side effect of carboplatin is thrombocytopenia. Leukopenia and anemia also occur but are less severe. Neurotoxicity and nephrotoxicity are less severe with carboplatin than with cisplatin. Other important side effects include alopecia and mucositis.

      (3) **Paclitaxel** acts as a mitotic spindle poison. Some patients exhibit hypersensitivity to paclitaxel. Other important side effects include myelosuppression, neuropathy, mucositis, diarrhea, alopecia, nausea, and vomiting.

   c. **Whole abdominal radiation** may be used as an alternative to chemotherapy, although it is not widely used as a first-line treatment in the United States. Radiotherapy is most effective in patients who have no macroscopic residual disease after primary debulking. Acute side effects include fatigue, nausea, and vomiting. Long-term side effects are more severe and include bowel damage resulting in obstruction that sometimes requires surgical therapy.

   d. **New therapies.** Disappointingly low lifetime survival rates in patients with advanced epithelial ovarian cancer have stimulated continued innovation in treatment approach. Experimental first-line postoperative treatments include concomitant chemotherapy and radiation therapy and dose-intensity strategies using autologous bone marrow transplant or peripheral stem cell support. Drugs undergoing phase II trials include Navelbine and Doxil, which is a liposomal doxorubicin, currently under investigation for salvage therapy. Other new chemotherapeutic ideas for salvage include weekly single-agent regimens of taxol or gemcitabine, as well as some new phase I drugs identified only by numbers. Alternative modalities, including biologic therapy using autologous tumor-infiltrating lymphocytes and monoclonal antibodies are also under investigation.

   e. **Second-look laparotomy** is performed in an experimental setting on patients with advanced epithelial ovarian cancer who have undergone primary debulking followed by a complete course of chemotherapy and who have no clinical evidence of disease. The technique is identical to that of the staging laparotomy and requires multiple peritoneal biopsies and washings if no gross disease is apparent. Biopsies of the peritoneal surfaces in the areas of previously documented tumor are most important to obtain because they are most likely to produce a positive result. In 50% of patients, clinically occult disease appears on surgical exploration. For these patients, further treatment is indicated. Patients with persistent gross disease may be candidates for secondary cytoreduction. Of patients with negative findings on second-look laparotomy, 20% to 50% experience recurrence of disease. Consolidation treatment should be considered in these patients. Patients with negative findings on second-look laparotomy have a 5-year survival rate of 50%, compared with a rate of 5% to 35% for patients with a positive finding on second-look laparotomy. The use of second-look laparotomy in the management of patients with advanced epithelial ovarian cancer remains controversial (9,10). Second-look laparotomy has not been shown to affect patient survival, and therefore should be performed only in the setting of a clinical trial, not as routine care for all patients.

f. **Second-line chemotherapy.** Patients with persistent gross disease should be treated with second-line chemotherapy. Unfortunately, response rates for second-line chemotherapy are only 10% to 30%. Depending on the initial chemotherapy, second-line chemotherapy may include platinum, paclitaxel, ifosfamide, or hexamethylmelamine. Regardless of the approach, chemotherapy in this setting is not curative.

g. **Second-look laparoscopy** may be performed as an alternative to second-look laparotomy. Visibility may be limited, however, by the presence of intraabdominal adhesions. In addition, in laparoscopy procedures the operator is unable to perform a manual exploration of the entire bowel or the peritoneal cavity. The role of second-look laparoscopy is still being defined.

h. **Appropriate follow-up for asymptomatic patients** after completion of primary surgery and a full course of chemotherapy should include routine history and physical examination, rectovaginal examination, and CA-125 testing. As discussed in sec. I.H.3.e, the role of second-look laparotomy is a subject of controversy. Patients should be seen every 3 months for the first 2 years. In patients whose CA-125 level was elevated preoperatively, CA-125 is a reliable marker of disease recurrence (although a negative CA-125 test result does not guarantee disease absence). The combination of thorough physical examination and CA-125 testing has been shown to detect recurrent disease in 90% of patients (3).

4. **Recurrent or persistent disease**

a. **Secondary debulking.** Patients with recurrent or persistent disease may be candidates for further surgical therapy, or secondary debulking. Surgery should be reserved for patients in whom therapy has a good chance of prolonging life or palliating symptoms; the majority of patients with persistent or progressive disease after primary therapy do not benefit from secondary debulking, and at this time no effective salvage treatment is available for patients with recurrent or persistent disease.

b. **Salvage chemotherapy.** Unfortunately, response rates for second-line chemotherapy are in the range of 10% to 30%. For women with recurrent disease resistant to platinum who have not received paclitaxel, it is the best salvage therapy currently available. Some interest in intraperitoneal (IP) chemotherapy has been shown; the complete response rate for IP chemotherapy, however, is only 10% to 20%. Most commonly, IP cisplatin is used. An IP catheter must be surgically placed for IP chemotherapy administration. Complications can occur with the catheter. In addition, patients with dense peritoneal adhesions are not candidates for IP therapy because the drug cannot be distributed evenly.

c. **Whole abdominal radiation** has been used as a salvage therapy. It may be effective in patients with microscopic disease, but it is associated with high intestinal morbidity. Thirty percent of patients develop intestinal obstruction after whole abdominal radiation. IP therapy with

^{32}P is under investigation in clinical trials for patients with microscopic residual disease at second-look laparotomy.

d. **Hormone therapy** has been used as salvage treatment. Both megestrol (Megace) and tamoxifen have been used in experimental protocols to treat recurrent disease. Response rates have been low: 15% and 45%, respectively.

e. **Experimental protocols**

(1) **Stem-cell therapy.** Clinical trials are under way using high-dose chemotherapy regimens followed by autologous bone marrow transplant.

(2) **Immunotherapy.** Interferon has been found to have some activity in patients with minimal residual disease. Studies are being done with cytokines, tumor necrosis factor, and interleukin-2. Vaccine trials are under way, but results are not yet available.

(3) **Genetic therapy.** Currently, experimental protocols are using adenovirus vectors, administered intraperitoneally, to deliver genes to patients.

5. **Complications of advanced ovarian cancer**

a. **Intestinal obstruction.** Many women with ovarian cancer develop intestinal obstruction, either at initial diagnosis or with recurrent disease. Obstruction may be related to mechanical blockage or carcinomatous ileus. Correction of intestinal obstruction at initial treatment is usually possible; obstruction associated with recurrent disease, however, is a more complex problem. Some of these obstructions may be treated conservatively with i.v. hydration, total parenteral nutrition, and gastric decompression. The decision to proceed with palliative surgery must be based on the physical condition of the patient and her expected survival. In one study, surgical treatment corrected the intestinal obstruction in 79% of patients; the remaining patients were deemed inoperable (11). Of the patients who underwent successful surgery, mean survival was only 6.8 months. If patients are unable to undergo surgery or are judged to be poor operative candidates, a percutaneous gastric tube may offer some relief.

b. **Ascites.** Initial ascites on presentation with ovarian cancer is almost always cured by debulking surgery and, possibly, several courses of chemotherapy. Persistent ascites is difficult to manage and is a very poor prognostic sign. Installation of bleomycin into the peritoneal cavity has been tried, with limited success. Ascites is best managed by repeated paracenteses as needed and appropriate treatment, if possible, for the patient's cancer.

I. **Survival**

1. **Borderline tumors.** Overall survival for borderline tumors is excellent. Unlike patients with epithelial malignancies, most patients with borderline tumors die with their disease rather than of their disease. Ten- and 20-year survival rates are 95% and 90%, respectively.

2. **Early-stage malignant disease.** The 5-year survival rates for patients who are appropriately surgically staged with stage I or stage II disease are 80% to 100%, depending on the tumor grade.

3. **Advanced disease.** The 5-year survival rate for patients with stage IIIA tumors is 30% to 40%. Patients with stage IIIB disease have a 5-year survival rate of 20%, and patients with stages IIIC and IV disease have a 5-year survival rate of 5%. Recall that approximately 80% of patients have at least stage III disease on presentation.

4. **Recurrent disease.** Patients with no evidence of disease at second-look laparotomy have a 5-year survival rate of 50% (recall that most patients who undergo second-look laparotomy initially presented with stage III or higher disease). In contrast, patients with microscopic residual disease have a 5-year survival rate of 35%, and those with macroscopic residual disease have a 5-year survival of 5%.

5. **Age.** Regardless of disease stage, patients younger than 50 years have a 5-year survival of 50%, versus 15% for patients older than 50 years.
6. **Performance status.** Patients whose Karnofsky index (KI) is low (less than 70) have a significantly shorter survival period than those with a KI higher than 70.

J. **Peritoneal carcinoma.** The primary malignant transformation of the peritoneum is termed *primary peritoneal carcinoma* or *primary peritoneal papillary serous carcinoma*, and clinically and pathologically resembles serous carcinoma of the ovary. A borderline or LMP variant of this tumor also exists, which behaves clinically similar to a serous borderline tumor of the ovary. Primary peritoneal carcinoma therefore can appear to cause ovarian cancer in patients with a history of oophorectomy or with pathologically normal-appearing or minimally involved ovaries. Extensive upper abdominal disease is common, and clinical course, management, and prognosis are similar to that for epithelial ovarian cancer.

K. **Ovarian cancer in pregnancy** is very rare. One study from Israel quoted an incidence of malignant ovarian tumors in pregnancy of 0.12 per 100,000 women (12). Borderline tumors were present in 35% of these cases, epithelial cancers in 30%, dysgerminoma in 17%, granuloma cell tumor in 13%, and undifferentiated carcinoma in 5%. Seventy-four percent of patients were diagnosed with stage I disease. Early-stage disease can be treated with conservative surgery in the second trimester of pregnancy, usually with good maternal and fetal results. Late-stage and high-grade disease should be treated aggressively after appropriate counseling of the patient.

II. **Nonepithelial tumors of the ovary** are rare, compared with epithelial tumors, accounting for 10% of cases of ovarian cancer.

A. **Germ cell tumors** (Fig. 38-4)

1. **Epidemiology.** Twenty percent to 25% of all benign and malignant tumors of the ovary are of germ cell origin, but only 3% of these are malignant. Germ cell malignancies account for fewer than 5% of all cases of ovarian cancers in the United States. In the first two decades of life, 70% of ovarian tumors are of germ cell origin and one-third are malignant. Germ cell tumors are quite rare after the third decade of life.

2. **Pathology.** Germ cell tumors are derived from the primordial germ cells of the ovary.

3. **Diagnosis.** Clinically, germ cell malignancies grow quickly and often are characterized by acute pelvic pain. The pain can be caused by distention of the ovarian capsule, hemorrhage, necrosis, or torsion. Adnexal masses that are 2 cm or larger in premenarchal girls or 8 cm or larger in premenopausal patients necessitate surgical exploration. Tumor markers may assist in the diagnosis of germ cell malignancies (see Figs. 38-3 and 38-4).

4. **Preoperative workup** should include serum hCG and alpha-fetoprotein (AFP) titers, a complete blood cell count, and liver function tests. A chest x-ray study is important to rule out pulmonary metastases. A preoperative computed tomographic scan should be considered to assess for the presence or absence of liver metastases and retroperitoneal lymphadenopathy.

5. **Specific tumor types**

a. **Dysgerminoma**

(1) **Incidence.** Dysgerminoma is the most common germ cell tumor, comprising 30% to 40% of ovarian cancers of germ cell origin. Among all age groups dysgerminoma accounts for 12% of all ovarian cancers but 5% to 10% of ovarian cancers in patients younger than 20 years. Seventy-five percent of dysgerminomas occur in the second and third decades of life. Five percent of dysgerminomas occur in phenotypic female patients with gonadal dysgenesis. In these patients, the dysgerminoma may arise in a gonadoblastoma. More than 50% of gonadoblastomas left *in situ* in patients with gonadal dysgenesis have been reported to develop into malignancies.

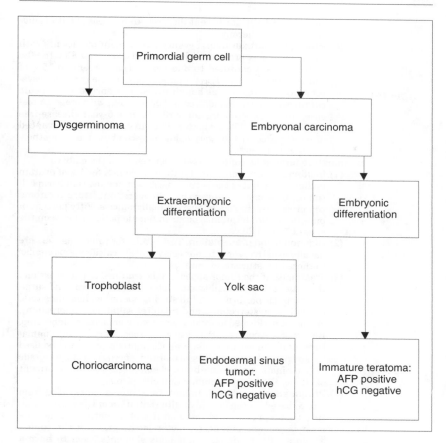

Figure 38-4. Origin of malignant germ cell tumors and their markers. AFP, alpha-fetoprotein; hCG, human chorionic gonadotropin.

(2) **Diagnosis and presentation.** The diagnosis and presentation of dysgerminoma is typical of the diagnosis and presentation of germ cell tumors in general.

(3) **Treatment.** Primary treatment is surgical, and should include proper surgical staging. A vertical midline incision should be used. Unilateral oophorectomy is performed. The remaining pelvic organs may be left *in situ* if maintenance of fertility is desired. A careful staging operation should rule out the presence of microscopic disease. Unilateral pelvic lymphadenectomy and paraaortic lymphadenectomy should be performed. Some authors advocate bisection of the contralateral ovary and excisional biopsy of any suspicious lesions because dysgerminoma may be bilateral. Biopsy, however, has been associated with adhesion formation and subsequent infertility. Dysgerminomas are very sensitive to radiation therapy; fertility, however, is lost as a consequence of radiation therapy. Therefore, chemotherapy is the first-line treatment. Usually, combination therapy with three agents is used [one example is bleomycin, etoposide, and

cisplatin (BEP)]. Recurrent disease can be treated with radiation or chemotherapy.

(4) Prognosis and survival. Seventy-five percent of patients with dysgerminomas present with stage I disease, and 85% to 90% of tumors are confined to one ovary. Ten percent to 15% of tumors are bilateral. The tumor spreads via the lymphatic system most commonly, although it also can spread via capsule rupture or via the bloodstream. For patients with stage IA disease, unilateral oophorectomy results in a 5-year, disease-free survival rate of 95% or better. The survival rate for advanced disease treated with surgery followed by combination chemotherapy is 85% to 90%.

b. **Immature teratomas** contain tissues derived from the embryo.
   (1) Incidence. Pure immature teratoma accounts for 1% of ovarian malignancies but is the second most common ovarian germ cell tumor. In women younger than 20 years, immature teratoma comprises 10% to 20% of ovarian malignancies. Fifty percent of pure immature teratomas occur in female patients between the ages of 10 and 20 years.
   (2) Diagnosis and presentation. Test results for tumor markers are usually negative; some tumors may contain calcifications similar to those in mature teratomas.
   (3) Treatment. If the tumor appears to be confined to one ovary and the patient desires fertility, a unilateral oophorectomy and surgical staging is performed. A full staging operation, including total abdominal hysterectomy and bilateral salpingo-oophorectomy, should be performed in women who have completed childbearing. Biopsy of the contralateral ovary is unnecessary because immature teratoma is rarely bilateral. Chemotherapy should be used for any patient who has disease more advanced than stage I, grade 1. Combination platinum-based chemotherapy is the treatment of choice. (BEP is the combination of choice.)
   (4) Prognosis and survival. Immature teratomas are graded from 1 to 3, based on the degree of differentiation of the most immature tissue present and the quantity of immature tissue. The most important prognostic factor is the grade of the tumor. Tumors with malignant squamous elements seem to have a poorer prognosis than tumors without malignant squamous elements. In addition, if the tumor is incompletely resected, survival drops from 94% at 5 years to 50%. The overall 5-year survival rate for patients with disease at all stages is 70% to 80%. The 5-year survival rate for grade 1 tumors is 82%, compared with 62% and 30% for grades 2 and 3, respectively.

c. **Endodermal sinus tumors** (yolk sac tumors) are derived from cells of the primitive yolk sac.
   (1) Incidence. Endodermal sinus tumors are the third most frequently encountered malignant germ cell tumor of the ovary. Median age of presentation is 18 years. One-third of patients are premenarchal.
   (2) Diagnosis and presentation. Abdominal and pelvic pain are the presenting symptoms in 75% of patients. Asymptomatic pelvic mass occurs in 10% of patients. Most endodermal sinus tumors secrete AFP.
   (3) Treatment consists of surgical exploration with unilateral salpingo-oophorectomy. Hysterectomy and contralateral salpingo-oophorectomy do not alter outcome. Gross metastatic disease should be resected; surgical staging, however, is not necessary because all affected patients require chemotherapy. Preferably, cisplatinum-based combination chemotherapy such as BEP is used for adjuvant therapy.

(4) Prognosis and survival. Most patients have early-stage disease at diagnosis. The 2-year survival rate is 60% to 70%.

d. Embryonal carcinoma

(1) Incidence. Embryonal carcinoma is extremely rare. Patients are very young, ranging in age from 4 to 28 years (median 14 years). Embryonal tumors may secrete estrogen.

(2) Presentation is similar to that of endodermal sinus tumors. Because embryonal tumors may produce estrogen, patients may present with precocious pseudopuberty or irregular vaginal bleeding. Primary lesions tend to be large, and two-thirds of lesions are confined to the ovary. Embryonal lesions secrete AFP and hCG.

(3) Treatment is unilateral oophorectomy, followed by combination platinum-based chemotherapy. Radiation is not useful.

e. Choriocarcinoma

(1) Incidence. Pure, nongestational choriocarcinoma of the ovary is extremely rare.

(2) Diagnosis and presentation. Almost all patients are premenarchal. The tumor often produces high levels of hCG. Isosexual precocious puberty is seen occasionally.

(3) Treatment is surgical excision, followed by combination chemotherapy.

(4) Prognosis is poor, because most patients have metastatic disease on presentation.

f. Mixed germ cell tumors contain two or more characteristics of the germ cell tumors discussed above. The most common component is dysgerminoma. Lesions should be managed with combination chemotherapy. Prognosis depends on the size of the initial tumor and the relative amount of the most malignant component of the lesion.

B. Sex cord stromal tumors are derived from the sex cords and mesenchyme of the embryonic gonad and account for 5% of all ovarian tumors and 2% of cases of ovarian cancer.

1. Granulosa cell tumor. The granulosa cell tumor is the most common malignant sex cord stromal tumor. Granulosa cell tumors account for 2% to 3% of all ovarian malignancies. In the majority of cases, the tumor is estrogenic. Two forms exist: an adult form and a much rarer juvenile form. The tumor is bilateral in only 2% of cases. Histologically, the likely origin of these tumors is the normal granulosa cells of the coelomic epithelium.

a. Incidence. Adult granulosa cell tumors occur in the perimenopausal years. Patients' mean age at presentation is 57 years. The highest incidence is in the immediate postmenopausal age group, women aged 51 to 60 years.

b. Diagnosis and presentation. Patients may present with abdominal distention, pain, or a mass. Because most granulosa cell tumors produce estrogen, patients may present with a variety of menstrual irregularities. The incidence of concurrent endometrial hyperplasia is 50%, and the incidence of concurrent endometrial adenocarcinoma is at least 5%. The majority of affected patients present with stage I disease, mainly because the hormonal effects of the tumor cause symptoms early in the disease.

c. Treatment. Surgery alone is usually sufficient treatment. Radiation, chemotherapy, or both are reserved for recurrent disease. If the patient desires to maintain fertility, a unilateral salpingo-oophorectomy is adequate for treating stage IA tumors, and a staging operation also should be performed. If the patient has completed her childbearing, a total abdominal hysterectomy and bilateral salpingo-oophorectomy should be performed. If the uterus is left *in situ*, dilatation and curettage should be performed to rule out endometrial hyperplasia or adenocarcinoma. Chemotherapy after surgery does not prevent recurrence of the disease.

d. Prognosis and survival. Granulosa cell tumors have a propensity for late recurrence, with recurrence reported as many as 30 years after treatment for primary tumor. The 10-year survival rate is 90%, and the 20-year survival rate drops to 75%.

2. **Sertoli-Leydig cell tumor**
   a. **Incidence.** Sertoli-Leydig cell tumors account for only 0.2% of cases of ovarian cancer. Sertoli-Leydig cell tumors are diagnosed most commonly in the third and fourth decades of life. Seventy-five percent of Sertoli-Leydig cell lesions are present in women younger than 40 years. The tumors are most frequently low-grade malignancies.
   b. **Diagnosis and presentation.** Sertoli-Leydig cell tumors often produce androgens. Seventy percent to 85% of patients demonstrate clinical virilization.
   c. **Treatment.** In young patients, unilateral salpingo-oophorectomy may be performed to preserve fertility. In older patients, a total abdominal hysterectomy and bilateral salpingo-oophorectomy should be performed.
   d. **Prognosis.** The 5-year survival rate is 70% to 90%.
C. **Sarcomas.** Malignant mixed-mesodermal tumors of the ovary are extremely rare. The lesions are very aggressive, and no effective treatment exists.
D. **Metastatic tumors** account for 5% to 8% of ovarian malignancies.
   1. **Metastatic gynecologic tumors** may involve the ovaries. Tubal carcinoma involves the ovaries by direct extension in 13% of cases. Cervical cancer very rarely spreads to the ovaries (less than 1% of cases). Endometrial cancer may metastasize to the ovaries; more often, however, synchronous endometrioid adenocarcinoma are the primary lesions that involve the ovary and the endometrium.
   2. **Metastatic breast cancer.** Of women who die of metastatic breast cancer, the ovaries are involved in 24% of cases. Most metastases to the ovaries from a primary breast cancer are bilateral.
   3. **Gastrointestinal cancers** may metastasize to the ovary. Krukenberg's tumor accounts for 30% to 40% of metastatic tumors to the ovary. The metastasis is almost always bilateral and is characterized histologically by signet-ring cells, in which the nucleus is flattened against the cell wall by the accumulation of cytoplasmic mucin. One percent to 2% of women with intestinal cancer have ovarian metastases at the time of presentation. In postmenopausal women undergoing evaluation for an adnexal mass, metastatic colon cancer should be ruled out if possible, using barium enema or a similar study.
   4. **Metastatic carcinoid tumors** are very rare. If an ovarian carcinoid tumor is diagnosed, it is necessary to search for an intestinal primary cancer.
   5. **Lymphomas** of the ovary are usually metastatic and bilateral. Burkitt's lymphoma may affect children or young adults. Rarely, ovarian lesions are the primary manifestation of disease in lymphoma patients.

III. **Fallopian tube cancers**
A. **Epidemiology.** Carcinoma of the fallopian tube is a very rare tumor, accounting for 0.3% to 1.0% of cases of genital tract cancer in women. Carcinoma of the fallopian tube is seen most often in the fifth and sixth decades of life, and affected patients present at a mean age of 55 to 60 years.
B. **Histology.** To confirm a diagnosis of fallopian tube cancer histologically, most of the tumor must be present in the fallopian tube, the mucosa of the tube must be involved, and a demonstrable transition from benign to malignant tubal epithelium must exist.
C. **Clinical presentation and diagnosis.** The classic triad of symptoms of fallopian tube carcinoma is watery vaginal discharge, pelvic mass, and pelvic pain. Most patients, however, do not present with this triad. Vaginal discharge or bleeding is the most common presenting symptom. As in ovarian cancer, presentation may be nonspecific. Ascites may be present if the disease is advanced. Unlike ovarian cancer, fallopian tube carcinoma more often presents at an early stage. In one study, 41% of patients presented with stage I or II disease (13).
D. **Natural history and patterns of spread.** Tubal cancers spread in a similar fashion to ovarian cancers. The main route of spread is transcoelomic.

Table 38-2. Surgical stage of fallopian tube cancer

Stage I	Carcinoma confined to fallopian tube(s)
Stage IA	Unilateral disease; no ascites
Stage IB	Bilateral disease; no ascites
Stage IC	Either A or B with ascites and/or neoplastic cells in peritoneal washings
Stage II	Carcinoma extends beyond fallopian tube(s) but confined to pelvis
Stage IIA	Extension to uterus and/or ovary
Stage IIB	Extension to other pelvic organs
Stage IIC	Either A or B with ascites and/or neoplastic cells in peritoneal washings
Stage III	Carcinoma extends beyond pelvis but confined to abdominal cavity
Stage IIIA	Tumor microscopic only
Stage IIIB	Tumor metastasis ≤2 cm
Stage IIIC	Tumor metastasis >2 cm
Stage IV	Carcinoma extends beyond abdominal cavity

From Podratz KC, Podczaski ES, Gaffey TA, et al. Primary carcinoma of the fallopian tube. *Am J Obstet Gynecol* 1986;154:1319. Modified with permission.

E. **Staging.** The ovarian cancer staging system has been adapted for the fallopian tube. Twenty percent to 25% of patients have stage I disease on presentation, 20% to 25% have stage II, 40% to 50% have stage III, and 5% to 10% have stage IV (Table 38-2).

F. **Treatment** is similar to that of ovarian cancer, with surgical debulking the mainstay of treatment, followed by combination platinum-based chemotherapy. Chemotherapy for early-stage disease is the subject of controversy. In addition, the use of second-look laparotomy for primary fallopian tube carcinoma is controversial and should occur only in the setting of clinical trials.

G. **Prognosis.** The overall 5-year survival rate for fallopian tube cancer is 40%. Prognosis is related to the stage of disease.

References

1. Landis SH, Murray T, Bolden S, Wingo PA. Cancer statistics, 1998. *CA Cancer J Clin* 1998;48:6–25.
2. Nguyen HN, Averette HE, Janicek M. Ovarian carcinoma: a review of the significance of familial risk factors and the role of prophylactic oophorectomy in cancer prevention. *Cancer* 1994;74:545–555.
3. Trimble EL. The NIH consensus conference on ovarian cancer: screening, treatment, and follow-up. *Gynecol Oncol* 1994;55:S1–S3.
4. Karlan BY, Platt LD. The current status of ultrasound and color Doppler imaging in screening for ovarian cancer. Gynecol Oncol 1994;55:S28–S33.
5. Gershenson DM, Tortolero-Luna G, Malpica A, et al. Ovarian intraepithelial neoplasia and ovarian cancer. *Gynecol Cancer Prev* 1996;23:475–543.
6. Hoskins WJ, McGuire WP, Brady MF, et al. The effect of diameter of largest residual disease on survival after primary cytoreductive surgery in patients with suboptimal residual epithelial ovarian carcinoma. *Am J Obstet Gynecol* 1994;170:974–980.
7. Barakat RR. Borderline tumors of the ovary. *Obstet Gynecol Clin North Am* 1994; 21:93–105.
8. Hoskins WJ. Epithelial ovarian carcinoma: principles of primary surgery. *Gynecol Oncol* 1994;55:S91–S96.
9. Creasman WT. Second-look laparotomy in ovarian cancer. *Gynecol Oncol* 1994;55: S122–S127.
10. Podratz KC, Cliby WA. Second-look surgery in the management of epithelial ovarian carcinoma. *Gynecol Oncol* 1994;55:S128–S133.

11. Rubin SC, Hoskins WJ, Benjamin I, Lewis JL Jr. Palliative surgery for intestinal obstruction in advanced ovarian cancer. *Gynecol Oncol* 1989;34:16–19.
12. Dgani R, Shoham (Schwartz) Z, Atar E, Zosmer A, Lancet M. Ovarian carcinoma during pregnancy: a study of 23 cases in Israel between years 1960 and 1984. *Gynecol Oncol* 1989;33:326–331.
13. Harrison CR, Averette HE, Jarrell MA. Carcinoma of the fallopian tube: clinical management. *Gynecol Oncol* 1989;32:357–359.

Gestational Trophoblastic Disease

Cecilia Lyons and
Robert J. Kurman

I. **General features.** Gestational trophoblastic disease (GTD) includes disorders of placental development, hydatidiform mole, neoplasms of the trophoblast, choriocarcinoma, and placental site trophoblastic tumor. A classification by the World Health Organization clearly defines the different histologic forms of GTD.

A. The reported **incidence** of hydatidiform mole and choriocarcinoma varies widely throughout the world; the incidence is greatest in Asia, Africa, and Latin America and significantly lower in North America, Europe, and Australia. Despite methodological differences in calculating the rate of GTD, it appears that developing countries have a substantially higher rate of GTD than Europe and North America. It has been suggested that low socioeconomic conditions or dietary factors may contribute to the development of GTD. One case-control study suggested that dietary deficiency of carotene, a vitamin A precursor, may predispose to molar pregnancy. Definite evidence linking possible etiologic factors with GTD, however, is lacking.

1. **Hydatidiform mole.** In the United States, hydatidiform moles are observed in approximately 1 in 600 therapeutic abortions and 1 in 1,000 to 2,000 pregnancies. Therefore, a practicing obstetrician or gynecologist encounters approximately one or two molar pregnancies per year. Approximately 20% of patients with primary hydatidiform mole develop malignant sequelae; the majority of these sequelae are invasive moles and do not metastasize.

2. **Choriocarcinoma.** In the United States, choriocarcinoma occurs in approximately 1 in 20,000 to 40,000 pregnancies; approximately 50% of gestational choriocarcinomas develop after term pregnancies, with 25% following molar gestations and 25% following nonmolar gestations. Estimates of incidence in Asia, Africa, and Latin America are generally higher than estimates of incidence in the United States, and as many as 1 in 500 to 1,000 pregnancies have been reported to be affected in those areas.

B. An increased risk of a complete hydatidiform mole is present at both extremes of **reproductive age.** In contrast, maternal age has no effect on the risk of a partial hydatidiform mole. Malignant sequelae occur more frequently in older patients.

C. An **obstetric history** of spontaneous abortion is more common in patients with GTD than in other women. Women who have had one hydatidiform mole are at increased risk of having another. Conversely, term pregnancies and live births have a protective effect; GTD is less common in patients who are parous than in nulliparous patients.

D. An association has been reported between ABO **blood groups** and choriocarcinoma, but not hydatidiform mole. Among patients with choriocarcinoma, blood group A is more prevalent and blood group O is less prevalent. The significance of these data is difficult to assess because the children of gestations associated with choriocarcinoma show no pattern in blood group distribution. In contrast to ABO blood group distribution, no consistent pattern in HLA distribution has been observed between women with choriocarcinoma and their partners.

II. **Morphology of normal trophoblast.** In normal placentation, the trophoblast associated with chorionic villi is referred to as *villous trophoblast*, whereas the trophoblast in all other locations is referred to as *extravillous trophoblast*. Three distinctive types of trophoblastic cells have been recognized: cytotrophoblast (CT), syncytiotrophoblast (ST), and intermediate trophoblast (IT). Villous trophoblast is composed for the most part of CT and ST, with small amounts of IT. In contrast, the extravillous trophoblast that infiltrates the decidua, myometrium, and spiral arteries of the placental site, also known as the *implantation site* or the *placental bed*, is composed mostly of IT, with a minor component of CT and ST. The cells of CT, or Langhans' cells, are germinative trophoblastic cells, whereas the ST consists of highly differentiated cells that interface with the maternal circulation and produce most of the placental hormones. The IT cell is a distinct form of trophoblastic cell that shares some of the morphologic and functional features of both CT and ST cells.

   A. **Cytotrophoblast.** In normal gestation, CT is composed of primitive epithelial cells that are uniform and polygonal to oval in shape. Cytotrophoblastic cells have a single nucleus, clear to granular cytoplasm, and well-defined cell borders. Mitotic activity is evident.

   B. **Syncytiotrophoblast** consists of large, multinucleate cells with dense, amphophilic cytoplasm containing vacuoles that vary in size, some of which form lacunae. A distinct brush border often lines the cell membrane. ST nuclei are dark and often appear pyknotic. ST cells do not show mitotic activity.

   C. **Intermediate trophoblast.** The cells of IT generally are mononucleate, but cells with several nuclei can be present. IT cells vary in shape, ranging from round to polyhedral to spindle shaped. Cytoplasm is abundant and is eosinophilic to amphophilic. Scattered small vacuoles may be present in IT cytoplasm. The nuclear morphology of these cells is highly characteristic. The nuclei of IT have highly irregular nuclear outlines and hyperchromatic, coarsely granular chromatin. Often, nuclei are lobulated or show multiple deep nuclear clefts. Nucleoli in IT are smaller and less prominent than those in CT, and cytoplasmic nuclear invaginations may be seen. The cytologic features that distinguish IT from CT cells include their larger size, more abundant amphophilic or clear cytoplasm, and coarse, granular chromatin with irregular nuclear membranes. IT, particularly in extravillous locations, shows infiltrative growth into decidua, myometrium, and blood vessels dissecting the normal cells. Intermediate trophoblastic cells characteristically invade the wall of large vascular channels until the wall is completely replaced. Eosinophilic fibrinoid material often is deposited around IT. The IT cell is the predominant cell of placental site trophoblastic tumors and exaggerated placental sites.

   D. A large number of **protein hormones, steroid hormones, and enzymes** such as human chorionic gonadotropin (hCG), human placental lactogen (hPL), estradiol, progesterone, and placental alkaline phosphatase (PLAP) have been localized in the placenta during various stages of development. Most of these products are confined to the syncytiotrophoblast. CT does not contain either hCG or hPL. IT contains abundant hPL, which appears as early as 12 days' gestation and reaches a peak at 11 to 15 weeks' gestation. In contrast, hCG is present only focally in IT, appearing as early as 12 days' gestation and remaining until 6 weeks' gestation, at which time it disappears. ST contains abundant hCG at least 12 days' gestation until 8 to 10 weeks' gestation, after which it diminishes. By 40 weeks' gestation, hCG is present only focally in ST. hPL also is localized in ST at 12 days' gestation but increases steadily thereafter.

III. **Hydatidiform mole** is a noninvasive abnormal placenta characterized by enlarged, edematous, and vesicular chorionic villi accompanied by variable amounts of proliferative trophoblast. The lesion is classified as either complete hydatidiform mole or partial hydatidiform mole.

   A. **Chromosomal abnormalities.** Cytogenetic studies have shown that chromosomal abnormalities play a key role in the development of both complete and partial moles. Although it is not known why certain chromosomal aberrations lead to the formation of molar pregnancies, experimental studies suggest that a relationship may exist between the molar phenotype and the ratio of paternal to maternal haploid sets of chromosomes. The higher the ratio of paternal to maternal chromosomes, the greater the molar change. Complete moles show a 2 to 0 ratio of paternal to maternal chromosomes, whereas partial moles show a 2 to 1 ratio.

1. Most **complete moles** are diploid, with a 46,XX karyotype, but rare examples are triploid or tetraploid. All the chromosome complements are paternally derived. In the diploid complete mole, both X chromosomes result from duplication of a haploid sperm pronucleus in an empty ovum that has lost its maternal chromosomal haploid set. Duplication of a 23,Y sperm results in a nonviable 46,YY cell. Three percent to 13% of complete moles have a 46,XY chromosome complement, presumably as a result of dispermy, in which an empty ovum is fertilized by two sperm pronuclei, one with an X and the other with a Y chromosome. An embryo or fetus is absent in cases of complete mole; cases in which a fetus is present represent twin gestations, one of which is molar.

2. Karyotypes of **partial moles** most frequently show triploidy (69 chromosomes), with two paternal sets and a maternal chromosome complement. Rarely, a partial mole with an identifiable fetus has a 46,XX karyotype. Rare examples of tetraploidy with three sets of chromosomes of paternal origin also have been reported. When triploidy is present in a partial mole, the chromosomal complement is XXY in 70% of cases, XXX in 27% of cases, and XYY in 3% of cases. The abnormal conceptus in these cases arises from the fertilization of an egg with a haploid set of chromosomes either by two sperms, each with a set of haploid chromosomes, or by a single sperm with a diploid 46,XY complement. A conceptus with a diploid maternal 46,XX genome and a haploid set of paternal chromosomes evolves into an abnormal triploid fetus that is usually a nonmolar pregnancy called a *digynic conceptus*; such pregnancies account for 15% to 20% of cases of triploidy. Therefore, most well-documented partial moles are triploid, but not all triploid conceptuses are associated with partial moles. Although many partial moles have a triploid karyotype and evidence of an embryo or fetus, no consensus has been reached that all partial moles have these features. Similarly, not all molar pregnancies with evidence of fetal development are partial moles, because fetal development may occur in rare instances of twin gestation in which one conceptus is a complete mole.

B. **Clinical features**

1. **Complete moles** typically present between 11 and 25 weeks' gestation, with an average gestational age of 16 weeks. Excessive uterine enlargement for dates and vaginal bleeding are common and are accompanied by severe vomiting (hyperemesis gravidarum) in 25% of cases, pregnancy-induced hypertension in 25% of cases, and hyperthyroidism in 7% of cases. In approximately one-third of patients, however, the uterus is small for dates. The cause of hyperthyroidism is not fully known. Intrinsic thyroid-stimulating activity of hCG is one possible mechanism, but some investigators suggest that trophoblast produces other, undefined substances that cause thyrotoxicosis. Often, patients with a complete mole abort spontaneously, presenting with vaginal bleeding and passage of molar vesicles. Ovarian enlargement caused by multiple theca-lutein cysts and pulmonary embolization occurs in some patients with a complete mole; hCG levels are markedly elevated, and ultrasound often discloses a classic "snowstorm" appearance.

2. **Partial moles** account for 25% to 74% of all molar pregnancies and occur between 9 and 34 weeks' gestation. Patients with partial moles may have signs and symptoms that are similar to those of complete moles, but usually such symptoms are absent. Uterine size is generally small for dates, and excessive uterine enlargement is rare. Usually, the patient presents with abnormal uterine bleeding and is believed to have experienced a

spontaneous or missed abortion. Serum hCG levels are in the normal or low range for gestational age. Hypertension or preeclampsia occur later with a partial mole than with complete moles but can be equally severe.

C. Pathologic findings

1. **Complete hydatidiform mole.** A complete mole is a hydatidiform mole in which hydropic swelling in the majority of villi is accompanied by a variable degree of trophoblastic proliferation. Fetal tissue usually is absent. Most hydatidiform moles have a 46,XX karyotype.

   a. **Gross findings** include massively enlarged, edematous villi that give the classic, grape-like appearance to the placenta. The swollen villi may range in diameter from a few millimeters to as large as 3 cm but usually average 1.5 cm. Molar specimens evacuated by suction curettage may lack vesicles because the evacuation procedure may lead to their collapse. Immersing the tissue in water can resuspend collapsed villi.

   b. **Microscopic features.** Two key features characterize complete mole: trophoblastic proliferation and villous edema. Many villi display central cisterns, characterized by a prominent central space that is completely acellular. The villi usually are avascular, and, typically, patchy villous calcification is present. All hydatidiform moles display some degree of trophoblastic proliferation on the villous surface. This proliferation is haphazard and circumferential around the villus. The proliferation may be significant and affect most villi, or it may be minimal and focal. Columns and streamers of cells, composed of a mixture of CT, ST, and IT, project randomly from the villous surface. Frequently, the trophoblasts show cytologic atypia, with nuclear enlargement, irregularity of the nuclear outline, and hyperchromasia. Mitotic figures may be evident.

2. **Partial hydatidiform mole.** The partial mole has two populations of chorionic villi, one of normal size and the other grossly hydropic.

   a. **Gross findings.** Generally, the amount of tissue found is less than that found in a complete mole, usually no more than 100 to 200 mm. The gross specimen contains large hydropic villi similar to those seen in a complete mole, but smaller and mixed with nonmolar placental tissue, which is an important distinguishing characteristic. A fetus is nearly always present, although it may require careful examination to detect because early fetal death is the rule (8 to 9 weeks' menstrual age). In some cases, the fetus may show gross developmental abnormalities.

   b. **Microscopic findings.** A mixture of edematous villi and small normal-sized villi is present. The chorionic villi often have a scalloped outline, compared with the typically round, distended appearance of the villi in a complete mole. These irregular outlines produce infoldings of the trophoblast into the villous stroma that, when prominent and sectioned tangentially, appear to be inclusions. In addition, the villous stroma of partial moles frequently undergo fibrosis, unlike that of complete moles. The capillaries of partial moles frequently contain nucleated fetal red cells (fetal red cells nucleated between 8 and 12 weeks' gestation). The trophoblasts covering the villi are typically only focally and mildly hyperplastic. As in the complete mole, the trophoblastic overgrowth is circumferential rather than polar. The cell population is composed of CT and ST. IT is rarely encountered.

D. Immunohistochemical findings. As a group, complete moles have widespread, diffuse staining for hCG; moderately diffuse staining for hPL; and focal staining for PLAP. In contrast, partial moles show focal to moderate staining for hCG and widespread, diffuse staining for hPL and PLAP.

E. Differential diagnosis. Studies indicate that no single criterion enables a definitive distinction between complete mole, partial mole, and hydropic abortus. For practical purposes, however, if an abortion specimen shows villous edema that is only evident microscopically and has minimal to no cistern formation, it should not be considered a molar pregnancy. In a hydropic abortus, the trophoblast proliferating from the villous surface characteristically shows polarity and is localized to the distal end of the villous that implants into the decidua.

F. **Clinical behavior**
1. **Complete mole.** Ten percent to 20% of evacuated complete moles are followed by persistent gestational trophoblastic disease that requires therapy, demonstrated by a plateau or rise in hCG titers or the presence of metastasis. Important clinical risk factors identified in more than 60% of patients who have required subsequent chemotherapy include large-for-dates uteri and ovarian enlargement due to theca-lutein cysts. Choriocarcinoma is the most serious form of persistent gestational trophoblastic disease and occurs in about 2% to 3% of complete moles. Currently, no morphologic or genetic markers that can be used to predict the behavior of a complete mole exist. Some studies have suggested that complete moles with a Y chromosome are more likely to undergo malignant transformation than those without a Y chromosome, but other studies have not confirmed this finding. Between 0.6% and 1.5% of patients who have had a complete hydatidiform mole are at risk of having a recurrent molar pregnancy. Some studies show that the need for chemotherapy is greater in recurrent disease than in single occurrences.
2. **Partial mole.** Because less risk of persistent gestational trophoblastic disease exists for partial moles than for complete moles, the percentage of patients requiring therapy after evacuation of a partial mole is no greater than 5%. In one large study, the risk of persistent gestational trophoblastic disease after a partial mole, based on the need for chemotherapy, was 1 in 200, compared with a risk of 1 in 12 after a complete mole. Choriocarcinoma is an extremely rare occurrence after a partial mole; only one well-documented case has been reported. The observed sequelae of a partial mole are persistent intrauterine disease or, in rare instances, an invasive mole. The magnitude of the risk of recurrent partial moles is not known, although recurrent partial mole does occur.
G. **Management.** Occasionally, the diagnosis of a hydatidiform mole is made on the basis of dilation and curettage for an incomplete abortion. In such cases, the patient should undergo serial quantitative measurements of β-hCG levels. A baseline chest radiograph (CXR) also should be obtained. In patients in whom hydatidiform mole is suspected before evacuation, the following laboratory studies should be done: hematologic evaluation, prothrombin time, partial thromboplastin time, a comprehensive panel of blood chemistries, including liver function tests, blood type and screen, and β-hCG level; and CXR.
1. **Complications**
   a. **Common medical complications** of hydatidiform mole include anemia, infection, hyperthyroidism, pregnancy-induced hypertension or preeclampsia, and coagulopathy.
   b. **Pulmonary complications** frequently are observed at the time of evacuation of a mole in patients with marked uterine enlargement. Although the syndrome of trophoblastic embolization has been emphasized as an underlying cause for respiratory distress syndrome, many other potential causes for respiratory distress syndrome have been identified in affected women, including high-output congestive heart failure caused by anemia or hyperthyroidism, preeclampsia, or iatrogenic fluid overload. In general, pulmonary complications should be treated aggressively with therapy directed by Swan-Ganz catheter monitoring and with assisted ventilatory support as required. Hyperthyroidism and pregnancy-induced hypertension usually abate promptly after evacuation of the molar pregnancy and may not require specific therapy. Theca-lutein cysts occur because of β-hCG stimulation and may take several months to resolve after molar evacuation.
2. **Evacuation.** As soon as any medical complications have been stabilized, the mole should be evacuated.
   a. **Suction curettage.** In most patients, the preferred method of evacuation is suction curettage. After dilatation of the cervix, uterine evacuation is accomplished with the largest cannula that can be introduced through the cervix. Intravenous oxytocin is begun after the cervix is

dilated and continued for several hours postoperatively. After completion of suction curettage, gentle sharp curettage may be performed.

b. **Hysterectomy** is an alternative to suction curettage in selected patients. The adnexa usually may be preserved. Although hysterectomy reduces the risk of malignant sequelae, the chance of malignant GTD after hysterectomy for hydatidiform mole remains approximately 3% to 5%. Therefore, patients who have undergone hysterectomy should be monitored with serial β-hCG levels as follows:

(1) hCG level should be determined 48 hours after evacuation.

(2) Patients should be followed with weekly β-hCG level determinations until results are normal for 3 consecutive weeks, then with monthly determinations until results are normal for 6 consecutive months.

(3) Pelvic examinations should be performed to monitor the involution of pelvic structures and to aid in early detection of metastasis.

(4) CXR is indicated if the β-hCG titer plateaus or rises.

H. Follow-up

1. **Contraception** is recommended for the entire interval of gonadotropin follow-up: 6 months to 1 year. If the patient does not require surgical sterilization, either oral contraceptives or barrier methods may be chosen. An intrauterine device should not be inserted until the patient achieves normal gonadotropin levels, because of the risk of uterine perforation.

2. Virtually all episodes of **malignant sequelae** occur within approximately 6 months after molar evacuation of a hydatidiform mole. If β-hCG values rise or plateau over more than 2 weeks, immediate workup and treatment for malignant postmolar GTD is indicated.

3. **Recurrence.** Patients who have had a partial or complete molar gestation have a tenfold increase in risk (1% to 2% incidence) of a second mole in subsequent pregnancies. Therefore, all future pregnancies should be evaluated by ultrasound early in their course.

IV. Invasive hydatidiform mole is a disorder in which hydropic chorionic villi are present within the myometrium or its vascular spaces, or at distant sites. The lesion was formerly known as chorioadenoma destruens, penetrating mole, malignant mole, or molar destruens. Invasive mole is a possible sequela of hydatidiform mole, complete or partial. It is unusual for patients to present with primary invasive mole, although invasive mole can occur simultaneously with intracavitary molar pregnancy. Pathologic diagnosis requires demonstration of molar villi invading the myometrium or deported to extrauterine sites. When metastases occur, they generally are found in the lungs, vagina, vulva, or broad ligament. The diagnosis usually is made from a hysterectomy specimen. Overall, invasive mole is a clinically significant sequela of about 15% of cases of hydatidiform mole.

A. Gross findings. In the uterus, invasive mole is an erosive, hemorrhagic lesion extending from the uterine cavity into the myometrium. Invasion can range from superficial penetration to extension through the wall, with perforation or involvement of the broad ligament. Molar vesicles often are grossly apparent.

B. Microscopic findings. The confirming diagnostic feature is the presence of molar villi along with trophoblast in the myometrium or at an extrauterine site. Hydropic swelling tends not to be as marked as in noninvasive mole. Molar villi usually are no more than 4 to 5 mm in diameter. Lesions at distant sites usually are composed of molar villi confined within blood vessels, without invasion into adjacent tissue. Trophoblastic atypia can vary from slight to extreme. The trophoblastic cells are predominantly of intermediate type.

C. Differential diagnosis

1. **Placenta accreta,** specifically placenta increta or percreta, represents normal placenta that has implanted without an intervening decidual layer and invaded the myometrium. In contrast to invasive mole, the villi in placenta accreta are not hydropic and the trophoblast does not show the proliferative activity found in a mole.

2. Invasive mole must be distinguished from **choriocarcinoma.** Both invasive mole and choriocarcinoma after a hydatidiform mole are detected by a

plateau or elevation in the hCG titer. Consequently, it is often impossible to distinguish between these lesions clinically. Invasive moles are differentiated from choriocarcinomas by the presence of chorionic villi in the former.
   3. **Noninvasive hydatidiform mole** is discussed extensively in sec. **III.**
D. **Clinical behavior.** Invasive mole is the most common form of persistent or metastatic GTD found after hydatidiform mole, occurring 6 to 10 times more frequently than choriocarcinoma. In histologically verified cases, the lesion most often is confined to the uterus, with spread outside the uterus occurring in 20% to 40% of cases. The risk of progression to choriocarcinoma is no greater than that of a complete mole.

V. **Choriocarcinoma** is a pure epithelial neoplasm, comprising both neoplastic ST and CT elements without chorionic villi. Choriocarcinoma may be associated with any form of gestation. Theoretically, choriocarcinoma may arise in the trophoblast of the primitive blastocyst before implantation, but most cases of choriocarcinoma appear to follow a recognizable gestational event. The more abnormal the pregnancy, the more likely that choriocarcinoma may supervene. An incidence of 1 in 160,000 normal gestations, 1 in 15,386 abortions, 1 in 5,333 ectopic pregnancies and 1 in 40 molar pregnancies has been found. Early systemic hematogenous metastasis tends to develop in gestational choriocarcinoma.
A. **Presenting symptoms.** Abnormal uterine bleeding is one of the most frequent symptoms of choriocarcinoma, but uterine lesions may be restricted to the myometrium and remain asymptomatic. Also, many cases of metastatic choriocarcinoma with no uterine tumor have been described. Apparently, the neoplasm undergoes regression in the uterus. The lungs are the most frequent site of blood-borne metastasis, and patients may present with hemoptysis. Symptomatology related to hemorrhagic events in the central nervous system, liver, gastrointestinal tract, or urinary tract also occur. Choriocarcinoma may have an unusually long latent period, manifesting 10 or more years after hysterectomy.
B. **Gross findings.** Uterine choriocarcinoma generally is a dark red, hemorrhagic mass with a shaggy, irregular surface. Rarely, a lesion may lack significant hemorrhage and appear as a fleshy, tan-gray mass with necrosis. The size of uterine lesions varies greatly, ranging from tiny microscopic foci to large necrotic tumors. Metastases outside the uterus appear to be well-circumscribed and hemorrhagic. Ill-defined infiltrative growth is unusual because of the rapid proliferation with hemorrhage and necrosis that characterize the neoplasm.
C. **Microscopic findings.** Choriocarcinoma is characterized by masses and sheets of trophoblastic cells without chorionic villi that invade surrounding tissue and permeate vascular spaces. Central hemorrhage and necrosis, with viable tumor constituting only a thin peripheral rim, is a characteristic feature. The interface with normal tissue, if preserved, is circumscribed. The cellular population of choriocarcinoma consists of a mixture of CT, IT, and ST. The CT and IT components tend to grow in clusters and sheets, separated by ST. Considerable cytologic atypia may appear in the IT and ST, with pleomorphic enlarged nuclei, abnormal mitotic figures, and bizarre cellular configurations. Nuclear chromatin is coarsely granular, with an uneven distribution, and multiple nuclei may be present. Choriocarcinoma has no intrinsic vascular stroma; the tumor receives its vascular supply by syncytial cells permeating and replacing host vessels. Histologic features that reportedly correlate with response to treatment include a marked lymphoid infiltrate, high mitotic activity, nuclear atypia, vascular invasions, and a compact growth pattern showing minimal differentiation into ST. These correlations may have prognostic value but are based only on a small number of cases, and further study is needed to determine their significance.
D. **Clinical behavior.** More than 90% of patients with extrauterine spread of gestational choriocarcinoma have lung metastasis. The frequency of involvement of other sites varies, depending on whether the frequency rates are based on autopsy studies and whether the patients have received chemotherapy. Brain and liver metastases occur in 20% to 60% of patients. The kidney and gastrointestinal tract are the other common sites for metastatic involvement, but almost any organ, including the skin, may be involved. Usually, the infant is free of disease.

VI. **Epithelioid trophoblastic tumors** are very rare, are associated with elevated serum hCG levels, and are composed predominantly of highly atypical mononucleate trophoblastic cells and indistinct ST. The tumors have a striking epithelioid appearance, both in their cytological features and in their pattern of invasion. The invasive pattern is characterized by diffusely infiltrating cords and nests of cells, typically surrounded by dense eosinophilic hyaline material. The hyaline material and necrotic debris simulate keratin; therefore, epithelioid trophoblastic tumors easily may be confused with poorly differentiated squamous carcinoma. Immunohistochemistry testing for hCG is helpful in identifying ST in epithelioid trophoblastic tumors. Because only a few cases have been described, it is difficult to draw any conclusions about the precise biological behavior of the tumor, but a few patients have died of the tumor.

VII. **Placental site trophoblastic tumors** form a variable cellular mass, occupying the endometrium and myometrium, that resembles a nonneoplastic trophoblastic infiltration of the placental site. This type of tumor is composed predominantly of intermediate trophoblast. It is generally benign but can be highly malignant. Placental site trophoblastic tumor (PSTT) is the rarest form of GTD.

    A. **Clinical features.** Patients are in the reproductive age group and can experience either amenorrhea or abnormal bleeding, often accompanied by uterine enlargement. The result of a pregnancy test depends on the type of test used, but is almost always positive with a sensitive immunologic assay.

    B. **Gross findings.** The appearance of the lesion varies from a mass that is barely grossly visible to a diffuse nodular enlargement of the myometrium. Most tumors are well circumscribed, but they can be poorly defined. A PSTT may be polypoid, projecting into the uterine cavity, or may predominantly involve the myometrium. The sectioned surface is soft and tan and contains only focal areas of hemorrhage or necrosis. Invasion frequently extends to the uterine serosa and in rare instances extends to adnexal structures.

    C. **Microscopic findings.** The predominant cells of PSTT are IT. PSTT also contains scattered syncytiotrophoblastic giant cells. The IT cells invade singly or in cords or sheets, separating individual muscle fibers or groups of fibers. Many of the IT cells assume a spindle shape and are closely apposed to myometrial cells. The IT cells have irregular, hyperchromatic nuclei and dense, eosinophilic to amphophilic cytoplasm, with occasional vacuoles. As it is in the normal placental implantation site, abundant extracellular eosinophilic fibrinoid is present in the tumor. The neoplasm has a characteristic form of vascular invasion, in which the blood vessel wall is extensively replaced by trophoblastic cells and fibrinoid material. Decidua or Arias-Stella reaction may be present in the adjacent, uninvolved endometrium. Villi are only rarely present.

    D. The **differential diagnosis** is choriocarcinoma.

    E. **Clinical behavior.** PSTTs tend to have an indolent behavior. In most cases, the tumor is confined to the uterus. Most placental site trophoblastic tumors are benign, but approximately 15% behave in a malignant fashion. In general, PSTTs with a rate of two or fewer mitotic figures per ten high-power fields behave in a benign fashion. In overtly malignant cases, lungs, liver, abdominal cavity, and brain have been involved by metastasis. Metastases usually develop rapidly after the initial diagnosis. Although serum hCG levels are very useful in monitoring disease, the baseline serum hCG level is typically low, despite a large tumor burden, because the predominant cellular population is IT, which secretes only small amounts of hCG.

VIII. **Nonneoplastic trophoblastic lesions**

    A. An **exaggerated placental site** is an exuberant infiltrative proliferation of intermediate trophoblast at the placental site. An exaggerated placental site may occur in association with normal pregnancy, abortion, or frequently, hydatidiform mole. The lesion is characterized by extensive trophoblastic invasion of the endometrium and underlying myometrium. Despite the extensive infiltration by IT, the overall architecture of the uterus is not disturbed. Distinguishing an exaggerated placental site from a PSTT in curettage specimens can be difficult. In an exaggerated placental site, the IT cells do not form confluent masses, no necrosis is present, and little or no mitotic activity is found. In addition, other components associated with normal pregnancy including decidua, villi, CT, and ST, are present in normal implantations but not in PSTT.

B. Placental site nodule and plaque. Placental site nodules are small, localized, circumscribed aggregates of IT that may be found in uterine curettage or hysterectomy specimens. Placental site nodules are also known as hyalinized implantation sites. In reported cases, patients range in age from 20 to 47 years, with their last gestational event ranging from 6 to 108 months before diagnosis. The lesions usually are microscopic abnormalities found on curettage performed for abnormal bleeding, and they often are admixed with proliferative or secretory endometrium. The lesions represent benign retention of a small area of placental implantation site from previous gestations. The nodules and plaques are circumscribed, microscopic foci of hyalin material that contain intermediate trophoblast. Often, these nodules have a thin rim of chronic inflammatory cells. The IT cells in the placental site nodule appear degenerate; their nuclei have granular chromatin and they lack defined cytoplasmic borders. Placental site nodules' microscopic size, circumscription, and extensive hyalinization differentiate them from PSTT.

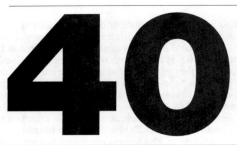

Chemotherapy and Radiation Therapy

Nicholas C. Lambrou,
Edward Trimble, and
Fredrick J. Montz

Chemotherapy

I. **Cell kinetic concepts**
   A. **Normal tissue growth**
      1. **Static population of cells** consists of relatively well-differentiated cells that, after initial proliferative activity in the embryonic and neonatal period, rarely undergo cell division (e.g., striated muscle, neurons).
      2. **Expanding population of cells** comprises normally quiescent cells (liver, kidney) that have the capacity to proliferate and grow when induced by special stimuli (tissue injury).
      3. **Renewing population of cells** is constantly in a proliferative state. Cell division, cell turnover, and cell loss are constant (e.g., bone marrow, epidermis, gastrointestinal mucosa).
      4. **Chemotherapy and tissue growth.** Generally, tissues with a static pattern of growth are rarely seriously injured by drug therapy, while renewing cells are commonly injured.
   B. **Tumor growth.** Although cell proliferation occurs continuously in human tumors, it does not occur more rapidly than in normal tissues. Therefore, it is not the speed of cell proliferation but the failure of the *regulated balance* between cell loss and cell proliferation that differentiates tumorous tissues from normal tissues.
      1. **Gompertzian growth** is governed by the principle that as a tumor's mass increases, the time required to double the tumor's volume also increases.
      2. **Doubling time** is the time it takes for the mass of a tumor to double its size. Considerable variation exists in doubling times of human tumors. Metastases generally have faster doubling times than primary lesions.
      3. **Clinical implications**
         a. Many tumor doublings take place before a tumor is clinically detectable (i.e., 30 doublings for a 1-cm mass).
         b. In late stages of tumor growth, a very few doublings in tumor mass have a dramatic impact on tumor size (e.g., a palpable tumor of 1 cm only takes three doublings to reach a size of 8 cm).
II. **Cell cycle.** The kinetic behavior of individual tumor cells has been well described, and a classic cell cycle model has been developed (Fig. 40-1).
   A. **Growth fraction** is the number of cells in the tumor mass that are actively undergoing cell division.
   B. **Generation time** is the duration of the cycle from M phase to M phase. The largest variation in generation time among tumors occurs in the G_1 phase.
   C. **Cell cycle–specific drugs** depend on the proliferative capacity of the cell and on the phase of the cell cycle for their action. Effective agents act against tumors with relatively long S phases, high growth fractions, and rapid proliferation rates.
   D. **Cell cycle–nonspecific drugs** kill cells in all phases of the cell cycle, and their effectiveness is not very dependent on a tumor's proliferative capacity.

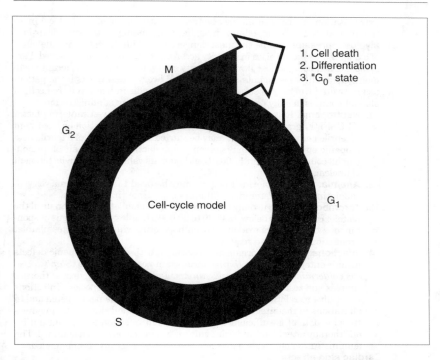

Figure 40-1. The cell cycle. The M phase (mitotic phase) of the cell cycle is the phase of cell division. The G_1 phase (postmitotic phase) is a period of variable duration when cellular activities and protein and RNA synthesis continue. These G_1 cells can differentiate or continue in the proliferative cycle. The S phase (DNA synthetic phase) is the period in which new DNA replication occurs. The G_2 phase (postsynthetic phase) is the period in which the cell has a diploid number of chromosomes and twice the DNA content of the normal cell. The cell remains in this phase for a relatively short time and then enters the mitotic phase again. G_0 phase (the resting phase) is the time during which cells do not divide. Cells may move in and out of the G_0 phase. After cell division, a cell can either die, differentiate, or enter a resting (G_0) phase. Cells that differentiate or enter a G_0 phase can reenter the cycle at G_1. (From Berek JS, Hacker NF. *Practical gynecologic oncology*, 2nd ed. Baltimore: Williams & Williams, 1994:7. Reprinted with permission.)

> **E. The log kill hypothesis** states that chemotherapeutic agents appear to work by first-order kinetics (they kill a constant fraction of cells rather than a constant number).
>
> This hypothesis helps explain the need for intermittent courses of chemotherapy to achieve the magnitude of cell kill necessary to produce tumor regression and cure. This hypothesis also supports the rationale for multiple drug therapy.
>
> **F. The Goldie-Coldman hypothesis** of drug resistance states that most mammalian cells start out with an intrinsic sensitivity to antineoplastic drugs but develop spontaneous resistance at variable rates by somatic mutation.

III. Common side effects of chemotherapy

> **A. Local and dermal side effects** include alopecia (which is reversible after treatment stops), photosensitivity, phlebitis, tissue necrosis, and local infiltration or

extravasation. Extravasation may be treated with topical steroids, local injection of hyaluronidase, or sodium thiosulfate, depending on the specific drug.

B. **Myelosuppression** can be the most dangerous and life-threatening side effect of chemotherapy and varies in severity according to the drug administered. Pancytopenia is the major dose-limiting toxicity associated with chemotherapy treatment. Generally, most agents can be repeated every 3 to 4 weeks if the patient has recovered from myelosuppressive effects. A nadir in white cell, red cell, or platelet count is usually observed 7 to 14 days after drug administration.

1. **Neutropenia.** Recombinant human granulocyte colony-stimulating factor (G-CSF) (Filgrastim, Neupogen) may be given for prevention or treatment of febrile neutropenia. G-CSF may be started after the onset of a febrile neutropenic episode and often is given prophylactically for an absolute neutrophil count of less than 1,500/μL, although its value as a prophylactic agent is unclear.

2. **Anemia.** Erythropoietin (Epogen) may be used to treat anemia. Erythropoietin is administered, 3,000 units s.q., three times a week.

3. **Thrombocytopenia** usually is not treated with platelet transfusion until the platelet count drops below 15,0000 to 20,000/μL unless clinical signs of spontaneous bleeding are evident. Thrombopoietin, which stimulates platelet production, is not used readily.

4. **Infections.** Infectious organisms associated with granulocytopenic defects include enteric gram-negative bacteria, gram-positive bacteria (*Staphylococcus epidermidis*, *Staphylococcus aureus*, and diphtheroid), viruses (herpes simplex and zoster), and fungi (*Candida* and *Aspergillus* species). Infections generally are related to the severity and duration of the neutropenia and to alterations in the integrity of mucous membranes and skin. Fever in a neutropenic patient is sufficient evidence of occult infection to warrant antibiotic therapy after blood and urine culture specimens have been obtained. The administration of broad-spectrum antibiotics is generally recommended.

C. **Cardiac side effects**

1. **Daunorubicin and doxorubicin** have significant cardiac toxic effects, including irreversible cardiomyopathies involving progressive congestive heart failure, pleural effusions, heart dilatation, and venous congestion. These side effects are generally cumulative; therefore, dosages of daunorubicin and doxorubicin are kept under the maximum. Commonly, multiple gated acquisition scans are obtained before treatment with cardiotoxic agents to obtain a baseline ejection fraction and may be repeated as necessary.

2. **Paclitaxel** (Taxol) may cause asymptomatic and transient bradycardia (40 to 60 beats/minute), ventricular tachycardia, and atypical chest pain during infusion. These symptoms resolve with slowing of infusion.

D. **Pulmonary side effects. Bleomycin** may cause significant pulmonary fibrosis, and careful attention should be given to the lung examination in patients receiving this agent. Generally, this side effect is both dose- and age-related, but it can be idiopathic. Pulmonary function tests (PFTs) are performed for baseline pulmonary capacity before the first dose of bleomycin is administered and are repeated as needed.

E. **Hepatic side effects.** Transient elevations in transaminase and alkaline phosphatase may occur with chemotherapy. However, cholangitis, hepatic necrosis, and hepatic veno-occlusive disease, although rare, must be considered.

F. **Gastrointestinal side effects**

1. **Stomatitis** and **mucositis** may occur most commonly with antimetabolites such as methotrexate and with paclitaxel. Treatment includes either Larry's solution [three equal parts diphenhydramine (Benadryl) elixir, magnesia and alumina oral suspension (Maalox), and viscous lidocaine] or nystatin, swish and swallow every 6 hours.

2. **Nausea and vomiting** are two of the most common and most distressing side effects of chemotherapy for cancer. The severity and incidence of nausea and vomiting vary greatly, but the inability to effectively control these symptoms often can result in patient refusal of further potentially curative treatment. Three patterns of nausea and vomiting exist: *acute, delayed,*

Table 40-1. Emetogenic potential of commonly used chemotherapeutic agents

Very high (>90%)	High (60% to 90%)	Moderate (30% to 60%)	Low (<30%)
Cisplatin	Carboplatin	Etoposide	Bleomycin
Cyclophosphamide	Cyclophosphamide	Ifosfamide	5-Fluorouracil
(high dose)	Dactinomycin	Topotecan	Methotrexate
			Paclitaxel
			Vincristine

and anticipatory. The incidence and severity of nausea and vomiting are related to the emetogenic potential of the drug, the dose, the route and time of day of administration, patient characteristics, and the combination of drugs. Emetogenic potential of commonly used chemotherapeutic agents is listed in Table 40-1.

   a. **Diagnosis.** Symptoms of nausea and vomiting temporally related to the administration of chemotherapy are usually diagnostic of chemotherapy-induced emesis. Gastrointestinal obstruction must be ruled out, however, especially if abdominal distention or obstipation is present.

   b. **Therapy.** Table 40-2 lists antiemetic drugs used to treat chemotherapy-induced emesis. Ondansetron and granisetron, both serotonin S_3 receptor-blocking agents, have been shown to be particularly effective in reducing acute emesis associated with cisplatin and other highly emetogenic drugs. It is important to recognize that antiemetic medications are effective in the treatment of acute nausea and vomiting that result from the pattern of serotonin release, which is not a major factor in delayed emesis. Prevention is the key to management of delayed-onset nausea and vomiting. Patients are encouraged to take antiemetics as prescribed for 3 to 4 days after chemotherapy to prevent delayed emesis (see Table 40-2).

   3. **Diarrhea** frequently accompanies stomatitis and, if temporally associated with the administration of chemotherapy, is most likely not infectious in origin. Patients are encouraged to increase their fluid intake to prevent postchemotherapy dehydration, with its risk of secondary side effects such as nephrotoxicity or electrolyte disturbances. If an infection is suspected, a stool specimen should be examined for the presence of white blood cells, enteric pathogens (e.g., *Salmonella, Shigella*), ova and parasites, and *Clostridium difficile* toxin. In particular, if the patient has been on broad-spectrum antibiotics, *C. difficile* pseudomembranous colitis must be suspected. For diarrhea associated with *C. difficile* infection, therapy consists of oral vancomycin or metronidazole.

   4. **Constipation** usually is seen in patients with neurogenic gastrointestinal atony who are being treated with vinca alkaloids. In severe cases of constipation, ileus may ensue. Treatment includes hydration, stool softeners (docusate sodium), laxatives (milk of magnesia), enemas, cathartics, and bulking agents.

G. Acute **allergic reactions** occasionally occur with the use of chemotherapeutic agents, most commonly etoposide. Acute pulmonary infiltrates have been known to occur with methotrexate and respond to steroid therapy. Bleomycin can cause anaphylaxis, skin reactions, fever, chills, and pulmonary fibrosis. Because of the high incidence of allergic reactions to bleomycin, patients are given a test dose of 2 to 4 units i.m. before the first dose of drug. Paclitaxel has been shown to cause hypersensitivity reactions in small numbers of patients within 2 to 3 minutes of infusion. The characteristic hypersensitivity reaction is bradycardia, diaphoresis, hypotension, cutaneous flushing, and abdominal pain. Premedications of diphenhydramine hydrochloride, dexamethasone, and ranitidine are given prophylactically.

Table 40-2. Antiemetic therapy

Drug	Dosage	Route
Histamine antagonists		
Hydroxyzine (Atarax)	50–100 mg q6h	i.v./p.o.
Diphenhydramine (Benadryl)	10–50 mg q6h	i.v./i.m./p.o.
Muscarine antagonists		
Scopolamine (Transderm-Scop)	0.5 mg q3d (apply hours before needed)	transdermal
Dopamine antagonists		
Metoclopramide (Reglan)	1–2 mg/kg q3h	i.v./i.m./p.o.
Droperidol (Inapsine)	0.5–2.5 mg q4h	i.v.
	2.5–10 mg q4h	i.m.
Haloperidol (Haldol)	0.5–5.0 mg q4h	i.m./p.o.
Prochlorperazine (Compazine)	2.5–10 mg q4h	slow i.v.
	5–10 mg q4h	i.m./p.o.
	25 mg q4h	p.r.
Chlorpromazine (Thorazine)	2–25 mg q4h	slow i.v.
	25–50 mg q4h	i.m.
	10–25 mg q4h	p.o.
	50–100 mg q4h	p.r.
Thiethylperazine (Torecan)	2 mg q8h	i.m.
	10 mg q8h	p.o.
Trimethobenzamide (Tigan)	200 mg	i.m./p.r.
	250 mg	p.o.
Corticosteroids		
Methylprednisolone (Solu-Medrol)	250–500 mg q6h	i.v.
Dexamethasone (Decadron)	4–25 mg q6h	i.v./p.o.
Benzodiazepines		
Lorazepam (Ativan)	1–2 mg q4h	i.v./p.o./s.l.
	1–4 mg q4h	i.m.
Cannabinoids		
Dronabinol (Δ^9-tetrahydro-cannabinol)	5–15 mg/m^2 q4h	p.o.
Nabilone (Cesamet)	1–2 mg q8h	p.o.
Serotonin antagonists		
Ondansetron (Zofran)	32 mg 30 min before treatment; 0.15 mg/kg q4h × 2 after treatment	i.v.
Granisetron (Kytril)	0.7–1.0 mg 30 min before treatment	i.v.

H. Hemorrhagic cystitis may occur with cyclophosphamide and ifosfamide. Preventive measures include hydration and diuretics, and treatment includes dose reduction or discontinuation of the drug. Mesna, a uroprotector, always is administered simultaneously with ifosfamide to protect against bladder toxicity. Mesna also may be given with cyclophosphamide for the same purpose.

I. Neurotoxicity. The vinca alkaloids in particular have been implicated in the development of peripheral, central, and visceral neuropathies. Neuropathies are cumulative side effects suggested by absent reflexes, constipation, and

Table 40-3. Alkylating agents used for gynecologic cancer

Drug	Route of administration	Common treatment schedules	Common toxicities	Diseases treated
Nitrogen mustard (Mustargen, HN_2)	i.v. Intracavitary	0.4 mg/kg as a single dose, or 0.1 mg/kg every day × 4 days 0.2–0.4 mg/kg	Nausea and vomiting, myelosuppression	Ovary, malignant pleural or pericardial effusions
Cyclophosphamide (Cytoxan)	p.o. i.v.	1.5–3.0 mg/kg/day 10–50 mg/kg every 1–4 wk	Myelosuppression, cystitis ± bladder fibrosis, alopecia, hepatitis, amenorrhea, azoospermia	Breast, ovary, soft tissue sarcomas
Chlorambucil (Leukeran)	p.o.	0.03–0.10 mg/kg/day	Myelosuppression, gastrointestinal distress, dermatitis, hepatotoxicity	Ovary
Melphalan (Alkeran, L-PAM)	p.o.	0.2 mg/kg/day × 5 days every 4–6 wk	Myelosuppression, nausea and vomiting (rare), mucosal ulceration (rare), second malignancies	Ovary, breast
Triethylene thiophosphoramide (TSPA, Thiotepa)	i.v. Intracavitary	0.8 mg/kg every 4–6 wk 45–60 mg	Myelosuppression, nausea and vomiting, headaches, fever (rare)	Ovary, breast; intracavitary for malignant effusions
Ifosfamide (Ifex)	i.v.	1.0 or 1.2 g/m²/day × 5 days With mesna, 200 mg/m² immediately before and 4 and 8 hr after ifosfamide	Myelosuppression, bladder toxicity, central nervous system dysfunction, renal toxicity	Cervix, ovary

From Berek JS, Hacker NF. *Practical gynecologic oncology,* 2nd ed. Baltimore: Williams & Wilkins, 1994:28. Adapted with permission.

ileus. Rarely, cranial nerve abnormalities may be seen with neurotoxicity. Other agents, such as cisplatin and carboplatin, may cause a peripheral neuropathy characterized by paresthesias of the extremities. Cisplatin is thought to be more neurotoxic than carboplatin. Paclitaxel also has been shown to produce peripheral neuropathies, especially in heavily pretreated patients. Treatment of neurotoxicity involves discontinuation of the offending agent if neuropathies become debilitating.

    J. Nephrotoxicity. Dose-related and cumulative renal insufficiency is the major dose-limiting toxic effect of cisplatin. Elevations may occur in blood urea nitrogen, serum creatinine, and serum uric acid within 2 weeks of treatment. Irreversible renal damage can occur. Prevention of nephrotoxicity with large amounts of i.v. hydration and diuretics is important during cisplatin treatment. Typically, 24-hour creatinine clearance is obtained to establish baseline renal function before infusion of drug.

    K. Ototoxicity. Tinnitus or high-frequency hearing loss may be observed in patients receiving cisplatin and may be more severe with repeated doses. It is unclear whether or not these effects are reversible. Audiograms may be obtained before treatment to acquire a baseline and throughout treatment to assess hearing loss.

IV. Chemotherapeutic agents. The agents commonly used for chemotherapy of cancers of the female reproductive system are listed in Tables 40-3 through 40-8.

Table 40-4. Alkylating-like agents used for gynecologic cancer

Drug	Route of administration	Common treatment schedules	Common toxicities	Diseases treated
Cis-dichloro-diamino-platinum (Cisplatin)	i.v.	10–20 mg/m^2/day × 5 days every 3 wk, or 50–75 mg/m^2 every 1–3 wk	Nephrotoxicity, tinnitus and hearing loss, nausea and vomiting, myelo-suppression, peripheral neuropathy	Ovarian and germ cell carcinomas, cervical cancer
Carboplatin	i.v.	300–400 mg/m^2 × 6 every 3–4 wk	Less neuropathy, ototoxicity, and nephrotoxicity than cisplatin; more hemato-poietic toxicity, especially throm-bocytopenia, than cisplatin	Ovarian and germ cell carcinomas
Dacarbazine (DTIC)	i.v.	2.0–4.5 mg/kg/day × 10 days every 4 wk	Myelosuppression, nausea and vomiting, flu-like syndrome, hepatotoxicity	Uterine sarco-mas, soft tis-sue sarcomas

From Berek JS, Hacker NF. *Practical gynecologic oncology*, 2nd ed. Baltimore: Williams & Wilkins, 1994:28. Adapted with permission.

Radiation Therapy

I. **Definitions and general concepts**
   A. **Teletherapy** is external-beam radiation. During external-beam radiation, the patient may be in either the prone or the supine position. The usual daily dose of radiation to the pelvis is 180 to 200 cGy, with a total dose generally ranging from 4,000 to 5,000 cGy.
   B. **Brachytherapy.** In brachytherapy, the radiation device is placed either within or close to the target tumor volume (i.e., interstitial and intracavitary irradiation). The radiation applicators are called intrauterine tandems or colpostats.
      1. **Intracavitary irradiation.** Intrauterine tandems are placed within the uterine cavity of a patient under anesthesia in an operating room. Their position is confirmed using x-ray studies. The hollow center of the tandem then is loaded with radioactive sources such as radium or cesium. Vaginal ovoids or colpostats are designed for placement into the vaginal vault. Vaginal, endometrial, and cervical cancers may require high or low dose-rate intracavitary implants. High dose-rate implants can be performed on an outpatient basis, whereas low dose-rate implants require hospitalization for 3 to 4 days.
      2. **Interstitial implants** are another form of brachytherapy. Various sources of radiation, such as ^{192}Ir, ^{125}I, and ^{182}Ta, may be configured as radioactive wires or seeds and placed directly within tissues. Hollow guide needles are placed in a geometric pattern to deliver a relatively uniform dose of radiation to a target tumor volume. After the position of the guide needles is confirmed radiologically, they can be threaded with the radioactive sources (loaded) and the hollow guides removed.
      3. **Inverse square law.** The inverse square law states that the dose of radiation at a given point is inversely proportional to the square of the distance

Table 40-5. Antitumor antibiotics used for gynecologic cancer

Drug	Route of administration	Common treatment schedules	Common toxicities	Diseases treated
Actinomycin D (Dactino-mycin, Cos-megen)	i.v.	0.3–0.5 mg/m² × 5 days every 3–4 wk	Nausea and vomiting, skin necrosis, mucosal ulceration, myelosuppression	Germ cell ovar-ian tumors, choriocarci-noma, soft tis-sue sarcoma
Bleomycin (Blenoxane)	i.v., s.q., i.m., i.p.	10–20 U/m² 1–2 times/ wk to total dose of 400 U; for effusions, 60–120 U	Fever, dermatologic reactions, pul-monary toxicity, anaphylactic reactions	Cervix, germ cell ovarian tumors, malignant effusions
Mitomycin-C (Mutamycin)	i.v.	10–20 mg/m² every 6–8 wk	Myelosuppression, local vesicant, nau-sea and vomiting, mucosal ulcera-tions, nephrotoxic-ity	Breast, cervix, ovarian tumors
Doxorubicin (Adriamycin)	i.v.	60–90 mg/m² every 3 wk or 20–35 mg/m² every day × 3 days every 3 wk	Myelosuppression, alopecia, cardio-toxicity, local vesi-cant, nausea and vomiting, mucosal ulcerations	Ovarian, breast, endometrium tumors
Mithramycin (Mithracin)	i.v.	20–50 mg/kg/day every 4–6 wk; hypercal-cemia, 25 mg/kg every 3–4 days	Nausea and vomiting, hemorrhagic diathesis, hepato-toxicity, renal toxicity, fever, myelosuppression, facial flushing	Hypercalcemia of malignancy

From Berek JS, Hacker NF. *Practical gynecologic oncology*, 2nd ed. Baltimore: Williams & Wilkins, 1994:30. Adapted with permission.

from the source of radiation. Therefore, in brachytherapy, the dose at a given distance from the source is determined largely by the inverse square law.

C. **Intracavitary radioisotopes.** In intracavitary radioisotope therapy, radioactive isotopes are placed within a body cavity such as the abdomen and pelvis. To treat epithelial ovarian cancer, ^{32}P has been used because its pattern of dissemination extends throughout the peritoneal cavity, theoretically irradiating all structures within the cavity. The half-life of ^{32}P is 14.3 days, and its pure beta decay with a mean energy of 0.698 MeV enables deeper penetration into tissues than other radioisotopes (approximately 8 mm penetration). After instillation, most of the isotope is absorbed onto the peritoneal surface, but some is phagocytosed by macrophages and taken up by lymphatics (Table 40-9).

II. **Toxicity.** The severity of normal tissue reactions to radiation depends on total dose, dose fractionation, treatment volume, and energy of radiation.

A. **Skin toxicity.** With megavoltage radiation, serious skin reactions are less fre-quent than with regular-voltage radiation. Late subcutaneous fibrosis can develop, especially with doses greater than 65 cGy. An acute skin reaction com-monly becomes evident during the third week of therapy. The reaction is char-acterized by erythema, desquamation, and pruritus and should resolve completely within 3 weeks of the end of treatment. Topical corticosteroids or moisturizing creams may be applied several times a day for symptomatic palli-ation and to promote healing. If the skin reaction worsens, it may be necessary to stop treatment and apply zinc oxide or silver sulfadiazine to the affected area

Table 40-6. Antimetabolites used for gynecologic cancer

Drug	Route of administration	Common treatment schedules	Common toxicities	Diseases treated
5-Fluorouracil (Fluorouracil, 5-FU)	i.v.	10–15 mg/kg/wk	Myelosuppression, nausea and vomiting, anorexia, alopecia	Breast, ovary
Methotrexate (MTX, amethopterin)	p.o. i.v. Intrathecal	15–40 mg/day × 5 days 240 mg/m² with leucovorin rescue 12–15 mg/m²/wk	Mucosal ulceration, myelosuppression, hepatotoxicity, allergic pneumonitis; with intrathecal, meningeal irritation	Choriocarcinoma, breast, ovary
Hydroxyurea (Hydrea)	p.o., i.v.	1–2 g/m²/day for 2–6 wk	Myelosuppression, nausea and vomiting, anorexia	Cervix

From Berek JS, Hacker NF. *Practical gynecologic oncology*, 2nd ed. Baltimore: Williams & Wilkins, 1994:31. Adapted with permission.

until it improves enough to continue treatment. The perineum is at greater risk for skin breakdown than other areas because of its increased warmth and moisture and lack of ventilation. The patient should be taught to keep the perineal area clean and dry in an effort to prevent skin breakdown.

B. Hematologic toxicity. The volume of marrow irradiated and the total radiation dose determine the severity of myelosuppression. In adults, 40% of active marrow is situated in the pelvis, 25% is in the vertebral column, and 20% is

Table 40-7. Plant alkaloids

Drug	Route of administration	Common treatment schedules	Common toxicities	Diseases treated
Vincristine (Oncovin)	i.v.	0.01–0.03 mg/kg/wk	Neurotoxicity, alopecia, myelosuppression, cranial nerve palsies, gastrointestinal	Ovarian germ cell, sarcomas, cervical cancer
Vinblastine (Velban)	i.v.	5–6 mg/m² every 1–2 wk	Myelosuppression, alopecia, nausea and vomiting, neurotoxicity	Ovarian germ cell, choriocarcinoma
Epipodophyllotoxin (Etoposide, VP-16)	i.v.	300–600 mg/m² divided over 3–4 days every 3–4 wk	Myelosuppression, alopecia, hypotension	Ovarian germ cell, choriocarcinoma
Paclitaxel (Taxol)	i.v.	135–250 mg/m² as a 3–24 hr infusion every 3 wk	Myelosuppression, alopecia, allergic reactions, cardiac arrhythmias	Ovarian cancer, breast cancer

From Berek JS, Hacker NF. *Practical gynecologic oncology*, 2nd ed. Baltimore: Williams & Wilkins, 1994:31. Adapted with permission.

Table 40-8. Miscellaneous agent

Drug	Route of administration	Common treatment schedules	Common toxicities	Diseases treated
Hexamethyl-melamine, Altretamine (Hexalen)	p.o.	120 mg/m^2/day × 14 days every 4 wk	Nausea and vomiting, myelo-suppression, neu-rotoxicity, skin rashes	Ovary, breast

From Berek JS, Hacker NF. *Practical gynecologic oncology*, 2nd ed. Baltimore: Williams & Wilkins, 1994:32. Adapted with permission.

in the ribs and skull. Extensive radiation of these sites may cause significant myelosuppression. Transfusions occasionally may be required to support the patient's hematological function during the recovery period.

   C. Gastrointestinal toxicity

     1. Acute complications. Nausea, vomiting, and diarrhea commonly occur 2 to 6 hours after abdominal or pelvic irradiation. The severity of the effect increases with the fraction size and treatment volume. Treatment involves supportive therapy with hydration, antiemetics, and antidiarrheals. Loperamide (Imodium) is generally used for first-line therapy, followed by

Table 40-9. Tolerance doses (TD 5/5 to TD 50/5) for whole organ irradiation

Single dose (cGy)		Fractionated dose (cGy)	
Lymphoid	200–500	Testes	200–1,000
Bone marrow	200–1,000	Ovary	600–1,000
Ovary	200–600	Eye (lens)	600–1,200
Testes	100–200	Lung	2,000–3,000
Eye (lens)	200–1,000	Kidney	2,000–3,000
Lung	700–1,000	Liver	3,500–4,000
Gastrointestinal	500–1,000	Skin	3,000–4,000
Colorectal	1,000–2,000	Thyroid	3,000–4,000
Kidney	1,000–2,000	Heart	4,000–5,000
Bone marrow	1,500–2,000	Lymphoid	4,000–5,000
Heart	1,800–2,000	Bone marrow	4,000–5,000
Liver	1,500–2,000	Gastrointestinal	5,000–6,000
Mucosa	500–2,000	VCTS	5,000–6,000
VCTS	1,000–2,000	Spinal cord	5,000–6,000
Skin	1,500–2,000	Peripheral nerve	6,500–7,700
Peripheral nerve	1,500–2,000	Mucosa	6,500–7,700
Spinal cord	1,500–2,000	Brain	6,000–7,000
Brain	1,500–2,500	Bone and cartilage	>7,000
Bone and cartilage	>3,000	Muscle	>7,000
Muscle	>3,000		

VCTS, vasculoconnective tissue systems.
From Rubin P. The law and order of radiation sensitivity, absolute vs. relative. In: Vaeth JM, Meyer JL, eds. *Radiation tolerance of normal tissues*, Vol 23. Basel: Karger, 1989. Adapted with permission.

diphenoxylate (Lomotil) if necessary. The usual dosage for both medications is one to two tablets after each loose stool, not to exceed eight doses per day. If the patient is having severe diarrhea, opiates may be used to decrease peristalsis. Opiate agents include opium tincture, 0.5 to 1.0 mL every 4 hours; paregoric elixir, 4 mL p.o. every 4 hours; or codeine, 15 to 30 mg p.o. every 4 hours. Occasionally, a reduction in fraction size or a break in treatment is necessary to control the acute gastrointestinal effects.

2. **Chronic complications.** Chronic diarrhea, obstruction caused by bowel adhesions, and fistula formation are serious complications of intestinal irradiation that occur in fewer than 1% of cases. Small bowel and rectovaginal fistulas can be caused by radiation effects on tissue or by recurrent disease. After recurrent disease is ruled out, the patient may require a temporary colostomy to allow healing of the affected bowel. Fistulas often are associated with a foul odor, and good hygiene is important in eliminating the odor. Items that may assist with odor control are charcoal-impregnated dressings, skin cleansers, and air deodorizers.

D. **Genitourinary toxicity**

1. **Cystitis** is characterized by inflammation of the bladder with associated symptoms of pain, urgency, hematuria, and urinary frequency. The bladder is relatively tolerant of radiation, but doses greater than 6,000 to 7,000 cGy over a 6- to 7-week period can result in cystitis. A diagnosis of radiation cystitis may be made after a normal urine culture result has been obtained. Hydration, frequent sitz baths, and possibly the use of antibiotics and antispasmodic agents may be necessary for treatment.

2. **Vesicovaginal fistulas and ureteral strictures** are possible long-term complications of radiation therapy. A urinary diversion or placement of ureteral stents may be necessary.

E. **Vulvovaginitis.** Pelvic irradiation often results in erythema, inflammation, mucosal atrophy, inelasticity, and ulceration of the vaginal tissue. Adhesions and stenosis of the vagina may occur, resulting in painful intercourse and pelvic examination. Treatment involves vaginal dilation, either by frequent sexual intercourse or by the use of a vaginal dilator. Vaginal dilation should be performed at least 2 to 3 times per week for up to 2 years. In addition, the use of estrogen creams is useful in promoting epithelial regeneration. Infections, including candidiasis, trichomoniasis, and bacterial vaginosis, may be associated with radiation-induced vaginitis.

F. **Fatigue.** During radiation therapy, many women report an overwhelming sense of exhaustion. The etiology of this fatigue is unclear but most likely involves a combination of physiologic, psychological, and situational factors. Close monitoring of blood count findings is necessary to ensure that the patient is not anemic. It is often helpful for patients to rest immediately after treatment and to enlist family and friends to assist with daily activities and chores. Fatigue may continue for several months after completion of therapy.

Treatment of Specific Cancer Types

I. **Cervical cancer**

A. **When to use radiation therapy.** Radiotherapy can be used to treat all stages of cervical squamous cell cancer, with cure rates of approximately 70% for stage I, 60% for stage II, 45% for stage III, and 18% for stage IV. The treatment plan usually includes a combination of external teletherapy to treat the regional nodes and to shrink the primary tumor, and intracavitary brachytherapy to boost the central tumor. In cases of early disease in which the risk of lymph node metastases is negligible, intracavitary therapy may be used alone. See also Chap. 36.

1. The **treatment sequence** depends on tumor volume. Stage IB lesions smaller than 2 cm may be treated first with an intracavitary source to treat the primary lesion, followed by external therapy to treat the pelvic nodes.

Table 40-10. Risk/benefit analysis of cervical cancer treatment modalities

	Surgery	Radiation
Survival	85%	85%
Serious complications	Urologic fistulas, 1–2%	Intestinal and urinary stricture and fistulas, 1.4–5.3%
Vagina	Initially shortened but may lengthen with regular intercourse	Fibrosis and possible stenosis, especially in postmenopausal patients
Ovaries	Can be conserved	Ablated
Chronic effects	Bladder atony in 3%	Radiation fibrosis of bowel and bladder in 6–8%
Applicability	Best candidates are <65 yr, <200 lb, and in good health	All patients are potential candidates, but more difficult to give adequate doses in obese patients
Surgical mortality	1%	<1% (intracavitary therapy)

From Berek JS, Hacker NF, eds. *Practical gynecologic oncology,* 2nd ed. Baltimore: Williams & Wilkins, 1994. Adapted with permission.

Tumors larger than 2 cm require external radiotherapy first to shrink the tumor and enable the therapist to achieve better intracavitary dosimetry.

2. **Posthysterectomy radiotherapy** has been recommended for patients with significant risk factors such as metastases to pelvic lymph nodes, paracervical tissue invasion, deep cervical invasion, or positive surgical margins. Of these risk factors, most authors agree that positive surgical margins warrant the use of radiotherapy. In patients with positive pelvic nodes, however, most studies show a reduction in pelvic recurrence but no significant changes in survival with radiotherapy.

3. For **stage IB or IIA cancer** of the cervix, the decision of whether surgery or radiation therapy should be used for primary treatment may be individualized to the patient. The risks and benefits of each modality when used to treat early cervical cancer are listed in Table 40-10.

B. **Extended-field radiotherapy.** Clinical staging fails to predict the spread of disease to the paraaortic nodes in 7% of patients with stage IB disease, 18% of patients with stage IIB disease, and 28% of patients with stage III disease. To avoid postsurgical adhesions and subsequent entrapment of bowel in the radiotherapy field, extraperitoneal dissection of the paraaortic nodes is recommended, and the radiotherapy dose should be 5,000 cGy or less. When this approach is used, postradiotherapy bowel complications occur in fewer than 5% of patients, and the 5-year survival rate is 15% to 26% in patients with positive paraaortic nodes. Survival appears to be related to the size of the primary tumor and to the amount of disease in the paraaortic nodes.

C. **Palliation.** Because cervical cancer is generally a radioresponsive lesion, radiation therapy has played an important role in palliation of metastatic disease. Short courses of palliative radiation, such as 2,000 cGy in five fractions or 3,000 cGy in ten fractions, usually relieve symptoms associated with bony metastases or paraaortic involvement.

D. **Method of radiation therapy**
1. **Dose.** Microscopic or occult tumor deposits from epithelial cancers require 4,000 to 5,000 cGy for local control. Clinically obvious tumor will require in excess of 6,000 cGy.
   a. Two reference points are commonly used to describe the dose prescription.

    (1) Point A is 2 cm lateral and 2 cm superior to the external cervical os.

    (2) Point B is 3 cm lateral to point A and corresponds to the pelvic sidewall.

  b. The summated dose to point A (from intracavitary and external radiation therapy) believed to be adequate for central control is usually between 7,500 and 8,500 cGy.

  c. The prescribed dose to point B is 4,500 to 6,500 cGy, depending on the bulk of parametrial and sidewall disease.

2. Treatment volume describes the tumor volume receiving the prescribed tumor dose, ±5%. The treatment volume is designed to encompass the primary tumor in the pelvis and its possible adjacent extensions, as well as the appropriate first- and second-echelon draining lymph nodes. The pelvis is usually treated to within acceptable tolerance of normal tissues.

3. The borders of the **treatment field** are as follows:

  a. The inferior border usually lies at the inferior aspect of the obturator foramina and encompasses the obturator nodes. If vaginal extension has occurred, the border is moved inferiorly to 2 cm below visible and palpable tumor.

  b. The superior border is usually between L4 and L5 or in the midvertebral level of L5. The reason to treat up to this level is to provide some dose to the common iliac nodes, although in most cases it is unclear whether additional therapeutic benefit results from taking the field up to the L5 level, as opposed to the L5 and S1 junction.

  c. The lateral borders are 1 cm lateral to the pelvic lymph nodes as visualized on a lymphogram or at least 1 cm (usually 2 cm) lateral to the margins of the bony pelvis, noted on a flat plate. Appropriate shielding along the common iliac nodes decreases the volume of normal tissue irradiated.

4. Procedure. In general, especially for bulky lesions, external radiation therapy is given first to decrease the size of the primary tumor. One or two applications of intracavitary irradiation are given after external radiation therapy to achieve the desired radiation dose levels. The amount of radiation delivered by each technique is determined by the tumor extent. When disease is mainly central, a higher proportion of the total dose is prescribed for intracavitary radiation and less external radiation is used because the lateral disease is microscopic. If bulky lateral parametrial or sidewall disease is present, a greater proportion of the dose will be delivered with the external beam.

E. Complications of radiation therapy. The incidence of late complications depends on the specific tolerance of the normal tissues irradiated, the dose they receive, and the volume of radiation.

1. Perforation of the uterus may occur at the time of insertion of the uterine tandem. When perforation is recognized, the tandem should be removed and the patient should be observed for signs of bleeding or of peritonitis.

2. Fever may occur after insertion of the uterine tandem and ovoids and is most often a result of infection of the necrotic tumor. Fever usually appears 2 to 6 hours after insertion. After ruling out perforation by ultrasound, broad-spectrum i.v. antibiotic coverage should be initiated. If fever persists, or if the patient shows signs of septic shock or of peritonitis, the intracavitary system should be removed.

3. Acute morbidity includes diarrhea, abdominal cramps, nausea, frequent urination, and occasionally, bleeding from the bladder or bowel mucosa.

  a. Bowel symptoms can be treated with a low-gluten, low-lactose, and low-protein diet. Antidiarrheal and antispasmodic agents may also help.

  b. Bladder symptoms are treated with antispasmodics. Severe symptoms may require a week of rest from radiotherapy.

4. Chronic morbidity results from vasculitis and fibrosis, usually occurring several months to several years after radiotherapy. The bowel and bladder fistula rate after pelvic radiotherapy for cervical cancer is 1.4% to 5.3%. Bowel bleeding, stricture, stenosis, or obstruction occurs in 6.4% to 8.1%.

a. **Proctosigmoiditis.** Bleeding caused by inflammation of the rectum and sigmoid colon should be treated with a low-residue diet, antidiarrheals, and steroid enemas.

b. **Rectovaginal fistula** occurs in fewer than 2% of patients and requires surgical repair.

c. **Small bowel complications.** Patients who previously have undergone abdominal surgery are more likely to have pelvic adhesions than patients who have not, and are subsequently at a higher risk of developing radiotherapy complications in the small bowel. The terminal ileum may sustain chronic damage because of its relatively fixed position at the cecum. Symptoms include a history of persistent, crampy abdominal pain; intestinal rushes; and distention characteristic of partial small bowel obstruction. Low-grade fever and anemia may accompany symptoms. Treatment includes nasogastric suction, total parenteral nutrition, and early surgery.

d. **Chronic urinary tract complications** occur in 1% to 5% of patients. Vesicovaginal fistulas are the most common of these complications and require supravesicular urinary diversion. Ureteral strictures are usually a sign of recurrent cancer and may require ureteral stent placement or ureterolysis.

F. **Posttreatment care.** Regression of tumor may be expected to continue for up to 3 months after treatment. If the disease obviously progresses during this time, surgery should be considered.

1. **Pelvic examination** should be performed regularly, noting the progressive shrinkage of the cervix and possible stenosis of the cervical os and surrounding upper vagina.

2. During **rectovaginal examination,** it is important to palpate carefully the uterosacral and cardinal ligaments for nodules.

3. **Fine-needle aspiration** of suspicious areas should be used to make an early diagnosis of persistent disease.

4. **Supraclavicular and inguinal lymph nodes** should be examined carefully.

5. **Cervical or vaginal cytology** should be studied every 3 months for 2 years, then every 6 months for 3 years. (Another approach is to perform a cytologic examination every 6 months and evaluate the findings based on symptoms.)

6. A **chest radiograph** should be obtained yearly for patients with advanced disease.

7. An **i.v. pyelogram** should be obtained if urinary symptoms warrant or if a pelvic mass is found.

II. **Endometrial cancer.** See also Chap. 37.

A. **When to use radiation therapy.** The cornerstone of treatment for endometrial cancer is total abdominal hysterectomy and bilateral salpingo-oophorectomy. Most patients present with early-stage disease and are cured with surgery alone; some patients, however, may benefit from adjuvant radiation therapy to help prevent vaginal vault recurrence and to treat any occult disease in lymph nodes. Treatment is determined best when all significant pathologic information is available; therefore, most adjuvant radiation is used postoperatively rather than preoperatively. At present, the most appropriate role for adjuvant pelvic radiation therapy appears to be in the prevention of pelvic recurrences in high-risk patients. The use of preoperative or postoperative irradiation decreases the overall incidence of recurrence at the vaginal vault, but no significant survival benefit has been demonstrated. In contrast to cervical cancer, patients with endometrial cancer who are treated with hysterectomy alone or with hysterectomy and radiation therapy fare significantly better than those treated with radiation alone; the data supporting this conclusion, however, are based on retrospective studies. In addition, patients treated with radiation alone generally have a higher degree of comorbidity than those treated with surgery. The recommended roles of radiation therapy in the treatment of endometrial carcinoma are as follows:

1. As an adjunct to surgery to prevent pelvic recurrence after bilateral salpingo-oophorectomy and hysterectomy in selected high-risk patients

      2. With curative intent in some patients whose preexisting medical problems preclude surgery

      3. With curative intent in patients with isolated vaginal or vaginal and pelvic recurrence; therapy is directed to the whole pelvis and the entire vagina, with the use of both external and intracavitary or interstitial radiation

      4. As palliative treatment or nonresectable intrapelvic or metastatic disease.

  B. Postoperative radiation. After primary surgery, adjuvant radiation therapy may be safely omitted for patients with tumors that carry favorable prognoses. For patients who may require postoperative radiation, however, treatment should be tailored to the needs of the individual patient. Patients should be advised that adjuvant radiation will not prolong survival.

    1. Vault irradiation

      a. Vault irradiation is indicated for patients with negative lymph nodes or one microscopically positive node.

      b. Colpostats alone are used to deliver a surface dose of 5,500 to 6,000 cGy.

      c. Cesium alone may be used for patients with negative lymph nodes after full surgical staging.

      d. Morbidity includes vaginal stenosis and dyspareunia, which are treated by routine vaginal dilatation.

    2. External pelvic radiation is indicated for the following patients:

      a. High-risk patients who have not undergone surgical staging

      b. All patients with grade 3 tumors

      c. All patients with invasion into the outer half of the myometrium or with cervical extension.

    3. Extended-field radiation is indicated in the following cases:

      a. Biopsy-proven paraaortic nodal metastases

      b. Grossly positive or multiple pelvic lymph nodes

      c. Grossly positive adnexal metastases

      d. Grade 2 or 3 tumor invasion of the outer half of myometrium.

    4. Whole abdominal radiation is indicated for patients with peritoneal or omental metastases that have been completely excised.

    5. Intraperitoneal ^{32}**P.** Investigators have reported favorable results with intraperitoneal ^{32}P used to treat patients with malignant peritoneal cytologic findings. Affected patients, however, are also at risk of developing vaginal vault and sidewall recurrence, which requires external radiation therapy and thus increases morbidity.

  C. Chemotherapy. Cytotoxic chemotherapy for endometrial cancer is used for palliation of symptoms. Single agents that act against endometrial cancer are doxorubicin (Adriamycin), cisplatin, carboplatin, paclitaxel, hexamethylmelamine, cyclophosphamide, and 5-fluorouracil. Doxorubicin appears to be the most active agent, with an overall response rate of 38% and a 26% complete response rate. The results of chemotherapy, however, are generally disappointing, with a median survival of complete responders of only 14 months.

III. Uterine sarcoma. The cornerstone of therapy for uterine sarcoma is total abdominal hysterectomy with or without bilateral salpingo-oophorectomy.

  A. Radiation therapy. The role of adjuvant radiation therapy has not been defined conclusively. It seems likely, however, that radiation improves tumor control in the pelvis without influencing final outcome. A high incidence of distant failure is associated with radiation therapy for uterine sarcoma, including persistent metastases to the lungs and upper abdomen. Whole abdominal radiation has been reported to prevent abdominal relapse.

  B. Chemotherapy. Most responses of uterine sarcoma to chemotherapeutic agents studied to date are partial and of short duration. The most active agents are doxorubicin, cisplatin, and ifosfamide. In a randomized Gynecologic Oncology Group (GOG) study of Adriamycin after total abdominal hysterectomy and bilateral salpingo-oophorectomy for stage I and stage II uterine sarcoma, no increase in survival or in progression-free interval resulted from treatment.

IV. Epithelial ovarian cancer. The cornerstone of therapy for epithelial ovarian cancer is total abdominal hysterectomy and bilateral salpingo-oophorectomy, with optimal cytoreductive surgery (less than 1 cm residual disease). Figure 40-2 is a proposed algorithm for treating epithelial ovarian cancer. See also Chap. 38.

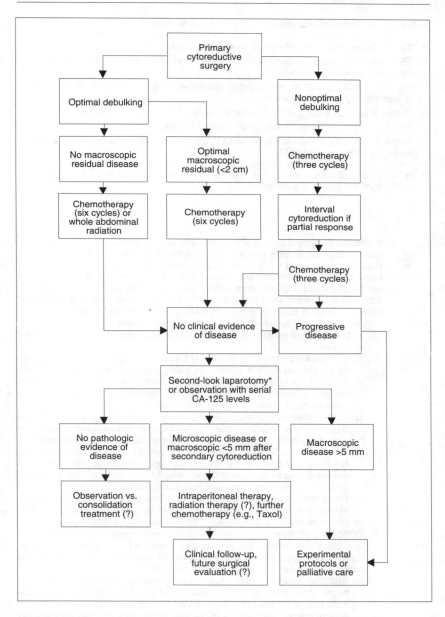

Figure 40-2. Treatment scheme for patients with advanced-stage ovarian cancer. *Under selected or experimental circumstances. (From Berek JS, Hacker NF. *Practical gynecologic oncology*, 2nd ed. Baltimore: Williams & Wilkins, 1994: 342. Modified with permission.)

Table 40-11. Technical principles of curative radiotherapy

1. The entire peritoneal cavity must be encompassed.
2. The moving-strip and open-field techniques are equally effective, but the open-field technique is preferred.
3. No liver shielding is used, which limits the upper abdominal dose to 2,500–2,800 cGy in 100–120 cGy daily fractions.
4. Partial kidney shielding is used to keep the renal dose at 1,800–2,000 cGy.
5. The true pelvis is given a boost dose in 180–220 cGy.
6. Parallel-opposing portals are used, with beam energy sufficient to ensure a dosage variation no greater than 5%.

From Dembo AJ. Epithelial ovarian cancer: the role of radiotherapy. *Int J Radiat Oncol Biol Phys* 1992;22:838. Adapted with permission.

A. **Radiation therapy.** The use of radiation therapy in ovarian cancer continues to be controversial, despite selected data supporting its use. The dose of radiation that can be delivered safely to the upper abdomen in such cases is considerably lower than that which would be considered optimal and sufficient for the successful treatment of solid tumors. Abdominal irradiation has little or no curative potential for patients with bulky disease in the upper abdomen. External-beam radiation therapy must be combined with systemic chemotherapy for patients with positive lymph nodes or lymph vascular involvement.
   1. **Techniques.** In general, two techniques have been used to treat the whole abdomen.
      a. The **moving-strip technique** employs a 10-cm high field that is moved in 2.5-cm increments, so that each strip receives 8 or 10 fractions. The rationale behind this method is to deliver a biologically higher dose than is possible with the open-field technique. The moving-strip method rarely, if ever, is used, however.
      b. In the **open-field technique,** the whole tumor volume is treated each day, usually in a single portal. This technique requires a reduction in the size of the daily dose. Variations include adding a T-shaped boost portal to the paraaortic nodes and medial domes of the diaphragm and treating the upper and lower abdomen through separate portals. The open-field technique has become the standard treatment method because of its shorter duration, simplicity, and reduced long-term toxicity.
      c. **Fractionation** schemes deliver 2 to 3 fractions per day of a fraction size of less than 100 cGy in an effort to increase the biologically effective dose without increasing radiation toxicity (Table 40-11).
   2. **Principles of curative radiotherapy.** A general principle exists that the less gross the disease, the greater the likelihood that it will respond to radiation therapy. Most studies demonstrate that success is impossible if more than 0.5 cm of gross disease is present.
      a. **Success rates.** At present, a curative role for whole abdominal and pelvic irradiation has been established for some subsets of patients with epithelial ovarian cancer by several independent investigators. Approximately 40% to 50% of patients with small residual lesions (less than 2 cm) who undergo radiation therapy after primary surgery are cured. Most curable residual lesions are derived from stage II tumors and are confined to the pelvis, where a higher radiation dose can be delivered. For patients with larger residual lesions (more than 2 cm), the probability of cure with radiotherapy falls to 5% to 15%.
      b. **Restrictions.** Because abdominopelvic radiotherapy encompasses only the peritoneal cavity and retroperitoneum, its use as primary treatment is restricted to stages I, II, and III disease. Radiotherapy should be used

only for patients with no macroscopic disease in the upper abdomen and small (less than 2 cm) or no macroscopic residual disease in the pelvis.
3. **Intraperitoneal ^{32}P.** Intraperitoneal administration of ^{32}P usually is reserved for patients with microscopic disease (second look) or minimal macroscopic disease because radiation from ^{32}P penetrates only 2 to 3 mm. A disadvantage of ^{32}P administration is that adhesive disease may prevent even distribution of radiation throughout the abdomen, resulting in inadequate dose to some areas and excessively toxic dose to others.
4. **Toxicity associated with radiation therapy**
   a. **Acute side effects** that resolve within 2 to 3 weeks of treatment include fatigue and gastrointestinal toxicity, with some degree of nausea, anorexia, and diarrhea. Ondansetron may be helpful in controlling the nausea.
   b. **Late effects** of radiation include asymptomatic basal pneumonitis or fibrosis, detectable in about 15% to 20% of patients on radiotherapy. About 50% of patients who have received upper abdominal doses develop transient elevations in alkaline phosphatase from hepatic irradiation a few months after radiation therapy. Fewer than 1% of patients develop jaundice or ascites from radiation.
   c. **Late gastrointestinal toxicity** is probably the greatest concern for patients after radiation therapy. If the technical principles of whole abdominal radiation are followed (see Table 40-11), the risk of serious bowel complications can be minimized. The frequency and severity of gastrointestinal toxic effects depend on the total dose of radiation, the dose per fraction, and the extent and number of previous surgical procedures. Generally, 10% to 15% of patients report some diarrhea or persistent bloating resulting from dietary intolerance, but frank malabsorption is rare. Bowel surgery necessitated by late complications of radiation therapy is required in approximately 5% to 6% of patients, and fewer than 0.5% of these patients die as a result of radiation-induced bowel injury.
5. **Survival rates.** The long-term survival rates for whole-abdominal irradiation and chemotherapy are very similar. The two modalities, however, have not been compared in phase III trials.
B. **Chemotherapy**
1. **Paclitaxel with a platinum compound** (cisplatin, carboplatin) currently constitutes the preferred regimen for previously untreated patients with advanced ovarian cancer.
   a. **Mechanism of action.** The cytotoxicity of paclitaxel (Taxol) is due to a unique effect on microtubules. Paclitaxel arrests cells in the G_2–M phase, primarily by disrupting mitosis.
   b. **Toxicity.** Major toxicities associated with paclitaxel include alopecia, myelosuppression (primarily neutropenia), myalgia, and peripheral neuropathy.
   c. **Clinical characteristics.** The regimen is based on a GOG study in which 385 patients with suboptimal stages III and IV disease were randomized to receive either cisplatin and cyclophosphamide or paclitaxel and cisplatin. The paclitaxel and cisplatin combination improved all outcome parameters in advanced ovarian cancer. Carboplatin is a cisplatin analogue that is less nephrotoxic, neurotoxic, and emetogenic than cisplatin and appears to have similar efficacy. The dose-limiting toxicity of carboplatin is myelosuppression (preferentially thrombocytopenia). Carboplatin is excreted rapidly by the kidney.
2. **Other chemotherapeutic regimens** used in ovarian cancer include the following:
   a. Cisplatin or carboplatin and cyclophosphamide
   b. H-CAP (hexamethylmelamine, cyclophosphamide, Adriamycin, cisplatin)
   c. PAC (cisplatin, Adriamycin, cyclophosphamide)
3. **Success rate**
   a. Approximately one-half of patients achieve a clinical complete remission after chemotherapy (i.e., no evidence of ovarian cancer on phys-

ical examination or in radiographic studies, and a CA-125 level in the normal range).

b. One-third of all patients with advanced ovarian cancer are free of disease at second-look laparotomy after cisplatin-based chemotherapy.

c. Patients with suboptimal residual disease after primary surgery have a four- to fivefold decreased likelihood of achieving a complete remission, compared with patients whose cytoreduction was optimal.

4. Toxicity associated with chemotherapy. Because of the highly emetogenic activity of cisplatin, both granisetron (Kytril) or ondansetron and dexamethasone (Decadron) are administered before cisplatin therapy to diminish acute nausea and vomiting. Prochlorperazine (Compazine) and Decadron also are administered for at least 3 days after cisplatin therapy to prevent delayed nausea and vomiting. The dosage of Compazine may need to be adjusted, or the drug discontinued, if signs of tardive dyskinesia develop. See Chemotherapy, sec. **III**, for a comprehensive discussion of toxicity of chemotherapy and its treatment.

V. Vulvar cancer. Historically, radiation therapy was delivered to the vulva using non–skin-sparing orthovoltage equipment in relatively high doses per fraction. This approach produced extensive acute morbidity with desquamation of the skin of the vulva and groin. Current approaches integrate limited surgery with adjunctive or primary radiation therapy for vulvar cancer. See also Chap. 35.

A. Multimodality treatment. The aims of integrated multimodality therapy including surgery, radiotherapy, and possible concurrent chemoradiation include the following:

1. To reduce the risks of postoperative locoregional failure in patients with advanced primary or nodal disease

2. To obviate the need for exenteration and to allow physiologic sphincter sparing in patients with disease involving the anus or proximal urethra.

B. Chemoradiation. The benefit of chemoradiation in the treatment of advanced vulvar cancer has yet to be proven in randomized phase III trials; chemoradiation has been investigated in several small trials, however, with promising results. In one study, 12 patients were treated with preoperative chemoradiation using cisplatin and 5-fluorouracil, and a 3-year survival rate of 83% was reported. Several studies by the GOG are investigating the use of 5-fluorouracil with or without cisplatin and radiation therapy as an alternative to extensive surgical resection.

VI. Vaginal cancer. Radiation therapy is the treatment of choice for most patients with vaginal cancer. Exceptions include patients with stage I disease involving the upper posterior vagina, patients with a central recurrence after radiation therapy, and patients with stage IVA disease, especially if a rectovaginal or vesicovaginal fistula is present.

A. Techniques of radiation therapy

1. For small, superficial lesions, intracavitary radiation is used alone.

2. For larger lesions, 5,000 cGy of external irradiation is used to shrink the primary tumor and treat pelvic nodes, followed by intracavitary treatment (tandem and ovoids).

3. If the lower one-third of the vagina is involved, the groin nodes are treated.

B. Toxicity associated with radiation therapy

1. Major complications of therapy are reported in 10% to 15% of patients and include radiation cystitis, rectovaginal and vesicovaginal fistulas, rectal strictures or ulcerations, and radiation necrosis.

2. Radiation-induced fibrosis and subsequent vaginal stenosis are a common concern, and patients who are sexually active should be encouraged to continue regular intercourse. Patients for whom sexual intercourse is too painful or who are not sexually active benefit from the use of topical estrogen and a vaginal dilator every second night.

VII. Ovarian germ cell tumors. Surgical resection and staging is the primary therapy for ovarian germ cell tumors.

A. Dysgerminoma is the female equivalent of seminoma. The majority of affected patients have stage I disease at diagnosis. These patients usually can be treated with unilateral salpingo-oophorectomy and, if fertility is an issue, can be followed carefully with regular pelvic examinations, computed tomography scans, and testing for tumor markers, including human chorionic gonadotropin (hCG), alpha-fetoprotein, and lactate dehydrogenase. In cases of more advanced disease, adjuvant therapy is recommended because of the significant risk of recurrence. Both chemotherapy and radiation are effective. Dysgerminoma is very responsive to cisplatin-based chemotherapy. The preferred therapy for most patients is BEP (bleomycin, etoposide, cisplatin). Nearly all patients with advanced disease experience a complete response to BEP therapy and retain their fertility. In unusual cases, such as for older patients or those with concomitant serious illness, radiation therapy may be preferable to chemotherapy.

B. Teratoma and other germ cell tumors. Most patients with grade 1, stage I immature teratoma survive free of disease progression after tumor resection. As many as 75% of patients with grade 3, stage I disease, however, experience recurrence after initial surgery. A similar recurrence rate after initial surgery is seen with endodermal sinus tumor, embryonal carcinoma, and mixed germ cell tumors. Adjuvant chemotherapy may play a significant role in reducing these rates of recurrence.

  1. Chemotherapeutic regimens. Because of the successes of cisplatin-based chemotherapy in treating testicular germ cell tumors and advanced-stage ovarian germ cell tumors, similar regimens have been used for patients with completely resected ovarian tumors. The largest study to date was conducted by GOG; other series, however, have also examined cisplatin-based chemotherapy.

  2. Success rates. Virtually all patients with early-stage, completely resected disease survive after careful surgical staging and cisplatin-based adjuvant chemotherapy. Over 50% to 80% of patients with disseminated disease also survive. Treatment should be initiated within 7 to 10 days of surgery because disease recurs very rapidly in some patients.

C. Advanced-stage disease. Patients with incompletely resected metastatic ovarian germ cell tumors should receive combination chemotherapy.

  1. Bleomycin, etoposide, and cisplatin is the preferred regimen. Patients should receive four courses of treatment given in full dose and on schedule. Treatment is given regardless of hematologic parameters on the scheduled day of treatment.

  2. Acute adverse effects of chemotherapy
    a. Twenty-five percent of patients have **febrile neutropenic episodes** during chemotherapy that require hospitalization and administration of broad-spectrum antibiotics.
    b. Cisplatin can be associated with **nephrotoxicity,** which can be avoided by ensuring adequate hydration during and immediately after chemotherapy and by avoiding aminoglycoside antibiotics.
    c. Bleomycin may cause **pulmonary fibrosis.** The best method of monitoring for pulmonary fibrosis is by physical examination of the chest; PFTs, however, are also useful. Any signs of pulmonary fibrosis (i.e., fine basilar rales that do not clear with cough, diminished expansion of one hemithorax) mandates immediate discontinuation of the drug.

VIII. Ovarian sex cord-stromal tumors. Granulosa cell tumors account for approximately 70% of malignant sex cord-stromal tumors. Definitive therapy begins with surgical exploration and staging. Generally, stage I disease does not warrant adjuvant therapy. The use of adjuvant therapy for resected primary advanced-stage disease is not clearly effective, but patients may benefit from a regimen of BEP. Other approaches include postoperative radiation therapy, hormonal therapy, or expectant follow-up. The management of patients with recurrent disease must be individualized. In some cases, granulosa cell tumors express steroid hormone receptors, and responses have been reported with the use of medroxyprogesterone acetate and gonadotropin-releasing hormone (GnRH) antagonists. Several chemotherapy regimens have also been detailed in the literature, with some responses reported with alkylating agents and doxorubicin and others with platinum-based chemotherapy.

IX. Carcinoma of the fallopian tube. Primary treatment of carcinoma of the fallopian tube is total abdominal hysterectomy and bilateral salpingo-oophorectomy, with attempts to surgically remove all evidence of disease. This cancer is generally staged and treated like ovarian cancer.

    A. Radiation therapy. Failure to irradiate the pelvis after cytoreductive surgery for stage I or II disease results in recurrence rates of 35% and 70%, respectively. Pelvic irradiation for local control is feasible; a high rate of metastatic recurrence, however, is associated with local approaches. Whole abdominal radiation and intraperitoneal ^{32}P therapy are the subjects of controversy and produce variable results.

    B. Chemotherapy. Cisplatin and doxorubicin or cyclophosphamide have been used as combination therapy for fallopian tube carcinomas, with a response rate and a survival rate similar to those of advanced ovarian cancer. Paclitaxel may improve cisplatin-based therapy, as has been shown in cases of advanced ovarian cancer.

X. Gestational trophoblastic neoplasia. See also Chap. 39.

    A. Molar pregnancies and risk of malignant gestational trophoblastic disease (GTD). The role of prophylactic chemotherapy, given at or before the time of molar evacuation, to prevent postmolar GTD is unclear. Using a limited course of methotrexate or dactinomycin may theoretically prevent metastatic invasion that might otherwise result from embolization of trophoblast at the time of dilatation and curettage. Patients with high-risk hydatidiform moles appear to benefit from chemotherapeutic prophylaxis but still require surveillance, with serial measurements of hCG levels. Methotrexate and folinic acid appear to be safe as a prophylactic regimen with minimal toxicity. For patients who are not receiving prophylactic chemotherapy, indications for initiating therapy after evacuation of mole include the following:

        1. A rise in hCG level

        2. A plateau in hCG level ($\pm 10\%$) for three or more consecutive measurements

        3. The appearance of metastases

        4. Histologic evidence of choriocarcinoma, placental site trophoblastic tumor, or invasive mole

    B. Management of nonmetastatic GTD and low-risk, good-prognosis metastatic GTD. The selection of treatment is based primarily on whether or not the patient desires to retain fertility.

        1. If the patient no longer wishes to preserve fertility, initial therapy is single-agent methotrexate, hysterectomy, or both.

        2. Single-agent chemotherapy alone is used for patients with stage I disease who wish to retain fertility; excellent remission rates have been achieved with single-agent chemotherapy in both nonmetastatic and low-risk GTD. In an effort to limit systemic toxicity, the administration of methotrexate and folinic acid may be advocated as an alternative (Table 40-12). The serum hCG level is measured weekly after each course of chemotherapy, and an adequate response is defined as a fall in the hCG level by 1 log. A second course of chemotherapy is administered if the hCG level plateaus for more than 3 consecutive weeks or begins to rise, or if the hCG level does not decline by 1 log within 18 days of completion of the first course.

        3. If the disease is resistant to single-agent chemotherapy and the patient wishes to preserve fertility, **combination chemotherapy** should be administered.

    C. Management of high risk, poor-prognosis metastatic GTD. Combination chemotherapy should be given as often as toxicity permits until three consecutive normal hCG levels have been obtained. At least two additional courses of chemotherapy then are given to reduce the risk of relapse.

        1. Etoposide, methotrexate, dactinomycin, cyclophosphamide, and vincristine is the preferred therapy because of its favorable response rate, toxicity profile, dose intensity for methotrexate and dactinomycin, and inclusion of etoposide (Table 40-13).

        2. Other regimens are methotrexate, dactinomycin, cyclophosphamide, doxorubicin, melphalan, hydroxyurea, and vincristine (CHAMMOMA) and methotrexate, folinic acid, dactinomycin, and cyclophosphamide (Cytoxan, MAC, or MACIII).

Table 40-12. Protocol for therapy with methotrexate and folinic acid "rescue"

Day	Time	Follow-up tests and therapy
1	8 a.m. 4 p.m.	CBC, platelet count, SGOT Methotrexate, 1.0 mg/kg
2	4 p.m.	Folinic acid, 0.1 mg/kg
3	8 a.m. 4 p.m.	CBC, platelet count, SGOT Methotrexate, 1.0 mg/kg
4	4 p.m.	Folinic acid, 0.1 mg/kg
5	8 a.m. 4 p.m.	CBC, platelet count, SGOT Methotrexate, 1.0 mg/kg
6	4 p.m.	Folinic acid, 0.1 mg/kg
7	8 a.m. 4 p.m.	CBC, platelet count, SGOT Methotrexate, 1.0 mg/kg
8	4 p.m.	Folinic acid, 0.1 mg/kg

CBC, complete blood cell count; SGOT, serum glutamic-oxaloacetic transaminase.
From Berkowitz RS, Goldstein DP, Bernstein MR. Ten years' experience with methotrexate and folinic acid as primary therapy for gestational trophoblastic disease. *Gynecol Oncol* 1986;23:111. Reproduced with permission.

Table 40-13. EMA-CO regimen for gestational trophoblastic neoplasm patients

Day	Regimen
Course 1 (EMA)	
Day 1	VP-16 mg/m^2, i.v. infusion in 200 mL of saline over 30 min Actinomycin D, 0.5 mg, i.v. push Methotrexate, 100 mg/m^2, i.v. push, followed by a 200 mg/m^2, i.v. infusion over 12 hr
Day 2	VP-16 mg/m^2, i.v. infusion in 200 mL of saline over 30 min Actinomycin D, 0.5 mg, i.v. push Folinic acid, 15 mg, i.m. or orally every 12 hr for 4 doses, beginning 24 hr after start of methotrexate
Course 2 (CO)	
Day 8	Vincristine, 1.0 mg/m^2, i.v. push Cytoxan, 600 mg/m^2, i.v. in saline

EMA-CO, etoposide, methotrexate, dactinomycin, cyclophosphamide, and vincristine; VP-16, etoposide.
This regimen consists of two courses; course 1 is given on days 1 and 2, and course 2 is given on day 8. Course 1 might require an overnight hospital stay; course 2 does not. These courses usually can be given on days 1 and 2, 8, 15, and 16, 22, and so forth; the intervals should not be extended without cause.
From Bagshawe KD. Treatment of high-risk choriocarcinoma. *J Reprod Med* 1984;29:813. Adapted with permission.

Appendix: Common Gynecologic and Obstetric Abbreviations

ABOG	American Board of Obstetrics and Gynecology
AC	abdominal circumference
a.c.	before meals
ACA	anticardiolipin antibody
ACE	angiotensin-converting enzyme
ACLS	advanced cardiac life support
ACOG	American College of Obstetricians and Gynecologists
AdenoCA	adenocarcinoma
ADH	antidiuretic hormone
ad lib	as desired
AF	amniotic fluid
AFB	acid-fast bacilli
AFI	amniotic fluid index
AFP	alpha-fetoprotein
AICD	automatic implantable cardiac defibrillator
ANA	antinuclear antibody
ANC	absolute neutrophil count
anti-HBC	antihepatitis B core
anti-HBS	antihepatitis B surface
ARF	acute renal failure
AROM	artificial rupture of membranes
ASD	atrial septal defect
AUC	area under the curve
AVC	atrioventricular canal
AVCD	atrioventricular conduction defect
AXR	abdominal x-ray
Ⓑ	bilateral
BBT	basal body temperature
BCG	bacillus Calmette-Guérin
BCLS	basic cardiac life support
BCP	birth control pill
BG	blood glucose
b.i.d.	twice a day
BMI	body mass index
BOA	birth out of asepsis, born on arrival
BPD	biparietal diameter
BPP	biophysical profile
BPS	bilateral partial salpingectomy
BRP	bathroom privileges
BSE	breast self-examination
BSO	bilateral salpingo-oophorectomy
BTL	bilateral tubal ligation
C&S	culture and sensitivities
CA	cancer
CBC	complete blood cell count

cc	with
CCU	clean-catch urine, cardiac care unit
CDDP	cis-diamino-dichloroplatinum (cisplatin)
CEA	carcinoembryonic antigen
CHO	carbohydrate
CI	cardiac index
cCirc	circumcision
CL	corpus luteum
CMV	cytomegalovirus
CNM	certified nurse midwife
CP	cerebral palsy
CPAP	continuous positive airway pressure
CPC	choroid plexus cyst
CPT	chest physical therapy
CRF	chronic renal failure
CRL	crown-rump length
c/s	cesarean section
CST	contraction stress test
CT	computed tomography
CVA	cerebrovascular accident
CVAT	costovertebral angle tenderness
c/w	consistent with
CXR	chest x-ray
D&C	dilation and curettage
D&E	dilation and evacuation
DAV	doxorubicin, adriamycin, vinblastine
d/c	discharge or discontinue
DCT	direct Coombs' test
DDx	differential diagnosis
DHEAS	dehydroepiandrosterone sulfate
DI	diabetes insipidus
DIC	disseminated intravascular coagulation
DKA	diabetic ketoacidosis
dL	decaliter
DMPA	depomedroxyprogesterone acetate
DNR	do not resuscitate
DPT	diphtheria, pertussis, and tetanus vaccine
DR	delivery room
DRCO	diffusion rate of carbon monoxide
D-stix	Dextrostix
DTR	deep tendon reflex
DUB	dysfunctional uterine bleeding
E_1	estrone
E_2	estradiol
E_3	estriol
EBV	Epstein-Barr virus
ECMO	extracorporeal membrane oxygenation
EDC	estimated date of confinement
EDD	estimated date of delivery
EIC	endometrial intraepithelial carcinoma
EMB	endometrial biopsy
EMC	endometrial curettage
epis	episiotomy
ER/PR	estrogen receptor/progesterone receptor
ESR	erythrocyte sedimentation rate
ET	embryo transfer
ETOH	ethyl alcohol
ex	culture
exlap	exploratory laparotomy

FAC	fetal assessment center
FB	fetal breathing
FDIU	fetal death *in utero*
FENa	fractional excretion of sodium
FEV_1	forced expiratory volume in 1 second
FL	femur length
FM	fetal movement
FOB	father of the baby
FRC	functional residual capacity
FSH	follicle-stimulating hormone
FT	fetal tone
FT_4	free thyroxine
FTA	fluorescent treponemal antigen
FTSVD	full-term spontaneous vaginal delivery
5-FU	5-fluorouracil
GBS	group B streptococcus
GC	gonococcus
GCT	glucose challenge test
GDM	gestational diabetes mellitus
GFR	glomerular filtration rate
GH	growth hormone
GIFT	gamete intrafallopian transfer
GNID	gram-negative intracellular diplococcus (e.g., GC)
GnRH	gonadotropin-releasing hormone
GOG	Gynecologic Oncology Group
G6PD	glucose-6-phosphate dehydrogenase
GTT	glucose tolerance test
H&E	hematoxylin and eosin
H&P	history and physical
HAV	hepatitis A virus
HBcAb	hepatitis B core antibody
HBcAg	hepatitis B core antigen
HBeAg	hepatitis B e antigen
HBIG	hepatitis B immune globulin
HBsAg	hepatitis B surface antigen
HBV	hepatitis B virus
HC	head circumference
hCG	human chorionic gonadotropin
HCTZ	hydrochlorothiazide
HCV	hepatitis C virus
HgA_{1c}	hemoglobin A_{1c}
HgEP	hemoglobin electrophoresis
HIV	human immunodeficiency virus
HLA	human leukocyte antigen
H/O	history of
HONK	hyperosmotic nonketotic coma
HPL	human placental lactogen
HPV	human papillomavirus
h.s.	at bedtime
HSG	hysterosalpingogram
HSV	herpes simplex virus
HUS	hemolytic uremic syndrome
hx	history
IACD	implantable automatic cardiac defibrillator
I&D	incision and drainage
IBD	inflammatory bowel disease
ICT	indirect Coombs' test
IDDM	insulin-dependent diabetes mellitus
I:E	inspiratory to expiratory ratio

IFN-α	interferon-alpha
IFOS	ifosfamide
Ig	immunoglobulin
IGF	insulin-like growth factor
IJ	internal jugular (catheter)
IMV	intermittent mandatory ventilation
INH	isoniazid
INR	international normalized ratio
ITP	idiopathic thrombocytopenic purpura
IUD	intrauterine device
IUFD	intrauterine fetal demise
IUGR	intrauterine growth retardation
IUP	intrauterine pregnancy
IVC	inferior vena cava
IVF	*in vitro* fertilization
IVH	intraventricular hemorrhage
IVP	intravenous pyelogram
IVPB	intravenous piggy-back
LATS	long-acting thyroid stimulator
LAVH	laparoscopic-assisted vaginal hysterectomy
LBW	low birth weight
LDH	lactate dehydrogenase
LDR	labor, delivery, recovery (room)
LDRP	labor, delivery, recovery, postpartum (room)
LFD	low-forceps delivery
LFVD	low-forceps vaginal delivery
LGA	large for gestational age
LH	luteinizing hormone
LMP	last menstrual period
LP	lumbar puncture
LR	labor room
L/RBBB	left/right bundle-branch block
L/RLQ	left/right lower quadrant
L/ROA	left/right occiput anterior
L/ROP	left/right occiput posterior
L/ROT	left/right occiput transverse
L/RUQ	left/right upper quadrant
L-S ratio	lecithin-sphingomyelin ratio
MAP	mean arterial pressure
MAS	meconium aspiration syndrome
MCA	middle cerebral artery
mCi	millicurie
MCV	mean corpuscular volume
MEN	multiple endocrine neoplasia
mEq	milliequivalent
MFM	maternal fetal medicine
MgGSO$_4$	magnesium sulfate
MHAA-TP	microhemagglutination assay for *Treponema pallidum*
MI	myocardial infarction
MIC	mean inhibitory concentration
MICU	medical intensive care unit
MIF/S	müllerian inhibitory factor/substance
MMR	measles, mumps, rubella
MMT	mixed müllerian tumor
MRI	magnetic resonance imaging
MRSA	methicillin-resistant *Staphylococcus aureus*
MSAFP	maternal serum alpha-fetoprotein
MSO$_4$	morphine sulfate
MTB	*Mycobacterium tuberculosis*

MTX	methotrexate
μ	micro
MVA	motor vehicle accident
NAS	National Academy of Sciences
N:C	nuclear to cytoplasmic ratio
NCI	National Cancer Institute
NEC	necrotizing enterocolitis
NED	no evidence of disease
NEFG	normal external female genitalia
NGT	nasogastric tube
NGU	nongonococcal urethritis
NIDDM	non–insulin-dependent diabetes mellitus
NOS	night of surgery
NPP	nursing pitocin protocol
NS	normal saline
NSAID	nonsteroidal antiinflammatory drug
NSSC	normal size, smooth contour
NST	nonstress test
NTD	nothing to do
ntg	nitroglycerine
N/V	nausea/vomiting
O&P	ova and parasites
OCP	oral contraceptive preparation
OFD	oral-facial-digital
OGTT	oral glucose tolerance test
OI	osteogenesis imperfecta
OOB	out of bed
OTC	over the counter
P	parity
p	after
$Paco_2$	partial pressure of carbon dioxide
para	parity
PAS	periodic acid–Schiff
PAWP	pulmonary artery wedge pressure
PCP	*Pneumocystis carinii* pneumonia
PCV	packed cell volume
PDA	patent ductus arteriosus
PDC	prenatal diagnostic center
PE	physical examination
PEEP	positive end-expiratory pressure
PFT	pulmonary function tests
PGA_1	prostaglandin A_1
PI	principle investigator
PID	pelvic inflammatory disease
PIH	pregnancy-induced hypertension
PLAP	placental alkaline phosphatase
PMN	polymorphonuclear leukocyte
PMP	previous menstrual period
PMS	premenstrual syndrome
PN	parenteral nutrition
p.o.	by mouth
POD	postoperative day
pp	postpartum
PPD	purified protein derivative
PPLND	pelvic and paraaortic lymph node dissection
PPPROM	premature, prelabor, prolonged rupture of membrane
PPROM	premature, prelabor rupture of membrane
p.r.	by rectum
PRBC	packed red blood cells
PRL	prolactin

p.r.n.	as needed
PROM	prelabor rupture of membrane
PT	prothrombin time
PTFE	polytetrafluoroethylene (Teflon)
p.v.	by vagina
q.h.s.	every night
q.i.d.	four times a day
q.o.d.	every other day
RAH	radical abdominal hysterectomy
RCM	Royal College of Midwives
RDS	respiratory distress syndrome
reg	regular insulin
ROM	rupture of membrane
RPR	reactive plasma reagin
RR	relative risk, R-R interval, respiratory rate
RSV	respiratory syncytial virus
RU486	mifepristone
s	without
SAB	spontaneous abortion
SaO_2	oxygen saturation
SBE	subacute bacterial endocarditis
SBFT	small bowel follow-through
SBO	small bowel obstruction
SBP	spontaneous bacterial peritonitis
SCA	squamous carcinoma
SCD	sequential compression devices
S/D ratio	systolic/diastolic ratio
SEM	standard error of measurement
SG	specific gravity
SGA	small for gestational age
SGI	Society of Gynecologic Investigation
SGO	Society of Gynecologic Oncologists
SIADH	syndrome of inappropriate antidiuretic hormone secretion
SICU	surgical intensive care unit
SIDS	sudden infant death syndrome
SLE	systemic lupus erythematosus
SMV	spontaneous mechanical ventilation
sono	sonogram
s.q.	subcutaneous
SROM	spontaneous rupture of membrane
STD	sexually transmitted disease
STS	serum test for syphilis
SVC	superior vena cava
SVR	systemic vascular resistance
T	testosterone
TAB	therapeutic abortion
TAH	total abdominal hysterectomy
TEDs	elastic antiembolism stockings
TEE	transesophageal echocardiogram
TEF	tracheoesophageal fistula
TFT	thyroid function tests
TGA	transposition of the great arteries
THC	tetrahydrocannabinol
TIBC	total iron-binding capacity
t.i.d.	three times a day
TMP-SMX	trimethoprim-sulfamethoxazole (Bactrim)
TOA	tubo-ovarian abscess
TPN	total parenteral nutrition
TRH	thyrotropin-releasing hormone
TSH	thyroid-stimulating hormone

TSIG	thyroid-stimulating immunoglobulins
TVH	total vaginal hysterectomy
TVU	transvaginal ultrasound
tx	treatment
TZ	transition zone
UA	urinalysis
UC	uterine contraction
U/S, US	ultrasound
VAIN	vaginal intraepithelial neoplasia
VCUG	voiding cystourethrogram
VD	venereal disease
VDRL	Venereal Disease Research Laboratory
VIN	vulvar intraepithelial neoplasia
VRE	vancomycin-resistant enterococcus
VSA	victim of sexual assault
VSD	ventricular septal defect
vtx	vertex
VZIG	varicella-zoster immune globulin
VZV	varicella-zoster virus
XX/XY	male/female
ZIFT	zygote intrafallopian transfer

Index